Robbins
Review of
PATHOLOGY

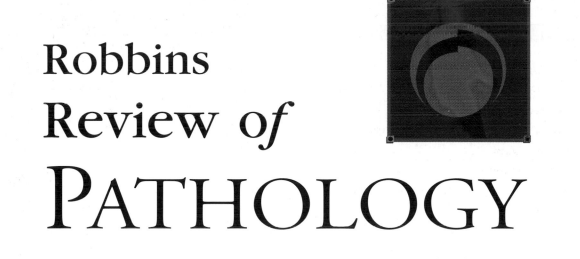

Edward C. Klatt, M.D.
Professor of Pathology
The University of Utah
Health Sciences Center
Salt Lake City, Utah

Vinay Kumar, M.D., F.R.C.Path.
Vernie A. Stembridge Chair in Pathology
Department of Pathology
The University of Texas
Southwestern Medical School
Dallas, Texas

W.B. SAUNDERS COMPANY
An Imprint of Elsevier Science
Philadelphia   London   New York   St. Louis   Sydney   Toronto

W.B. SAUNDERS COMPANY
An Imprint of Elsevier Science

The Curtis Center
Independence Square West
Philadelphia, Pennsylvania 19106

Library of Congress Cataloging-in-Publication Data

Klatt Edward C.
Robbins review of pathology/Edward C. Klatt, Vinay Kumar—1st ed.

p. cm.

ISBN 0–7216–8259–6

I. Pathology—Examinations, questions, etc.   I. Title: Review of pathology.   II. Robbins,
  Stanley L. (Stanley Leonard)   III. Kumar, Vinay.   IV. Title.   DNLM: 1. Pathology. QZ 4 K63r
2000]

RB119 .K56 2000   616.07′076—dc21   99-057050

Acquisitions Editor: William Schmitt
Developmental Editor: Hazel Hacker
Project Manager: Agnes Hunt Byrne
Production Manager: Pete Faber
Illustration Specialist: Peg Shaw
Book Designer: Paul Fry

ROBBINS REVIEW OF PATHOLOGY   ISBN 0–7216–8259–6

Printed in China

Last digit is the print number: 9   8   7   6

To our students, for constant challenge and stimulation

Preface

This book is designed to provide a comprehensive review of pathology through multiple choice questions and explanations of the answers. The source materials are the sixth editions of Cotran, Kumar, Collins: *Robbins Pathologic Basis of Disease* (PBD6) and Kumar, Cotran, Robbins: *Basic Pathology* (BP6). It is intended to be a useful resource for students at a variety of levels, including those in the allied health professions.

In keeping with the style used by the USMLE, only two question formats are used: single best answer and extended matching. The majority of the questions contain a clinical vignette that is followed by a series of homogenous choices. This approach emphasizes an understanding of mechanisms and manifestations of disease in a clinical context. Wherever possible, we have incorporated relevant laboratory, radiologic, and physical diagnostic findings in the questions to emphasize clinicopathologic correlations. For each question, the correct answer is provided with a brief explanation of why the correct answer is "correct" and why the other choices are "incorrect." Each answer is referenced to *Robbins Pathologic Basis of Disease* and to *Basic Pathology* to facilitate and encourage a more complete reading of the topic. Pathology is a visually oriented discipline and hence we have used full color images in many of the questions. The illustrations are taken from the Robbins textbooks, so students can reinforce their study of the illustrations in the text with questions that utilize the same images.

The questions are intentionally fairly difficult, with the purpose of "pushing the envelope" of student understanding of pathology. We hope, therefore, that this text will be useful not only prior to examinations but also during the course. We must hasten to add that no review book is a substitute for the textbooks and other course material provided by individual instructors. The best use of this book will be after a thorough study of *Robbins Pathologic Basis of Disease* and/or *Basic Pathology*. Finally, we hope that students and instructors will find this review book to be a useful adjunct to the learning of pathology.

EDWARD C. KLATT
VINAY KUMAR

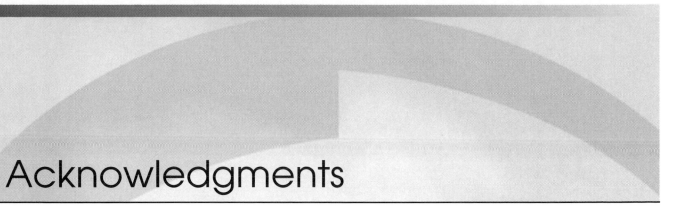

Acknowledgments

We are very grateful to our editorial assistants, Beverly Shackelford and Carolyn Osterman, for their invaluable help in the production of the manuscript. Thanks are also due to Hazel Hacker, our Developmental Editor, and William Schmitt, Editor-in-Chief, Medical Textbooks, W.B. Saunders Company, for their support of this project. Last but not least, we are grateful to our families and colleagues for graciously accepting this additional demand on our time.

EDWARD C. KLATT
VINAY KUMAR

Contents

PART 1
GENERAL PATHOLOGY

1. Cellular Pathology 3

2. Acute and Chronic Inflammation 11

3. Tissue Repair: Cellular Growth, Fibrosis, and Wound Healing 18

4. Hemodynamic Disorders, Thrombosis, and Shock 21

5. Genetic Disorders 29

6. Diseases of Immunity 36

7. Neoplasia 51

8. Infectious Diseases 64

9. Environmental and Nutritional Pathology ... 78

10. Diseases of Infancy and Childhood 89

PART 2
DISEASES OF ORGAN SYSTEMS

11. Blood Vessels 101

12. The Heart 110

13. Red Cells and Bleeding Disorders 123

14. White Cells, Lymph Nodes, Spleen, and Thymus 136

15. The Lung 153

16. Head and Neck 168

17. The Gastrointestinal Tract 173

18. The Liver and the Biliary Tract 190

19. The Pancreas 203

20. The Kidney and the Lower Urinary Tract 210

21. The Male Genital Tract 229

22. The Female Genital Tract 236

23. The Breast 249

24. The Endocrine System 255

25. The Skin 267

26. Bones, Joints, and Soft Tissue Tumors 274

27. Peripheral Nerve and Skeletal Muscle 286

28. The Central Nervous System 290

29. The Eye 305

PART 1

GENERAL PATHOLOGY

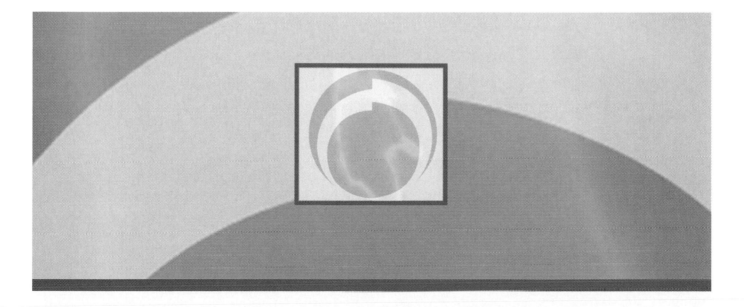

Cellular Pathology

PBD6 Chapter 1 - Cellular Pathology I
PBD6 Chapter 2 - Cellular Pathology II
BP6 Chapter 1 - Cell Injury, Death, and
Adaptation

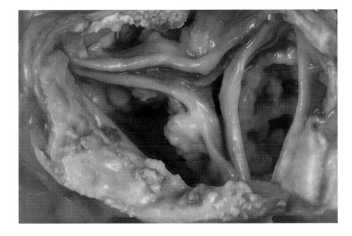

1. A 17-year-old male infected with hepatitis A experiences some mild nausea for about a week and has very mild scleral icterus. Laboratory findings include elevations in the levels of the hepatic enzymes aspartate transaminase (AST) and alanine transaminase (ALT). The increase in the enzyme levels in the serum results from which of the following changes in the hepatocytes?

○ (A) Dispersion of ribosomes
○ (B) Autophagy by lysosomes
○ (C) Swelling of the mitochondria
○ (D) Clumping of nuclear chromatin
○ (E) Defects in the cell membrane

2. A 54-year-old male experienced the onset of severe chest pain. An electrocardiogram demonstrated changes consistent with an acute myocardial infarction. He was given thrombolytic therapy with tissue plasminogen activator (tPA). However, his serum creatine kinase increased after this therapy. Which of the following events most likely occurred?

○ (A) Reperfusion injury
○ (B) Cellular regeneration
○ (C) Chemical injury
○ (D) Increased synthesis of creatine kinase
○ (E) Myofiber atrophy

3. A 51-year-old male has a blood pressure of 150/95 mm Hg. If this condition remains untreated for years, which of the following cellular alterations will be seen in the heart?

○ (A) Atrophy
○ (B) Hyperplasia
○ (C) Metaplasia
○ (D) Hemosiderosis
○ (E) Hypertrophy

4. The aortic valve seen in the figure was discovered at the autopsy of a 72-year-old male. The heart weighed 580 g, with marked left ventricular hypertrophy and minimal coronary arterial atherosclerosis. A serum chemistry panel revealed no abnormalities prior to death from congestive heart failure. Which of the following pathologic processes accounts for the appearance of the valve?

○ (A) Amyloidosis
○ (B) Dystrophic calcification
○ (C) Lipofuscin deposition
○ (D) Hemosiderosis
○ (E) Fatty change

5. A right carotid endarterectomy is performed on a 69-year-old female who had an audible bruit on auscultation of the neck. Examination of the curetted atheromatous plaque reveals a grossly yellow-tan, firm appearance. Microscopically, which of the following materials can be found in abundance in the form of crystals producing long, cleftlike spaces?

○ (A) Glycogen
○ (B) Lipofuscin
○ (C) Hemosiderin
○ (D) Immunoglobulin
○ (E) Cholesterol

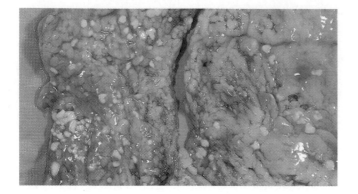

6. A 38-year-old woman experienced severe abdominal pain with hypotension and shock that led to her death within 36 hours. From the gross appearance of the mesentery, seen in the figure, which of the following events has most likely occurred?

○(A) Hepatitis B virus infection
○(B) Small intestinal infarction
○(C) Tuberculous lymphadenitis
○(D) Gangrenous cholecystitis
○(E) Acute pancreatitis

7. Absorption of radiant energy, such as x-rays, can result in cell injury by causing hydrolysis of water. Which of the following cellular enzymes protects cells from this type of injury?

○(A) Phospholipase
○(B) Glutathione peroxidase
○(C) Endonuclease
○(D) Lactate dehydrogenase
○(E) Proteases

8. In patients with emphysema due to α_1-antitrypsin deficiency, the molecular mechanism responsible for the accumulation of α_1-antitrypsin in hepatocytes is

○(A) Excessive hepatic synthesis of α_1-antitrypsin
○(B) Retention in the endoplasmic reticulum because of poorly folded α_1-antitrypsin
○(C) Decreased catabolism of α_1-antitrypsin in lysosomes
○(D) Inability to metabolize α_1-antitrypsin
○(E) Impaired dissociation from chaperones

9. A 63-year-old man experienced diaphoresis and substernal chest pain after thrombosis of the left anterior descending artery. His serum creatine kinase level was elevated. Which of the following patterns of tissue injury was most likely?

○(A) Liquefactive necrosis
○(B) Caseous necrosis
○(C) Coagulative necrosis
○(D) Fat necrosis
○(E) Gangrenous necrosis

10. After several weeks of immobilization of the leg in a plaster cast, the diameter of the calf often decreases. This change results from which of the following alterations in the calf muscles?

○(A) Aplasia
○(B) Hypoplasia
○(C) Atrophy
○(D) Dystrophy
○(E) Hyalin change

11. Which of the following cells have the highest telomerase activity?

○(A) Endothelial cells
○(B) Germ cells
○(C) Neurons
○(D) Neutrophils
○(E) Erythrocytes

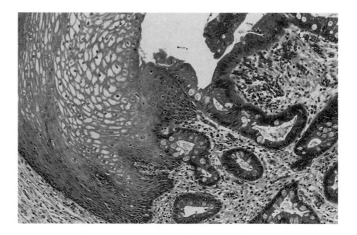

12. A 32-year-old male experiences "heartburn" with substernal pain from reflux of gastric contents into the lower esophagus. After many months, the esophageal epithelium exhibits the microscopic appearance shown here. Which of the following pathologic alterations has occurred?

○(A) Squamous metaplasia
○(B) Mucosal hypertrophy
○(C) Columnar epithelial metaplasia
○(D) Atrophy of lamina propria
○(E) Goblet cell hyperplasia

13. On day 28 of the menstrual cycle in a 23-year-old female, there is menstrual bleeding that lasts for a few days. She has had these regular cycles for many years. Which of the following processes is most likely happening in the endometrium just before the onset of bleeding?

○(A) Apoptosis
○(B) Caseous necrosis
○(C) Heterophagocytosis
○(D) Atrophy
○(E) Liquefactive necrosis

14. Many drugs that are used to treat cancer cause death of tumor cells by apoptosis. Mutational inactivation of which of the following genes can render tumor cells resistant to the effects of such chemotherapeutic drugs?

○ (A) *bcl-2*
○ (B) *p53*
○ (C) NF-κB
○ (D) P450
○ (E) Granzyme B

15.   After the birth of her first child, a 19-year-old female began breast feeding the baby. She continued breast-feeding for almost a year. Which of the following processes that occurred in the breast during pregnancy allowed her to nurse the infant?

○ (A) Stromal hypertrophy
○ (B) Lobular hyperplasia
○ (C) Epithelial dysplasia
○ (D) Intracellular accumulation of fat
○ (E) Ductal epithelial metaplasia

16.   A 22-year-old female has a congenital anemia that required multiple transfusions of red blood cells for many years. She now has no significant findings on physical examination. However, her liver function test results are abnormal. Which of the following findings would most likely appear in a liver biopsy?

○ (A) Steatosis in hepatocytes
○ (B) Bilirubin in canaliculi
○ (C) Glycogen in hepatocytes
○ (D) Amyloid in portal triads
○ (E) Hemosiderin in hepatocytes

For each of the clinical histories in questions 17, 18, and 19, match the most closely associated lettered description of a form of cellular change or injury:

(A) Apoptosis
(B) Atrophy
(C) Caseous necrosis
(D) Coagulative necrosis
(E) Dysplasia
(F) Dystrophic calcification
(G) Fat necrosis
(H) Fatty change
(I) Gangrenous necrosis
(J) Hydropic change
(K) Hyperplasia
(L) Hypertrophy
(M) Liquefactive necrosis
(N) Metaplasia
(O) Metastatic calcification

17.   A 3-cm, right middle lobe lung nodule was seen on a chest radiograph of an asymptomatic 37-year-old male. The nodule was excised with a pulmonary wedge resection by the thoracic surgeon. On sectioning by the pathologist, the nodule was sharply circumscribed and had a soft, white center. Culture of tissue from the nodule grew *Mycobacterium tuberculosis.* (   )

18.   A 69-year-old male has difficulty with urination. A digital rectal examination reveals that the prostate gland is palpably enlarged to about twice normal size. A transurethral resection of the prostate is performed, and the microscopic appearance of the prostate "chips" obtained is that of nodules of glands with intervening stroma. (   )

19.   Blunt trauma to the abdomen of a 16-year-old male occurred during a vehicular accident in which he lost control of the vehicle at high speed and struck a bridge abutment. He is found to have a hemoperitoneum, and at laparotomy, a small portion of the left lobe of the liver was resected because of the injury. Weeks later, the liver had regained its normal size. (   )

20.   Accumulation of lipofuscin granules in cells is typically seen in which of the following conditions?

○ (A) Atrophy
○ (B) Hypertrophy
○ (C) Hyperplasia
○ (D) Metaplasia
○ (E) Apoptosis

21.   A 40-year-old male was diagnosed with an undifferentiated carcinoma of the lung. Despite treatment with chemotherapy, he died of widespread metastases. At autopsy, tumor was found in many organs. Histologic examination revealed many foci in which individual tumor cells appeared shrunken and deeply eosinophilic. Their nuclei showed condensed aggregates of chromatin under the nuclear membrane. The process affecting these shrunken tumor cells was triggered by the release of which of the following proteins into the cytosol?

○ (A) Lipofuscin
○ (B) Cytochrome *c*
○ (C) Catalase
○ (D) Phospholipase
○ (E) *bcl 2*

22.   Metastatic calcification is most likely to occur in which of the following conditions?

○ (A) Tuberculosis of the lung
○ (B) Acute hemorrhagic pancreatitis
○ (C) Aortic stenosis in a 70-year-old man
○ (D) Vitamin D intoxication
○ (E) Amyloidosis

23.   A 68-year-old female suddenly lost consciousness and, on awakening an hour later, could not speak or move her right arm and leg. Two months later, a head computed tomography (CT) scan showed a large cystic area in her left parietal lobe. Which of the following pathologic processes most likely occurred in the brain?

○ (A) Fat necrosis
○ (B) Coagulative necrosis
○ (C) Apoptosis
○ (D) Liquefactive necrosis
○ (E) Karyolysis

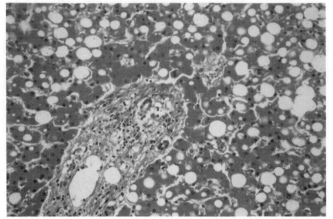

Courtesy of Dr. James Crawford, Department of Pathology. Brigham and Women's Hospital, Boston.

24. At autopsy, a 40-year-old male has an enlarged (2200 g) liver with a yellow cut surface. The microscopic appearance of this liver is shown in the figure. Before death, his total serum cholesterol and triglyceride levels were normal, but he had a decreased serum albumin concentration and increased prothrombin time. Which of the following activities by this man most likely led to these findings?

○ (A) Injecting heroin
○ (B) Playing basketball
○ (C) Drinking beer
○ (D) Smoking
○ (E) Ingesting aspirin

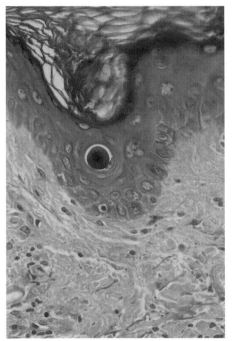

Courtesy of Dr. Scott Granter, Brigham and Women's Hospital, Boston.

25. The cellular change in the epidermal cell located in the midepidermis, in the figure, results from which of the following biochemical reactions?

○ (A) Activation of caspases
○ (B) Reduced ATP synthesis
○ (C) Increased glycolysis
○ (D) Activation of lipases
○ (E) Lipid peroxidation

26. At autopsy, the heart of a 63-year-old male is only 250 g, with small right and left ventricles. The myocardium is firm, with a dark chocolate brown color throughout. The coronary arteries demonstrate very little atherosclerosis. Which of the following substances will most likely be found in the myocardial fibers of this heart?

○ (A) Melanin
○ (B) Hemosiderin
○ (C) Glycogen
○ (D) Lipofuscin
○ (E) Bilirubin

27. A pneumonectomy is performed for lung cancer diagnosed in a 69-year-old female. Examination of the hilar lymph nodes reveals a uniform dark black cut surface. What is most likely to account for this appearance of these lymph nodes?

○ (A) Smoking
○ (B) A bleeding disorder
○ (C) Liver failure
○ (D) Aging
○ (E) Metastases

28. Deposition of calcium in the renal tubular epithelium in patients with primary hyperparathyroidism is the result of which of the following processes?

○ (A) Dystrophic calcification
○ (B) Renal tubular atrophy
○ (C) Autophagocytosis
○ (D) Metastatic calcification
○ (E) Cellular aging

29. A renal biopsy is performed on a 33-year-old female who has had increasing renal failure for the past week. Which of the following changes seen with electron microscopy most likely suggests a diagnosis of acute tubular necrosis?

○ (A) Mitochondrial swelling
○ (B) Plasma membrane blebs
○ (C) Chromatin clumping
○ (D) Nuclear fragmentation
○ (E) Ribosomal disaggregation from endoplasmic reticulum

30. Reperfusion of ischemic tissues, as may occur after therapeutic use of thrombolytic agents, sometimes leads to cell death after the blood flow resumes. The biochemical basis for cell death under these circumstances is most likely which of the following?

○ (A) Reduction in protein synthesis
○ (B) Increased generation of oxygen-derived free radicals

○ (C) Increased activity of catalase
○ (D) Reduced oxidative phosphorylation
○ (E) Release of calcium from endoplasmic reticulum

31. A 50-year-old male experienced several episodes of chest pain before his death. A histologic section of left ventricular myocardium taken at autopsy showed a deeply eosinophilic staining area with loss of nuclei and cross-striations in myocardial fibers. There was no hemorrhage or inflammation. Which of the following conditions most likely produced these myocardial changes?

○ (A) Viral infection
○ (B) Coronary artery thrombosis
○ (C) Blunt chest trauma
○ (D) Antibodies directed against myocardium
○ (E) A protein-deficient diet

32. The nonpregnant uterus of a 20-year-old female measured 7 × 4 × 3 cm. She became pregnant, and just before delivery of a term infant, the uterus measured 34 × 18 × 12 cm. Which of the following cellular processes was the major reason for the increase in the size of the uterus?

○ (A) Endometrial glandular hyperplasia
○ (B) Myometrial fibroblast proliferation
○ (C) Endometrial stromal hypertrophy
○ (D) Myometrial smooth muscle hypertrophy
○ (E) Vascular endothelial hyperplasia

33. A 40-year-old female with chronic congestive heart failure has a cough productive of rust-colored sputum. A sputum cytology specimen shows numerous hemosiderin-laden macrophages. Which of the following subcellular structures in macrophages is most important for the accumulation of this pigment?

○ (A) Lysosome
○ (B) Endoplasmic reticulum
○ (C) Ribosome
○ (D) Golgi apparatus
○ (E) Chromosome

ANSWERS

1. **(E)** Irreversible cell injury is associated with loss of membrane integrity. This allows intracellular enzymes to leak into the serum. All other morphologic changes listed are associated with reversible cell injury, in which the cell membrane remains intact.
BP6 6–8 PBD6 7–9

2. **(A)** The restoration of blood flow is helpful if the existing cell damage is not great, and further damage can be prevented. However, the reperfusion of damaged cells results in generation of oxygen-derived free radicals to produce a reperfusion injury. The elevation in the creatine kinase level is indicative of myocardial cell necrosis, not

regeneration or atrophy. The tPA does not produce a chemical injury but induces thrombolysis to restore blood flow.
BP6 9–10 PBD6 12–13

3. **(E)** The pressure load on the left ventricle results in an increase in myofilaments in the existing myofibers. The result of continued stress from hypertension is eventual heart failure with decreased contractility, but the cells do not decrease in size. Metaplasia of muscle does not occur, although loss of muscle occurs with aging, with replacement by fibrous tissue and adipose tissue. Hemosiderin deposition in heart is a pathologic process resulting from increased iron stores in the body.
BP6 22 PBD6 33–35

4. **(B)** The valve is stenotic because of nodular deposits of calcium. The process is "dystrophic" because calcium deposition occurs in damaged tissues. The damage here results from wear and tear of aging. Amyloid deposition in the heart typically occurs within the myocardium and the vessels. The amount of lipofuscin increases within myocardium with aging. With a genetic defect in iron absorption known as hereditary hemochromatosis, there is extensive myocardial iron deposition. Fatty change is uncommonly seen in myocardium, but infiltration of fat cells can occur.
BP6 20 PBD6 43–44

5. **(E)** Cholesterol is a form of lipid commonly deposited within atheromas in arterial walls, imparting a yellow color to these plaques. Glycogen is a storage form of carbohydrate seen mainly in liver and muscle. Lipofuscin is a brown pigment that increases with aging in cell cytoplasm, mainly in cardiac myocytes and in hepatocytes. Hemosiderin is a storage form of iron that appears in tissues of the mononuclear phagocyte system (e.g., marrow, liver, spleen) but can be widely deposited with hereditary hemochromatosis. Immunoglobulin occasionally may be seen as rounded globules in plasma cells (i.e., Russell bodies).
BP6 18 PBD6 40

6. **(E)** The focal chalky-white deposits are areas of fat necrosis resulting from the release of pancreatic lipases in patients with acute pancreatitis. Viral hepatitis does not cause necrosis in other organs, and hepatocyte necrosis from viral infections occurs mainly by means of apoptosis. Intestinal infarction is a form of coagulative necrosis. Tuberculosis produces caseous necrosis. Gangrenous necrosis is mainly coagulative necrosis but occurs over an extensive area.
BP6 12–13 PBD6 16–17

7. **(B)** Intracellular mechanisms exist that deal with free radical generation, as can occur with radiant injury from irradiation. Glutathione peroxidase reduces such injury by catalyzing the breakdown of H_2O_2. Phospholipases decrease cellular phospholipids and promote cell membrane injury. Proteases can damage cell membranes and cytoskeletal proteins. Endonucleases damage nuclear chromatin. Lactate dehydrogenase (LDH) is present in a variety of cells, and its elevation in the serum is an indicator of cell death.
BP6 9–11 PBD6 12–14

8. **(B)** Mutations in the α_1-antitrypsin gene give rise to α_1-antitrypsin molecules that cannot fold properly. The partially folded molecules accumulate in the endoplasmic reticulum (ER) and cannot be secreted. Impaired dissociation of the cystic fibrosis transmembrane conductance regulator (CFTR) protein from chaperones is the cause of many cases of cystic fibrosis. There is no abnormality in the synthesis or metabolism of α_1-antitrypsin in patients with α_1-antitrypsin deficiency.
PBD6 41

9. **(C)** He has an acute myocardial infarction. An ischemic injury to most internal organs produces a pattern of cell death called coagulative necrosis. Liquefactive necrosis occurs following ischemic injury to brain and is also the pattern seen with abscess formation. Caseous necrosis can be seen in various forms of granulomatous inflammation, typified by tuberculosis. Fat necrosis is usually seen in pancreas and breast tissue. Gangrenous necrosis is a form of coagulative necrosis that usually results from ischemia and affects limbs.
BP6 12-13   PBD6 16-18

10. **(C)** Reduced workload causes shrinkage of cell size because of loss of cell substance, a process called atrophy. Aplasia refers to lack of embryonic development; hypoplasia is used to describe poor or subnormal development. Dystrophy of muscles refers to inherited disorders of skeletal muscles that lead to muscle weakness and wasting. Hyaline change is the name given to a nonspecific, pink, glassy eosinophilic appearance of cells.
BP6 21-22   PBD6 35-36

11. **(B)** Germ cells have the highest telomerase activity, and the telomere length therefore can be stabilized in these cells. This allows germ cells to retain the ability to divide. Normal somatic cells have no telomerase activity, and telomeres progressively shorten with each cell division until growth arrest occurs.
PBD6 47

12. **(C)** Inflammation has resulted in replacement of normal squamous epithelium by intestinal-type columnar epithelium with goblet cells. Such conversion of one adult cell type to another type is called metaplasia. The thickness of the mucosa is normal. The lamina propria has some inflammatory cells but is not atrophic.
BP6 22-23   PBD6 36-37

13. **(A)** This is an example of orderly, programmed cell death (apoptosis) through hormonal stimuli. The endometrium breaks down, sloughs off, and then regenerates. Caseous necrosis is typical of granulomatous inflammation, resulting most commonly from mycobacterial infection. Heterophagocytosis is typified by the clearing of an area of necrosis through macrophage ingestion of the necrotic cells. With cellular atrophy, there is often no visible necrosis, but the tissues shrink in size, something that would happen to the endometrium after menopause. Liquefactive necrosis can occur in any tissue after acute bacterial infection or in the brain after ischemia.
BP6 13-14   PBD6 18-19

14. **(B)** On DNA damage induced by chemotherapeutic drugs (or other agents), normal *p53* genes trigger the cells to undergo apoptosis. When *p53* is inactivated, this pathway of cell death can be blocked, rendering the chemotherapy less effective. *bcl-2* and NF-κB favor cell survival. Cytochrome P450 does not affect apoptosis. Granzyme B is found in cytotoxic T cells and not tumor cells. It triggers apoptosis.
BP6 155-156   PBD6 25

15. **(B)** Lobules increase under hormonal influence to provide for lactation. The breast stroma plays no role in lactation and may increase in pathologic processes. Epithelial dysplasia denotes disordered growth and maturation of epithelial cells that may progress to cancer. Accumulation of fat within the cells is a common manifestation of sublethal cell injury or, uncommonly, because of inborn errors in fat metabolism. Epithelial metaplasia in the breast is a pathologic process.
BP6 22   PBD6 32-33

16. **(E)** Each unit of blood contains 250 mg of iron. The body has no mechanism for getting rid of excess iron. A small amount of iron is lost with normal desquamation of epithelia, and menstruating women lose a bit more. The excess iron becomes storage iron, or hemosiderin. Over time, hemosiderosis involves more and more tissues of the body, particularly the liver. Initially, the hemosiderin deposits are found in Kupffer cells in the liver and other mononuclear phagocytes in the bone marrow, spleen, and lymph nodes. With great excess of iron, liver cells also accumulate iron. Steatosis usually occurs with ingestion of hepatotoxins such as alcohol. Bilirubin, a breakdown product of blood, can be passed out in the bile so that a person does not become jaundiced. Amyloid is an abnormal protein derived from a variety of precursors such as immunoglobulin light chains.
BP6 19   PBD6 42-43

17. **(C)** The cheeselike appearance gives this form of necrosis its name—caseous necrosis. In the lung, tuberculosis and fungal infections are most likely to produce this pattern of tissue injury.
BP6 13   PBD6 17

18. **(K)** Nodular prostatic hyperplasia (also-known as benign prostatic hyperplasia, or BPH) is a common condition in older males that results from proliferation of both prostatic glands and stroma. The prostate becomes more sensitive to androgenic stimulation with age. This is an example of pathologic hyperplasia.
BP6 22   PBD6 32-33

19. **(K)** The liver is one of the few organs that can at least partially regenerate itself in the human body. This is a form of compensatory hyperplasia. The stimuli to hepatocyte mitotic activity cease when the liver has attained its normal size.
BP6 22   PBD6 32-33

20. **(A)** Atrophy is often associated with increased destruction of subcellular components by autophagy. The cellular components (e.g., mitochondria, endoplasmic reticulum) are digested by the lysosomal enzymes. Some of the cell debris resist digestion and persist as insoluble material in the lysosomes. Lipofuscin granules represent undigested material that results from lipid peroxidation.
BP6 19   PBD6 26, 36

21. **(B)** This histologic picture is typical of apoptosis produced by chemotherapeutic agents. The release of cytochrome from the mitochondria is a key step in many forms of apoptosis, and it leads to the activation of caspases. *bcl-2* is an antiapoptotic protein that prevents cytochrome *c* release and prevents caspase activation. Lipofuscin is a pigmented residue representing undigested cellular organelles in autophagic vacuoles. Catalase is a scavenger of H_2O_2. Phospholipases are activated during necrosis and cause cell membrane damage.
BP6 13-15   PBD6 22-24

22. **(D)** Metastatic calcification of tissues occurs when there is marked hypercalcemia, and calcium is precipitated within interstitial tissues, particularly the lung, kidney, and stomach. Hypercalcemia can have a variety of causes, including hyperparathyroidism, bone destruction due to metastases, paraneoplastic syndromes, and, less commonly, vitamin D intoxication or sarcoidosis. Tuberculosis of the lung results in caseous necrosis and dystrophic calcification in the damaged tissues. Pancreatitis may be the result of hypercalcemia, but the pancreas demonstrates fat necrosis that may develop dystrophic calcification. So-called senile calcific aortic stenosis is a form of dystrophic calcification in a person whose serum calcium level is normal. With amyloidosis, there is deposition of the amyloid protein in a variety of tissues, but calcification does not occur, and hypercalcemia is not a complication.
BP6 20   PBD6 45

23. **(D)** The high lipid content of central nervous system (CNS) tissues results in liquefactive necrosis as a consequence of ischemic injury, as in this case of a "stroke." Fat necrosis is seen in breast and pancreas tissues. Coagulative necrosis is the typical result of ischemia in most solid organs. Apoptosis affects single cells and typically is not grossly visible. Karyolysis refers to fading away of cell nuclei in dead cells.
BP6 12-13   PBD6 16-17

24. **(C)** This is fatty change (steatosis) of the liver, with lipid vacuoles seen in many of the hepatocytes. Abnormalities in lipoprotein metabolism can lead to steatosis. Alcohol is a hepatotoxin that produces hepatic steatosis. Decreased serum albumin levels and increased prothrombin time suggest alcohol-induced liver damage. Drug abuse with heroin has surprisingly few organ-specific pathologic findings. Exercise has little direct effect on hepatic function. Smoking directly damages lung tissue but has no direct effect on the liver. Aspirin has a significant effect on platelet function, not on hepatocytes.
BP6 17-18   PBD6 39-40

25. **(A)** This cell is shrunken and converted into a dense eosinophilic mass. The surrounding cells are normal, and there is no inflammatory reaction. This pattern is typical of apoptosis. Caspase activation is a universal feature of apoptosis, regardless of the initiating cause. Reduced ATP synthesis and increased glycolysis occur when a cell is subjected to anoxia. These changes are reversible. Lipases are activated in enzymatic fat necrosis. Lipid peroxidation occurs when the cell is injured by free radicals.
BP6 13-14   PBD6 18-20

26. **(D)** Lipofuscin is a "wear and tear" pigment that increases with aging, particularly in liver and in myocardium. The pigment has minimal effect on cellular function in most cases. Rarely, there is marked lipofuscin deposition in a small heart, a so-called brown atrophy. Melanin pigment is responsible for skin tone: the more melanin, the darker the skin. Hemosiderin is the breakdown product of hemoglobin that contains the iron. Hearts with excessive iron deposition tend to be large. Glycogen is increased with some inherited enzyme disorders and, when the heart is involved, increases heart size. Bilirubin, another breakdown product of hemoglobin, imparts a yellow appearance (icterus) to tissues.
BP6 19   PBD6 42

27. **(A)** Anthracotic pigmentation is common in lung and hilar lymph nodes. This is carbon pigment inhaled from polluted air. The tar in cigarette smoke is a good source of such carbonaceous pigment. Hemorrhage can resolve, with formation of hemosiderin pigmentation that imparts a brown color to tissues. Hepatic failure may result in jaundice, with a yellow color. Older persons generally have more anthracotic pigment, but this is not inevitable with aging—persons living in rural areas will have less. Metastases impart a tan to white appearance to tissues.
BP6 19   PBD6 42

28. **(D)** Deposition of calcium in normal healthy tissues from prolonged hypercalcemia is called metastatic calcification. This may occur in hyperparathyroidism. Dystrophic calcification refers to calcium deposition in injured tissues, with normal serum calcium levels.
BP6 20   PBD6 45

29. **(D)** The loss of the nucleus results in cell death. All other cellular morphologic changes represent reversible cellular injury. The plasma membrane and intracellular organelles remain functional unless severe damage causes loss of membrane integrity.
BP6 11-12   PBD6 8-10

30. **(B)** Reperfusion injury is clinically important in myocardial infarction and stroke. Paradoxically, the oxygen that flows in with blood can be converted to free radicals by parenchymal and endothelial cells and infiltrating leukocytes. Catalase is a scavenger of free radicals. All other changes listed occur in sublethal cell injury.
BP6 11   PBD6 14-15

31. **(B)** The deep eosinophilic staining, loss of nuclei, and the loss of cell structure suggest an early ischemic

injury, resulting in coagulative necrosis. This is typically caused by loss of blood flow. Viral infection could cause necrosis of the myocardium, but this is usually accompanied by an inflammatory infiltrate consisting of lymphocytes and macrophages. Blunt trauma produces hemorrhage. An immunologic injury may produce focal cell injury but not widespread ischemic injury. Lack of protein leads to a catabolic state with gradual decrease in cell size but it does not cause ischemic changes.

BP6 6–7 **PBD6** 7

32. **(D)** The increase in uterine size is primarily the result of an increase in myometrial smooth muscle cell size. The endometrium also increases in size, but it remains just a lining to the muscular wall and does not contribute as much to the size change. There is little stroma in myometrium and a greater proportion in endometrium, but this contributes a smaller percentage to the size gain than does muscle. The vessels are a minor but essential component to this process.

BP6 22 **PBD6** 33–35

33. **(A)** Heterophagocytosis by macrophages requires that endocytosed vacuoles fuse with lysosomes to degrade the engulfed material. With congestive failure, extravasation of red blood cells (RBCs) into alveoli occurs, and pulmonary macrophages must phagocytose the RBCs, breaking down the hemoglobin and recycling the iron by hemosiderin formation.

BP6 15–16 **PBD6** 25–26

Acute and Chronic Inflammation

PBD6 Chapter 3 - Acute and Chronic Inflammation
BP6 Chapter 2 - Acute and Chronic Inflammation

1. The products of the complement system are involved in all of the following steps or phases of the inflammatory response *except*

- (A) Chemotaxis
- (B) Increased vascular permeability
- (C) Neutrophil activation
- (D) Phagocytosis
- (E) Killing of bacteria in the phagocytic vacuole

2. After the leukocytes leave the vasculature, their migration in tissues to the site of infection or injury is mediated by which of the following substances acting as a chemotactic factor?

- (A) Bradykinin
- (B) Chemokines
- (C) Histamine
- (D) Prostaglandins
- (E) Complement C3a

3. A 53-year-old female has had a high fever with cough productive of yellowish sputum for the past 2 days. Auscultation of the chest reveals a few crackles in both lung bases. A chest radiograph reveals bilateral patchy pulmonary infiltrates. Which of the following inflammatory cell types will be seen in greatly increased numbers in a sputum specimen?

- (A) Macrophages
- (B) Neutrophils
- (C) Mast cells
- (D) Small lymphocytes
- (E) Langhans giant cells

4. Two weeks after an acute myocardial infarction, the necrotic myocardium has largely been replaced by capil-laries, fibroblasts, and collagen. A variety of inflammatory cells are present. Which of the following inflammatory cell types in such a lesion plays an important part in the healing process?

- (A) Macrophages
- (B) Plasma cells
- (C) Neutrophils
- (D) Eosinophils
- (E) Epithelioid cells

5. Aspirin is often used for its anti-inflammatory effects. Which of the following features of the inflammatory response is affected by aspirin?

- (A) Vasodilation
- (B) Chemotaxis
- (C) Phagocytosis
- (D) Emigration of leukocytes
- (E) Release of leukocytes from the bone marrow

6. A 6-year-old male child presents with a history of recurrent infections with pyogenic bacteria (e.g., *Staphylococcus aureus, Streptococcus penumoniae*). After infections, there is an expected increase in the total white blood cell (WBC) count and neutrophilic leukocytosis. However, histologic examination of tissues reveals very few neutrophils. An analysis of patient's neutrophil function in specially constructed tubes lined with human endothelium shows a defect in rolling. A defect or deficiency affecting which of the following molecules is likely to be responsible for the increased susceptibility to infection in this patient?

- (A) Selectins
- (B) Integrins
- (C) Leukotriene B_4
- (D) C3b
- (E) NADPH oxidase

7. A 32-year-old female has had a chronic cough with fever for the past month. A chest radiograph shows many small, ill-defined nodular opacities in all lung fields. A transbronchial biopsy reveals interstitial infiltrates with lymphocytes, plasma cells, and epithelioid macrophages.

Which of the following infectious agents most likely caused this appearance?

○ (A) *Staphylococcus aureus*
○ (B) *Plasmodium falciparum*
○ (C) *Candida albicans*
○ (D) *Mycobacterium tuberculosis*
○ (E) *Klebsiella pneumoniae*

8. A 36-year-old male has experienced mid-epigastric abdominal pain for the past 3 months. Upper endoscopy reveals a 2-cm ulceration of the gastric antrum. A biopsy of the ulcer shows angiogenesis with fibrosis and mononuclear cell infiltrates with lymphocytes, macrophages, and plasma cells. The best term for this pathologic process is

○ (A) Acute inflammation
○ (B) Serous inflammation
○ (C) Granulomatous inflammation
○ (D) Fibrinous inflammation
○ (E) Chronic inflammation

For each of the descriptions of an inflammatory response in questions 9, 10, and 11, match the most closely associated lettered chemical mediator involved with the response.

(A) Bradykinin
(B) Chemokines
(C) Complement C3b
(D) Complement C5a
(E) Leukotrienes
(F) Histamine
(G) Interferon-γ
(H) Interleukin-1
(I) Myeloperoxidase
(J) Nitric oxide
(K) Oxygen metabolites
(L) Phospholipase C
(M) Platelet-activating factor
(N) Substance P
(O) Tumor necrosis factor

9. Lymphocytes are activated by contact with antigen and then begin to produce a substance that is a major stimulator of monocytes and macrophages. (   )

10. A 41-year-old man has a severe headache. A lumbar puncture is performed, and the cerebrospinal fluid obtained has a cell count of 910 WBCs/mm^3, with differential count of 94% neutrophils and 6% lymphocytes. Inflammatory mediators are released that cause him to develop a fever with temperature of 39.7°C. (   )

11. A woman who dislikes cats because she is allergic to them visits her neighbor, who has several cats in the house. Of course, one of the cats immediately jumps into her lap. The cat dander is inhaled, and within minutes, she is sneezing and develops nasal stuffiness with abundant nasal secretions. The mast cells have released a mediator to produce these findings. (   )

12. A month after an appendectomy, a 25-year-old woman palpates a small nodule beneath the skin at the site of the healed right lower quadrant incision. The nodule is excised and microscopically shows macrophages, collagen, a few small lymphocytes, and giant cells. Polarizable, refractile material is in the nodule. Which of the following complications of her surgery best accounts for these findings?

○ (A) Chronic inflammation
○ (B) Abscess formation
○ (C) Suture granuloma
○ (D) Ulceration
○ (E) Edema

13. A defect in which of the following steps of inflammatory response is responsible for the increased susceptibility to infection seen in patients with chronic granulomatous disease?

○ (A) Activation of macrophages by interferon-γ
○ (B) Oxygen-dependent killing of bacteria by neutrophils
○ (C) Firm adhesion between leukocytes and endothelial cells
○ (D) Synthesis of lysozyme in neutrophil granules
○ (E) Opsonization of bacteria by immunoglobulins

14. During acute inflammation, there is a "burst" of oxygen consumption (respiratory burst) in neutrophils. This is an essential step for which of the following events?

○ (A) Increased production in the bone marrow
○ (B) Attachment to the endothelial cells
○ (C) Opsonization of bacteria
○ (D) Phagocytosis of bacteria
○ (E) Generation of microbicidal activity

15. A 20-year-old, sexually promiscuous female experiences lower abdominal pain of 24 hours' duration. There is no previous history of pain. She is febrile and has a markedly tender lower abdomen on palpation. The total WBC is 29,000/mm^3, with 75% neutrophils. Laparotomy reveals a distended, fluid-filled, reddened left fallopian tube that is about to rupture. The tube is removed. Histologic examination of the fallopian tube is likely to reveal all of the following *except*

○ (A) Neutrophilic infiltrate
○ (B) Fibroblastic proliferation
○ (C) Exudation of fibrin
○ (D) Necrosis of mucosa
○ (E) Dilated blood vessels full of red cells

16. A chest radiograph of a 9-year-old male infected with *Mycobacterium tuberculosis* reveals enlargement of hilar lymph nodes. There is granulomatous inflammation within the nodes, marked by the presence of Langhans giant cells. The mediator that most aids in this giant cell formation is

○ (A) Tumor necrosis factor
○ (B) Complement C3b
○ (C) Leukotriene B$_4$
○ (D) Interferon-γ
○ (E) Interleukin-1

17. A patient with recurrent bacterial infections is diagnosed to have a genetic deficiency in myeloperoxidase. The

cause of increased susceptibility to infections is

○ (A) Defective neutrophil degranulation
○ (B) Defective production of prostaglandins
○ (C) An inability to produce hydroxy-halide radicals
○ (D) Decreased oxygen consumption after phagocytosis
○ (E) An inability to produce hydrogen peroxide

18. A 78-year-old female suffers a stroke, with loss of movement on the right side of her body. She is found to have an occlusion of the left middle cerebral artery. To prevent further ischemic injury, which of the following mediators would be most beneficial?

○ (A) Thromboxane A$_2$
○ (B) Bradykinin
○ (C) Nitric oxide
○ (D) Platelet activating factor
○ (E) Leukotriene E$_4$

For the clinical histories in questions 19 and 20, match the most closely associated lettered inflammatory response.

(A) Abscess
(B) Caseating granuloma
(C) Chronic inflammation
(D) Edema
(E) Fibrinous inflammation
(F) Fibrosis
(G) Foreign body granuloma
(H) Lymphadenitis
(I) Purulent exudate
(J) Regeneration
(K) Serous effusion
(L) Ulceration

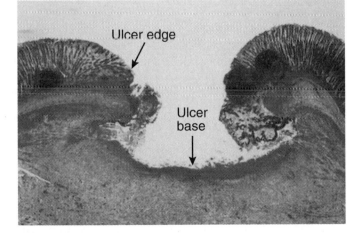

19. A 50-year-old man who has experienced midabdominal pain for several weeks is found to have occult blood–positive stool. On upper endoscopy, he is found to have the duodenal lesion depicted microscopically in the figure. (   )

20. Thoracentesis is performed on a 70-year-old woman, and 800 mL of cloudy yellow fluid is obtained from the left pleural cavity. A cell count on this fluid reveals 2500 white blood cells/mm³, with a differential count of 98% neutrophils and 2% lymphocytes. A Gram stain of this fluid reveals gram-positive cocci in clusters. (   )

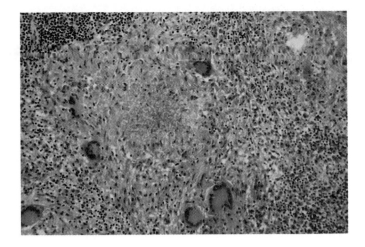

21. A 43-year-old male has had a cough with fever for the previous 2 months. A chest radiograph reveals nodular densities, some with calcification, located mainly in the upper lobes. The microscopic appearance of a lung biopsy is shown. Which of the following chemical mediators is most important in the pathogenesis of this lesion?

○ (A) Complement C5a
○ (B) Interferon-γ
○ (C) Bradykinin
○ (D) Nitric oxide
○ (E) Prostaglandin

22. A 59-year-old male has had a cough with fever for the past week. A chest radiograph reveals a right pleural fluid collection. A right thoracentesis yields 500 mL of cloudy yellow fluid. Which of the following cell types is most likely to be abundant in this fluid?

○ (A) Macrophages
○ (B) Neutrophils
○ (C) CD4 lymphocytes
○ (D) Plasma cells
○ (E) Eosinophils

23. A 5-year-old child reaches up to the stove and touches a pot of boiling soup. Within several hours, there is marked erythema of the skin of the fingers on the right hand, and small blisters appear on the finger pads. Which of the following terms best describes this process?

○ (A) Fibrinous inflammation
○ (B) Purulent inflammation
○ (C) Serous inflammation
○ (D) Ulceration
○ (E) Granulomatous inflammation

24. Two weeks after a 90-year-old female with *Staphylococcus aureus* pneumonia received a course of antibiotic therapy, she no longer has a productive cough, but she still has a fever. A chest radiograph reveals a 3-cm, rounded

density in the right lower lobe whose liquefied contents form a central air-fluid level. There are no surrounding infiltrates. What is the best description for this outcome of her pneumonia?

○ (A) Complete resolution
○ (B) Regeneration
○ (C) Fibrosis
○ (D) Abscess formation
○ (E) Progression to chronic inflammation

25. A 30-year-old female who has a history of congenital heart disease with a ventricular septal defect presents with persistent fever and headache. A head computed tomography scan reveals an abscess in the right parietal lobe that is 3 cm in diameter. Which of the following actions by inflammatory cells best accounts for abscess formation?

○ (A) Formation of nitric oxide by macrophages
○ (B) Production of interferon-γ by lymphocytes
○ (C) Formation of TGF-β by macrophages
○ (D) Generation of prostaglandin by endothelium
○ (E) Release of lysosomal enzymes from neutrophils

26. A chest radiograph of a 35-year-old male demonstrates large, bilateral pleural effusions that have accumulated in the past 24 hours. Thoracentesis is performed, and 500 mL of slightly cloudy yellow fluid is removed. Cytologic examination of the fluid reveals many neutrophils but no lymphocytes or red blood cells. Which of the following mechanisms contributes to the accumulation of the fluid in the pleural space?

○ (A) Arteriolar vasoconstriction
○ (B) Neutrophil release of lysosomes
○ (C) Endothelial contraction
○ (D) Inhibition of platelet adherence
○ (E) Lymphatic obstruction

27. A 12-month-old child with a 6-month history of repeated infections presents with a lung infection and elevated numbers of neutrophils in peripheral blood. Aspiration of a lung abscess shows accumulation of neutrophils. Laboratory studies demonstrate that his neutrophils phagocytose and kill organisms normally in the presence of normal human serum (but not patient's serum). They migrate normally in a chemotaxis assay. Which of the following is the most likely cause for the increased susceptibility to infection?

○ (A) Deficiency of integrins
○ (B) Neutrophil microtubular protein defect
○ (C) Immunoglobulin deficiency
○ (D) Defective neutrophil H_2O_2 generation
○ (E) Deficiency of selectins

28. A 35-year-old female takes aspirin for her arthritis. Although her joint pain is reduced with this therapy, the inflammatory process continues. The aspirin therapy alleviates her pain mainly through reduction in the synthesis of which of the following mediators?

○ (A) Complement C1q
○ (B) Prostaglandins

○ (C) Leukotriene E_4
○ (D) Histamine
○ (E) Nitric oxide

29. A patient with right ventricular failure (congestive heart failure) develops fever and accumulation of fluid in the pleural space. The fluid has a high specific gravity (1.030), and it contains degenerating neutrophils. The most likely cause of fluid accumulation is an *increase* in

○ (A) Colloid osmotic pressure
○ (B) Lymphatic pressure
○ (C) Vascular permeability
○ (D) Renal retention of sodium and water
○ (E) Leukocytes

30. A 5-year-old child who presents with history of recurrent infections with gram-positive bacteria such as *Staphylococcus aureus* is found to have a genetic lack of β_2-integrins. Which of the following abnormalities of neutrophil function is responsible for his clinical symptoms?

○ (A) Neutrophils show normal "rolling" but inadequate sticking on cytokine-activated endothelial cells
○ (B) Failure of the neutrophils to migrate to the site of infection after leaving the vasculature
○ (C) Reduced respiratory burst in neutrophils after phagocytosis of bacteria
○ (D) Diminished phagocytosis of bacteria opsonized with immunoglobulin G
○ (E) Failure to generate hydroxy-halide radicals (HOCl)

ANSWERS

1. **(E)** Complement components are not involved in the killing of bacteria within leukocytes. The components of complement circulate in plasma and can be found in exuded plasma at sites of inflammation, but these components are not found intracellularly. The membrane attack complex formed by C5-9 can kill bacteria extracellularly. C5a is a powerful chemotactic agent, and it causes neutrophil activation. C3a and C5a increase vascular permeability by causing release of histamine from mast cells. C3b is an opsonin.
BP6 35–36   PBD6 67–69

2. **(B)** Chemokines include a number of molecules that are chemotactic for neutrophils, eosinophils, lymphocytes, monocytes, and basophils. Bradykinin causes pain and increased vascular permeability. Histamine causes vascular leakage, and prostaglandins have multiple actions, but they do not cause chemotaxis. C3a causes increased vascular permeability by releasing histamine from mast cells.
BP6 31   PBD6 61

3. **(B)** The signs and symptoms suggest an acute bacterial pneumonia. Such infections induce an acute inflammation dominated by neutrophils, which gives the sputum the yel-

lowish, purulent appearance. Macrophages become more numerous after the acute events and clean up the debris through phagocytosis. Mast cells are better known as participants in allergic and anaphylactic responses. Lymphocytes are a feature of chronic inflammation. Langhans giant cells are seen with granulomatous inflammatory responses.
BP6 26   PBD6 51

4. **(A)** Macrophages, present in such lesions, play a prominent role in the healing process. Activated macrophages can secrete a variety of cytokines that promote angiogenesis and fibrosis, including platelet-derived growth factor, fibroblast growth factor, interleukin-1, and tumor necrosis factor. Plasma cells can secrete immunoglobulins and are not instrumental to healing of an area of tissue injury. The neutrophils are most numerous within the initial 48 hours after infarction but are not numerous after the first week. Eosinophils are most prominent in allergic inflammations and in parasitic infections. Epithelioid cells, which are aggregations of activated macrophages, are typically seen with granulomatous inflammation. The healing of acute inflammatory processes does not involve granulomatous inflammation.
BP6 41-42   PBD6 79-81

5. **(A)** Aspirin (acetylsalicylic acid) blocks the cyclooxygenase pathway of arachidonic acid metabolism, which leads to reduced prostaglandin generation. Prostaglandins promote vasodilation at sites of inflammation. Chemotaxis is a function of various chemokines, and complement C3b may promote phagocytosis, but neither is affected by aspirin. Leukocyte emigration is aided by various adhesion molecules. Leukocyte release from the marrow can be driven by the cytokines interleukin-1 and tumor necrosis factor (TNF).
BP6 37   PBD6 71-72

6. **(A)** The patient has a defect in leukocyte rolling, the first step in transmigration of neutrophils from the vasculature to the tissues. Rolling depends on interaction between selectins (P- and E-selectins on endothelial cells, and L-selectin on neutrophils) and their sialyated ligand molecules (e.g., sialyated Lewis X). Integrins are involved in the next step of transmigration, during which there is firm adhesion between neutrophils and endothelial cells. Leukotriene B_4 is a chemotactic agent, C3b facilitates phagocytosis, and NADPH oxidase is involved in microbicidal activity.
BP6 28-29   PBD6 58-63

7. **(D)** Her disease has features of granulomatous inflammation, and tuberculosis is a common cause. Bacteria such as *Staphylococcus* and *Klebsiella* are more likely to produce acute inflammation. *Plasmodium* produces malaria, which is a parasitic infection without a significant degree of lung involvement. *Candida* is often a commensal organism in the oropharyngeal region and rarely causes a pneumonia in healthy (nonimmunosuppressed) individuals.
BP6 42-43   PBD6 82-83

8. **(E)** One of the outcomes of acute inflammation with ulceration is chronic inflammation. This is particularly true when the inflammatory process continues for weeks to months. Chronic inflammation is characterized by tissue destruction, mononuclear cell infiltration, and repair. In acute inflammation, the healing process with fibrosis and angiogenesis has not started. Serous inflammation refers to an inflammatory process involving a mesothelial surface (e.g., lining of the pericardial cavity), with an outpouring of fluid having little protein or cellular content. Granulomatous inflammation is a special form of chronic inflammation in which epithelioid macrophages form aggregates. With fibrinous inflammation, typically involving a mesothelial surface, there is an outpouring of protein-rich fluid that results in precipitation of fibrin.
BP6 41   PBD6 79

9. **(G)** Interferon-γ secreted from lymphocytes stimulates monocytes and macrophages, which then secrete their own cytokines that further activate lymphocytes. Interferon-γ is also important in transforming macrophages into epithelioid cells in a granulomatous inflammatory response.
BP6 42-43   PBD6 82-83

10. **(H or O)** Fever is produced by a variety of inflammatory mediators, but the major cytokines that produce fever are interleukin-1 and tumor necrosis factor, produced by macrophages and other cell types. Interleukin-1 and tumor necrosis factor can have autocrine, paracrine, and endocrine effects. They mediate the acute phase responses, such as fever, nausea, and neutrophil release from marrow.
BP6 40   PBD6 78

11. **(F)** Histamine is found in abundance in mast cells, normally present in connective tissues next to blood vessels beneath mucosal surfaces in airways. Binding of an antigen (i.e., allergen) to IgE antibodies that have previously attached to the mast cells by the Fc receptor triggers mast cell degranulation, with release of histamine. This response causes increased vascular permeability and mucous secretions.
BP6 34   BPD6 66

12. **(C)** The polarizable material is the suture, and a giant cell reaction, typically with foreign body giant cells, is characteristic for a granulomatous reaction to foreign material. Chronic inflammation alone is not likely to produce a localized nodule with giant cells. An abscess, typically from a wound infection, should have liquefactive necrosis and numerous neutrophils. An ulceration involves loss of epidermis or other epithelial layer. Edema refers to accumulation of fluid in the interstitial space. It does not produce a cellular nodule.
BP6 42-43   PBD6 83

13. **(B)** Chronic granulomatous disease is characterized by reduced killing of ingested microbes because of inherited defects in the NADPH oxidase system. This system generates superoxide anions (O_2^-), essential for the subsequent production of microbicidal products such as H_2O_2, OH, and $HOCl^-$. Firm adhesions between leukocytes and

endothelium are impaired in leukocyte adhesion deficiency type 1, in which there is a mutation in the beta chain of integrins. Lysozyme contained in neutrophil granules is responsible for oxygen-independent killing of bacteria. Impaired opsonization can lead to infections in states of immunoglobulin deficiency.
BP6 32-33   PBD6 62-65

14.   **(E)** The oxidative burst generates the reactive oxygen species (i.e., superoxide anion) that are important in destruction of engulfed bacteria. Myelopoiesis does not depend on generation of superoxide. Endothelial attachment of neutrophils is aided by adhesion molecules on the endothelium and the neutrophil surface. These molecules include selectins and integrins. Bacteria are opsonized by complement C3b and immunoglobulin G, allowing the bacteria to be more readily phagocytosed.
BP6 32-33   PBD6 62-64

15.   **(B)** This is an acute inflammatory response, with edema, erythema, and pain of short duration. Fibroblasts are more likely participants in chronic inflammatory responses and in healing responses, generally appearing beyond a week after the initial event.
BP6 40-41   PBD6 78-79

16.   **(D)** Interferon-γ is secreted by activated T cells and is an important mediator of granulomatous inflammation. It causes activation of macrophages and their transformation into epithelioid cells and giant cells. Tumor necrosis factor can be secreted by activated macrophages and induces activation of lymphocytes and proliferation of fibroblasts, other elements of a granuloma. Complement C3b acts as an opsonin in acute inflammatory reactions. Leukotriene B_4 induces chemotaxis in acute inflammatory processes. Interleukin-1 can be secreted by macrophages to produce a variety of effects, including fever, leukocyte adherence, fibroblast proliferation, and cytokine secretion.
BP6 42   PBD6 82-83

17.   **(C)** Myeloperoxidase is present in the azurophilic granules of neutrophils. It converts H_2O_2 into $HOCl^-$, a powerful oxidant and antimicrobial agent. Degranulation occurs when phagolysosomes are formed with engulfed bacteria in phagocytic vacuoles within the neutrophil cytoplasm. In contrast, prostaglandin production depends on a functioning cyclooxygenase pathway of arachidonic acid metabolism. Oxygen consumption with an oxidative burst after phagocytosis is aided by glucose oxidation and activation of neutrophil NADPH oxidase, resulting in generation of superoxide that is converted by spontaneous dismutation to H_2O_2.
BP6 32-33   PBD6 62-64

18.   **(C)** Endothelial cells can release nitric oxide to produce vasodilation. Nitric oxide can also be administered to patients to promote vasodilation in areas of ischemic injury. Thromboxane A_2, platelet activating factor, and leukotriene E_4 have vasoconstrictive properties. Bradykinin mainly increases vascular permeability and produces pain.
BP6 38-39   PBD6 75

19.   **(L)** Inflammation involving an epithelial surface may produce enough necrosis so that the surface becomes eroded and is lost. This forms an ulcer. If the inflammation continues, the ulcer can continue to penetrate downward into submucosa and muscularis. Alternatively, the ulcer may heal or may remain chronically inflamed.
BP6 45   PBD6 85

20.   **(I)** Some bacteria evoke an acute inflammatory response dominated by neutrophils. The extravasated neutrophils attempt to phagocytose and kill the bacteria. In the process, some neutrophils die, and the release of their lysosomal enzymes can cause liquefactive necrosis of the tissue. This liquefied tissue debris and the live and dead neutrophils comprise "pus," or purulent exudate. Such an exudate is typical for bacterial infections that involve body cavities. This infection probably spread from the lung.
BP6 45   PBD6 84-85

21.   **(B)** This is a granuloma with many epithelioid cells and prominent large Langhans giant cells. Macrophage stimulation and transformation to epithelioid cells and giant cells are characteristic of granuloma formation. Interferon-γ promotes the formation of epithelioid cells and giant cells. Complement C5a is chemotactic for neutrophils. Although occasional neutrophils are seen in granulomas, neutrophils do not form a major component of granulomatous inflammation. Bradykinin, released in acute inflammatory responses, results in pain. Macrophages can release nitric oxide to destroy other cells, but nitric oxide does not stimulate macrophages to form a granulomatous response. Prostaglandins are mainly involved in the causation of vasodilation and pain in acute inflammatory responses.
BP6 42-43   PBD6 83-84

22.   **(B)** His findings suggest an acute inflammatory process, dominated by the presence of neutrophils. As this process resolves, the number of macrophages will increase. Chronic inflammatory cells, including lymphocytes and plasma cells, may be few in number but are not necessarily absent from acute inflammatory processes. Eosinophils form the minority of acute inflammatory infiltrates unless allergic or parasitic stimuli are present.
BP6 45   PBD6 84-85

23.   **(C)** Serous inflammation represents the mildest form of acute inflammation. A blister is a good example of serous inflammation. It is associated primarily with exudation of fluid into the subcorneal or subepidermal space. Because the injury is mild, the fluid is relatively protein poor. A protein-rich exudate results in fibrin accumulation. Acute inflammatory cells, mainly neutrophils, exuded into a body cavity or space form a purulent (suppurative) exudate, typically associated with liquefactive necrosis. Loss of the epithelium leads to ulceration. Granulomatous inflammation is characterized by collections of transformed macrophages called epithelioid cells.
BP6 44   PBD6 84

24.   **(D)** The formation of a fluid-filled cavity after an infection with *S. aureus* suggests that liquefactive necrosis has occurred. The cavity is filled with tissue debris and

viable and dead neutrophils (i.e., pus). Localized, pus-filled cavities are called abscesses. Some bacterial organisms, such as *S. aureus*, are more likely to be pyogenic, or pus forming. With complete resolution, the structure of the lung remains almost unaltered. Lung tissue, unlike liver, is not capable of regeneration. Scarring or fibrosis may follow acute inflammation as the damaged tissue is replaced by fibrous connective tissue. Most bacterial pneumonias resolve, and progression to continued chronic inflammation is uncommon.
BP6 40-41   PBD6 78-79, 85

25. **(E)** The tissue destruction that accompanies abscess formation as part of acute inflammatory processes occurs from lysosomal enzymatic destruction, aided by release of reactive oxygen species. Nitric oxide generated by macrophages aids in destruction of infectious agents. The interferon-γ released from lymphocytes plays a major role in chronic and granulomatous inflammatory responses. Transforming growth factor-β formed by macrophages promotes fibrosis. Prostaglandins produced by endothelium promote vasodilation.
BP6 33   PBD6 64-65

26. **(C)** Exudation of fluid from venules and capillaries is a key component of the acute inflammatory process. There are several proposed mechanisms of increased vascular permeability. They include formation of interendothelial gaps by contraction of endothelium. This is caused by mediators such as histamine and leukotrienes. The vessels then become more "leaky," and the fluid leaves the intravascular space. Arteriolar vasoconstriction is a transient response to injury that diminishes blood loss. After neutrophils reach the site of tissue injury outside of the vascular space, they release lysosomal enzymes. Platelets adhere to damaged endothelium and promote hemostasis. Lymphatic obstruction results in the accumulation of protein-rich lymph and lymphocytes, producing a chylous effusion.
BP6 27-28   PBD6 53-54

27. **(C)** The patient has immunoglobulin deficiency, which prevents opsonization and phagocytosis of microbes. Deficiency of integrins and selectins and a defect in microtubules would prevent adhesion and locomotion of neutrophils. H_2O_2 production is part of the oxygen-dependent killing mechanism. This is intact in this patient, because his neutrophils are able to kill bacteria when immunoglobulins in normal serum allow phagocytosis.
BP6 32   PBD6 62-64

28. **(B)** Prostaglandins are produced through the cyclooxygenase pathway of arachidonic acid metabolism. Aspirin and nonsteroidal anti-inflammatory drugs block the synthesis of prostaglandins, which can produce pain. Complement C1q is generated in the initial stage of complement activation, which can result in cell lysis. Leukotrienes are generated by the lipooxygenase pathway, which is not blocked by aspirin. Histamine is mainly a vasodilator. Nitric oxide elaborated by endothelium is a vasodilator.
BP6 37   PBD6 70-71

29. **(C)** The formation of an exudate containing a significant amount of protein and cells depends on the "leakiness" of blood vessels, principally venules. The extravascular colloid osmotic pressure increases when exudation has occurred and the protein content of the extravascular space increases. The lymphatics serve to scavenge exuded fluid with protein and lower the amount of extravascular and extracellular fluid. Sodium and water retention helps drive transudation of fluid. Leukocytosis alone is not sufficient for exudation, because the leukocytes must be driven to emigrate from the vessels by chemotactic factors.
BP6 26-28   PBD6 52-54

30. **(A)** During acute inflammation, neutrophils extravasate from the blood vessels. This process depends on adhesion molecules expressed on the neutrophils and endothelial cells. In the first stage of extravasation, the neutrophils roll over the endothelium. At this stage, the adhesion between the neutrophils and endothelial cells is not very strong. Rolling is mediated by binding of selectins to sialyated oligosaccharides. The next step, firm adhesion, is mediated by binding of integrins on the leukocytes to their receptors intracellular adhesion molecule-1 or vascular cell adhesion molecule-1 (VCAM-1) on endothelial cells. Integrins have two chains, α and β. A genetic lack of β chains prevents firm adhesion of leukocytes to endothelial cells.
BP6 28-29   PBD6 57-59

Tissue Repair: Cellular Growth, Fibrosis, and Wound Healing

CHAPTER 3

PBD6 Chapter 4 - Tissue Repair: Cellular
          Growth, Fibrosis, and
          Wound Healing
BP6 Chapter 5 - Repair: Cell Regeneration,
          Fibrosis, and Wound
          Healing

1. Neutralization of transforming growth factor-β (TGF-β) is most likely to affect which of the following steps in the inflammatory-repair response?

O (A) Leukocyte extravasation
O (B) Increased vascular permeability
O (C) Production of collagen
O (D) Chemotaxis of lymphocytes
O (E) Migration of epithelial cells

2. A 60-year-old female suffered an acute myocardial infarction that involved a 3×4 cm area of the posterior left ventricular free wall. Creatine kinase was elevated to 600 U/L in her serum. She was treated for arrhythmias and decreased cardiac output while in the hospital. A month later, which of the following pathologic findings would you most expect to find in her left ventricle?

O (A) Abscess
O (B) Complete resolution
O (C) Coagulative necrosis
O (D) Nodular regeneration
O (E) Fibrous scar

3. After viral hepatitis, there is usually complete recovery of the normal liver architecture. In contrast, a healed liver abscess caused by bacteria leaves a scar in the liver. Which of the following factors best explains the difference in outcome with these two different forms of liver injury?

O (A) The nature of the etiologic agent
O (B) The extent of liver cell injury
O (C) The injury to the connective tissue framework
O (D) The location of the lesion
O (E) The extent of damage to the bile ducts

4. A 23-year-old female receiving chronic corticosteroid therapy for an autoimmune disease underwent minor surgery for incision and drainage of an abscess on her upper outer right arm. The wound healed poorly over the next month. Which of the following aspects of wound healing is most likely to be deficient?

O (A) Re-epithelization
O (B) Fibroblast growth factor elaboration
O (C) Collagen deposition
O (D) Serine proteinase production
O (E) Neutrophil infiltration

5. A cesarean section was performed on a 20-year-old female to deliver a term baby, and the lower abdominal incision was sutured. The sutures were removed a week later. Which of the following statements regarding the wound site at the time of suture removal is most appropriate?

O (A) Granulation tissue is still present
O (B) Collagen degradation exceeds synthesis
O (C) Wound strength is 80% of normal tissue
O (D) There is a predominance of type IV collagen
O (E) No more wound strength will be gained

For each of the descriptions of the wound healing process in questions 6 and 7, match the most closely associated lettered substance:

(A) Collagenase
(B) Cyclin B
(C) Epidermal growth factor
(D) Fibronectin
(E) Integrin
(F) Interleukin-1
(G) Platelet-derived growth factor
(H) Plasmin
(I) Tumor necrosis factor
(J) Type IV collagen
(K) Vascular endothelial cell growth factor
(L) Zinc

6. During remodeling of scars, metalloproteinases degrade extracellular matrix components. This action of metalloproteinases is diminished because of the lack of this substance. (   )

7. Intracytoplasmic cytoskeletal elements, including actin, interact with the extracellular matrix through this molecule to provide cell attachment and migration in wound healing. (   )

8. Release of epidermal growth factor in an area of denuded skin causes mitogenic stimulation of the skin epithelial cells. Which of the following proteins is involved in transducing the mitogenic signal from the epidermal cell membrane to the nucleus?

○ (A) G proteins
○ (B) ras proteins
○ (C) Cyclin D
○ (D) cAMP
○ (E) Cyclin-dependent kinase

9. During growth factor–induced cellular regeneration, which of the following transitions during cell cycle is controlled by the phosphorylation of the retinoblastoma (Rb) protein:

○ (A) G_0 to G_1
○ (B) G_1 to S
○ (C) S to G_2
○ (D) G_2 to M
○ (E) M to G_1

10. Which of the following molecules synthesized by fibroblasts can bind to cellular integrins and to extracellular collagen and can attach epidermal basal cells to basement membrane?

○ (A) Heparin
○ (B) Dermatan sulfate
○ (C) Procollagen
○ (D) Fibronectin
○ (E) Hyaluronic acid

11. A laceration to the left hand of an 18-year-old male was sutured, and after the sutures were removed a week later, healing continued. However, the site of the wound became disfigured by a prominent raised, nodular scar that developed over the following 2 months. What process occurred?

○ (A) Organization
○ (B) Dehiscence
○ (C) Resolution
○ (D) Keloid formation
○ (E) Secondary union

12. During the healing of a skin ulcer, which of the following factors is most effective in promoting angiogenesis?

○ (A) Platelet-derived growth factor (PDGF)
○ (B) Epidermal growth factor (EGF)
○ (C) Basic fibroblast growth factor (bFGF)
○ (D) Endostatin
○ (E) Interleukin-1

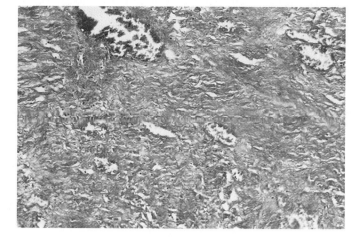

13. The appearance of the trichrome-stained section of a surgical wound site in the figure is most likely to be seen how long after surgery?

○ (A) 1 day
○ (B) 2 to 3 days
○ (C) 4 to 5 days
○ (D) 2 weeks
○ (E) 1 month

14. In a 50-year-old woman found to be positive for hepatitis A antibody, the serum aspartate aminotransferase (AST) level was 275 U/L and that of alanine aminotransferase (ALT) was 310 U/L. A month later, these enzyme levels have returned to normal. At the end of the month after infection, in which part of the cell cycle are most of the hepatocytes going to be?

○ (A) G_0
○ (B) G_1
○ (C) S
○ (D) G_2
○ (E) M

15. A 40-year-old male underwent laparotomy for a perforated sigmoid colon diverticulum. A wound infection complicated the postoperative course, and surgical wound dehiscence occurred. Six weeks later, the wound was only 10% of its original size. Which of the following processes best accounts for the decrease in wound size?

○ (A) Greater synthesis of collagen
○ (B) Myofibroblast contraction
○ (C) Inhibition of metalloproteinases
○ (D) Diminished subcutaneous edema
○ (E) Elaboration of adhesive glycoproteins

ANSWERS

1. **(C)** TGF-β stimulates many steps in fibrogenesis— fibroblast chemotaxis, production of collagen by fibroblasts—while inhibiting degradation of collagen. All other steps are unaffected by TGF-β.
BP6 51 PBD6 98

2. **(E)** The enzyme elevation indicates that myocardial necrosis occurred. The destruction of myocardial fibers precludes complete resolution. The area of myocardial necrosis is gradually replaced by a fibrous scar. Liquefactive necrosis with abscess formation is not a feature of ischemic myocardial injury. Coagulative necrosis is typical for myocardial infarction, but after a month a scar will be present. Nodular regeneration is typical for hepatocyte injury, because hepatocytes are stable cells.
BP6 58 PBD6 111

3. **(C)** Hepatocytes are stable cells with extensive ability to regenerate. However, the ability to restore normal architecture of an organ such as liver depends on the viability of the supporting connective tissue framework. If the connective tissue cells are not injured, hepatocyte regeneration can restore normal liver architecture. This happens in many cases of viral hepatitis. A liver abscess is associated with liquefactive necrosis of hepatocytes and the supporting connective tissue. It heals by scarring.
BP6 48-49 PBD6 91

4. **(C)** Glucocorticoids inhibit wound healing by impairing collagen synthesis. This is a desirable side effect if the amount of scarring is to be reduced, but results in the delayed healing of surgical wounds. Re-epithelization, in part driven by epidermal growth factor, is not affected by corticosteroid therapy. Serine proteinases are important in wound remodeling. Neutrophil infiltration is not prevented by glucocorticoids.
BP6 57-58 PBD6 110

5. **(A)** At 1 week, wound healing is still not complete, and more collagen will be synthesized in the coming weeks. Granulation tissue will still be present. Wound strength will top out at about 80% by 3 months. Type IV collagen is found in basement membranes.
BP6 56-57 PBD6 108-109

6. **(L)** Zinc is a trace element in the diet that aids wound healing because of its effect in promoting the activity of metalloproteinases.
BP6 55 PBD6 106-107

7. **(E)** Integrins interact with the extracellular matrix proteins (e.g., fibronectin). Engagement of integrins by extracellular matrix proteins leads to the formation of focal adhesions where integrins link to intracellular cytoskeletal elements such as actin. These interactions lead to intracellular signals that modulate cell growth, differentiation, and migration during wound healing.
BP6 52 PBD6 100-101

8. **(B)** ras proteins transduce signals from growth factor receptors, such as epidermal growth factor, that have intrinsic tyrosine kinase activity. G proteins perform a similar function for G-protein–linked, seven spanning receptors. cAMP is an effector in the G-protein signaling pathway. Cyclins and cyclin-dependent kinases regulate the cell cycle in the nucleus.
BP6 51 PBD6 93-94

9. **(B)** Rb proteins control an extremely important check point, the G_1 to S transition during the cell cycle. The other check points are regulated by a distinct set of proteins.
BP6 50 PBD6 96

10. **(D)** Fibronectin is a key component of the extracellular matrix. Fibronectin can be synthesized by monocytes, fibroblasts, and endothelium.
BP6 52-53 PBD6 100-103

11. **(D)** The healing process may sometimes result in an exuberant production of collagen, giving rise to a keloid. This tendency may run in families. Organization occurs as granulation tissue is replaced by fibrous tissue. When a wound pulls apart, dehiscence has occurred. If normal tissue architecture is restored, then resolution of inflammation has occurred. Secondary union describes the process by which large wounds fill in and contract.
BP6 58 PBD6 110

12. **(C)** Basic fibroblast growth factor is a potent inducer of angiogenesis. It can participate in all steps of angiogenesis. Endostatin is an inhibitor of angiogenesis. Platelet-derived growth factor plays a role in vascular remodeling. Epidermal growth factor and interleukin-1 have no angiogenic activity.
BP6 51 PBD6 104-105

13. **(E)** This is dense collagen with some remaining dilated blood vessels, typical of the final phase of wound healing. By day 1, the wound is filled only with fibrin and inflammatory cells. Macrophages and granulation tissue are seen by 2 to 3 days postoperatively. Neovascularization is most prominent on days 4 and 5. By the second week, collagen is prominent, and fewer vessels and inflammatory cells are seen.
BP6 56 PBD6 104,108

14. **(A)** Hepatocytes are quiescent (stable) cells that can re-enter the cell cycle and proliferate in response to hepatic injury. The liver can partially regenerate itself. Acute hepatitis results in hepatocyte necrosis, marked by AST and ALT elevations. After the acute process has ended, the cells return to G_0, and the liver becomes quiescent again.
BP6 48-49 PBD6 90-91

15. **(B)** Wound contraction is a characteristic feature of healing by second intention that occurs in larger wounds. Collagen synthesis helps fill the defect but not contract it. The inhibition of metalloproteinases leads to decreased degradation of collagen and impaired connective tissue remodeling in wound repair. Edema does diminish over time, but this does not result in much contraction. Adhesive glycoproteins such as fibronectin help to maintain a cellular scaffolding for growth and repair but do not contract.
BP6 56 PBD6 108-109

Hemodynamic Disorders, Thrombosis, and Shock

PBD6 Chapter 5 - Hemodynamic Disorders,
Thrombosis, and Shock
BP6 Chapter 4 - Hemodynamic Disorders,
Thrombosis, and Shock

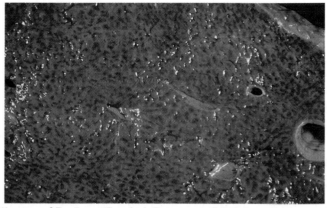

Courtesy of Dr. James Crawford, Department of Pathology, Brigham and Women's Hospital, Boston.

1. While shaving one morning, a 23-year-old male nicks his upper lip with the razor. Within a second after this injury, blood loss from a small dermal arteriole is reduced through

- (A) Activated protein C
- (B) Vasoconstriction
- (C) Platelet aggregation
- (D) Neutrophil chemotaxis
- (E) Fibrin polymerization

2. In which of the following organs is an arterial thromboembolus *least* likely to produce an infarct?

- (A) Brain
- (B) Liver
- (C) Kidney
- (D) Heart
- (E) Spleen

3. A 21-year-old female sustains multiple injuries, including fractures of the right femur, right tibia, and left humerus. These fractures are stabilized at surgery soon after admission to the hospital. She is in stable condition. However, 2 days after admission, she suddenly becomes severely dyspneic. What most likely happened to produce her sudden respiratory difficulty?

- (A) Right hemothorax
- (B) Pulmonary edema
- (C) Fat embolism
- (D) Cardiac tamponade
- (E) Pulmonary infarction

4. The serum aspartate aminotransferase and alanine aminotransferase are observed to be increasing in a 61-year-old man over the past week. He also has increasing lower leg swelling with grade 2+ pitting edema to the knees. He has prominent jugular venous distention in neck veins to the level of the mandible. Which of the following underlying conditions is he most likely to have, based on the gross appearance of the liver seen in the figure?

- (A) Thrombocytopenia
- (B) Portal vein thrombosis
- (C) Chronic renal failure
- (D) Common bile duct obstruction
- (E) Congestive heart failure

5. A 55-year-old female has had discomfort with swelling of her left leg for the past week. The leg is slightly difficult to move, but there is no pain on palpation. A venogram reveals thrombosis of deep left leg veins. Which of the following conditions is most likely to promote this event?

- (A) Turbulent blood flow
- (B) Nitric oxide
- (C) Ingestion of aspirin
- (D) Hypercalcemia
- (E) Immobilization

History for questions 6 through 8: A 56-year-old diabetic male presented with left-sided chest pain that radiated to the arm. Serial measurements of serum creatine kinase isoenzyme MB (CK-MB) levels revealed an elevated level 24 hours after the onset of pain. Coronary angiography revealed occlusion of the left anterior descending artery.

6. In this setting, the most likely cause of thrombosis is

- (A) Stasis of blood flow
- (B) Damage to endothelium
- (C) Decreased production of tissue plasminogen activator (t-PA) by intact endothelial cells
- (D) A decreased level of antithrombin III
- (E) Mutation in factor V gene

7. This patient was then given thrombolytic therapy. Which of the following drugs did he most likely receive?

- (A) t-PA
- (B) Aspirin
- (C) Heparin
- (D) Nitric oxide
- (E) Vitamin K

8. After this treatment, the patient remained stable for 3 days but then developed severe breathlessness and was diagnosed to have acute left ventricular failure. He died 2 hours later. At autopsy, the lungs would most likely show which of the following histologic changes?

- (A) Congestion of alveolar capillaries with fibrin and neutrophils in alveoli
- (B) Congestion of alveolar capillaries with transudate in the alveoli
- (C) Fibrosis of alveolar walls with heart failure cells in alveoli
- (D) Multiple areas of subpleural hemorrhagic necrosis
- (E) A purulent exudate in the pleural space

9. A 27-year-old male is on a scuba diving trip to the Caribbean. After descending to 50 m in the Blue Hole, he returns to the boat. About an hour later, he develops severe, painful myalgias and arthralgias. These symptoms abate over the next day. His symptoms are most likely the result of

- (A) Disseminated intravascular coagulation
- (B) Systemic vasodilation
- (C) Venous thrombosis
- (D) Tissue nitrogen emboli
- (E) Fat globules in arterioles

10. The left breast of a 39-year-old female is slightly enlarged compared with the right. The skin overlying this breast is thickened, reddish-orange, and pitted. Mammography reveals a 3-cm underlying density. A fine-needle aspirate of this mass reveals carcinoma. How is the gross appearance of the left breast best explained?

- (A) Venous thrombosis
- (B) Lymphatic obstruction
- (C) Ischemia
- (D) Chronic passive congestion
- (E) Chronic inflammation

11. Patients with an inherited deficiency of von Willebrand factor have spontaneous bleeding under the skin. A derangement in which of the following steps in hemostasis is most likely affected in such individuals?

- (A) Vasoconstriction
- (B) Platelet adhesion
- (C) Platelet aggregation
- (D) Prothrombin generation
- (E) Fibrin polymerization

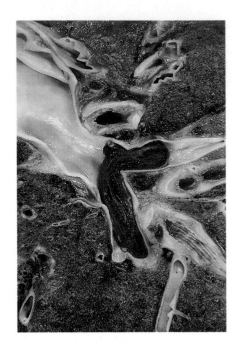

12. A 70-year-old male is ambulating for the first time in 3 weeks after hospitalization for a cerebral infarction. Within minutes of returning to his hospital room, he has a sudden onset of dyspnea. He cannot be resuscitated. At autopsy, the gross appearance of the left lung at the hilum is depicted in the figure. Which of the following risk factors contributed the most to this finding?

- (A) Venous stasis
- (B) Pulmonary arterial atherosclerosis
- (C) Lupus anticoagulant
- (D) Bronchopneumonia
- (E) Factor V Leiden mutation

13. A 25-year-old female has had multiple episodes of deep venous thrombosis in the past 10 years. She has had one episode of pulmonary thromboembolism. Which of the following risk factors has most likely contributed to her condition?

- (A) Factor V Leiden mutation
- (B) Antithrombin III deficiency
- (C) Mutation in protein C
- (D) Hypercholesterolemia
- (E) Smoking

14. A 76-year-old female fell and fractured her left femoral trochanter. After 2 weeks in the hospital, her left leg is swollen, particularly her lower leg below the knee. She experiences pain on movement of this leg, and there is tenderness to palpation. Which of the following complications is most likely to occur after these events?

○ (A) Gangrenous necrosis of the foot
○ (B) Hematoma of the thigh
○ (C) Disseminated intravascular coagulation
○ (D) Pulmonary thromboembolism
○ (E) Fat embolism

15. Patients with hemophilia A (i.e., factor VIII deficiency) have a bleeding disorder. Bleeding occurs because factor VIII

○ (A) Acts as a reaction accelerator (cofactor) during the activation of a coagulation factor
○ (B) Provides the phospholipid necessary for assembly of coagulation factors, cofactors, and calcium
○ (C) Promotes platelet aggregation
○ (D) Neutralizes antithrombin III
○ (E) Causes platelets to release thromboxane A_2

16. Within an hour after a gunshot wound to the abdomen, a 16-year-old male begins to exhibit tachycardia. His skin is cool and clammy to touch. His blood pressure is 80/30 mm Hg. Which of the following organ-specific changes would you most expect to occur over the next 2 days after this injury?

○ (A) Acute hepatic infarction
○ (B) Cerebral basal ganglia hemorrhage
○ (C) Renal passive congestion
○ (D) Pulmonary diffuse alveolar damage
○ (E) Gangrenous necrosis of the lower legs

For each of the clinical histories in questions 17 and 18, match the most closely associated lettered substance that plays a role in coagulation:

(A) Adenosine diphosphate
(B) Antithrombin III
(C) Extracellular matrix
(D) Factor V Leiden
(E) Fibrinogen
(F) Lupus anticoagulant
(G) Plasminogen
(H) Prostaglandin
(I) Thrombomodulin
(J) Thromboxane A_2
(K) Tissue factor
(L) von Willebrand factor

17. A 25-year-old female presents with a stroke resulting from cerebral arterial embolism. In the past 3 years she has had an episode of pulmonary embolism, and her last pregnancy ended in a miscarriage. She is found to have a false-positive serologic test for syphilis. (   )

18. Platelet dense bodies (delta granules) release their contents, and platelets aggregate to form a primary plug within an arterial lumen after a small cut to the forehead in a young boy. (   )

19. After a thrombus is formed in an area of vascular injury, the propagation of the thrombus to normal arteries is prevented in part by the action of

○ (A) Tumor necrosis factor
○ (B) Platelet factor 4
○ (C) Calcium
○ (D) Thrombomodulin
○ (E) Fibrin

20. A 44-year-old male suffers an acute myocardial infarction. After this event, his ejection fraction is only 30%, with reduced cardiac output. He develops increasing pulmonary edema. How does this edema occur?

○ (A) Lymphatic obstruction
○ (B) Decreased plasma osmotic pressure
○ (C) Decreased central venous pressure
○ (D) Increased hydrostatic pressure
○ (E) Acute inflammation

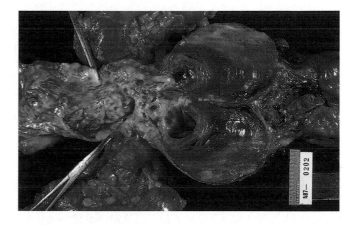

21. A 70-year-old male with a history of diabetes mellitus died of an acute myocardial infarction. The appearance at autopsy of his aorta opened longitudinally is seen in the figure. Which of the following complications of his aortic disease would you most expect to have been present during his life?

○ (A) Renal infarction
○ (B) Pulmonary thromboembolism
○ (C) Edema of the left leg
○ (D) Thrombocytopenia
○ (E) Popliteal arterial occlusion

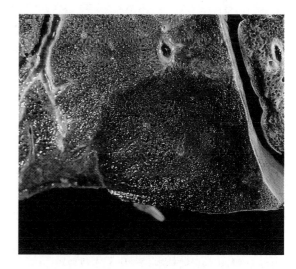

22. A 49-year-old male has congestive heart failure. He develops pneumonia after a bout of influenza, and he spends 2 weeks recuperating. Later, he develops pleuritic chest pain due to the development of the lesion depicted in the figure. Which of the following events has most likely happened?

○ (A) Pulmonary infarction
○ (B) Pulmonary chronic congestion
○ (C) Pulmonary edema
○ (D) Pulmonary acute congestion
○ (E) Pulmonary venous thrombosis

For each of the clinical histories in questions 23, 24, 25, and 26, match the most closely associated lettered pathologic finding.

(A) Air embolus
(B) Amniotic fluid embolus
(C) Anasarca
(D) Cholesterol embolus
(E) Chronic passive congestion
(F) Fat embolus
(G) Mural thrombus
(H) Organization with recanalization
(I) Petechial hemorrhage
(J) Phlebothrombosis
(K) Red infarct
(L) Sacral pitting edema
(M) Septic infarct
(N) Vegetation
(O) White infarct

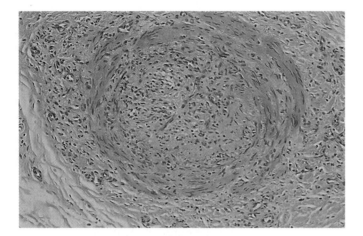

23. The small artery depicted in the figure is present in the epicardium of a 58-year-old male with severe atherosclerosis who experienced some anginal pain 2 weeks ago; there was no increase in troponin I or CK-MB. (   )

24. A 60-year-old female has been hospitalized for 3 weeks after an auto accident in which she sustained fractures to the right femur, pelvis, and left humerus. Physical examination reveals swelling and warmth in her left leg, with local pain and tenderness in her left thigh. She is otherwise asymptomatic. (   )

25. A heart murmur is auscultated in a 73-year-old male with adenocarcinoma of the pancreas. Echocardiography reveals a 1-cm nodular lesion located on the superior aspect of the anterior mitral valve leaflet. The valve leaflet appears to be intact. The blood culture result is negative. (   )

26. A 58-year-old female underwent a left mastectomy with axillary lymph node dissection for breast cancer. She then developed marked swelling of her left arm that persisted for several months. The arm was not tender or erythematous and was not painful to move or touch. She was afebrile. (   )

27. A 61-year-old febrile female has a blood pressure of 85/40 mm Hg. Her serum lactic acid level is 6.8 mg/dL. She also has marked peripheral vasodilation. Which of the following laboratory findings is most likely to be related to the cause of her clinical condition?

○ (A) Elevated serum creatine kinase
○ (B) Decreased PO_2 on blood gas measurement
○ (C) Blood culture positive for *Escherichia coli*
○ (D) Increased blood urea nitrogen
○ (E) Decreased hematocrit

28. A section through a branch of the right main pulmonary artery at autopsy reveals a band of fibrous connective tissue that extends across the lumen. Which of the following events best explains the presence of this finding?

○ (A) Hemorrhage
○ (B) Passive congestion
○ (C) Ischemia
○ (D) Hypertension
○ (E) Thromboembolism

29. Low doses of aspirin are commonly used to reduce the risk of arterial thrombosis in patients who have suffered myocardial infarction. Which one of the following steps in hemostasis is inhibited by aspirin?

○ (A) Adhesion of platelets to collagen
○ (B) Aggregation of platelets
○ (C) Production of tissue factor
○ (D) Synthesis of von Willebrand factor
○ (E) Synthesis of antithrombin III

30. After falling in the bathtub and striking her head, a 78-year-old female becomes increasingly somnolent. A day later, a head computed tomography scan demonstrates an accumulation of fluid beneath the dura, compressing the left cerebral hemisphere. What is the best term for this fluid collection?

○ (A) Hematoma
○ (B) Purpura
○ (C) Congestion
○ (D) Petechia
○ (E) Ecchymosis

31. A 45-year-old female is in good health, with no medical problems. She takes no medications. At the end of an 8-hour shift working at her job as a bank teller, she notices that there is swelling of her lower legs and feet, even though there was no swelling at the beginning of the day. There is no pain or erythema associated with this swelling. Which of the following mechanisms best explains how this phenomenon occurred?

○ (A) Increased hydrostatic pressure
○ (B) Lymphatic obstruction
○ (C) Secondary aldosteronism
○ (D) Hypoalbuminemia
○ (E) Excessive water intake

32. During routine vaginal delivery of a term infant, a 23-year-old female with an uncomplicated pregnancy develops sudden dyspnea with cyanosis and hypotension. She then suffers a generalized seizure, followed by coma. Her condition does not improve over the next few days. What is most likely to be present in her peripheral pulmonary arteries?

○ (A) Gas bubbles
○ (B) Thromboemboli
○ (C) Fat globules
○ (D) Aggregates of red blood cells
○ (E) Amniotic fluid

ANSWERS

1. **(B)** The initial response to injury is arteriolar vasoconstriction, but this is transient, and the coagulation mechanism must be initiated to maintain hemostasis. Protein C is involved in anticoagulation to counteract clotting. Platelet aggregation occurs with release of factors such as ADP, but this takes several minutes. Neutrophils are not essential to hemostasis. Fibrin polymerization is part of secondary hemostasis after the vascular injury is initially closed.
BP6 65–66   PBD6 119

2. **(B)** The liver has a dual blood supply, with a hepatic arterial circulation and a portal venous circulation. Therefore, infarction of the liver caused by occlusion of hepatic artery is not common. Cerebral infarction typically produces liquefactive necrosis. Infarcts of most solid parenchymal organs such as the kidney, heart, and spleen demonstrate coagulative necrosis.
BP6 76   PBD6 133

3. **(C)** The mechanism for fat embolism is unknown, particularly the reason why the onset of symptoms is delayed from 1 to 3 days (or even a week for cerebral symptoms) after the initial injury. The cumulative effect of many small fat globules filling peripheral pulmonary arteries is the same as one large pulmonary thromboembolus. Hemothorax and cardiac tamponade should be immediate complications after traumatic injury, not delayed events. Pulmonary edema severe enough to cause dyspnea should not occur because of fluid status monitoring in the hospital. Pulmonary infarction may cause dyspnea, but pulmonary thromboembolus from deep venous thrombosis is typically a complication of a longer hospitalization.
BP6 74   PBD6 130–131

4. **(E)** This is a "nutmeg" liver from chronic passive congestion. The enzyme level elevations suggest that the process is so severe that hepatic centrilobular necrosis has also occurred. His findings suggest right heart failure. This regular pattern of red lobular discoloration is not likely to occur with hemorrhage from decreased platelets with petechiae and ecchymoses. A portal vein thrombus diminishes blood flow to the liver but is not likely to cause necrosis, because there is a dual blood supply. Hepatic congestion is not directly related to renal failure; there is no characteristic gross appearance with hepatorenal syndrome. Biliary tract obstruction should produce bile stasis (cholestasis) with icterus.
BP6 63–64   PBD6 116–117

5. **(E)** The most important and the most common cause of venous thrombosis is vascular stasis. Turbulent blood flow is another risk for thrombosis, but it is more of a factor in fast flowing arterial circulation. Nitric oxide is a vasodilator and an inhibitor of platelet aggregation. Aspirin inhibits platelet function and limits thrombosis. Calcium is a cofactor in the coagulation pathway, but an increase in calcium has minimal effect on the coagulation process.
BP6 69   PBD6 124–125

6. **(B)** Atherosclerotic damage to vascular endothelium is the most common cause of arterial thrombosis. Stasis of blood flow is important in the low-pressure venous circulation. Decreased production of t-PA from intact endothelial cells may occur with anoxia of the endothelial cells in veins with sluggish circulation. Decreased levels of antithrombin and mutation in factor V gene are inherited causes of hypercoagulability. They are far less common than atherosclerosis of coronary vessels.
BP6 69 PBD6   124–125

7. **(A)** The thrombolytic agent t-PA causes the generation of plasmin, which cleaves fibrin to dissolve the clot. Aspirin prevents formation of new thrombi by inhibiting platelet aggregation. Heparin prevents thrombosis by activating antithrombin III. Nitric oxide is a vasodilator. Vitamin K is required for synthesis of certain clotting factors.
BP6 65–66   PBD6 118–120

8. **(B)** Acute left ventricular failure after a myocardial infarction causes venous congestion in the pulmonary capillary bed and increase in hydrostatic pressure, which causes pulmonary edema by transudation in the alveolar space. Neutrophils and fibrin are found in cases of acute inflammation (i.e., pneumonia) of the lung. Fibrosis and hemosiderin-filled macrophages (heart failure cells) are found with long-standing, not acute, left ventricular failure. Subpleural hemorrhagic necrosis occurs if there are pulmonary thromboemboli. They can cause right heart failure. Purulent exudate in the pleural space (empyema) results from bacterial infection, not heart failure.
BP6 61–64   PBD6 113–116

9. **(D)** He has the "bends" from decompression sickness. At high pressures during the deep scuba dive, nitrogen is dissolved in blood and tissues in large amounts. Ascending too quickly does not allow for slow release of the gas, and small gas blubbles are formed. Hemorrhage or thrombosis from disseminated intravascular coagulation is more likely to occur with underlying diseases such as sepsis, and recovery is not so fast. Systemic vasodilation is a feature of some forms of shock. Venous thrombosis is more typically a complication of stasis, something that does not occur in a physically active person. Fat globules in pulmonary arteries are a feature of fat embolism, which usually follows trauma.
BP6 74   PBD6 131

10. **(B)** The cancer spreads to the dermal lymphatics to produce the gross peau d'orange appearance. There is an extensive venous drainage of the breast, and cancer or other focal mass lesions are not likely to cause significant congestion and edema of the breast. Ischemia is rare in breast because of the abundant arterial supply. Passive congestion does not involve breast. Chronic inflammation is rare in breast tissue and not associated with cancer.
BP6 62   PBD6 115

11. **(B)** von Willebrand factor acts as a glue between platelets and the exposed extracellular matrix of the vessel wall after vascular injury. None of the other steps listed here depends on von Willebrand factor.
BP6 65-67   PBD6 118-120

12. **(A)** This is a large pulmonary thromboembolus. The most common risk factor is immobilization leading to venous stasis. These thrombi form in the large deep leg or pelvic veins, not in the pulmonary arteries. Coagulapathies from acquired or inherited disorders, such as those from the lupus anticoagulant or factor V mutation, are possible causes for thrombosis but usually are manifested at a younger age and are far less common than venous stasis as risks for pulmonary thromboembolism. Local inflammation from a pneumonia may result in thrombosis of small vessels in affected areas.
BP6 73-74   PBD6 130

13. **(A)** The recurrent thrombotic episodes at such a young age strongly suggest an inherited coagulopathy, and the factor V mutation affects 2% to 15% of the population. More than one half of persons with a history of recurrent deep venous thrombosis have such a defect. Inherited deficiencies of the anticoagulant proteins antithrombin III and protein C can cause hypercoagulable states, but these are much less common than factor V mutation. She is unlikely to have cancer at such a young age, but some cancers do elaborate factors that promote thrombosis. Hypercholesterolemia is a risk factor for atherosclerosis that predisposes to arterial thrombosis.
BP6 69-70   PBD6 125-126

14. **(D)** She has deep and superficial venous thrombosis as a consequence of venous stasis from immobilization.

The large, deep thrombi can embolize to the lungs and lead to death. Gangrene occurs from arterial, not venous, occlusion in the leg. Vessels with thrombi typically stay intact; if she had a hematoma as a consequence of the trauma from the fall, it should be organizing and decreasing in size after 2 weeks. Disseminated intravascular coagulation (DIC) is not a common complication with thrombosis of extremities or during recuperation from an injury. Fat embolism can occur with fractures, but pulmonary problems typically appear 1 to 3 days after the traumatic event.
BP6 71-72   PBD6 127-129

15. **(A)** Factor VIII, tissue factor, and factor V act as cofactors or reaction accelerators in the clotting cascade. Factor VIII acts as a reaction accelerator for the conversion of factor X and Xa. The platelet surface provides phospholipid for assembly of coagulation factors. Platelet aggregation is promoted by thromboxane A_2 and ADP. Thromboxane A_2 is released when platelets are activated during the process of platelet adhesion.
BP6 68   PBD6 121

16. **(D)** He is going into shock quickly after trauma. So-called shock lung, with diffuse alveolar damage, is a common occurrence in this situation. The liver is difficult to infarct because of its dual blood supply. Basal ganglia hemorrhages are more typical with hypertension, not hypotension with shock. Passive congestion is less likely with diminished blood volumes and tissue perfusion from shock. Gangrene requires much longer to develop and is not a common complication with shock.
BP6 78-79   PBD6 136-137

17. **(F)** This woman has a hypercoagulable state, and she has antibodies that react with cardiolipin, a phospholipid antigen used for the serologic diagnosis of syphilis. These so-called antiphospholipid antibodies are directed against phospholipid-protein complexes and are sometimes called lupus anticoagulant because they are present in some patients with systemic lupus erythematosus (SLE). However, lupus anticoagulant may occur in persons without any evidence of SLE. Patients with lupus anticoagulant have recurrent arterial and venous thrombosis and repeated miscarriages. In vitro, these antibodies inhibit coagulation by interfering with the assembly of phospholipid complexes. In contrast, the antibodies in vivo induce a hypercoagulable state by unknown mechanisms.
BPD6 126   BP6 70

18. **(A)** The adenosinediphosphate (ADP) is released from the dense bodies and is a potent stimulator of platelet aggregation. ADP also stimulates ADP release from other platelets. Thromboxane A_2, another powerful aggregator of platelets, is synthesized by the cyclooxygenase pathway; it is not stored in dense bodies. Many other substances involved in hemostasis (e.g., fibrinogen, von Willebrand factor, and factor V) are stored in the alpha granules of platelets.
BP6 67,   PBD6 120-121

19. **(D)** Thrombomodulin is present on intact endothelium and binds thrombin, which inhibits coagulation by activating protein C. Tumor necrosis factor is not significantly involved in coagulation. Platelet factor 4 is released from platelet alpha granules and promotes platelet aggregation during the coagulation process. Calcium is a cofactor that assists clotting in the coagulation cascade (the ethylenediaminetetraacetic acid [EDTA] in some blood collection tubes binds calcium to prevent clotting). Fibrin protein forms a meshwork that is essential to thrombus formation.
BP6 66–67   PBD6 119–120

20. **(D)** There is greater hydrostatic pressure in the pulmonary capillary bed from his left heart failure. Plasma oncotic pressure is mainly diminished by decreased synthesis of protein in the liver or by loss of protein through the kidney (proteinuria). With right heart failure, there is increased central venous pressure. Acute inflammation of the lung (pneumonia) can give rise to alveolar exudate. This occurs only if infection supervenes. It is not caused by a myocardial failure.
BP6 62–64   PBD6 114–117

21. **(E)** A mural thrombus fills an atherosclerotic aortic aneurysm below the renal arteries. One of the complications of mural thrombosis is embolization when a small piece breaks off. The embolus is carried distally and may occlude the popliteal artery. Because this thrombus is in the arterial circulation, an embolus will not go to the lungs. A venous thrombus produces leg swelling from edema. Although platelets contribute to the formation of thrombi, the platelet count does not drop appreciably with formation of a localized thrombus, and a generalized process such as disseminated intravascular coagulation (DIC) is needed to use up enough platelets to cause thrombocytopenia.
BP6 71–72   PBD6 127–129

22. **(A)** This is a hemorrhagic infarct based on the pleura, typical of what may happen when a medium-sized thromboembolus lodges in a pulmonary artery branch. The infarct is hemorrhagic because the bronchial arterial circulation in the lung, which is from the systemic arterial circulation and is separate from the pulmonary arterial circulation, continues to supply a small amount of blood to the affected area of infarction. Passive congestion, whether acute or chronic, is a diffuse process, as is edema, which does not impart a red color. Pulmonary venous thrombosis is rare.
BP6 75   PBD6 132–133

23. **(H)** There is an organizing thrombus in this small artery with several small recanalized channels. Such a peripheral arterial occlusion was not sufficient to produce infarction, as evidenced by the lack of enzyme elevation. Thrombi become organized over time if they are not dissolved by fibrinolytic activity.
BP6 71–73   PBD6 127–129

24. **(J)** Venous stasis favors the development of phlebothrombosis (venous thrombosis) particularly in the leg veins and the pelvic veins. The obstruction may produce local pain and swelling, although it may be asymptomatic. Such deep thrombi in large veins create a risk for pulmonary thromboembolism.
BP6 72–73   PBD6 129

25. **(N)** A thrombotic mass that forms on a cardiac valve is known as a vegetation. Such vegetations may produce thromboemboli. Vegetations on the right-sided heart valves may embolize to the lungs; those on the left embolize systemically to organs such as brain, spleen, and kidney. A "paradoxical embolus" occurs when a right-sided cardiac thrombus crosses a patent foramen ovale and enters the systemic arterial circulation. Persons with cancer may have a hypercoagulable state (Trousseau syndrome) that favors the development of arterial and venous thrombosis.
PBD6 127

26. **(L)** The surgery disrupted lymphatic return, resulting in functional lymphatic obstruction and lymphedema of the arm. The lymphatic channels are important in scavenging fluid and protein that have leaked into the tissues from the intravascular space. Although the amount of fluid that is drained through lymphatics is not great, it can gradually build up over time.
BP6 62   PBD6 115

27. **(C)** She has septic shock, with poor tissue perfusion evidenced by the high lactate level. Vasodilation is a feature of septic shock, typically from gram-negative endotoxemia. An elevated creatine kinase level suggests an acute myocardial infarction, which produces cardiogenic shock. A decreased PO_2 suggests a problem with lung ventilation or perfusion. An increased blood urea nitrogen concentration is a feature of renal failure, not the cause of renal failure. A decreased hematocrit suggests hypovolemic shock from blood loss.
BP6 77   PBD6 134

28. **(E)** Organization with recanalization occurs in a vessel after thrombosis or thromboembolism. A small fibrous band may be all that remains. Hemorrhage alone cannot result in fibrosis. Passive congestion of surrounding lung tissue has a negligible effect on arteries. Ischemia could result from the same thromboembolus but would produce a hemorrhagic infarct of the lung. Pulmonary hypertension could occur from the decreased vascular bed resulting from recurrent, widespread thromboembolism to small peripheral pulmonary arteries.
BP6 71   PBD6 127–128

29. **(B)** Aspirin blocks the cyclooxygenase pathway of arachidonic acid metabolism and generation of eicosanoids, including thromboxane A_2, which causes vasoconstriction and promotes platelet aggregation. Platelet adhesion to extracellular matrix is mediated by interactions with von Willebrand factor. Tissue factor (thromboplastin) is released

with tissue injury and is not platelet dependent. Endothelial cells produce von Willebrand factor independent of platelet action. Antithrombin III has anticoagulant properties because it inactivates several coagulation factors, but its function is not affected by aspirin.

BP6 37,66–67   PBD6 71,120–122

30. **(A)** She has a subdural hematoma. A hematoma is a collection of blood in a potential space or within tissue. Purpura denotes blotchy hemorrhage on skin, serosal, or mucous membrane surfaces, and areas larger than 1 to 2 cm are often call ecchymoses. Petechiae are pinpoint areas of hemorrhage. Congestion occurs when there is vascular dilation with pooling of blood within an organ.

BP6 64   PBD6 117–118

31. **(A)** The hydrostatic pressure exerted from standing leads to edema in dependent parts of the body. Lymphatic obstruction from infection or tumor can lead to lymphedema, but this is a chronic process. Secondary aldosteronism results from congestive heart failure and renal hypoperfusion, but this is a generalized process. Hypoalbuminemia leads to more generalized edema as well, although the effect is more pronounced in dependent areas. If she is healthy, normal renal function is sufficient to clear free water from oral intake.

BP6 61–62   PBD6 114–115

32. **(E)** Amniotic fluid embolism is a rare event in pregnancy but carries a high mortality rate. The fluid reaches torn uterine veins through ruptured fetal membranes. Gas bubbles in vessels from air embolism can be a rare event with some obstetric procedures, but it is not likely with natural deliveries. Peripheral pulmonary thromboemboli are most likely to produce chronic pulmonary hypertension and develop over weeks to months. Fat globules are seen with fat embolism, usually after severe trauma.

BP6 74–75   PBD6 131–132

Genetic Disorders

BP6 Chapter 7 - Genetic and Pediatric
Diseases
PBD6 Chapter 6 - Genetic Disorders

1. An absence of low-density lipoprotein (LDL) receptors on liver cells, inherited as an autosomal dominant condition, is best characterized by which of the following laboratory test findings in a 22-year-old male who has had a myocardial infarction:

○ (A) Abetalipoproteinemia
○ (B) Hypertriglyceridemia
○ (C) Ketonuria
○ (D) Hypoglycemia
○ (E) Hypercholesterolemia

2. A 25-year-old male has a work-up for infertility and is found to have oligospermia. Physical examination findings include bilateral gynecomastia, reduced testicular size, and reduced body hair. Karyotypic analysis will most likely reveal which of the following abnormalities?

○ (A) 46,X,i(Xq)
○ (B) 47,XYY
○ (C) 47,XXY
○ (D) 46XX/47XX,+21
○ (E) 46,XY,del(22q11)

For the descriptions of a patient with a genetic disease in questions 3, 4, and 5, select the most closely associated lettered gene product that is likely to be abnormal or absent with that disease:

(A) Adenosine deaminase
(B) Alpha$_1$-antitrypsin
(C) Alpha-L-iduronidase
(D) Dystrophin
(E) Factor VIII
(F) Fibrillin
(G) Globin chains
(H) Glucocerebrosidase
(I) Glucose-6 phosphatase
(J) Hexosaminidase
(K) Homogentisic oxidase
(L) Lysosomal acid maltase
(M) Muscle phosphorylase
(N) Spectrin
(O) Sphingomyelinase

3. Male children over several generations in a family have been affected by a progressive disorder involving multiple organ systems. These children have had coarse facial features, corneal clouding, joint stiffness, hepatosplenomegaly, and mental retardation. Laboratory testing reveals increased urinary excretion of mucopolysaccharides. The accumulated mucopolysaccharides are found in macrophages ("balloon cells" filled with minute vacuoles) on bone marrow biopsy. Some of the children at autopsy have had subendothelial coronary arterial deposits that produced myocardial infarction. (   )

4. An apparently healthy 25-year-old female drops out of her aerobic exercise class because of severe muscle cramps during every session for the past 2 months. Several hours after each of these sessions, she has noticed that her urine has a brown color. (   )

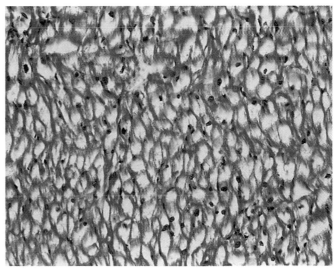

Courtesy of Dr. Trace Worrell, Department of Pathology, University of Texas Southwestern Medical Center, Dallas, TX.

5. A 6-month-old infant has failure to thrive, with muscle weakness and enlargement of liver and spleen. A chest

radiograph reveals marked cardiomegaly. The child dies with congestive heart failure at 19 months of age. At autopsy, the myocardial fibers and liver cells are seen microscopically to have the appearance shown in the figure. ( )

6. Multifactorial inheritance is most likely to play a significant role in the appearance of

○ (A) Marfan syndrome
○ (B) Tay-Sachs disease
○ (C) Erythroblastosis fetalis
○ (D) Cleft lip
○ (E) Polycystic kidneys

For each of the patients with genetic disorders in questions 7 and 8, match the most characteristic cause of death from the list:

   (A) Acute leukemia
   (B) Aortic dissection
   (C) Bronchiectasis
   (D) Chronic renal failure
   (E) Heart failure caused by thickness of coronary artery endothelium and valve leaflets
   (F) Heart failure caused by myocardial glycogen accumulation
   (G) Intracerebral hemorrhage
   (H) Malignant transformation of a subcutaneous tumor
   (I) Myocardial infarction
   (J) *Pneumocystis carinii* pneumonia
   (K) Severe diarrhea and liver failure
   (L) Severe congenital heart malformation

7. An infant born to a 36-year-old mother was observed at birth to have microcephaly, a cleft lip and palate, and six fingers on each hand. ( )

8. An otherwise normal 12-year-old female with fatty deposits under the skin (i.e., xanthomas) of her elbows collapsed suddenly while playing volleyball. ( )

9. A 10-year-old male, although mentally retarded, is able to carry out activities of daily living, including feeding and dressing himself. On physical examination, he has brachycephaly and oblique palpebral fissures with prominent epicanthal folds. On the palm of each hand is seen a transverse crease. On auscultation of the chest, there is a grade III/VI systolic murmur. Which of the following diseases will he most likely have by the age of 20?

○ (A) Acute leukemia
○ (B) Hepatic cirrhosis
○ (C) Chronic renal failure
○ (D) Acute myocardial infarction
○ (E) Aortic dissection

10. The left hand of a baby born at 38 weeks' gestation has the appearance shown in the figure. Which of the following chromosomal abnormalities is most likely to be present?

○ (A) 45,X
○ (B) 47,XX,+21
○ (C) 47,XY,+18
○ (D) 69,XXY
○ (E) 47,XXY

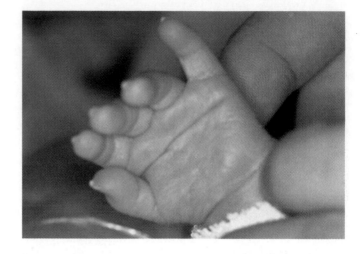

11. A young man's ophthalmologist refers him to a neurologist because, in addition to failing eyesight, he complains of progressive muscle weakness. The neurologist takes a careful history and finds that several of this young man's male and female relatives are similarly affected. His mother, her brother and sister, and two of his aunt's children are affected, but his uncle's children seem to be fine. His genetic disorder is an example of

○ (A) Trinucleotide repeat expansion
○ (B) Genetic imprinting
○ (C) X-linked inheritance pattern
○ (D) A mitochondrial mutation
○ (E) Uniparental disomy

12. Which of the following karyotypic abnormalities in a liveborn baby is most likely to be found in a parent?

○ (A) Robertsonian translocation
○ (B) Ring chromosome
○ (C) Isochromosome
○ (D) Paracentric inversion
○ (E) A q arm deletion

For each of the clinical histories in questions 13 and 14, match the most closely associated lettered karyotype:

   (A) 46,XX
   (B) 47,XX,+18
   (C) 45,X/46,XX
   (D) 47,XYY
   (E) 47,XY,+13
   (F) 47,XXY
   (G) 23,X
   (H) 47,XXX
   (I) 46,X,X(fra)
   (J) 46,XY,der(14;21)(q10;q10),+21
   (K) 47,XX,+21
   (L) 47,XY,+16

13. A 25-year-old female with amenorrhea is 146 cm tall and is found on physical examination to have a webbed neck. An abdominal magnetic resonance scan shows "streak ovaries" that are small, long, and thin. ( )

14. A 25-year-old male, a professional hockey player who has never won the Lady Byng trophy, is 195 cm tall. There are no abnormal findings on a physical examination, other than some prominent facial acne scars and some missing teeth. He is married and has two children who show normal development for age. (   )

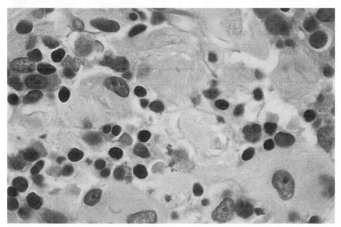

Courtesy of Dr. Matthew Fries, Department of Pathology, University of Texas Southwestern Medical Center, Dallas, TX.

15. A 10-year-old neurologically normal child has hepatosplenomegaly along with anemia and leukopenia. A bone marrow biopsy is performed and shows at high magnification the findings depicted in the figure. Therapy for this condition can be accomplished by infusion of

○ (A) Glucocerebrosidase
○ (B) Acid maltase
○ (C) Glucose-6-phosphatase
○ (D) Sphingomyelinase
○ (E) Hexosaminidase A

16. Mental retardation has affected several generations of a family. Only male family members manifest this condition. In general, it appears that the severity of mental retardation has increased with each passing generation. By which of the following mechanisms is this genetic condition most likely to be produced?

○ (A) Trinucleotide repeat mutation
○ (B) Frameshift mutation
○ (C) Missense mutation
○ (D) Point mutation
○ (E) Mitochondrial DNA mutation

17. About a dozen pale brown macules averaging 2 to 5 cm in diameter and having irregular borders are observed on the trunk and extremities of a 15-year-old female. Examination of her eyes with a slit lamp reveals pigmented nodules in the iris. Other family members are similarly affected. Which of the following neoplasms is she most likely to develop?

○ (A) Dermatofibroma
○ (B) Leiomyoma
○ (C) Neurofibroma
○ (D) Lipoma
○ (E) Hemangioma

18. A fetus is most likely to be carried to term with which of the following chromosomal abnormalities?

○ (A) Triploidy
○ (B) Monosomy
○ (C) Aneuploidy
○ (D) Tetraploidy
○ (E) Mosaicism

19. A baby born at term has ambiguous external genitalia. The parents want to know the baby's sex, but the physician is hesitant to assign a sex without further information. A chromosome analysis is performed, and the karyotype is 46,XX. An abdominal computed tomography (CT) scan reveals bilaterally enlarged adrenal glands, and the internal genitalia appear to consist of uterus, tubes, and ovaries. This is most likely to be an example of

○ (A) Female pseudohermaphroditism
○ (B) Testicular femininization
○ (C) A nondisjunctional event with loss of a Y chromosome
○ (D) Excessive trinucleotide repeats
○ (E) Mitochondrial DNA mutation

20. A 1-year-old female is brought to attention because of failure to thrive, mental retardation, and poor motor function. Examination of the retina reveals a cherry red spot in the macula. Both parents and a brother and sister are normal. However, one brother died, with a similar condition, at the age of 18 months. This genetic disorder most likely resulted from which of the following underlying abnormalities?

○ (A) Mutation in a mitochondrial gene
○ (B) Mutation in a gene encoding a lysosomal enzyme
○ (C) Mutation in a gene encoding a receptor protein
○ (D) Mutation in a gene encoding a structural protein
○ (E) Genomic imprinting

21. A 10-year-old male presents with recurrent infections. Physical examination reveals a cleft palate and murmur suggestive of congenital heart disease. A thoracic CT scan reveals a smaller than normal thymus. Results of laboratory investigations suggest mild hypoparathyroidism. Which of the following tests is most likely to be helpful in arriving at the diagnosis?

○ (A) Human immunodeficiency virus (HIV) type 1 RNA level
○ (B) Fluorescence in situ hybridization (FISH) analysis with a probe for chromosome 22q11
○ (C) Polymerase chain reaction (PCR) analysis for trinucleotide repeats affecting the X chromosome
○ (D) Assay for the enzyme adenosine deaminase in lymphocytes
○ (E) Lymph node biopsy

22. A 2-year-old child demonstrates failure to thrive. Hepatomegaly and ecchymoses of the skin are found on physical examination. The child exhibits convulsions, and the blood glucose is found to be only 31 mg/dL. Liver biopsy shows cells filled with clear vacuoles that stain

positively for glycogen. Which of the following conditions best explains these findings?

○ (A) McArdle syndrome
○ (B) von Gierke disease
○ (C) Tay-Sachs disease
○ (D) Hurler syndrome
○ (E) Pompe disease

23. An 8-year-old female can bend her thumb back to touch her forearm. She can pull her skin out from her abdomen about 8 cm, and a cut to her skin gapes open and is difficult to repair. Her underlying disease process results from an inherited defect in

○ (A) Alpha₁-antitrypsin
○ (B) Retinoblastoma (Rb) protein
○ (C) LDL receptor
○ (D) Collagen
○ (E) Factor VIII

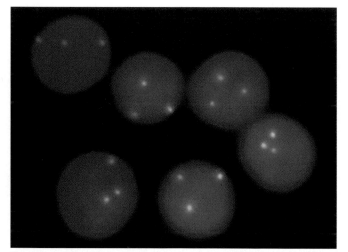

Courtesy of Dr. Vijay Tonk, Department of Pathology, University of Texas Southwestern Medical Center, Dallas, TX.

24. An ultrasound examination performed at 18 weeks reveals that this male fetus is mildly growth retarded. Multiple congenital anomalies are observed, including a ventricular septal defect, atrial septal defect, horseshoe kidney, and omphalocele. An amniocentesis is performed, and the fetal cells are examined with FISH. Based on the findings shown in the figure, the most likely karyotypic abnormality is

○ (A) 46,XY,der(14;21)(q10;q10),+21
○ (B) 47,XY,+18
○ (C) 47,XXY
○ (D) 46,XY,del(22q11)
○ (E) 45,X/46,XX

25. A 4-year-old child demonstrates severe neurologic deterioration. Examination reveals marked hepatosplenomegaly, and a bone marrow biopsy shows numerous foamy vacuolated macrophages. Which of the following tests is likely to reveal the diagnosis of this condition?

○ (A) The number of LDL receptors on hepatocytes
◉ (B) The level of sphingomyelinase in splenic macrophages

○ (C) The rate of synthesis of collagen
○ (D) The level of glucose-6-phosphatase in liver cells
○ (E) The level of α₁-antitrypsin in the liver

26. A fetus is delivered stillborn at 19 weeks' gestation. The macerated fetus shows marked hydrops fetalis. There is a large posterior cystic hygroma of the neck. Autopsy reveals internal anomalies, including aortic coarctation and a horseshoe kidney. Which of the following karyotypes is most likely to be found on chromosome analysis of fetal cells?

○ (A) 47,XX,+18
○ (B) 48,XXXY
○ (C) 47,XX,+21
○ (D) 47,XYY
○ (E) 45,X

27. A 13-year-old male has been drinking large quantities of fluids and has an insatiable appetite, even for a teenager. However, he is losing weight and has become more tired and listless over the past month. A complete blood count is normal, but he is found to have a fasting serum glucose of 175 mg/dL. A diagnosis of type 1 diabetes is made. What is the probable inheritance pattern of his underlying disease?

○ (A) Autosomal dominant
○ (B) Multifactorial
○ (C) X-linked recessive
○ (D) Mitochondrial DNA
○ (E) Autosomal recessive

28. A pregnant woman with a family history of fragile X syndrome wants prenatal diagnosis of her fetus. Amplification of the appropriate region of the *FMR1* gene by PCR is attempted on DNA from amniotic fluid cells, but no amplified products are obtained. What is the best next step?

○ (A) Routine karyotype of the amniotic fluid cells
○ (B) Routine karyotype of the unaffected father
○ (C) Southern blot of the DNA from the amniotic fluid cells
○ (D) PCR analysis of the mother's *FMR*1 gene
○ (E) No further tests necessary

29. A 3-year-old child with developmental delay, ataxia, seizures, and inappropriate laughter has a normal karyotype (46,XY), but DNA analysis shows that he has inherited both of his number 15 chromosomes from his father. His genetic disorder is an example of

○ (A) X-linked inheritance pattern
○ (B) Maternal inheritance pattern
○ (C) Mutation of mitochondrial DNA
○ (D) Genetic imprinting
○ (E) Trinucleotide repeat expansion

30. A 34-year-old male has loss of vision from a subluxation of the crystalline lens of the right eye. A mid-systolic click is audible on auscultation of the chest, and an echocardiogram reveals a floppy mitral valve. The aortic arch is also dilated. His brother and his cousin are also affected. Which of the following genes is probably involved in his underlying disease process?

○ (A) Dystrophin
○ (B) Collagen
○ (C) Fibrillin
○ (D) NF1 protein
○ (E) Spectrin

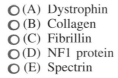

ANSWERS

1. **(E)** Familial hypercholesterolemia results from mutations in the LDL receptor gene such that LDL cholesterol is increased in the blood because it is not catabolized or taken up by the liver. Triglycerides are not primarily affected. Ketonuria can occur with starvation or insulin deficiency. The LDL receptors do not play a direct role in gluconeogenesis.
BP6 182–183   PBD6 150–153

2. **(C)** He has Klinefelter syndrome, one of the more common chromosomal abnormalities, which occurs in about 1 of 850 liveborn males. The findings can be subtle. The 46,X,i(Xq) is a variant of Turner syndrome (seen only in females), caused by a defective second X chromosome. The 47,XYY karyotype is not uncommon—about 1 in 1000 liveborn males—and is associated with taller than average stature. A person with a mosaic such as 46,XX/47,XX,+21 has milder features of Down syndrome than persons with the more typical 47,XX,+21 karyotype. The 22q11 deletion syndrome is associated with congenital defects affecting the palate, face, and heart, and in some cases, T-cell immunodeficiency.
BP6 196   PBD6 174

3. **(C)** This is Hunter syndrome, one of the mucopolysaccharidoses (MPS) that result from deficiencies of lysosomal enzymes, such as α-L-iduronidase. The glycosaminoglycans that accumulate in MPS include dermatan sulfate, heparan sulfate, keratan sulfate, and chondroitin sulfate. All of the MPS variants are autosomal recessive, except for Hunter syndrome, which is an X-linked recessive.
BP6 187–188   PBD6 159–160

4. **(M)** She has McArdle syndrome, a form of glycogen storage disease with an onset in young adulthood and in which there is a deficiency of muscle phosphorylase enzyme. As a consequence, glycogen accumulates in skeletal muscle. Because strenuous exercise requires glycogenolysis and use of anaerobic metabolism, muscle cramps ensue and the blood lactate level does not rise. Myoglobinuria is seen in about one half of cases.
BP6 188–189   PBD6 160,163

5. **(L)** This is Pompe disease, a form of glycogen storage disease that results from a deficiency in lysosomal glucosidase (acid maltase). The glycogen stored in the myocardium results in massive cardiomegaly and heart failure within 2 years.
BP6 188–189   PBD6 160,163

6. **(D)** Cleft lip and most congenital malformations are not determined by a single gene, and they may be conditioned by environmental influences (multifactorial inheritance). Marfan syndrome is an autosomal dominant disorder affecting fibrillin. Tay-Sachs disease, a lysosomal storage disorder, is inherited as an autosomal recessive trait. Erythroblastosis fetalis results from maternal sensitization to fetal red blood cells and formation of antibody that can cross the placenta in future pregnancies to produce hemolysis. Polycystic kidneys may be caused by dominant, recessive, or sporadic mutations.
BP6 190   PBD6 165

7. **(L)** Cleft lip and palate, along with microcephaly and polydactyly, are features of trisomy 13. These patients also have severe heart defects.
BP6 194   PBD6 172

8. **(I)** This patient has homozygous familial hypercholesterolemia, characterized by severe hypercholesterolemia that gives rise to xanthomas and premature coronary artery disease leading to myocardial infarction.
BP6 182–183   PBD6 151–152

9. **(A)** He has Down syndrome, or trisomy 21. This is one of the trisomies that can result in a liveborn baby. However, there are often many associated congenital anomalies, particularly congenital heart disease, including ventricular septal defect. These are happy children who can function fairly well. However, there is a 10- to 20-fold increased risk for acute leukemia. If persons with Down syndrome live to the age of 40, virtually all of them will have evidence for Alzheimer disease. Hepatic cirrhosis is a feature of galactosemia. Chronic renal failure may be seen with genetic disorders that produce polycystic kidneys. Myocardial infarction at a young age suggests familial hypercholesterolemia. Aortic dissection is seen in persons with Marfan syndrome.
BP6 193–195   PBD6 170–172

10. **(B)** There is a single palmar flexion crease and a single flexion crease on the fifth digit. These are features of trisomy 21. Monosomy X may be marked by a short fourth metacarpal. With trisomy 18, the fingers are often clenched, with digits 2 and 5 overlapping 3 and 4. Triploidy may be marked by syndactyly of digits 3 and 4. There are no characteristic features of the hand of a male with Klinefelter syndrome.
BP6 193–194   PBD6 170–172

11. **(D)** This is a classic pattern of maternal inheritance, resulting from a mutation in mitochondrial DNA. Males and females are affected, but affected males cannot transmit the disease to their offspring. Because mitochondrial DNA encodes many enzymes involved in oxidative phosphorylation, mutations in mitochondrial genes exert their most deleterious effects on organs most dependent on oxidative phosphorylation, including the central nervous system (CNS) and muscles.
BP6 178   PBD6 6 179–180

12. **(A)** Nearly all of the normal genetic material is present in the case of a robertsonian translocation, because only a small amount of p arm from each chromosome is lost. Statistically, one of six fetuses in a mother who car-

ries a robertsonian translocation will also be a carrier. In balanced reciprocal translocation, the same possibility of inheriting the defect exists. However, other structural abnormalities are likely to result in loss of significant genetic material, reducing survivability, or to interfere with meiosis.
BP6 192-193   PBD6 168-170

13. **(C)** The features are those of classic Turner syndrome. Patients who grow to adulthood are usually mosaics, karyotype of 45,X/46,XX.
BP6 196-197   PBD6 174-176

14. **(D)** The extra Y chromosome is seen in about 1 of 1000 liveborn males. There is a tendency for such persons to be tall and prone to severe acne. The missing teeth are specific to hockey, not to an extra Y chromosome. There is a controversy about whether such individuals exhibit more aggressive behavior. However, the behavior of virtually all 46,XYY males is indistinguishable from that of other males.
BP6 196   PBD6 174

15. **(A)** Gaucher disease has three forms. Type 1 accounts for 99% of cases and does not involve the CNS, as in this child. It is caused by a deficiency of glucocerebrosidase, and infusion with this enzyme reduces severity and progression. Type 2 involves the CNS and is lethal in infancy. Type 3 also involves the CNS, although not as severely as type 2. A deficiency of acid maltase is a feature of Pompe disease. Von Gierke disease results from deficiency of glucose-6-phosphatase. Sphingomyelinese deficiency leads to Niemann-Pick disease types A and B. Type A, the more common form, is associated with severe neurologic deterioration. Type B, the less common form, may resemble this case, but the appearance of macrophages is different: they contain many small vacuoles. In Tay-Sachs disease, there is a deficiency of hexosaminidase A. It is also associated with severe mental retardation and death before 10 years of age.
BP6 187   PBD6 158-159

16. **(A)** This is fragile X syndrome, a condition in which there are 250 to 4000 tandem repeats of the trinucleotide sequence CGG. In general, the more repeats, the worse is the disease or the earlier the onset in conditions caused by trinucleotide repeats. The trinucleotides are dynamic; because their size increases during oogenesis, the male offspring have more severe disease compared with, for example, their grandfathers. With a frameshift mutation, one, two, or three nucleotide base pairs are inserted or deleted. The protein transcribed is abnormal. A missense mutation results from a single nucleotide base substitution, resulting in an abnormal protein being elaborated. Abnormalities of mitochondrial DNA are transmitted on the maternal side.
BP6 176-178   PBD6 143, 177-178

17. **(C)** She has neurofibromatosis type 1. Neurofibromas are most numerous in the dermis but may occur in visceral organs as well. Dermatofibromas are also subcutaneous masses, but they are typically small and solitary and not seen with neurofibromatosis. Leiomyomas are most fre-

quent in the uterus and are not typically part of a genetic disorder. Lipomas can occur just about anywhere but are sporadic in occurrence. Hemangiomas may occur sporadically on the skin. They are not part of neurofibromatosis type 1.
BP6 189-190   PBD6 162-164

18. **(E)** There are a greater number of potentially normal cells having the proper chromosomal complement with mosaicism, and this may allow babies with abnormalities of chromosome number to make it to term and beyond. Triploid fetuses rarely go past the second trimester and are virtually never liveborn. Likewise, tetraploidy accounts for many first-trimester fetal losses and is not survivable. Loss of a chromosome is devastating; the only monosomy in which there is possible survival to term is Turner syndrome (monosomy X). Most aneuploid conditions (trisomies and monosomies) lead to fetal demise. Trisomy 21 is the most likely to go to term.
BP6 191   PBD6 168

19. **(A)** It is important to be careful in assigning sex; changing your opinion of the sex is about as popular as an umpire changing the call. True hermaphoditism, with ovarian and testicular tissue present, is rare. This patient has female pseudohermaphroditism, resulting from exposure of the fetus to excessive androgenic stimulation, as can occur with congenital adrenal hyperplasia. Both the gonadal and karyotypic sex is female. Male pseudohermaphroditism has a variety of forms, but the most common is testicular feminization that results from androgen insensitivity, and the affected persons are phenotypically females but have testes and a 46,XY karyotype. Nondisjunctional events lead to monosomies or trisomies. Trinucleotide repeats are seen with fragile X syndrome in males. Abnormalities of mitochondrial DNA have a maternal transmission pattern and do not involve sex chromosomes or sexual characteristics.
PBD6 176

20. **(B)** This patient seems to have a severe inherited neurologic disease that gives rise to a cherry red spot in the retina. The pattern of inheritance (e.g., normal parents, an affected sib) is consistent with autosomal recessive inheritance. This is most likely Tay-Sachs disease, caused by mutations in the gene that encodes a lysomal enzyme hexosaminidase A. Mutations in genes affecting receptor proteins and structural proteins typically give rise to an autosomal dominant pattern of inheritance. Mitochondrial genes have a maternal pattern of transmission. Genomic imprinting is characterized by a parent of origin effect.
BP6 186   PBD6 148, 155-156, 179, and 180

21. **(B)** This patient has an immunodeficiency characterized by infection and a small thymus, congenital malformations, and hypoparathyroidism. This cluster is characteristic of the 22q11 deletion syndrome, readily diagnosed by FISH. HIV infection can lead to acquired immunodeficiency syndrome, but there are no congenital anomalies associated with this condition. Trinucleotide repeats of the X chromosome are seen with the fragile X syndrome, which manifests with mental retardation in males. Adenosine deaminase deficiency can also cause immunodefi-

ciency, but it is not associated with congenital malformations. A lymph node biopsy may show a reduction in T or B cells associated with various forms of immunodeficiency, but this is not a specific test to help confirm a specific diagnosis.
PBD6 173

22.   **(B)** This patient has von Gierke disease. Because of the deficiency of glucose-6-phosphatase, glycogen is not metabolized readily to glucose; and the patients have severe hypoglycemia, leading to convulsions. Intracytoplasmic accumulations of glycogen occur mainly in liver and kidney. Another form of glycogen storage disease, McArdle syndrome, results from a deficiency of muscle phosphorylase and leads to muscle cramping. Tay-Sachs disease is characterized by a deficiency in hexosaminidase A and results in severe neurologic deterioration. In Hurler syndrome, the enzyme α-L-iduronidase is deficient. Affected children have skeletal deformities and buildup of mucopolysaccharides in endocardium and coronary arteries, leading to heart failure. Cardiomegaly and heart failure mark Pompe disease, another form of glycogen storage disease.
BP6 188-189   PBD6 160-163

23.   **(D)** She has Ehlers-Danlos syndrome, which results from a collagen defect that makes connective tissues weak and fragile. A deficiency of α_1-antitrypsin leads to liver and lung disease. A mutated Rb protein is associated with development of retinoblastoma and osteosarcoma. Inherited defects in the number of LDL receptors result in early and advanced atherosclerosis. A deficiency of factor VIII occurs in hemophilia A.
BP6 182   PBD6 149-150

24.   **(B)** The baby has findings associated with trisomy 18. In the FISH analysis, the chromosomes in each cell have been painted with a marker to chromosome 18, and there are three markers per cell, consistent with a trisomy. In reality, many cells would have to be counted to allow for artifacts in preparation. Trisomy 18 results from nondisjunctional events in most cases. Most trisomy 18 cases are stillborn, and survival beyond 4 months is rare.
BP6 194   PBD6 172

25.   **(B)** The clinical features of this child—neurologic involvement, hepatosplenomegaly, and accumulation of foamy macrophages—suggest a lysosomal storage disorder. One such disorder, with which the clinical history is quite compatible, is Niemann-Pick disease type A. It is characterized by lysosomal accumulation of sphingomyelin due to a severe deficiency of sphingomyelinase. Reduced numbers of LDL receptors on hepatocytes can be seen with familial hypercholesterolemia. Collagen synthesis is impaired with Ehlers-Danlos syndrome. The glycogen storage disease known as von Gierke disease results from glucose-6-phosphatase deficiency. Globules of α_1-antitrypsin are seen in liver cells with inherited deficiency of α_1-antitrypsin.
BP6 186-187   PBD6 156-158

26.   **(E)** These are findings of Turner syndrome. The hygroma is quite suggestive. Such affected babies are rarely liveborn. Turner syndrome accounts for a considerable portion of first trimester losses. Trisomy 18 can be marked by multiple anomalies as well, but overlapping fingers and a short neck are more typical features. Additional X chromosomes may not have a serious effect, because all but one X chromosome is inactive. Down syndrome (47,XX,+21) may be accompanied by a hygroma and hydrops, but ventricular septal defect is more frequent than coarctation, and horseshoe kidney is uncommon. 47,XXY does not result in stillbirth. These males have no congenital defects.
BP6 196-197   PBD6 174-176

27.   **(B)** He has type 1 diabetes mellitus, which has an increased frequency in some families, but the exact mechanism for inheritance is unknown. The risk is about 6% for offspring when first-order relatives are affected. HLA-linked genes and other genetic loci along with environmental factors are considered important. This pattern of inheritance is multifactorial.
BP6 190, 564-565   PBD6 165, 915-916

28.   **(C)** Failure to find amplified product by PCR in such a case could mean that the fetus is not affected or that there is a full mutation that is too large to be picked up by PCR. The next logical step is a Southern blot analysis of genomic DNA from fetal cells. Routine karyotype of the amniotic fluid cells is much less sensitive than a Southern blot. Karyotype of the unaffected father cannot provide information on the status of the *FMR1* gene in the fetus, because amplification of the trinucleotide occurs during oogenesis. For the same reason, PCR of mother's *FMR1* gene is of no value.
PBD6 183-184, Fig. 6-36

29.   **(D)** These are features of Angelman syndrome. The DNA analysis shows uniparental disomy. The Angelman gene encoded on chromosome 15 is subject to genomic imprinting. It is silenced on the paternal chromosome 15 but is active on the maternal chromosome 15. If the child lacks maternal chromosome 15, there is no active Angelman gene in the somatic cells. This gives rise to the abnormalities typical of this disorder. The same effect occurs when there is a deletion of the Angelman gene from the maternal chromosome 15.
BP6 199   PBD6 180-181

30.   **(C)** He has Marfan syndrome, an autosomal dominant condition that is caused by quantitative and qualitative defects in fibrillin from mutations in the fibrillin gene. Genetic mutations in the dystrophin gene are involved in Duchenne and Becker muscular dystrophies. An abnormal collagen gene can account for osteogenesis imperfecta and Ehlers-Danlos syndrome. The NF1 protein is abnormal in neurofibromatosis type I. Disordered spectrin leads to hereditary spherocytosis.
BP6 181   PBD6 148-149

Diseases of Immunity

CHAPTER

6

PBD6 Chapter 7 - Diseases of Immunity
BP6 Chapter 5 - Disorders of the Immune
System

1. A 25-year-old female has pancytopenia, proteinuria, and a false-positive serologic test for syphilis. A chest radiograph reveals bilateral pleural effusions. A friction rub is auscultated over the chest. Which of the following historical findings is most likely?

- (A) Photosensitivity
- (B) Urethritis
- (C) Esophageal dysmotility
- (D) Xerostomia
- (E) Congenital heart disease

2. A 30-year-old female presents with fever, arthritis, and rash. She also has a history of recurrent thrombosis and infections. Initial laboratory investigations reveal that anti-nuclear antibodies are positive at 1:1600 and that anti–double-stranded DNA antibodies are positive at 1:3200. The serum creatinine level is markedly elevated, and levels of serum complement are decreased. A VDRL test for syphilis is positive, and in vitro tests for coagulation (prothrombin time and partial thromboplastin time) are prolonged. Which of the following clinical features is most likely caused by antibodies that interfere with the coagulation test?

- (A) Arthritis
- (B) Recurrent thrombosis
- (C) Rash
- (D) Renal failure
- (E) Fever

3. In epidemiologic studies of human immunodeficiency virus (HIV) infection and acquired immunodeficiency syndrome (AIDS), it was noticed that certain individuals failed to develop HIV infection despite known exposure to the virus under conditions that caused HIV disease in all other individuals similarly exposed. When the CD4+ lymphocytes from resistant individuals are incubated with HIV-1, they fail to be infected. Such a resistance to infection by

HIV is most likely caused by a mutation affecting which of the following genes?

- (A) T-cell receptor
- (B) Chemokine receptor
- (C) Interleukin-2 receptor
- (D) CD28 receptor
- (E) Fc receptor

4. A 20-year-old female has an erythematous rash over her face on both cheeks and across the bridge of her nose. This rash is made worse by sunlight exposure when she is outdoors. Along with the rash, she has had muscle and joint pains for several months. However, radiographs of the joints do not show any abnormalities, and she has normal joint mobility without deformity. Which of the following laboratory test findings is most characteristic of the disease?

- (A) Elevated anti-streptolysin O (ASO) titer
- (B) HLA-B27 genotype
- (C) Markedly decreased serum level of immunoglobulin G (IgG)
- (D) Increased rheumatoid factor titer
- (E) Antibodies to double-stranded DNA

5. A 15-year-old female has the sudden onset of difficulty breathing within minutes after a bee sting. She also manifests marked urticaria, and there is marked edema of the hand that was stung. Which of the following pharmacologic agents is best for treating these signs and symptoms?

- (A) Cyclosporine
- (B) Epinephrine
- (C) Penicillin
- (D) Glucocorticoids
- (E) Methotrexate

For each of the clinical histories in questions 6 and 7, match the most closely associated immunologically mediated pathologic process that can occur in the affected patients:

- (A) Angioedema of skin
- (B) Bronchoconstriction
- (C) Cerebral lymphoma
- (D) Contact dermatitis
- (E) Hemolytic anemia
- (F) Keratoconjunctivitis

(G) Localized amyloidosis of thyroid
(H) Parathyroid hypoplasia
(I) Sacroiliitis
(J) Sclerodactyly

6. A 31-year-old female has a positive antinuclear antibody test with a titer of 1:2048 and a diffuse homogeneous staining pattern. When she is outside in the sun for more than an hour, she develops a rash over her face. A urinalysis reveals proteinuria. (   )

7. A 28-year-old female has had severe psoriasis involving the skin of her face, trunk, and extremities. She is found by serologic testing to be positive for HLA-B27. She has been diagnosed with uveitis. Her antinuclear antibody and rheumatoid factor tests are negative. (   )

8. A 48-year-old male has a total white blood cell (WBC) count of 6900/μL, with a differential count of 72 segmented neutrophils, 3 band neutrophils, 18 lymphocytes, and 7 monocytes. Serum immunoglobulin levels show 1.9 g/dL IgG, 0.3 g/dL IgM, and 0.01 g/dL IgA. His antinuclear antibody test result is negative. His skin test result for mumps and *Candida* antigens is positive. Which of the following infectious agents is most likely to produce an illness in this patient?

(A) *Pneumocystis carinii*
(B) *Streptococcus pneumoniae*
(C) Hepatitis B virus
(D) *Aspergillus flavus*
(E) Herpes simplex

9. A 37-year-old male known to be HIV positive has noticed the appearance of multiple, 0.5- to 1.2-cm, plaque-like, reddish purple skin lesions on his face, trunk, and extremities. Some of the larger lesions appear to be nodular. These lesions have appeared over the past 6 months and have slowly enlarged. Molecular analysis of the spindle cells found in the lesion is likely to reveal the genome of which of the following viruses?

(A) Cytomegalovirus
(B) Epstein-Barr virus
(C) Adenovirus
(D) Human herpesvirus-8
(E) HIV-1

10. During the induction of immediate (type I) hypersensitivity response, which of the following cells secretes cytokines that stimulate IgE production by B cells, promotes mast cell growth, and recruits and activates eosinophils?

(A) CD4+ lymphocytes
(B) Natural killer (NK) cells
(C) Macrophages
(D) Dendritic cells
(E) Neutrophils

11. A 52-year-old female presents with diffuse pain in her thighs and shoulders bilaterally, difficulty in rising from a chair and climbing steps, and a rash with a violaceous color around the orbits and on the knuckles. Antinuclear antibodies are positive at 1:160. Which of the follow-

ing tests is most specific for the diagnosis of this condition?

(A) Anti–double-stranded DNA antibodies
(B) Rheumatoid factor latex test
(C) Anti–U1-ribonucleoprotein antibodies
(D) Antihistone antibodies
(E) Anti–Jo-1 antibodies

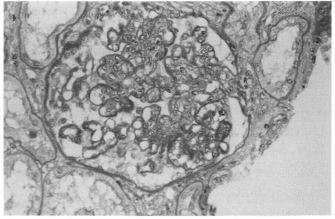

Courtesy of Dr. Helmut Renké, Department of Pathology, Brigham and Women's Hospital, Boston, MA.

12. A renal biopsy is performed on a 31-year-old female who presents with increasing edema, chest pain, and a rash for the past 6 months. She has an increasing serum creatinine level, and proteinuria with red blood cell casts is found on urinalysis. The light microscopic appearance of the renal biopsy is seen in the figure. It is stained with periodic acid–Schiff stain. Which of the following antibodies, if present, is diagnostic of this condition?

(A) Scl-70
(B) Anti-Sm
(C) Jo-1
(D) Anti–HLA-B27
(E) Anti-centromere

13. Larvae of *Trichinella spiralis* are present within the skeletal muscle fibers of the diaphragm of a 23-year-old male. He has a fever and peripheral blood eosinophilia. Years later, a chest radiograph shows only a few small calcifications in the diaphragm. Which of the following immunologic mechanisms probably contributed to the destruction of the larvae?

(A) Antibody-dependent cellular cytotoxicity (ADCC)
(B) Complement-mediated cell lysis
(C) Formation of Langhans giant cells
(D) Abscess formation with neutrophils
(E) Synthesis of leukotriene C_4 in mast cells

14. A 45-year-old male received a kidney from his brother 42 months ago. For the first three years, he did well with the allograft, with minor episodes of rejection that were controlled. However, he has had increasing renal failure for the past 6 months. He is afebrile. A urinalysis specimen examined microscopically shows no WBCs. A computed tomography scan of the pelvis shows that the

allograft is reduced in size. Which of the following immunologic processes is probably happening in this transplanted kidney?

○ (A) Macrophage-mediated cell lysis
○ (B) Vascular intimal fibrosis
○ (C) Granulomatous vasculitis
○ (D) Release of leukotriene C_4 from mast cells
○ (E) Complement-mediated cell lysis

15. A young male walks into an elevator full of people who are coughing and sneezing, all of whom appear to have colds or the flu. The influenza viral particles that he inhales attach to respiratory epithelium, and viral transformation reduces the class I major histocompatibility complex (MHC) molecules on these epithelial cells. Which of the following cells then responds to destroy the infected cells?

○ (A) NK cell
○ (B) Neutrophil
○ (C) Macrophage
○ (D) CD4 cell
○ (E) Dendritic cell

16. A 35-year-old male has a history of mild infections of the upper respiratory tract. He also has had diarrhea for most of his life, although not severe enough to have malabsorption with weight loss. After an episode of trauma with blood loss, he receives a blood transfusion complicated by an anaphylactic reaction. Which of the following underlying conditions best explains these findings?

○ (A) Severe combined immunodeficiency
○ (B) HIV infection
○ (C) DiGeorge syndrome
○ (D) Wiskott-Aldrich syndrome
○ (E) Selective IgA deficiency

17. A laboratory worker who was known to be "allergic" to fungal spores was accidentally exposed to culture of the incriminating fungus on a Friday afternoon. Within 60 minutes, he developed bouts of sneezing, watering of eyes, and nasal discharge. He decided to take the day off, and the symptoms seemed to subside in a few hours. However, the next morning, while he was still at home, his symptoms reappeared, although the laboratory fungus was not present in his environment. His symptoms persisted through the weekend, and he went to see a doctor on Monday morning. If the physician examines a nasal discharge under the microscope, which of the following cells are likely to be seen?

○ (A) Mast cells and neutrophils
○ (B) Lymphocytes and macrophages
○ (C) Neutrophils, eosinophils, and CD4+ lymphocytes
○ (D) Neutrophils and CD8+ lymphocytes
○ (E) Mast cells, lymphocytes, and macrophages

18. A 30-year-old male known to be infected with HIV begins to have difficulty with activities of daily living. He has memory problems and decreased ability to perform functions that require fine motor control, such as writing or painting. His CD4 lymphocyte count is 150/μL. Which of the following cell types is most important for the dissemination of the infection into the central nervous system?

○ (A) NK cell
○ (B) Macrophage
○ (C) Neutrophil
○ (D) CD8 lymphocyte
○ (E) Langerhans cell

19. A vasculitis affects arteries in many visceral organs of a 29-year-old male. There is focal fibrinoid necrosis of the small arterial and arteriolar vascular media along with intravascular microthrombi. Scattered neutrophils are seen in these areas of necrosis. Which of the following laboratory test findings would you most expect for this patient?

○ (A) Increased IgE
○ (B) Neutropenia
○ (C) Decreased C3 complement
○ (D) Tuberculin skin test positivity
○ (E) CD4 lymphocytosis

20. A 63-year-old male with chronic rheumatoid arthritis presents with proteinuria and the nephrotic syndrome. A rectal biopsy is performed, which demonstrates amyloid deposition. Amyloid deposition in this setting

○ (A) Is within the cytoplasm
○ (B) Contains mainly (>50%) P component
○ (C) Is derived from an acute-phase reactant (SAA)
○ (D) Does not show birefringence after Congo red staining
○ (E) Is derived from lambda light chains

For each of the clinical histories in questions 21 and 22, match the most closely associated lettered immunologically mediated disease process:

(A) Ankylosing spondylitis
(B) Dermatomyositis
(C) Diffuse systemic sclerosis
(D) Discoid lupus erythematosus
(E) Juvenile rheumatoid arthritis
(F) Limited scleroderma
(G) Mixed connective tissue disease
(H) Polymyositis
(I) Reiter syndrome
(J) Rheumatoid arthritis
(K) Sjögren syndrome
(L) Systemic lupus erythematosus (SLE)

21. A 41-year-old male has xerostomia, myalgias, rashes over his face, and arthralgias. An antinuclear antibody test result is positive with a speckled pattern. He also has high titers of antibodies to U1 ribonucleoprotein. He has no evidence of renal disease. (   )

22. A 42-year-old female is bothered by tightening of the skin of her fingers, making them difficult to bend. She has increasing difficulty swallowing, and her fingers become cyanotic and painful on exposure to cold. An x-ray film of the chest shows prominent interstitial markings, and lung

function tests reveal moderately severe restrictive pulmonary disease. Laboratory testing reveals a positive DNA topoisomerase I antibody test. (   )

23.   A 3-month-old boy presented with recurrent infections. The infectious agents included *Candida albicans, P. carinii, Pseudomonas aeruginosa*, and cytomegalovirus. Despite intensive treatment with antibiotics and antifungal drugs, he died at the age of 5 months. At autopsy, lymph nodes were found to be small with very few lymphocytes and no germinal centers. The thymus was hypoplastic, as were the Peyer patches and tonsils. There is a history of other males in the family who presented in a similar manner. The most common cause for this form of immunodeficiency is

○ (A) Maternal HIV infection
○ (B) Loss of chromosome 22q11
○ (C) Mutation in the common γ chain of cytokine receptors
○ (D) Mutation in the Bruton tyrosine kinase *(btk)* gene
○ (E) Mutation in CD40 ligand

24.   A 34-year-old female has experienced increasing muscular weakness over several months. This weakness is most pronounced in muscles that are used repetitively, such as the levator palpebrae of the eyelids. The most likely mechanism for muscle weakness in this case is

○ (A) Secretion of cytokines by activated macrophages
○ (B) Lysis of muscle cells by CD8+ T cells
○ (C) Antibody-mediated dysfunction of neuromuscular junction
○ (D) Deposition of immune complexes in the muscle capillaries
○ (E) A delayed hypersensitivity reaction against muscle antigens

25.   A 45-year-old female has experienced difficulty in swallowing that has increased in severity over the past year. She has also experienced malabsorption, demonstrated by a 10-kg weight loss in the past 6 months. She reports increasing dyspnea. Echocardiography demonstrates a large pericardial effusion. Her antinuclear antibody test is positive at 1:512 with a nucleolar pattern. Which of the following serious complications of her underlying autoimmune disease is most likely to occur?

○ (A) Meningitis
○ (B) Glomerulonephritis
○ (C) Perforated duodenal ulcer
○ (D) Adrenal failure
○ (E) Malignant hypertension

26.   Soon after birth, a female neonate developed tetany from hypocalcemia. Within the next year, this infant had bouts of *P. carinii* pneumonia, *Aspergillus fumigatus* pneumonia, and parainfluenza virus and herpes simplex virus upper respiratory infections. Which of the following mechanisms is responsible for the clinical features seen in this case?

○ (A) Malformation of third and fourth pharyngeal pouches
○ (B) Failure of maturation of B cells into plasma cells
○ (C) Lack of adenine deaminase
○ (D) Acquisition of maternal HIV infection at delivery
○ (E) Failure of differentiation of pre-B cells into B cells

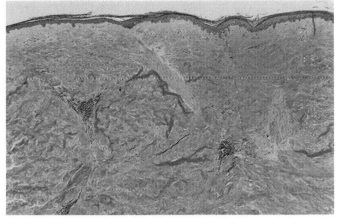

Courtesy of Dr. Trace Worrell, Department of Pathology, University of Texas Southwestern Medical School, Dallas, TX.

27.   A 39-year-old female has fingers that are tapered and clawlike, with decreased motion at the small joints. The microscopic appearance of the skin is shown in the figure. She also has diffuse interstitial fibrosis of the lungs, with pulmonary hypertension and cor pulmonale. Which of the following dermal inflammatory cells is considered the most likely initiator of the process that results in her skin disease?

○ (A) CD4 lymphocyte
○ (B) Macrophage
○ (C) Mast cell
○ (D) Neutrophil
○ (E) NK cell

28.   A 19-year-old female presented with fever, myalgia, sore throat, and mild erythematous rash over her abdomen and thighs. These symptoms abated in a month, and she remained healthy until 8 years later, when decreased visual acuity and pain in her right eye led to a finding of cytomegalovirus retinitis on funduscopy. Assuming that her initial illness and the ocular problem are a part of the same disease process, which of the following laboratory test findings is most likely to be found in this patient after her ocular problems began to appear?

○ (A) Antinuclear antibody titer of 1:1024
○ (B) Total serum globulin level of 650 mg/dL
○ (C) Positive HLA-B27 antigen
○ (D) Anticentromere antibody titer of 1:512
○ (E) CD4 lymphocyte count of 102/μL

29.   A 32-year-old female with a 10-year history of intravenous drug use developed a chronic watery diarrhea. Examination of the stool revealed cysts of *Cryptosporidium parvum*. She then developed a cryptococcal meningitis that

was successfully treated. A diagnosis of oral candidiasis was made a month later. Which of the following neoplasms is she at greatest risk for developing?

○ (A) Non-Hodgkin lymphoma
○ (B) Adenocarcinoma of the lung
○ (C) Leiomyosarcoma of retroperitoneum
○ (D) Cervical squamous carcinoma
○ (E) Cerebral astrocytoma

30. An inflamed mucosal surface makes an ideal location for the transmission of HIV during sexual intercourse. Which of the following cells is instrumental in transmitting HIV to CD4+ T lymphocytes?

○ (A) CD8+ cells
○ (B) NK cells
○ (C) Dendritic cells
○ (D) Neutrophils
○ (E) Plasma cells

31. A 35-year-old hospitalized female has developed an extensive, scaling rash during the past week. A skin biopsy shows keratinocyte apoptosis along the dermal-epidermal junction, with upper dermal lymphocytic infiltrates. She also has jaundice. Which of the following procedures has she recently undergone?

○ (A) Tuberculin skin testing
○ (B) Chemotherapy for malignant lymphoma
○ (C) Allogeneic bone marrow transplantation
○ (D) Penicillin therapy for pneumonia
○ (E) Patch testing for allergen detection

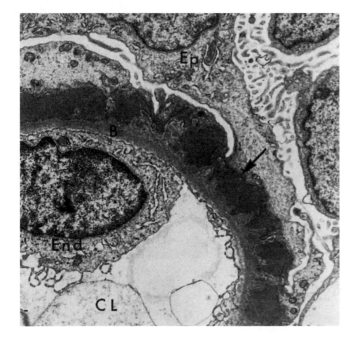

32. A 20-year-old female presents with acute renal failure over the past week. A renal biopsy shows immunofluorescent staining positive for Ig and complement C3 within the glomeruli. The electron microscopic appearance of the biopsy is shown in the figure. By which of the following immunologic mechanisms has this renal damage occurred?

○ (A) Antibody-dependent cell-mediated cytotoxicity
○ (B) Type III hypersensitivity
○ (C) Localized anaphylaxis
○ (D) Granulomatous inflammation
○ (E) T-cell–mediated cytotoxicity

33. A patient with multiple myeloma develops proteinuria, and you suspect a diagnosis of amyloidosis. Which of the following tests or procedures is most likely to establish the diagnosis of systemic amyloidosis?

○ (A) X-ray film of the skull to detect bone destruction
○ (B) Serum level of calcium
○ (C) Serum level of immunoglobulin light chains
○ (D) Rectal biopsy stained with Congo red
○ (E) Serum level of total immunoglobulins

For each of the clinical histories in questions 34 and 35, match the most closely associated lettered sign, symptom, or physical finding:

(A) Arthralgia
(B) Bony ankylosis
(C) Endocarditis
(D) Lymphadenopathy
(E) Myositis
(F) Pericarditis
(G) Photosensitivity
(H) Raynaud phenomenon
(I) Sclerodactyly
(J) Subcutaneous nodules
(K) Urethritis
(L) Xerophthalmia

34. A 29-year-old female has difficulty climbing a single flight of stairs. She has little difficulty in writing or typing. Laboratory tests reveal the presence of Jo-1 antibodies and a serum creatine kinase level of 458 U/L. (   )

35. A 52-year-old female is found to have a chronic, dry cough and a perforated nasal septum. A mild interstitial nephritis is present, as are antibodies to SS-A and SS-B. (   )

36. A 26-year-old female has had bouts of joint pain over the past 2 years. She also has a skin rash on the cheeks and bridge of the nose. On physical examination, she is found to have no joint swelling or deformity, although she has generalized lymphadenopathy. On laboratory testing, she is found to have anemia, leukopenia, a polyclonal gammopathy, and proteinuria. Her serum antinuclear antibody test result is positive at a titer of 1:1024, with a rim pattern identified by immunofluorescence. What advice would you give this patient?

○ (A) Blindness is likely to occur in the next 5 years.
○ (B) Avoid exposure to cold environments.
○ (C) Joint deformities will eventually occur.
○ (D) Chronic renal failure is likely to occur.
○ (E) A cardiac valve replacement will eventually be required.

37. In response to infection with *Mycobacterium tuberculosis*, a granuloma forms in the lung. Within the granuloma are cells expressing class II MHC antigens. These cells elaborate cytokines that promote fibroblastic production of collagen within the granuloma. From which of the following peripheral blood leukocytes are these class II antigen-bearing cells derived?

○ (A) Neutrophil
○ (B) Monocyte
○ (C) B cell
○ (D) NK cell
○ (E) Basophil

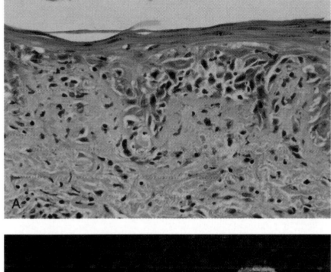

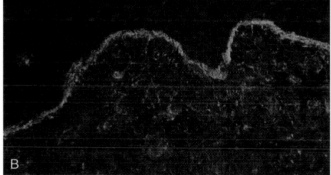

Courtesy of Dr. Richard Sontheimer, Department of Dermatology, University of Texas Southwestern Medical School, Dallas, TX.

38. A 17-year-old female has several disc-shaped, slightly raised, erythematous lesions located over her trunk and thighs. The light microscopic and immunofluorescent (with antibody to IgG) appearances of a skin biopsy are shown here. Which of the following conditions does the patient most likely have?

○ (A) Limited scleroderma
○ (B) Sjögren syndrome
○ (C) SLE
○ (D) Rheumatoid arthritis
○ (E) Dermatomyositis

39. Laboratory tests are ordered for two patients on a hospital ward. However, during the phlebotomy procedure, the Vacutainer tubes drawn from these two patients are mislabeled. One of these patients receives a blood transfusion later that day. Within an hour after starting the transfusion of red blood cells, the patient becomes tachycardic and hypotensive and passes pink-colored urine. How is this reaction mediated?

○ (A) Release of tumor necrosis factor-α into the circulation
○ (B) Antibody-dependent cellular cytotoxicity by NK cells
○ (C) Antigen-antibody complex deposition in glomeruli
○ (D) Complement-mediated lysis of red blood cells
○ (E) Mast cell degranulation

40. A 45-year-old male presents with fever, cough, and dyspnea worsening over the past few days. A bronchoalveolar lavage shows cysts of *P. carinii*. His CD4 lymphocyte count is $135/\mu L$, total serum globulin concentration is 2.5 g/dL, and WBC count is $7800/\mu L$, with a differential count of 75 segmented neutrophils, 8 band neutrophils, 6 lymphocytes, 10 monocytes, and 1 eosinophil. Which of the following positive serologic laboratory findings would you most expect?

○ (A) Antineutrophil cytoplasmic autoantibody
○ (B) Rheumatoid factor
○ (C) Antibodies to human immunodeficiency virus
○ (D) Antistreptolysin O
○ (E) Antinuclear antibody

41. "The boy in the bubble" was a famous experiment in the treatment of a primary immunodeficiency disorder by isolating the patient from potential pathogens. This boy started life with a hypoplastic thymus. He had small lymph nodes that lacked germinal centers, and gut-associated lymphoid tissue was scant. His total lymphocyte count was very low, and his total serum globulin concentration was diminished. How is this disorder now treated?

○ (A) Chemotherapy
○ (B) Allogeneic bone marrow transplantation
○ (C) Corticosteroid therapy
○ (D) Intravenous immunoglobulin therapy
○ (E) Antibiotic therapy

42. A 9-year-old girl had pain and swelling of her elbows and knees for a month, with fever to 38°C. Her peripheral WBC count was elevated. She had a positive antinuclear antibody test result but negative results for rheumatoid factor, Scl-70, and SS-A serologies. Several years later, her symptoms abated, never to recur again. She most likely had

○ (A) Systemic sclerosis
○ (B) Juvenile rheumatoid arthritis
○ (C) Psoriatic arthropathy
○ (D) Ankylosing spondylitis
○ (E) Reiter syndrome

43. A 9-month-old child presents with a history of recurrent infections with multiple agents, including cytomegalovirus, *Candida* (a fungus), and staphylococci. A careful family history and pedigree analysis reveals this to be a genetic disorder that is inherited in an autosomal recessive

pattern. Of the laboratory tests listed (all of which are relevant), which one is likely to be the *most useful* in establishing the underlying mechanism of immunodeficiency?

○ (A) Quantitative serum immunoglobulin levels
○ (B) Enumeration of B cells in the blood
○ (C) Enumeration of CD3+ cells in blood
○ (D) Tests of neutrophil function
○ (E) Adenosine deaminase (ADA) levels in leukocytes

44. An acute pharyngitis is diagnosed in a 12-year-old girl, and throat culture grows group A β-hemolytic streptococcus. The pharyngitis resolves, but 3 weeks later, she develops chest pain with fever. Her antistreptolysin O (ASO) titer is 1:512. By which of the following immunologic mechanisms has the carditis developed?

○ (A) Breakdown of T-cell anergy
○ (B) Polyclonal lymphocyte activation
○ (C) Release of sequestered antigens
○ (D) Molecular mimicry
○ (E) Failure of T-cell–mediated suppression

45. A 32-year-old male has experienced nausea and vomiting for the past week and is mildly icteric. His serum aspartate aminotransferase level is 208 U/L and alanine aminotransferase level is 274 U/L. A liver biopsy shows focal death of hepatocytes with a portal infiltrate composed mainly of lymphocytes. Serologic findings indicate positivity for hepatitis B surface antigen (HBsAg) and hepatitis B core antibody (HBcAb). The most likely mechanism by which the liver cell injury occurs under these conditions is

○ (A) Recognition of HBsAg by the CD8 molecule of T cells
○ (B) Recognition of an antigenic peptide presented by MHC class I molecules to NK cells
○ (C) Recognition of an antigenic peptide presented by MHC class I molecule to CD8+ cells
○ (D) Destruction of HBs antigen-expressing cells by anti-HBs IgG antibody
○ (E) Apoptosis of the liver cells by cytokines released by activated macrophages

For each of the clinical scenarios in questions 46 and 47, select the most likely antibody that will be positive:

(A) Anti–double-stranded DNA antibodies
(B) Antibody to Sm antigen
(C) Anti-histone antibody
(D) Anti–Jo-1 antibody
(E) Anti–U1-riboneucleoprotein antibody
(F) Anti-centromere antibody
(G) Anti-SSA antibody
(H) Anti–basement membrane antibody
(I) Anti-phospholipid antibody
(J) Antibodies against desmosomes

46. A 60-year-old female is being treated with hydralazine for long-standing hypertension when she develops some clinical features suggestive of lupus erythematosus. Initial laboratory findings include antinuclear antibody titers of 1:2560 in a diffuse pattern. Anti–double-stranded DNA antibodies are not present. (   )

47. A 28-year-old male presents with a 2-day history of hemoptysis and blood in urine (i.e., hematuria). He develops acute renal failure. Renal biopsy shows glomerular damage and linear immunofluorescence with labeled anti-complement antibody. (   )

For each of the clinical histories in questions 48 and 49, match the most closely associated lettered cell that participates in an immunologic response.

(A) CD4+ lymphocyte
(B) CD8+ lymphocyte
(C) Eosinophil
(D) Epithelioid cell
(E) Fibroblast
(F) Follicular dendritic cell
(G) Macrophage
(H) Mast cell
(I) Neutrophil
(J) NK cell
(K) Plasma cell
(L) Pre-B cell
(M) Pro-T cell
(N) Stem cell
(O) Type 1 helper T cells (T_H1)

48. A 40-year-old male is known to have been infected with HIV for the past 10 years. He has been bothered in the past with oral candidiasis but has had no major illnesses. He is diagnosed with Kaposi sarcoma involving the skin. He has experienced a 20-kg weight loss in the past 6 months. His HIV-1 RNA viral load is 60,000 copies/mL. Which type of cell is depleted the most in his lymph nodes? (   )

49. As a 4-year-old child, this patient had recurrent sinopulmonary infections with *Staphylococcus aureus* and *Streptococcus pneumoniae*; he also developed an arthritis that cleared with immunoglobulin therapy. The germinal centers of his lymph nodes are rudimentary, and he has developed SLE. Which type of cell failed to differentiate? (   )

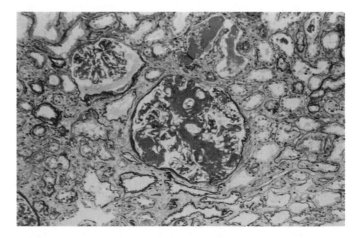

50. A 61-year-old male presents with decreasing renal function marked by rising concentrations of serum creatinine and urea nitrogen. A renal biopsy reveals the micro-

scopic appearance shown in the figure and urinalysis demonstrates Bence Jones proteinuria. Which of the following underlying conditions is he most likely to have?

○ (A) Rheumatic fever
○ (B) Multiple myeloma
○ (C) Ankylosing spondylitis
○ (D) Systemic sclerosis
○ (E) Common variable immunodeficiency

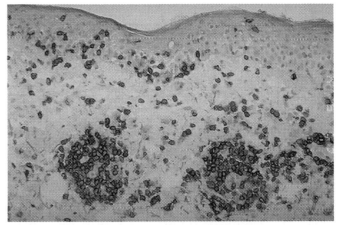

Courtesy of Dr. Louis Picker, Department of Pathology, University of Texas Southwestern Medical School, Dallas, TX.

51.   The skin of a 40-year-old male laboratory technician is shown here with immunostaining using antibody to CD4. A 10-mm-diameter area of red, indurated skin has persisted for the past 2 days after accidental injection of a chemical. Which of the following immunologic reactions is most consistent with this appearance?

○ (A) Systemic anaphylaxis
○ (B) Arthus reaction
○ (C) Graft-versus-host disease
○ (D) Delayed-type hypersensitivity
○ (E) Serum sickness

52.   A 19-year-old female with chronic renal failure received a cadaveric renal transplant. A month later, she experienced acute renal failure, and a renal biopsy was performed. She was then treated with corticosteroids, and her renal function improved. Which of the following changes was most likely seen in the biopsy before corticosteroid therapy?

○ (A) Interstitial infiltration by CD3+ lymphocytes and tubular epithelial damage
○ (B) Extensive fibrosis of the interstitium and glomeruli with markedly thickened blood vessels
○ (C) Fibrinoid necrosis of renal arterioles with thrombotic occlusion
○ (D) Interstitial infiltration by eosinophils with tubular epithelial damage
○ (E) Deposition of pink hyaline material in the glomeruli, which stains red with Congo red and shows green birefringence under polarized light

53.   A 35-year-old female has had bouts of severe pain and swelling of the small joints of both hands and feet for

the past 10 years, although she has had remissions with each of her three pregnancies. She has been bedridden for the past 2 months. A joint aspirate shows turbid fluid with many neutrophils containing phagocytized immune complexes. She has no myositis or rash. A painless subcutaneous nodule is present behind the elbow joint over the olecranon process. Which of the following long-term outcomes of her disease is most likely?

○ (A) Chronic renal failure
○ (B) Aortic dissection
○ (C) Vertebral kyphosis
○ (D) Adenocarcinoma of the colon
○ (E) Joint deformities

54.   A 48-year-old female has keratoconjunctivitis. She also has oral mucosal atrophy with buccal mucosal ulceration. A biopsy of her lip reveals marked lymphocytic and plasma cell infiltrates in minor salivary glands. Which of the following antibodies is most likely to be found for this patient?

○ (A) Anti–double-stranded DNA
○ (B) Anti-centromere antibody
○ (C) SS-B
○ (D) Scl-70
○ (E) Jo-1

55.   Within minutes after an injection of penicillin G, a 22-year-old male develops itching and erythema of his skin. This is quickly followed by severe respiratory difficulty with wheezing and stridor. Which of the following immunoglobulins has become attached to the penicillin G and mast cells to produce these symptoms?

○ (A) IgA
○ (B) IgG
○ (C) IgM
○ (D) IgD
○ (E) IgE

56.   A 4-year-old boy has had recurrent respiratory infections with multiple bacterial and viral pathogens. He also has eczema involving trunk and extremities. Laboratory findings include a platelet count of 71,000/μL, IgG level of 1422 mg/dL, IgM concentration of 11 mg/dL, and IgA level of 672 mg/dL. The WBC count is 3800/μL, with a differential count of 88 segmented neutrophils, 6 bands, 3 lymphocytes, and 3 monocytes. This patient is at an increased risk of developing

○ (A) Hypocalcemia
○ (B) Rheumatoid arthritis
○ (C) Glomerulonephritis
○ (D) Malignant lymphoma
○ (E) Dementia

57.   A 17-year-old boy is found to have a positive serologic test result for HIV. He is currently well. He is not an injection drug user, but he has been sexually active for 3 years. What is the best advice for this patient?

○ (A) You should not have unprotected sex with other persons.

○ (B) You will probably develop AIDS within the next year.

○ (C) Your HIV test may become negative within the next year.

○ (D) As long as you are clinically well, you can donate blood.

○ (E) The course of your infection is best followed by titers of anti-HIV antibodies.

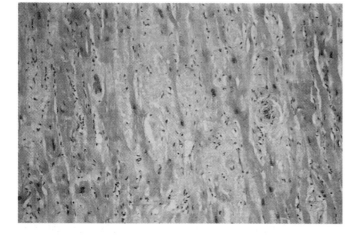

58. A 79-year-old male has experienced worsening congestive heart failure with pulmonary edema and peripheral edema. Echocardiography reveals cardiomegaly with four-chamber dilation. All laboratory tests, including serum protein electrophoresis and examination of bone marrow smear, are normal. An endomyocardial biopsy shows the histologic appearance represented in the figure. Which of the following proteins is most likely to be found in this lesion?

○ (A) Alpha-fetoprotein
○ (B) Beta$_2$-microglobulin
○ (C) Transthyretin
○ (D) Calcitonin
○ (E) IgE

59. A 2-year-old boy has had almost continuous infections since 6 months of age. These infections have included otitis media, pneumonia, and impetigo. Organisms cultured have included *Haemophilus influenzae*, *S. pneumoniae*, and *S. aureus*. He has also had diarrhea, with *Giardia lamblia* cysts identified in stool specimens. Family history reveals that an older brother who presented with a similar condition died because of overwhelming infections. His two sisters and both parents are normal. Which of the following laboratory findings is most likely for this boy?

○ (A) Absent IgA
○ (B) Decreased complement C3
○ (C) High titer of HIV-1 RNA
○ (D) Markedly decreased immunoglobulins
○ (E) Positive antinuclear antibody test

ANSWERS

1. **(A)** She has features of SLE. Patients with SLE often have a skin rash on sun-exposed areas. A urethritis is more characteristic of Reiter syndrome, one of the spondyloarthropathies. Difficulty in swallowing is a feature of scleroderma. Xerostomia suggests Sjögren syndrome. Though SLE has genetic associations with complement deficiencies or HLA-DQ, malformations are not a feature of SLE. Congenital heart disease may be seen with DiGeorge syndrome.
BP6 103   PBD6 217

2. **(B)** This patient has clinical and serologic features of SLE. She also has a false-positive test result for syphilis, indicating the presence of anticardiolipin antibodies. These antibodies against phospholipid-protein complexes are also called lupus anticoagulants because they interfere with in vitro clotting tests. However, in vivo, they are thrombogenic. Hence, these patients can have recurrent thrombosis. Lupus anticoagulants can also occur in the absence of lupus in some patients.
BP6 103   PBD6 218

3. **(B)** Entry of HIV into cells requires binding to the CD4 molecule and co-receptor molecules such as CCR5 and CXCR4. These HIV co-receptors are receptors for chemokines on the surface of T cells and macrophages. Mutations in genes encoding these co-receptor molecules make individuals resistant to the effects of HIV infection because HIV cannot enter lymphocytes and macrophages. The other cell surface receptors are not relevant for HIV entry into cells.
BP6 119-120   PBD6 242

4. **(E)** She has features of SLE. The antinuclear antibody test result is nearly always positive for persons with SLE. The presence of anti-double-stranded DNA or anti-Smith antibodies is more specific for SLE than for other autoimmune diseases. An elevated ASO titer indicates a previous group A streptococcal infection. HLA-B27 is strongly associated with spondyloarthropathies, such as ankylosing spondylitis. Most persons with SLE have a polyclonal gammopathy with increased serum IgG. Rheumatoid factor is seen with rheumatoid arthritis, which is unlikely to be accompanied by a malar rash and, more importantly, is associated with joint destruction and fibrosis.
BP6 102-104   PBD6 216-218

5. **(B)** She has experienced a systemic anaphylactic reaction from a type I hypersensitivity reaction. Epinephrine is the fastest acting agent to treat this life-threatening condition. Cyclosporine is used to minimize transplant rejection. Penicillin is an antibiotic that often induces a type I hypersensitivity reaction. Glucocorticoids can reduce immune reactions, although over days to weeks. Methotrexate is useful to treat graft-versus-host disease.
BP6 87-89   PBD6 197-199

6. **(E)** She has SLE. These patients can develop anti–red cell antibodies that can cause a hemolytic anemia. Cytopenias, including leukopenia, thrombocytopenia, and anemia, are common with SLE.
BP6 103   PBD6 217

7. **(I)** She has psoriatic arthropathy. The arthritis in this condition can clinically and pathologically resemble rheumatoid arthritis. Like other spondyloarthropathies, sacroiliitis occurs in patients with psoriatic arthropathy.
BP6 112   PBD6 1252

8. **(B)** He has a selective IgA deficiency. Such persons are bothered by minor recurrent sinopulmonary infections and by diarrhea. *Pneumocystis* infections are seen in patients with more severe acquired or inherited immunodeficiency disorders affecting cell-mediated immunity, particularly AIDS. Hepatitis infections are not directly related to immunodeficiency states, although AIDS patients with a history of injection drug use are often infected with hepatitis B or C. Resistance against fungal and viral infection is mediated by T cells.
BP6 116   PBD6 234

9. **(D)** He has AIDS with Kaposi sarcoma of the skin. Kaposi sarcoma is associated with a herpesvirus agent that is sexually transmitted: human herpesvirus 8 (HHV-8), also called the Kaposi sarcoma herpesvirus. Other herpesviruses are not involved in the pathogenesis of Kaposi sarcoma, although they can be frequent with AIDS. HIV, although present in the lymphocytes and monocytes, is not detected in the spindle cells that proliferate in Kaposi sarcoma. Other than the varicella zoster virus, which is associated with the appearance of dermatomally distributed skin vesicles known as *shingles*, skin lesions are not common for cytomegalovirus, Epstein-Barr virus, or adenovirus infections.
BP6 125   PBD6 248

10. **(A)** CD4 cells of the T_H2 type are essential to the induction of type I hypersensitivity because they can secrete cytokines such as interleukin (IL)-4, IL-5, IL-3, and granulocyte-macrophage colony-stimulating factor, which are required for the growth, recruitment, and activation of mast cells and eosinophils. NK cells can lyse other cells, such as virus-infected cells, without prior sensitization. Macrophages can secrete a variety of cytokines, but they are not essential to type I hypersensitivity. Dendritic cells trap antigen and aid in antigen presentation. Neutrophils are recruited by cytokines to participate in acute inflammatory reactions.
BP6 87   PBD6 196

11. **(E)** She has dermatomyositis, a form of inflammatory myopathy in which capillaries are the primary target for antibody and complement-mediated injury. Anti-Jo-1 antibodies, although not present in most cases, are quite specific for inflammatory myopathies. The perivascular and perimysial inflammatory infiltrates result in peripheral muscle fascicular myocyte necrosis. The process is mediated by CD4+ cells and B cells. The heliotrope rash is a characteristic feature of dermatomyositis. Anti–double-stranded DNA is specific for SLE, in which there can be a myositis

without significant inflammation or necrosis. Rheumatoid arthritis is accompanied by inflammatory destruction of joints, not muscle, although muscle may atrophy secondary to diminished movement. The anti–U1-ribonucleoprotein antibodies suggest a diagnosis of mixed connective tissue disease, a condition that can overlap with polymyositis. Anti-histone antibodies are associated with drug-induced SLE.
BP6 114–115   PBD6 230–232

12. **(B)** These are the "wire loop" glomerular capillary lesions of lupus nephritis. Anti-Sm and anti–double-stranded DNA are specific for SLE. However, anti-Sm is present in only 25% of cases. Scl-70 is a marker for diffuse systemic sclerosis. Jo-1 is most specific for polymyositis. HLA-B27 is seen with ankylosing spondylitis. Anti-centromere antibody is seen most often with limited scleroderma.
BP6 104, 108   PBD6 218, 222

13. **(A)** This is an example of antibody-dependent cell-mediated cytotoxicity directed at a parasitic infection. IgG and IgE antibodies bearing Fc receptors coat the parasite. Macrophages, NK cells, and neutrophils can recognize the Fc receptor and lyse the antibody-coated target cells. Complement-mediated lysis is most typical for immune destruction of red blood cells with hemolysis. Langhans giant cells are seen in granulomatous inflammation, a form of type IV hypersensitivity. Acute inflammatory reactions have little effect against tissue parasites. Leukotriene C_4 is a potent agent that promotes vascular permeability and bronchial smooth muscle contraction in type I hypersensitivity reactions.
BP6 90–91   PBD6 200–201

14. **(B)** This is chronic rejection. The progressive renal failure results from ischemic changes with vascular narrowing. Cell lysis with macrophages is typical for antibody-dependent cell-mediated cytotoxicity that does not play a key role in chronic rejection. Granulomatous inflammation is not typical for transplant rejection. Release of leukotriene C_4 from mast cells is a feature of type I hypersensitivity. Complement-mediated cell lysis can occur when anti-donor antibodies are preformed in the host, as occurs in hyperacute rejection.
BP6 98   PBD6 210

15. **(A)** NK cells have the ability to respond without prior sensitization. They carry receptors for MHC class I molecules that inhibit their lytic function. When expression of class I MHC molecules is reduced on the cell surface, the inhibitory receptors on NK cells do not receive a negative signal. The cell is killed. NK cells are often the first line of defense against viral infection. Neutrophils provide a nonspecific immune response, primarily to bacterial infections and not to intracellular viral infections. Macrophages can process antigen and can phagocytize necrotic cells. CD4 cells are helper T cells that assist other cells, such as NK cells, macrophages, and B cells, in the immune response. Dendritic cells help in antigen presentation.
BP6 83   PBD6 191

16. **(E)** There is a failure of terminal differentiation of B cells into IgA-secreting plasma cells. Lack of IgA in mucosal secretions leads to increased risk for respiratory and gastrointestinal infections. There are IgA antibodies in serum that can lead to a transfusion reaction with IgA in donor serum. Persons with severe combined immunodeficiency (SCID) do not live this long with such mild infections. HIV infection is marked by failure of cell-mediated immunity. The DiGeorge syndrome manifests in infancy with failure of cell-mediated immunity from lack of functional T cells. Wiskott-Aldrich syndrome is associated with eczema and thrombocytopenia.
BP6 116 PBD6 234

17. **(C)** This history is typical of the late-phase reaction in type I hypersensitivity. The initial rapid response is largely caused by degranulation of mast cells. The late-phase reaction follows without additional exposure to antigen and is characterized by more intense infiltration by inflammatory cells such as neutrophils, eosinophils, basophils, monocytes, and CD4+ lymphocytes. There is more tissue destruction in this late phase.
BP6 88–89 PBD 196–198

18. **(B)** Macrophages can become infected with HIV and are not destroyed like CD4 cells. Instead, macrophages survive to carry the infection to tissues throughout the body, particularly the brain. HIV infection of the brain can result in encephalitis and dementia. NK cells and neutrophils play no significant role in HIV infection. CD8 lymphocytes cannot be infected with HIV. Langerhans cells in mucosal surfaces may aid in initial HIV infection of CD4 lymphocytes.
BP6 120–121 PBD6 241–243

19. **(C)** This is a localized immune-complex reaction (i.e., Arthus reaction), which activates and depletes complement C3 and C4. IgE concentration is increased in persons with atopy and the potential for type I hypersensitivity. Although neutrophils are being recruited locally to the inflammatory reaction in this case, they are not depleted systemically, and they may be increased in the circulation. Skin tests are measures of type IV hypersensitivity when antigens such as tuberculin are used. CD4 lymphocytes assist in a variety of antibody and cell-mediated immune reactions, but their numbers in peripheral blood do not change appreciably.
BP6 93–94 PBD6 204

20. **(C)** In chronic inflammatory conditions such as rheumatoid arthritis, the SAA precursor protein forms the major amyloid fibril protein AA. Amyloid is deposited in interstitial locations, not intracellularly. The P component is a minor component of the amyloid. All amyloid demonstrates the characteristic "apple green" birefringence under polarized light microscopy after Congo red staining — anything else would not be amyloid. Amyloid derived from light chains in association with multiple myeloma has AL fibrils.
BP6 126–128 PBD6 251–253

21. **(G)** Mixed connective tissue disease has features of SLE, polymyositis, and Sjögren syndrome. Unlike SLE, serious renal disease is unlikely.
BP6 115 PBD6 231

22. **(C)** This patient has cutaneous and visceral manifestations of diffuse systemic sclerosis (i.e., diffuse scleroderma). Raynaud phenomenon, skin changes, and esophageal dysmotility can also occur in limited scleroderma (i.e., CREST syndrome), but lung involvement does not.
BP6 114 PBD6 227–228

23. **(C)** This patient has severe combined immunodeficiency (SCID). Because the T- and B-cell arms of the immune system are deficient, there are severe and recurrent infections with bacteria, viruses, and fungi. With the family history of males being affected, the patient most likely has X-linked SCID. This form results from mutations in the common γ chain that is a part of many cytokine receptors such as IL-2, IL-4, IL-7, and IL-15. These cytokines are needed for normal B- and T-cell development. Loss of chromosome 22q11 is seen in DiGeorge syndrome. *btk* gene mutations give rise to Bruton agammaglobulinemia. Mutation in CD40 ligand is responsible for hyper IgM syndrome.
BP6 117 PBD6 234–236

24. **(C)** She has features of myasthenia gravis, a form of type II hypersensitivity reaction in which antibody is directed against cell surface receptors. Antibodies to acetylcholine receptors impair the function of skeletal muscle motor end plates. Antibodies are produced by B cells, and macrophages are not a significant part of this hypersensitivity reaction; there is little or no inflammation of the muscle with myasthenia gravis. Muscle lysis by CD8+ T cells occurs in polymyositis. Immune complex–mediated injury is a feature of dermatomyositis. Delayed hypersensitivity reactions are more likely in parasitic infestations of muscles.
BP6 90 PBD6 201

25. **(E)** She has diffuse systemic sclerosis (i.e., scleroderma). The small arteries of the kidney are involved with a hyperplastic arteriolosclerosis, which can be complicated by very high blood pressure and renal failure. Meningitis and adrenal failure are not typical features of autoimmune diseases. With scleroderma, the gastrointestinal tract undergoes fibrosis, without any tendency to perforation or ulceration. Glomerulonephritis is a more typical complication for SLE.
BP6 112–114 PBD6 226–229

26. **(A)** This is DiGeorge syndrome. The thymus, parathyroids, aorta, and heart can be involved. T-cell function is deficient, resulting in recurrent and multiple fungal, viral, and protozoal infections. Failure of B-cell maturation to plasma cells is one mode of development of common variable immunodeficiency. Some cases of SCID are caused by lack of ADA. HIV infection does not explain the hypocalcemia at birth. Failure of pre-B cell maturation results in Bruton agammaglobulinemia.
BP6 116–117 PBD6 235

27. **(A)** Although not proved, the CD4 lymphocytes are thought to respond to some unknown antigenic stimulation, releasing cytokines that further activate macrophages and mast cells. The result is extensive dermal fibrosis that produces the clinical appearance of sclerodactyly with scleroderma. Neutrophils and NK cells do not participate in this process. Despite scleroderma being an autoimmune disease, inflammation is minimal. The major finding is progressive fibrosis of skin, lung, and gastrointestinal tract.
BP6 113-114   PBD6 228-229

28. **(E)** Her original symptoms, although nonspecific, are seen in more than one half of adults with acute HIV infection. The average time to development of AIDS is 8 to 10 years, with the onset of opportunistic infections as the CD4 cell count falls below $200/\mu L$. Spondyloarthropathies and autoimmune diseases such as SLE or scleroderma are not likely to have such a long interval between illnesses and are not as likely to have opportunistic infections without immunosuppressive therapy. Persons with AIDS may have a polyclonal gammopathy but not marked hypogammaglobulinemia.
BP6 122-124   PBD6 245-246

29. **(A)** Opportunistic infections in an intravenous drug abuser suggest a diagnosis of AIDS. The most common neoplasms seen in association with AIDS are B-cell non-Hodgkin lymphoma and Kaposi sarcoma. A rare tumor associated with AIDS in children is leiomyosarcoma. Cervical dysplasias and carcinomas are increased in women with HIV infection, but such lesions are less frequent than lymphoma. Lung cancers at her age are not common in any circumstance. Opportunistic infections of the brain are common in AIDS, as are central nervous system lymphomas but not glial neoplasms.
BP6 124-126   PBD6 247-250

30. **(C)** Three types of cells can carry HIV: dendritic cells, monocytes, and CD4+ T cells. Mucosal dendritic cells (i.e., Langerhans cells) can bind to the virus and transport it to CD4+ cells in the lymph nodes. Whether the virus is internalized by mucosal dendritic cells is not clear. Monocytes and CD4+ T cells express CD4 and the co-receptors (CCR5 and CXCR4), and therefore HIV can enter these cells. Follicular dendritic cells are distinct from mucosal or epithelial dendritic cells; they trap antibody-coated HIV virions by means of their Fc receptors. The other listed cells cannot be infected by HIV.
BP6 83   PBD6 191

31. **(C)** This is graft-versus-host disease. The engrafted marrow contains immunocompetent cells that can proliferate and attack host tissues, usually skin, liver, and gastrointestinal epithelium. Tuberculosis skin testing is a form of delayed-type hypersensitivity. Some chemotherapy agents can produce a drug reaction with more acute inflammation. Urticaria with type I hypersensitivity is a typical reaction to penicillin therapy. Patch testing is done to determine the type of allergens to which atopic persons may react.
BP6 99   PBD6 210-211

32. **(B)** This is immune complex-mediated glomerulonephritis. The immune complexes activate complement and result in acute inflammation. Antibody-dependent cell-mediated cytotoxicity is initiated by IgG or IgE coating a target to attract cells that affect lysis, and immune complexes do not form. Localized anaphylaxis is a type I hypersensitivity mediated by IgE antibody. Granulomatous inflammation and T-cell cytotoxicity are features of type IV hypersensitivity.
BP6 92-93   PBD6 201-203

33. **(D)** The diagnosis of amyloidosis is based on light microscopic demonstration of amyloid in tissues with Congo red staining. Multiple myeloma can produce lytic skull lesions, although not in all cases, and such lesions are not always accompanied by amyloidosis. Hypercalcemia occurs frequently with myeloma because of the lytic skeletal lesions, but it does not predict amyloid deposition. The concentration of light chains in serum or urine can be elevated without amyloidosis, as can the total serum immunoglobulin.
BP6 126-128   PBD6 251-253

34. **(E)** She has polymyositis. Muscle weakness in polymyositis tends to be symmetric and proximal. This condition differs from dermatomyositis in that there is no skin involvement, and typically polymyositis affects adults. Her skeletal muscle on biopsy shows infiltration by lymphocytes along with degeneration and regeneration of muscle fibers. The lymphocytes are cytotoxic CD8+ cells.
BP6 115   PBD6 229-231

35. **(L)** She has Sjögren syndrome. This is characterized by immunologically mediated destruction of salivary and lacrimal glands, as well as other exocrine glands, lining the respiratory and gastrointestinal tracts. Dryness and crusting of the nose can lead to perforation of nasal septum. In 25% of cases, extraglandular tissues such as lung, skin, kidney, and muscles may be involved.
BP6 111-112   PBD6 225-226

36. **(D)** She has SLE. Many persons with SLE have glomerulonephritis and eventually develop renal failure. Blindness is uncommon with SLE. Raynaud phenomenon can be seen with many autoimmune diseases but is most troublesome with scleroderma. Although synovial inflammation is common with SLE, joint deformity is rare. The Libman-Sacks endocarditis of SLE tends to be nondeforming and limited. It is uncommon these days because of the use of corticosteroid therapy.
BP6 106-108   PBD6 220-222

37. **(B)** Blood monocytes express MHC class II antigens and can migrate into tissues to become macrophages. In tuberculosis, these macrophages transform into epithelioid cells, thus forming a granuloma. Macrophages play an important role in delayed hypersensitivity reactions with cell-mediated immunity. Neutrophils are important mainly in acute inflammatory responses, although there may be some of them in a granulomatous reaction. B cells form plasma cells that secrete immunoglobulin on stimulation and are essential to humoral immunity. NK cells can function without prior sensitization. Basophils may play a role in IgE-mediated responses.
BP6 83   PBD6 190-191

38. **(C)** With SLE, skin lesions can be seen on any area of the body but are worse in sun-exposed areas. Immune complexes are trapped at the epidermal basement membrane. The skin with scleroderma shows marked collagenous fibrosis and no detectable immune complexes. Skin involvement with Sjögren syndrome and rheumatoid arthritis is uncommon. The rash of dermatomyositis has lymphocytic infiltrates but not usually immune complex deposition.
BP6 105–106   PBD6 222–223

39. **(D)** This is a major transfusion reaction, resulting from a type II hypersensitivity reaction. The patient's serum contains naturally occurring antibodies to the incompatible donor red blood cells. They attach to the recipient red blood cells and induce complement activation that results in generation of the C5-9 membrane attack complex. Major transfusion reactions are rare, and most result from clerical errors. NK cell lysis is seen with antibody-dependent cell-mediated cytotoxicity. Antigen-antibody complex formation is typical for a type III hypersensitivity reaction. Mast cells degranulate with antigen attachment to IgE in type I hypersensitivity reactions.
BP6 90   PBD6 199–200

40. **(C)** *Pneumocystis* pneumonia is a common finding in persons with AIDS. His low CD4 count is characteristic for AIDS. Antineutrophil cytoplasmic autoantibody (i.e., C-ANCA or P-ANCA) can be seen with vasculitis. Persons with rheumatoid arthritis do not have significant immunosuppression unless they are treated with highly potent immunosuppressive drugs such as cyclosporine. The ASO titer is elevated with rheumatic fever, but there is no serious immunosuppression. The antinuclear antibody test result is positive in a variety of autoimmune diseases, but the decrease in CD4 count is not typical for such conditions.
BP6 124–125   PBD6 247–248

41. **(B)** He had SCID, which is treated with allogeneic bone marrow transplantation. The transplanted stem cells in the bone marrow give rise to normal T and B cells. Chemotherapy is used to treat malignancies, such as lymphoma or leukemia, that are causes for secondary immunodeficiency. Corticosteroid therapy helps to alleviate inflammation by reducing lymphocyte function and number. Intravenous immunoglobulin is helpful in conditions such as common variable immunodeficiency, in which IgG is deficient. Antibiotic therapy can aid in treatment of infections complicating immunodeficiency states but cannot treat the underlying problem.
BP6 117   PBD6 235–236

42. **(B)** She had juvenile rheumatoid arthritis. About 70% to 90% of cases resolve without joint deformity. Unlike rheumatoid arthritis, juvenile rheumatoid arthritis tends to involve lower and larger joints, and rheumatoid factor is often absent. Systemic sclerosis is disease of adults that may have features resembling early rheumatoid arthritis, but joint destruction is rare. Psoriatic arthritis is a disease of adults with features similar to rheumatoid arthritis, but joint involvement is more irregular. Ankylosing spondylitis in older adults affects principally the vertebral column. The major features of Reiter syndrome are urethritis, arthritis, and conjunctivitis in young to middle-aged adults.
BP6 115   PBD6 1251–1252

43. **(E)** This patient is susceptible to bacterial, fungal, and viral infections and most likely has SCID. The autosomal recessive pattern of inheritance implicates adenosine deaminase (ADA) deficiency rather than mutations in the γ chain of cytokine receptors. Low ADA levels in the leukocytes are diagnostic.
BP6 117   PBD6 235

44. **(D)** Streptococcal M proteins cross-react with cardiac glycoproteins, resulting in rheumatic heart disease, a form of autoimmunity. Breakdown of T-cell anergy usually occurs when localized tissue damage and inflammation cause up-regulation of costimulatory molecules on the target tissues. This is a possible mechanism of autoimmunity in the brain and pancreatic β cells. Polyclonal lymphocyte activation may be caused by microbial products such as endotoxin or bacterial superantigens. Release of sequestered antigens can cause autoimmunity. This mechanism is likely in autoimmune uveitis; failure of T-cell–mediated suppression has not yet been shown to cause any autoimmune disease. It remains a potential mechanism.
BP6 100–102   PBD6 214–215

45. **(C)** Virus-infected cells are recognized and killed by cytotoxic CD8+ T cells. The T-cell receptor on the CD8 T cells binds to the complex of viral peptide and MHC class I molecules on the surface of the infected cell. NK cells also recognize MHC class I molecules with self-peptides. This recognition inhibits NK cell killing.
BP6 96   PBD6 206

46. **(C)** This patient has a drug-induced SLE-like condition. Procainamide, isoniazid, and other drugs can cause this condition. Test results for the antinuclear antibody are often positive, but those for the anti–double-stranded DNA are negative. Anti-histone antibodies are present in many cases. Characteristic signs and symptoms of SLE are often lacking. Renal involvement is uncommon. This condition remits when the patient stops taking the drug.
PBD6 218, 224–225

47. **(H)** He has Goodpasture syndrome, in which there is an antibody directed against type IV collagen in basement membranes of glomeruli and in lung. This is a form of type II hypersensitivity reaction. The antibodies attach to the basement membrane and fix complement, thus damaging the glomeruli.
BP6 90   PBD6 201

48. **(A)** As HIV infection progresses, there is continuing, gradual loss of CD4 cells. The stage of clinical AIDS is reached when the peripheral CD4 count drops below 200/μL. This usually takes an average of 7 to 10 years. At this point, the risk for development of opportunistic infections and neoplasms typical for AIDS increases greatly. The extent of viremia also gives an indication of the progression of HIV infection, with increasing HIV-1 RNA levels as immunologic containment of HIV fails.
BP6 122–124   PBD6 245–247

49. **(L)** He has features of X-linked agammaglobulinemia of Bruton. In this condition, B-cell maturation stops after the rearrangement of heavy-chain genes, and light chains are not produced. Complete immunoglobulin molecules with heavy and light chains are not assembled and transported to the cell membrane. The lack of immunoglobulins predisposes the child to recurrent bacterial infections. Because T-cell function remains intact, viral, fungal, and protozoal infections are uncommon.
BP6 115–116   PBD6 232–233

50. **(B)** Amyloidosis is most often caused by excessive light chain production with plasma cell dyscrasias such as multiple myeloma (AL amyloid). Chronic inflammatory conditions may also result in amyloidosis (AA amyloid) but not in secretion of light chains in urine (i.e., Bence Jones proteinuria). Immunoglobulin levels are generally reduced in patients with common variable immunodeficiency.
BP6 127, 130   PBD6 252–255

51. **(D)** Perivascular accumulation of T cells, particularly CD4+ cells, is typical of delayed hypersensitivity skin reactions. Systemic anaphylaxis typically occurs within minutes after an encounter with the antigen. Systemic and localized immune complex diseases (serum sickness and Arthus reactions) are type III hypersensitivity reactions; they often demonstrate a vasculitis. Graft-versus-host disease is characterized by epidermal apoptosis and rash.
BP6 94–95   PBD6 204–205

52. **(A)** Acute rejection of kidney transplants occurs weeks, months, or even years after transplantation. It is characterized by infiltration with CD3+ T cells that include the CD4+ and CD8+ subsets. These cells damage tubular epithelium by direct cytotoxicity and by release of cytokines, such as interferon-γ, that activate macrophages. The reaction is called acute cellular rejection, and it can be readily treated with corticosteroids. Interstitial and glomerular fibrosis, along with blood vessel thickening, occur in chronic rejection. Fibrinoid necrosis and thrombosis are more typical of hyperacute rejection that occurs within minutes of placement of the transplant into the recipient. Eosinophils accumulate in acute interstitial nephritis due to drug reactions. Material that stains with Congo red and shows green birefringence is amyloid.
BP6 96–98   PBD6 207–209

53. **(E)** She has rheumatoid arthritis. The pannus of rheumatoid arthritis leads to joint destruction and ankylosis with marked deformity. There are few other organ-specific lesions, though rheumatoid nodules can be found under the skin over bony prominences and in organs such as lung and heart. Renal failure is more likely with SLE. Aortic dissection is more likely with Reiter syndrome. Ankylosing spondylitis is marked by kyphosis. The risk for malignancies is increased with autoimmune diseases, although not by a great degree, and not by much with rheumatoid arthritis.
BP6 109–111   PBD6 1248–1251

54. **(C)** She has Sjögren syndrome, which primarily involves salivary and lacrimal glands. Antibodies to SS-B are found in 60–90% of patients. Anti–double-stranded DNA is a specific autoantibody for SLE. Anti-centromere antibody is seen in systemic sclerosis. Scl-70 is a marker for diffuse systemic sclerosis. Jo-1 is a marker for polymyositis.
BP6 111–112   PBD6 225–226

55. **(E)** This is a systemic anaphylactic reaction, a form of type I hypersensitivity. IgE is bound to mast cells, after previous sensitization, so that a repeat encounter with the antigen results in mast cell degranulation and the release of mediators, such as histamine, that lead to anaphylaxis. IgE is also important in mediating more localized inflammatory reactions such as allergic rhinitis (i.e., hay fever). Other immunoglobulins do not bind so readily to mast cells.
BP6 87–88   PBD6 196–198

56. **(D)** The findings point to the X-linked disorder known as Wiskott-Aldrich syndrome. As with many immunodeficiency disorders, there is an increased risk for lymphoma. Hypocalcemia is seen in neonates with DiGeorge syndrome. Rheumatoid arthritis can complicate isolated IgA deficiency and common variable immunodeficiency, conditions with survival to adulthood. A deficiency of complement component C3 may be complicated by immune-complex glomerulonephritis. Dementia can be seen with AIDS.
PBD6 236

57. **(A)** Persons infected with HIV are infected for life. They can pass the virus to others by sexual intercourse even if they appear to be well. The average time for the development of AIDS after HIV infection is 8 to 10 years. Seroreversion in HIV infection does not occur. Screening questionnaires and serologic testing can prevent this person from being a blood donor. HIV infection affects mainly CD4 lymphocytes, with declining CD4 counts presaging the development of clinically apparent AIDS. Antibody titers do not predict clinical illness or complications. Progression of HIV disease is monitored by levels of HIV-1 mRNA in the blood and by CD4+ cell counts.
BP6 122–125   PBD6 245–248

58. **(C)** This is cardiac amyloidosis. At his age, a senile cardiac amyloidosis, resulting from deposition of transthyretin, is most likely. Alpha-fetoprotein is seen in fetal life, but is best known in adults as a serum tumor marker. Beta$_2$-microglobulin contributes to the development of amyloidosis associated with long-term hemodialysis. Calcitonin forms the precursor for amyloid deposited in thyroid medullary carcinomas. Amyloidosis associated with plasma cell dyscrasias results from light-chain production. Although the heart is commonly involved in light-chain amyloidosis, the normal laboratory values and absence of plasma cell collections in the marrow argue against a plasma cell dyscrasia.
BP6 127–130   PBD6 252–253, 256

59. **(D)** He most likely has Bruton agammaglobulinemia, an X-linked primary immunodeficiency marked by recurrent bacterial infections that begin after maternal antibody levels diminish. Selective IgA deficiency is marked by a more benign course, with sinopulmonary infections and

diarrhea that are not severe. Deficiency of C3 is rare and leads to greater numbers of infections in children and young adults, but *Giardia* infections are not a feature of this disease. Lack of cell-mediated immunity is more likely to be seen with childhood HIV infection. Although some patients with Bruton agammaglobulinemia can develop features of SLE, they generally do not have a positive test result for antinuclear antibody.

BP6 115   **PBD6** 232–233

Neoplasia

BP6 Chapter 6 - Neoplasia
PBPD6 Chapter 8 - Neoplasia

1. Patients with chronic hepatitis B virus (HBV) or hepatitis C virus (HCV) infection are at greatly increased risk of developing hepatocellular carcinomas. This predisposition is best explained by

○ (A) The consistent integration of these viruses in the vicinity of protooncogenes

○ (B) The ability of these viruses to capture protooncogenes from the host DNA

○ (C) Virus-induced injury to liver cells followed by extensive regeneration

○ (D) The ability of viral genes to inactivate *Rb* and *p53* expression

○ (E) The ability of these viruses to cause immunosuppression of the host

2. A mastectomy with axillary lymph node dissection was performed on a 48-year-old female diagnosed with infiltrating ductal carcinoma of the left breast. Which of the following factors is most responsible for the presence of her lymph node metastases?

○ (A) Increased laminin receptors on tumor cells
○ (B) Presence of keratin in tumor cells
○ (C) Diminished apoptosis of tumor cells
○ (D) Tumor cell monoclonality
○ (E) Lymphadenitis

3. A 30-year-old sexually promiscuous female presents with vaginal bleeding and discharge. Colposcopic examination reveals an ulcerated lesion arising from the squamocolumnar junction of the uterine cervix. Biopsy results show an invasive tumor containing areas of squamous epithelium in which pearls of keratin can be seen. In situ hybridization reveals the presence of human papillomavirus type 16 (HPV-16) DNA within the tumor cells. Which of the following molecular abnormalities in this tumor is most likely related to infection with HPV-16?

○ (A) Trapping of the *ras* protein in a GTP-bound state
○ (B) Increased expression of laminin receptor genes

○ (C) Inability to repair DNA damage
○ (D) Functional inactivation of the *Rb1* protein
○ (E) Increased expression of epidermal growth factor receptor

4. A 47-year-old male has a peripheral blood WBC count of $167,500/\mu L$, with mature and immature neutrophilic cells predominating. Cytogenetic analysis of cells obtained through bone marrow aspiration reveals a t(9;22) translocation. This has resulted in formation of a hybrid gene, causing potent tyrosine kinase activity. Which of the following genes was translocated from chromosome 9?

○ (A) *p53*
○ (B) *Rb*
○ (C) NF-1
○ (D) K-*ras*
○ (E) c-*abl*

5. Right axillary lymphadenopathy is palpable in a 44-year-old female on physical examination. These nodes are painless but firm. Which of the following conditions is most likely to be present?

○ (A) Ductal carcinoma of the breast
○ (B) Acute mastitis with breast abscess
○ (C) Leiomyosarcoma of the uterus
○ (D) Cerebral glioblastoma multiforme
○ (E) Squamous dysplasia of the larynx

For each of the clinical histories in questions 6 and 7, match the most closely related lettered environmental agent that is causally related to development of neoplasia in humans:

(A) Arsenic
(B) Asbestos
(C) Benzene
(D) Beryllium
(E) Cadmium
(F) Chromium
(G) Ethylene oxide
(H) Nickel
(I) Radon
(J) Vinyl chloride
(K) Naphthalene
(L) Gamma rays

6. A 51-year-old male who works in a factory producing plastic pipe experiences weight loss, nausea, and vomiting. His serum alkaline phosphatase level is 405 U/L. An abdominal computed tomography (CT) scan reveals a 12-cm right liver lobe mass. Liver biopsy reveals an angiosarcoma. (   )

7. For years, grandfather sprayed the orchard each spring with insecticide. After 20 years, grandfather notices a rough, erythematous area of skin on his right shoulder that becomes ulcerated and does not heal. The excised lesion is a squamous cell carcinoma. (   )

8. A 30-year-old male presents with multiple benign subcutaneous tumors that are attached to nerves. Further examination reveals numerous pigmented skin lesions. Ophthalmoscopic examination shows hamartomatous nodules on the iris. Which of the following mechanisms of transformation is most likely related to the mutation that this patient inherited?

O (A) Persistent activation of the *ras* gene
O (B) Increased production of epidermal growth factor
O (C) Decreased susceptibility to apoptosis
O (D) Impaired functioning of mismatch repair genes
O (E) Inactivation of the *Rb* gene

9. The major mechanism by which repeated application of croton oil (phorbol ester), after a single application of a mutagenic agent on the skin, promotes carcinogenesis is

O (A) Induction of chromosome breaks
O (B) Inhibition of DNA repair
O (C) Activation of protein kinase C
O (D) Activation of endogenous viruses
O (E) Amplification of growth factor receptor genes

10. An isolated polyp is found by colonoscopy in the sigmoid colon of a 50-year-old female. The excised polyp histologically reveals well-differentiated glands with no invasion of the stalk. Which of the following investigational research procedures can *most clearly* distinguish whether the polyp represents hyperplasia of the colonic mucosa or a tubular adenoma?

O (A) Histochemical staining for mucin
O (B) Flow cytometry to determine the frequency of cells in the S phase (growth fraction)
O (C) Determination of clonality by pattern of X chromosome inactivation
O (D) Immunoperoxidase staining for keratin
O (E) Immunoperoxidase staining for factor VIII

11. A 66-year-old female, who has worked all of her life on a small family farm on the Kanto plain near Tokyo, has a peripheral white blood cell (WBC) count of 64,000/μL. Immunophenotyping reveals that 90% of these WBCs are T lymphocytes that are CD4 positive. She has had no previous major illnesses. Which of the following viral agents is most likely involved in this process?

O (A) HPV
O (B) Human immunodeficiency virus type 1 (HIV-1)

O (C) Epstein-Barr virus (EBV)
O (D) Human T-cell lymphotropic virus type I (HTLV-I)
O (E) HBV

12. A 50-year-old female presents with a mass in her right breast. Physical examination reveals a single mass 2 cm in diameter that is fixed to the underlying tissues and three lymph nodes are palpable in the axilla. There is no family history of cancer. Histologic examination of a breast biopsy showed a well-differentiated ductal carcinoma. Over the next 6 months, additional lymph nodes became enlarged, and metastases appeared in the lung, liver, and brain. The patient dies 9 months after diagnosis. Which of the following molecular abnormalities is most likely to be found in this setting?

O (A) Inactivation of one copy of the BRCA-1 gene in fibroblasts cultured from the normal skin
O (B) Deletion of one copy of the *p53* gene in all cells of the clinically normal parent
O (C) Amplification of the c-*erb B2* (HER2) gene in breast cancer cells
O (D) Deletion of the *Rb* locus in the normal somatic cells of the patient
O (E) Fusion of *bcr* and c-*abl* genes in the cancer cells

13. Two of five children in a family are affected by a disorder that results in the development of multiple skin cancers with sun exposure. The parents and other relatives are not affected. Which of the following mechanisms is most likely operative to produce neoplasia in these children?

O (A) HPV infection
O (B) Failure of nucleotide excision repair of DNA
O (C) Ingestion of food contaminated with *Aspergillus flavus*
O (D) Inactivation of *p53*
O (E) Chromosomal translocation

14. Which of the following conditions is *least* likely to give rise to a subsequent carcinoma in the affected tissues?

O (A) Macronodular cirrhosis
O (B) Chronic atrophic gastritis
O (C) Oral leukoplakia
O (D) Atypical endometrial hyperplasia
O (E) Multiple skin nevi

15. A child is born with a single functional copy of a tumor suppressor gene. At the age of 5 years, the remaining normal allele is lost through mutation. As a result, the ability to control the transition from G_1 to the S phase of cell cycle is lost. Which of the following neoplasms is most likely to arise by means of this mechanism?

O (A) Retinoblastoma
O (B) Breast carcinoma
O (C) Adenocarcinoma of colon
O (D) Cerebral astrocytoma
O (E) Chronic myeloid leukemia

16. A biopsy of an enlarged, nontender posterior cervical lymph node from a 66-year-old female reveals effacement

of the nodal architecture by a monomorphous population of large cells with large, dark blue nuclei and scant cytoplasm. The peripheral blood smear and bone marrow biopsy are normal. This process is most likely to be a

○ (A) Lymphangioma
○ (B) Reactive hyperplasia
○ (C) Lymphoma
○ (D) Myeloma
○ (E) Leukemia

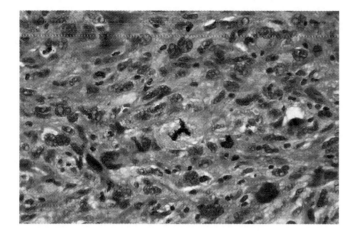

17. The high-power microscopic appearance of a neoplasm from a 58-year-old female is shown in the figure. All areas of the tumor have similar morphology. This neoplasm is best described as a(an)

○ (A) Adenoma
○ (B) Well-differentiated adenocarcinoma
○ (C) Squamous cell carcinoma
○ (D) Leiomyoma
○ (E) Anaplastic carcinoma

18. A 59-year-old male recently noticed some blood in his urine. A cystoscopy reveals a 4-cm exophytic mass involving the right bladder mucosa. A radical cystectomy is performed. Examination of the excised specimen shows that he has a grade IV transitional cell carcinoma that has infiltrated through the bladder wall. Which of the following statements regarding these findings is most appropriate?

○ (A) This neoplasm is a metastasis.
○ (B) He has a poorly differentiated neoplasm.
○ (C) A paraneoplastic syndrome is likely.
○ (D) The stage of this neoplasm is low.
○ (E) He is probably cured of his cancer.

19. Which of the following diagnostic screening techniques used in health care has had the greatest impact on reduction in cancer deaths in developed nations?

○ (A) Chest radiograph
○ (B) Stool guaiac
○ (C) Pap smear
○ (D) Serum carcinoembryonic antigen assay
○ (E) Urinalysis

20. A 46-year-old male is found to have an enlarged, nontender supraclavicular lymph node palpable on physical examination. The lymph node is excised and found to be 2 cm in diameter. Histologically, the nodal architecture is effaced by a monomorphous population of small lymphocytes. Which of the following procedures is best to confirm that he has a malignancy?

○ (A) Peripheral white blood cell count and differential cell count
○ (B) Flow cytometry of nodal tissue for DNA content
○ (C) Electron microscopy to determine cellular ultrastructure
○ (D) Southern blot analysis to demonstrate monoclonality
○ (E) Determination of the serum lactate dehydrogenase level

21. Which of the following principles of carcinogenesis is best illustrated by the study of molecular alterations that occur during the evolution of a sporadic colonic adenoma into an invasive carcinoma?

○ (A) Protooncogenes can be activated by chromosomal translocation.
○ (B) Malignant transformation involves accumulation of mutations in protooncogenes and tumor suppressor genes in a step-wise fashion.
○ (C) Extensive regeneration of tissues increases the risk of cancer-causing mutations.
○ (D) Inherited defects in DNA repair increase the susceptibility to the development of cancers.
○ (E) Overexpression of growth factor receptor genes is associated with poor prognosis.

For each of the patient histories in questions 22 through 26, match the most likely gene that is affected during the neoplastic process:

(A) p53 (DNA damage response gene)
(B) APC (tumor suppressor gene)
(C) IL-2 (growth factor gene)
(D) Lyn (tyrosine kinase gene)
(E) K-ras (GTP-binding protein gene)
(F) p16 (cyclin-dependent kinase inhibitor, INK4a)
(G) c-myc (transcription factor gene)
(H) bcl-2 (anti-apoptosis gene)
(I) EGF (epidermal growth factor gene)
(J) bcl-1 (cyclin gene)
(K) NF-1 (GPTase-activating protein)
(L) N-myc (transcription factor gene)
(M) BRCA-1 (DNA repair gene)
(N) hst-1 (fibroblast growth factor gene)
(O) c-erb B2 (growth factor receptor gene)

22. A patient is diagnosed with follicular lymphoma. Karyotypic analysis reveals a chromosomal translocation, t(14;18), involving the immunoglobulin heavy chain gene. (   )

23. A patient presents with cough and hemoptysis (i.e., blood in sputum). A lung biopsy reveals small cell lung carcinoma. Family history reveals three first-degree mater-

nal relatives who developed leukemia, sarcoma, and carcinoma before the age of 40. (   )

24. A 5-year-old child presents with an abdominal mass that is diagnosed as neuroblastoma. Cytogenetic analysis of tumor cells shows many double minutes and homogeneously staining regions. (   )

25. A 26-year-old female presents with carcinoma of the breast. Her 30-year-old sister was recently diagnosed with ovarian cancer, and her maternal aunt had a mastectomy 3 years earlier for ductal carcinoma of the breast. (   )

26. A 20-year-old male presents with a raised, irregular pigmented lesion on his forearm. Biopsy reveals a deeply infiltrating malignant melanoma. Family history reveals that his paternal uncle died of metastatic melanoma that spread to the liver after excision of a primary lesion on the foot. His grandfather required enucleation of the left eye because of a "dark brown" mass in the eyeball. (   )

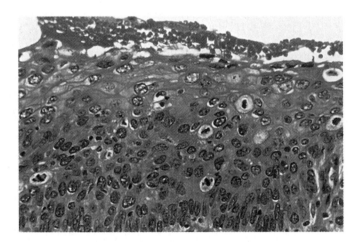

27. The medium-power magnification microscopic appearance of a lesion from a 39-year-old female is shown. She had an abnormal Pap smear, and a cervical biopsy of a 1-cm, red, slightly raised lesion on the anterior ectocervix at 2 o'clock was performed. Which of the following statements best characterizes her condition?

○ (A) A primary site should be sought.
○ (B) This is a high-grade lesion.
○ (C) The cell of origin is a fibroblast.
○ (D) A chest radiograph will show nodules.
○ (E) Local excision will be curative.

28. An immunoperoxidase stain for the protease cathepsin D is performed on the microscopic tissue section from a breast carcinoma in a 61-year-old female. There is pronounced cytoplasmic staining in the tumor cells. The presence of this marker is most likely to predict tumor:

○ (A) Angiogenesis
○ (B) Invasiveness
○ (C) Differentiation
○ (D) Heterogeneity
○ (E) Aneuploidy

29. A 22-year-old female works as a secretary for an accounting firm. She has a palpable nodule in the right lobe of her thyroid gland. A fine-needle aspirate of the nodule reveals cells consistent with a carcinoma of the thyroid. No other family members are affected by this disorder. Which of the following would you consider relevant in her past history?

○ (A) Chronic alcoholism
○ (B) Ataxia telangiectasia
○ (C) Radiation therapy in childhood
○ (D) Blunt trauma from a fall
○ (E) Exposure to arsenic compounds

30. A Pap smear reveals the presence of severe cervical dysplasia in a 35-year-old female. Which of the following viruses binds to pRb to increase the risk for this lesion?

○ (A) EBV
○ (B) HBV
○ (C) HIV
○ (D) Cytomegalovirus
○ (E) HPV

31. A 62-year-old male with a history of chronic alcoholism has an elevated serum α-fetoprotein level. There are no masses or lymphadenopathy palpable anywhere on physical examination. A stool guaiac test is negative. Which of the following neoplasms is most likely?

○ (A) Prostatic adenocarcinoma
○ (B) Pulmonary squamous cell carcinoma
○ (C) Multiple myeloma
○ (D) Pancreatic adenocarcinoma
○ (E) Hepatocellular carcinoma

32. A 49-year-old male has an episode of hemoptysis. A chest radiograph reveals a 5-cm right upper lobe lung mass. A fine-needle aspirate of this mass yields cells consistent with small cell anaplastic carcinoma. On careful examination, the patient is found to have puffiness of the face, some pedal edema, and systolic hypertension. A bone scan shows no metastases. Immunohistochemical staining of the tumor cells is likely to be positive for which of the following?

○ (A) Parathyroid hormone (PTH)–related protein
○ (B) Erythropoietin
○ (C) Corticotropin
○ (D) Insulin
○ (E) Gastrin

33. A routine checkup for a 40-year-old male included a stool guaiac test, which was positive. A sigmoidoscopy revealed a 1.5-cm, circumscribed, pedunculated mass on a short stalk located in the upper rectum. The best term for this lesion is

○ (A) Adenoma
○ (B) Hamartoma
○ (C) Sarcoma
○ (D) Choristoma
○ (E) Nevus

34. A 40-year-old male develops generalized lymph node enlargement and hepatosplenomegaly. Lymph node biopsy reveals a malignant tumor of lymphoid cells. Immunoperoxidase staining of the tumor cells with antibody to *bcl-2* is positive in the lymphocytic cell nuclei. By which of the following mechanisms has this lymphoma occurred?

○ (A) Increased tyrosine kinase activity
○ (B) Lack of apoptosis
○ (C) Gene amplifications
○ (D) Reduced DNA repair
○ (E) Loss of cell cycle inhibition

35. A 70-year-old female had a 4-month history of weight loss and increasing generalized icterus. An abdominal CT scan revealed a mass in the head of the pancreas. Molecular analysis revealed that the neoplastic cells showed continued activation of cytoplasmic kinases because a mutation greatly reduced the ability to hydrolyze GTP after growth factor stimulation. Which of the following oncogenes is most likely to be involved in this process?

○ (A) *myc*
○ (B) *abl*
○ (C) *ras*
○ (D) *neu*
○ (E) *sis*

For each of the patient histories in questions 36 through 38, match the most closely associated lettered neoplasm:

(A) Adenocarcinoma
(B) Adenoma
(C) Carcinoma in situ
(D) Fibroadenoma
(E) Fibroma
(F) Glioma
(G) Hamartoma
(H) Hemangioma
(I) Hepatocellular carcinoma
(J) Leiomyoma
(K) Lipoma
(L) Lymphoma
(M) Melanoma
(N) Meningioma
(O) Mesothelioma
(P) Nevus
(Q) Osteosarcoma
(R) Renal cell carcinoma
(S) Rhabdomyosarcoma
(T) Small cell anaplastic carcinoma
(U) Teratoma

36. A 23-year-old female has a 0.5-cm-diameter, nontender, raised nodule on the skin of her upper chest. This nodule has a smooth surface and is dark red. She states that the nodule has been present for many years and has not changed in size. (   )

37. A 29-year-old female has a cervical biopsy after a Pap smear that is abnormal. She is asymptomatic. She has a history of multiple sexual partners. The microscopic appearance of the biopsy is shown in the figure. (   )

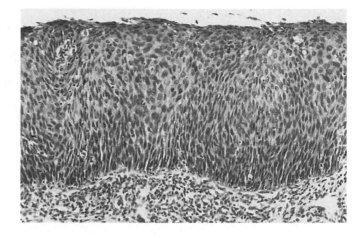

38. A 32-year-old female has had some dull pelvic pain for the last 2 months. An abdominal ultrasound reveals a mass involving the right ovary that is 8 cm in diameter. The mass is surgically excised. The surface of the mass is smooth, and it is not adherent to surrounding pelvic structures. Grossly, the mass is seen to be cystic and filled with hair. Microscopically, there is squamous epithelium, tall columnar glandular epithelium, cartilage, and fibrous connective tissue. (   )

39. A patient with malignant melanoma is treated by infusion of autologous CD8+ T cells that are known to kill his melanoma cells but not normal cells. The target antigen recognized by these CD8+ T cells is most likely composed of

○ (A) Class I major histocompatibility complex (MHC) molecules plus a peptide produced by normal melanocytes and melanoma cells
○ (B) Class I MHC molecules plus a peptide derived from carcinoembryonic antigen
○ (C) Class II MHC molecules plus a peptide derived from melanoma cells
○ (D) Class I MHC molecules plus a peptide produced by melanoma cells
○ (E) A peptide secreted by melanoma cells and presented by laminin receptors on melanoma cells

40. Several episodes of hematuria in the previous week were noticed by a 62-year-old male. His urologist performed a cystoscopy and observed a 4-cm sessile mass with a nodular, ulcerated surface in the dome of the bladder. How would you best describe this lesion?

○ (A) Papilloma
○ (B) Carcinoma
○ (C) Adenoma
○ (D) Sarcoma
○ (E) Fibroma

41. A 66-year-old male with chronic cough and recent hemoptysis has a chest radiograph that shows a 6-cm right lung mass. A sputum cytologic analysis reveals cells consistent with squamous cell carcinoma. Where are metastases from this neoplasm most likely to be found?

○ (A) Chest wall muscle
○ (B) Splenic red pulp
○ (C) Hilar lymph nodes
○ (D) Vertebral bone marrow
○ (E) Cerebrum

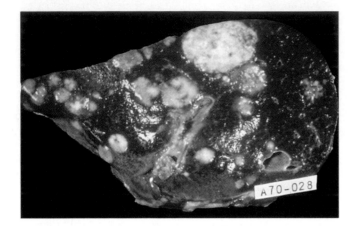

42. The liver at autopsy of a 69-year-old female is shown. Which of the following statements best characterizes this process?

○ (A) A liver biopsy would have shown a dysplasia.
○ (B) This is a multifocal hepatic adenoma.
○ (C) A hepatocellular carcinoma has invaded locally.
○ (D) Colonic adenocarcinoma with metastases was present.
○ (E) Resection of these lesions should have been done.

43. A surgeon is performing a partial colectomy on a 75-year-old female who has a 5-cm sessile mass in the lower sigmoid colon. Which of the following techniques performed during surgery best aids the surgeon in determining whether the resection is adequate to reduce the probability of a recurrence?

○ (A) Fine-needle aspiration
○ (B) Serum carcinoembryonic antigen assay
○ (C) Frozen section
○ (D) Electron microscopy
○ (E) Flow cytometry

44. A 12-cm mass is found in the uterine wall of a 60-year-old female who has smoked cigarettes for most of her life. This mass on removal has the microscopic appearance of a well-differentiated leiomyosarcoma. A year later, a chest radiograph reveals a 4-cm right lower lung nodule. A biopsy of a lung nodule reveals a poorly differentiated sarcoma. These findings are best explained by

○ (A) Development of a second primary neoplasm
○ (B) Inheritance of a defective *Rb* gene
○ (C) Continued smoking by the patient
○ (D) Loss of an oncogene
○ (E) Metastasis from an aggressive subclone of the primary tumor

45. If you were Sir Percival Pott, signing the death certificate for Bert the chimney sweep in London more than 200 years ago, what would be the most likely underlying cause of death?

○ (A) Kaposi sarcoma of the leg
○ (B) Infiltrating ductal carcinoma of breast
○ (C) Adenocarcinoma of the lung
○ (D) Squamous cell carcinoma of scrotum
○ (E) Osteosarcoma of the tibia

46. Which of the following principles of carcinogenesis is *best illustrated* by the study of humans with hereditary nonpolyposis colon cancer (HNPCC)?

○ (A) Tumor initiators are mutagenic.
○ (B) Tumor promoters induce proliferation.
○ (C) Many oncogenes are activated by translocations.
○ (D) Inability to repair DNA predisposes to development of cancer.
○ (E) Carcinogenesis is a multistep process.

47. A 38-year-old female presents with abdominal distention, and a CT scan demonstrates bowel obstruction with a 6-cm mass in the jejunum. A Burkitt lymphoma of the small bowel is resected, and a portion of the tumor sent for flow cytometry analysis shows a high S phase. Mutational activation of which of the following nuclear oncogenes is likely to be present in this tumor?

○ (A) *c-erb B2*
○ (B) *p53*
○ (C) *ras*
○ (D) *myc*
○ (E) APC

48. In taking a history, you record your 40-year-old female's previously diagnosed medical conditions. Although she currently is asymptomatic, which of the following pre-existing conditions is most likely to increase her risk for cancer?

○ (A) Fibroadenoma of the breast
○ (B) Bronchial asthma
○ (C) Degenerative osteoarthritis
○ (D) Chronic ulcerative colitis
○ (E) Leiomyomas of the uterus

49. A 33-year-old female has a routine physical examination. There are no abnormal findings. As part of the pelvic examination, a Pap smear is obtained. Cytologically, the cells obtained on the smear from the cervix demonstrate severe epithelial dysplasia. What would you advise this patient regarding the Pap smear diagnosis?

○ (A) This lesion could progress to invasive cervical carcinoma.
○ (B) An ovarian teratoma is present.
○ (C) There has been regression of a cervical carcinoma.
○ (D) Antibiotic therapy will cure the lesion.
○ (E) Your female relatives are at risk for the same problem.

50. A change in bowel habits prompted a 53-year-old female to see her physician, who found that she has a positive test result for stool guaiac. A colonoscopy revealed a 3-cm sessile mass in the cecum. A biopsy of this mass

demonstrated a moderately differentiated adenocarcinoma that was confined to the mucosa. How should a surgeon deal with this information?

- (A) Perform a limited excision to "shell out" the lesion from its surrounding capsule
- (B) Assume that this represents a metastasis and search for a primary elsewhere
- (C) Resect the tumor and some of the normal surrounding tissue
- (D) Remove the entire colon to prevent a recurrence
- (E) Observe the lesion for further increase in size

51. An 18-year-old boy has had multiple basal cell and squamous cell carcinomas of his sun-exposed skin on the trunk and extremities. He also has a sister who is similarly affected. This disease is most likely to be the result of defective genes that

- (A) Control apoptosis
- (B) Regulate repair of damaged DNA
- (C) Encode transcription factors
- (D) Inhibit the cell cycle
- (E) Regulate secretion of growth factors

52. A family history of colon cancer is elicited from a 36-year-old male. Based on this history, a screening colonoscopy is performed, and the ascending colon is found to contain five polyps from 0.5 to 2 cm in diameter. They are excised and examined microscopically. The 2-cm polyp is found to have a focus of adenocarcinoma. Inheritance of which of the following types of genes is most likely to be involved in the causation of this tumor?

- (A) Growth factor receptors
- (B) Growth factors
- (C) DNA mismatch repair
- (D) Cyclins
- (E) Inhibitors of apoptosis

53. A 56-year-old female has a granulosa-theca cell tumor of the left ovary producing excessive estrogen. She also has an endometrial carcinoma. The coexistence of these tumors is an example of

- (A) Promotion of carcinogenesis
- (B) Tumor heterogeneity
- (C) A paraneoplastic syndrome
- (D) Genetic susceptibility to tumorigenesis
- (E) Mutation of a tumor suppressor gene

54. A 67-year-old male has had a chronic cough for several months. A chest radiograph reveals a right lung mass, and a fine-needle aspirate of the mass shows cells consistent with squamous cell carcinoma. If staging of this neoplasm is denoted as T2 N1 M1, which of the following statements is most accurate?

- (A) A head CT scan shows a 2-cm right parietal mass.
- (B) Serum chemistry reveals an elevated corticotropin level.
- (C) The mass had infiltrated the chest wall.
- (D) This cancer is poorly differentiated.
- (E) The tumor is obstructing the left mainstem bronchus.

55. A 33-year-old male has had occasional headaches for the past 3 months. He suddenly has a generalized seizure. A head CT scan reveals a periventricular 3-cm mass in the region of the right thalamus. A stereotactic biopsy of the mass yields cells diagnostic for a B-cell malignant lymphoma. Which of the following underlying diseases is he most likely to have?

- (A) Diabetes mellitus
- (B) Acquired immunodeficiency syndrome (AIDS)
- (C) Hypertension
- (D) Multiple sclerosis
- (E) Tuberculosis

56. A serum chemistry panel on a 76-year-old male reveals an alkaline phosphatase level of 290 U/L with no other abnormalities identified. After a serum prostate-specific antigen level is found to be elevated, he has a prostate needle biopsy that reveals a moderately differentiated adenocarcinoma. Which of the following mechanisms best accounts for these findings?

- (A) Tumor extension to rectum
- (B) Paraneoplastic syndrome
- (C) High tumor grade
- (D) Metastases to vertebrae
- (E) Tumor angiogenesis

For each of the statements in questions 57 and 58, match the most closely associated lettered malignancy:

- (A) Angiosarcoma of liver
- (B) Breast carcinoma
- (C) Bronchogenic carcinoma
- (D) Cervical squamous cell carcinoma
- (E) Colonic adenocarcinoma
- (F) Gastric adenocarcinoma
- (G) Glioma of brain
- (H) Leukemia
- (I) Lymphoma of lymph nodes
- (J) Melanoma of the skin
- (K) Pancreatic adenocarcinoma
- (L) Prostatic adenocarcinoma

57. In the last half of the 20th century, the number of deaths from this cancer increased markedly in developed nations. In 1998, more than 30% of male cancer deaths and more than 24% of female cancer deaths were caused by this neoplasm. (   )

58. The incidence of this neoplasm has been decreasing in developed nations in the latter half of the 20th century, despite the absence of widespread screening programs. (   )

59. A 1.2-cm, darkly pigmented skin lesion is excised from the dorsum of the right hand of a 42-year-old male, who notices that the lesion had become larger during the previous month. Microscopically, a malignant melanoma is present. Which of the following factors presents the greatest risk for development of this neoplasm?

- (A) Smoking
- (B) Ultraviolet radiation
- (C) Chemotherapy

○ (D) Asbestos exposure
○ (E) Allergy to latex

ANSWERS

1. **(C)** Although the HBV and HCV genomes do not encode for any transforming proteins, the regenerating hepatocytes are more likely to develop mutations such as inactivation of *p53*. HBV does not have a consistent site of integration in the liver cell nuclei, nor does it contain viral oncogenes. Many DNA viruses, such as HPV, inactivate tumor suppressor genes, but there is no convincing evidence that HBV or HCV can bind to *p53* or *Rb* proteins.
BP6 167   PBD6 313-314

2. **(A)** Several pathologic mechanisms play a role in development of tumor metastases. The tumor cells must first become discohesive and detach from the primary site and then attach elsewhere to become metastases. Tumor cells tend to have many more laminin receptors than normal cells, allowing them to more readily attach to basement membranes at distant sites. A reduction in apoptosis allows greater proliferation but not necessarily metastases. Monoclonality is a feature of neoplasia, but further tumor heterogeneity helps increase the chance for metastases to occur. Inflammation probably does not play a major role in metastasis. Keratin is a marker of epithelial differentiation, not metastatic ability.
BP6 161-162   PBD6 302-304

3. **(D)** The oncogenic potential of HPV, a sexually transmissible agent, is related to products of two early viral genes—E6 and E7. E7 binds to *Rb* protein to cause displacement of normally sequestered transcription factors. This nullifies tumor suppressor activity of the *Rb* protein. E6 binds to and inactivates the *p53* gene product. Trapping of GTP-bound ras protein can occur in many tumors but is not related to HPV infection. Laminin receptor expression correlates with metastatic potential of a malignant neoplasm. Increased epidermal growth factor (EGF) receptor expression is a feature seen in many pulmonary squamous cell carcinomas, and the related c-*erb* B2 (HER2) receptor is seen in some breast carcinomas.
BP6 167   PBD6 311

4. **(E)** This is the Philadelphia chromosome of chronic myelogenous leukemia. The t(9;22) causes c-*abl* on chromosome 9 to fuse with *bcr* on chromosome 22. Both *p53* and *Rb* are tumor suppressor genes, and loss of both alleles is needed to promote cell proliferation. The NF-1 gene is a signal transducer seen in schwannomas. The *ras* oncogenes are involved with GTP binding and become activated from point mutations.
BP6 150-151   PBD6 285-286

5. **(A)** Lymphatic spread, especially to regional lymph nodes draining from the primary site, is typical for a carcinoma. Infection from a breast abscess can spread to the lymph nodes, but the resulting nodal enlargement is typically associated with pain—a cardinal sign of acute inflammation. Sarcomas uncommonly metastasize to lymph nodes. Central nervous system (CNS) malignancies rarely metastasize outside of the CNS. Dysplasias do not metastasize, because they are not malignancies.
BP6 139-142   PBD6 269-272

6. **(J)** Vinyl chloride is a rare cause of liver cancer. However, this causal relationship was easy to demonstrate, because hepatic angiosarcoma is a rare neoplasm.
BP6 144   PBD6

7. **(A)** Arsenic can cause skin cancer. However, lead arsenate has not been in widespread use for years, and occupational safety measures have reduced risks to workers from use of chemicals in agriculture and industry.
BP6 144   PBD6 274, 309

8. **(A)** This patient has clinical features of neurofibromatosis type 1. The NF-1 gene encodes a GTPase-activating protein that facilitates the conversion of active (GTP-bound) *ras* to inactive (GDP-bound) *ras*. Loss of NF-1 prevents such conversion and traps *ras* in the active signal-transmitting stage. All other genes are also involved in carcinogenesis, although in different tumors.
BP6 153   PBD6 293a

9. **(C)** Phorbol esters cause tumor promotion by activating protein kinase C. This enzyme phosphorylates several substrates in signal transduction pathways, including those activated by growth factors, and the cells divide. Forced cell division predisposes the accumulation of mutations in cells previously damaged by exposure to a mutagenic agent (i.e., initiator).
BP6 165   PBD6 309

10. **(C)** A true neoplasm is a monoclonal proliferation of cells, whereas a reactive proliferation of cells is not monoclonal. Reactive and neoplastic cellular proliferations may have similar histochemical and immunohistochemical staining patterns based on the type of cells that are present. Flow cytometry is good at indicating the DNA content, aneuploidy, and growth fraction but does not indicate clonality.
BP6 145-146   PBD6 277

11. **(D)** She has a T-cell leukemia, which develops in approximately 1% of persons infected with HTLV-I. HPV is best known for causing squamous epithelial dysplasias and carcinomas. HIV-1 infection is the cause for AIDS. EBV infection is associated with a variety of cancers, including Burkitt lymphoma and nasopharyngeal carcinoma. HBV infection may result in hepatic cirrhosis, in which hepatocellular carcinoma may arise.
BP6 166   PBD6 314

12. **(C)** Increased expression of c-*erb* B2 (HER-2) can be detected immunohistochemically in the biopsy specimen. Up to a third of breast cancers may demonstrate this change. Such amplification is associated with a poorer prognosis. Detection of a specific gene product in the tis-

sue has value for determination of prognosis. BRCA-1 and *p53* mutations, if inherited in the germ line, can predispose to breast cancer and other tumors. However, with BRCA-1 there is family history of breast cancer, and *p53* mutation predisposes to many types of cancers. An inherited deletion of *Rb* gene predisposes to retinoblastoma. The *bcr-c-abl* fusion product is seen in chronic myeloid leukemia. It results from t(9;22).
BP6 151 PBD6 286

13. **(B)** These children have the autosomal recessive condition known as xeroderma pigmentosum (XP). Affected persons have extreme photosensitivity, with a 2000-fold increase in the risk for skin cancers. The DNA damage is initiated by exposure to ultraviolet light, but nucleotide excision repair cannot occur normally in XP. HPV is a sexually transmitted agent that is associated with development of genital squamous cell carcinomas. The *Aspergillus flavus* on moldy peanuts and other foods produces the potent hepatic carcinogen aflatoxin B1. Inactivation of the *p53* tumor suppressor gene is found in many sporadic human cancers and in some familial cancers, but the cancers are not limited to the skin. Chromosomal translocations are often involved in development of hematologic malignancies, although not often in skin cancers.
BP6 165 PBD6 310

14. **(E)** There are preneoplastic conditions from which cancers are more likely to arise. Macronodular cirrhosis from hepatitis B infection can give rise to hepatocellular carcinoma. Gastric adenocarcinoma can arise in chronic atrophic gastritis. Oral squamous carcinomas arise in oral leukoplakia, and atypical hyperplasias of endometrium give rise to endometrial adenocarcinomas. It is a good thing that skin malignancies do not tend to arise from nevi, because many people have nevi.
BP6 144 PBD6 276

15. **(A)** The *Rb* gene is the classic example of the two-hit mechanism for loss of tumor suppression. About 60% of these tumors are sporadic. Others are familial, and there is inheritance of a mutated copy of the *Rb* gene. Loss of the second copy in retinoblasts leads to the occurrence of retinoblastoma in childhood. Why patients who inherit a mutant *Rb* gene through the germ line develop retinoblastoma and not most other tumors is unknown. The *Rb* gene controls the G_1 to S transition of the cell cycle; with loss of both copies, this important checkpoint in the cell cycle is lost.
BP6 151-154 PBD6 289-290

16. **(C)** Lymphomas are malignant neoplasms of lymphoid tissues. They have no benign equivalent. Monomorphous proliferations that destroy the nodal architecture suggest a neoplasm. A lymphangioma is composed mostly of a proliferation of lymphatics. A myeloma is composed of plasma cells and most often involves bone marrow. A leukemia is a neoplasm that arises in the bone marrow and spills over into peripheral blood.
BP6 135 PBD6 263

17. **(E)** These cells demonstrate marked pleomorphism and hyperchromatism (i.e., anaplasia). A bizarre tripolar mitotic figure is present. This degree of anaplasia is consistent with a malignancy. An adenoma is a benign tumor of glandular origin. Adenocarcinomas and squamous cell carcinomas show differentiation into glandular or squamous tissues. Leiomyomas are benign mesenchymal tumors of smooth muscle origin.
BP6 135-137 PBD6 264-266

18. **(B)** Cancer grading systems are typically denoted by I to III or I to IV, increasing with worse differentiation (i.e., more anaplasia). A transitional cell carcinoma would be expected at this site. Bladder cancers are not commonly associated with paraneoplastic syndromes. Infiltration through the wall makes the stage high. This high-grade, high-stage cancer has a poor cure rate.
BP6 171 PBD6 321-322

19. **(C)** Because Pap smear screening can detect dysplasias and in situ carcinomas that can be treated before progression to invasive lesions, deaths from cervical carcinoma have steadily decreased in the last half of the twentieth century. A chest radiograph is an insensitive technique for finding early lung cancers. Use of stool guaiac has not affected rates of death from colorectal carcinomas that much, but do not put "rectal deferred" on your physical examination report, or you will contribute to the problem. Serum tumor markers have not proved useful as general screening techniques, although they are useful in selected circumstances. Urine cytology is better than urinalysis for detection of urothelial malignancies but does not have a high sensitivity.
BP6 142 PBD6 272

20. **(D)** Monoclonality is the hallmark of a malignancy. In the diagnosis of a leukemia, WBC count is helpful but not definitive. The DNA content analysis alone cannot define a malignancy; Southern blot analysis for T- or B-cell receptor gene rearrangements can define monoclonality. Electron microscopy is an adjunct to diagnosis of the type of tumor. Lactate dehydrogenase levels are often increased with lymphoid proliferations but are not diagnostic of the type of proliferation.
BP6 171-174 PBD6 322-325

21. **(B)** Development of colonic adenocarcinoma typically takes years, during which time a number of mutations occur within the mucosa, including mutations involving such genes as APC (adenomatous polyposis coli), hMSH2 (human mismatch repair), K-*ras,* DCC (deleted in colon cancer), and *p53.* The accumulation of mutations, rather than their occurrence in a specific order, is most important for the development of a carcinoma. Activation of protooncogenes, extensive regeneration, faulty DNA repair genes, and amplification of growth factor receptor genes all contribute to the development of malignancies but are not sufficient by themselves to produce a carcinoma from a colonic adenoma.
BP6 157, 509 PBD6 296-297, 832

22. **(G)** This is an example of chromosomal translocation that brings a protooncogene (c-*myc*) close to another gene (immunoglobulin heavy chain gene). The c-*myc* gene be-

comes subject to continuous stimulation by the adjacent enhancer element of the immunoglobulin gene, leading to c-*myc* overexpression.
BP6 150 PBD6 285

23. (A) *p53* is the most common target for genetic alterations in human tumors. Most of these are sporadic mutations, although some are inherited. The inheritance of one faulty *p53* suppressor gene predisposes to a "second hit" that knocks out the remaining *p53* gene. Homozygous loss of the *p53* genes dysregulates the repair of damaged DNA, predisposing individuals to multiple tumors, as in this case.
BP6 153-154 PBD6 290-292

24. (L) Double minutes and homogeneously staining regions seen on a karyotype represent gene amplifications. Amplification of the N-*myc* gene occurs in 30% to 40% of neuroblastomas, and this change is associated with a poor prognosis.
BP6 151 PBD6 286

25. (M) Approximately 5% to 10% of breast cancers are familial, and 80% of these result from mutations in the BRCA-1 and BRCA-2 genes. The onset of these familial cancers is earlier in life than the sporadic cancers. The protein products of these genes are involved in DNA repair.
BP6 153, 156, 630 PBD6 292, 1106

26. (F) This patient has a family history of malignant melanoma. Familial tumors are often associated with inheritance of a defective copy of one of several tumor suppressor genes. In the case of melanomas, the implicated gene is called *p16,* or INK4a. The product of the *p16* gene is an inhibitor of cyclin-dependent kinases. With loss of control over cyclin-dependent kinases, the cell cycle cannot be regulated, and neoplastic transformation is favored.
PBD6 920

27. (E) This is an in situ carcinoma of the squamous cervical epithelium, with neoplastic growth above the basement membrane. Such cancers, limited to the epithelium, are noninvasive, and local excision has a virtual 100% cure rate. In situ lesions do not give rise to metastases. Lesions limited to the epithelium are low grade. Because of its origin in the epithelium, this neoplasm is not derived from fibroblasts.
BP6 136-138 PBP6 265-268

28. (B) The elaboration of a variety of enzymes by tumor cells aids in degradation of extracellular matrix and invasiveness. Cathepsin D is a cysteine proteinase that cleaves a variety of substrates such as fibronectin and laminin. High levels of this enzyme in tumor cells are associated with greater invasiveness. Angiogenesis is mediated mainly by basic fibroblast growth factor and vascular endothelial cell growth factor. Differentiation, aneuploidy, and heterogeneity are regulated by protooncogenes and tumor suppressor genes.
BP6 162 PBD6 303-304

29. (C) Radiation is oncogenic. Cancers of thyroid and bone often develop following radiation exposure. Leukemias can occur as well. Hepatocellular carcinomas can arise in cirrhosis from chronic alcoholism. Ataxia telangiectasia is an inherited syndrome that carries an increased risk for development of leukemias and lymphomas. Trauma is not a risk for cancer, but everyone remembers traumatic episodes and makes an association with them and subsequent health problems. Arsenic exposure is uncommon, and it leads to lung and skin cancers.
BP6 165 PBD6 310

30. (E) HPV types 16, 18, and 31 encode proteins that bind pRb with high affinity, resulting in loss of tumor suppressor activity. Seventy-five to nearly 100% of squamous epithelial dysplasias and carcinomas of the cervix are associated with HPV infection. EBV is associated with some malignant lymphomas and nasopharyngeal carcinomas. HBV is associated with hepatocellular carcinomas arising in the setting of regeneration in chronic liver injury. HIV does not affect pRb, but the loss of immune regulation promotes development of lymphomas and Kaposi sarcoma. Cytomegalovirus does not participate directly in carcinogenesis.
BP6 167 PBD6 311

31. (E) Alpha-fetoprotein (AFP) is a tumor marker for hepatocellular carcinomas and some testicular carcinomas. The serum prostate-specific antigen is a helpful marker for prostate adenocarcinoma. Squamous cell carcinomas of any site do not have good specific tumor markers. A serum immunoglobulin level with protein electrophoresis helps to diagnosis myeloma. Gastrointestinal tract adenocarcinomas may be accompanied by elevations in the serum carcinoembryonic antigen.
BP6 173-174 PBD6 325

32. (C) He has Cushing syndrome from ectopic corticotropin production by the tumor, a form of paraneoplastic syndrome common to small cell carcinomas of the lung. Hypercalcemia from a PTH-related protein is more typically associated with pulmonary squamous cell carcinomas. Erythropoietin production with polycythemia is more likely to be associated with a renal cell carcinoma. Insulin and gastrin production are most often seen with islet cell tumors of the pancreas.
BP6 171 PBD6 320-321

33. (A) A discrete small mass such as this is probably benign. Adenomas arise from epithelial surfaces. A hamartoma is rare and is a benign mass composed of tissues usually found at the site of origin. A sarcoma is a malignant neoplasm arising in mesenchymal tissues. A choristoma is a benign mass composed of tissues not found at the site of origin. A nevus arises in the skin.
BP6 133-134 PBD6 261-262

34. (B) Overexpression of the *bcl-2* gene prevents apoptosis, allowing accumulation of cells in lymphoid tissues. Increased tyrosine kinase activity results from mutations

affecting the *abl* oncogene. Gene amplifications are typically seen to affect the c-*erb B2* and *myc* oncogenes. Reduced DNA repair occurs in the inherited disorder xeroderma pigmentosa. Loss of cell cycle inhibition results from loss of tumor suppressor genes such as *p53*.
BP6 154–155   PBD6 294–295

35. **(C)** The *ras* oncogene is the most common oncogene involved in development of human cancers. Mutations of the *ras* oncogene reduce GTPase activity, and *ras* is trapped in an activated GTP-bound state. It then signals the nucleus through cytoplasmic kinases. The *myc* oncogene is a transcriptional activator that is overexpressed in many tumors. Mutations of the *abl* oncogene cause greatly increased tyrosine kinase activity, but this is not related to the hydrolysis of GTP. The *neu* oncogene encodes growth factor receptors that are amplified in certain tumors. The *sis* oncogene encodes platelet-derived growth factor receptor-β, which is overexpressed in certain astrocytomas.
BP6 147–148   PBD6 279–281

36. **(H)** The small, discrete nature of this mass and the fact that it has changed little suggests a benign neoplasm. The red color suggests vascularity. A hemangioma is a common benign lesion of the skin.
BP6 135 BPD6 263

37. **(C)** Notice that the disorderly, atypical epithelial cells involve the entire thickness of the epithelium but that the underlying basement membrane is intact, with no invasion. Carcinoma in situ is confined to the epithelium; if the basement membrane is breached, the lesion is no longer in situ but rather invasive.
BP6 137   PBD6 267

38. **(U)** A teratoma is a neoplasm derived from totipotential germ cells that differentiate into tissues that represent all three germ layers—ectoderm, endoderm, and mesoderm. When the elements are all well differentiated, the neoplasm is "mature" (i.e., benign).
BP6 135   PBD6 263–264

39. **(D)** CD8+ T cells recognize peptides presented by MHC class I antigens. In many tumors, especially melanomas, the tumor cells produce peptides that can be presented by MHC class I molecules. If such peptides are not produced by other cells, the CD8+ T cells specific for such peptides lyse melanoma cells but not normal melanocytes or other normal cells.
BP6 168   PBD6 315–317

40. **(B)** Such a large, irregular, ulcerated mass is most likely malignant, and the epithelium of the bladder gives rise to carcinomas. A papilloma is a benign, localized mass that has an exophytic growth pattern. An adenoma is a benign epithelial neoplasm of glandular tissues. A sarcoma is derived from cells of mesenchymal origin; sarcomas are much less common than carcinomas. A fibroma is a benign mesenchymal neoplasm.
BP6 133–134   PBD6 261–262

41. **(C)** Carcinomas like to metastasize through lymphatics most often, usually to regional nodes first. However, hematogenous metastases are always possible. About one half of all cerebral metastases come from lung. Soft tissue metastases are rare, as are splenic metastases.
BP6 140, 162   PBD6 269–270, 305

42. **(D)** This is the appearance of metastatic lesions from a malignant neoplasm, with multiple tumor masses present. Dysplastic lesions do not produce large masses. Although some benign tumors such as leiomyomas of the uterus can be multiple, this is not the rule in liver, and hepatic adenomas are rare. Though hepatocellular carcinomas can have "satellite" nodules, widespread nodules such as those seen here are more characteristic of metastases. Resection of multiple metastases is usually fruitless.
BP6 139–140   PBD6 268

43. **(C)** The rapid frozen section of resection margins helps determine whether enough colon has been resected. Fine-needle aspiration is used for preoperative diagnosis. Serum tumor markers may aid in preoperative diagnosis or postoperative follow-up of neoplasms. Electron microscopy takes at least a day to perform and helps determine the cell type. Flow cytometry can be done in several hours but is useful mainly for prognostic information and is not a "stat" procedure.
BP6 171–173   PBD6 322–325

44. **(E)** Although neoplasms begin their careers as monoclonal proliferations, additional mutations occur over time, leading to subclones of neoplastic cells with various properties. This may allow metastases, greater invasiveness, resistance to chemotherapy, and morphologic differences to occur over time. Because sarcomas are rare in the lung, the lung mass is statistically a metastasis. Inheritance of a mutant *Rb* gene is most likely to lead to childhood retinoblastomas. Pulmonary sarcomas are not related to smoking. Loss of tumor suppressor genes, not oncogenes, is related to tumor development.
BP6 160   PBD6 320

45. **(D)** Squamous cell carcinomas of the scrotal skin in chimney sweeps was the first documentation of an occupational risk for cancer. Endemic Kaposi sarcoma is rare, and epidemic Kaposi sarcoma was not seen with any frequency until AIDS became widespread in the late twentieth century. Breast cancers are rare in men. The great increase in lung cancer was not seen until the rise in popularity of cigarette smoking in the twentieth century. Many adenocarcinomas of lung are not related to smoking. Osteosarcomas may occur at sites of bone subjected to previous irradiation.
BP6 163   PBD6 306

46. **(D)** Patients with hereditary nonpolyposis colon carcinoma (HNPCC) inherit one defective copy of mismatch repair genes. Any of several human mismatch repair genes are involved in the development of HNPCC. Mutations in mismatch repair genes can be detected by the presence of microsatellite instability.
BP6 508   PBD6 295–296,831–833

47. **(D)** The *myc* oncogene is commonly activated in Burkitt lymphoma because of a t(8;14) translocation. The *myc* gene binds DNA to cause transcriptional activation of growth-related genes such as that for cyclin D1, resulting in activation of the cell cycle. *p53* and APC are tumor suppressor genes that are inactivated in many cancers, including colon cancer (APC). *ras* oncogene encodes a GTP-binding protein that is located under the cell membrane. c-*erb* B2 (also known as HER2) encodes growth factor receptor located on the cell surface.
BP6 149   PBD6 282

48. **(D)** There is an increased risk for colorectal carcinoma with ulcerative colitis. Benign neoplasms, even if multiple, do not tend to become malignant. Asthma is a sporadic condition without a significant risk for cancer. Degenerative changes with aging are not a risk for cancer, although the risk for cancer increases with aging because of other factors.
BP6 144–145   PBD6 276

49. **(A)** Epithelial dysplasias, especially those that are severe, can be the precursors of carcinomas, and this is a key reason for Pap smear screening. The incidence of cervical carcinoma decreases when routine Pap smears are performed. Teratomas show well-differentiated elements derived from all the germ cell layers, and they do not manifest as epithelial dysplasias. Severe dysplasias are not amenable to antibiotic therapy. Cervical dysplasias are not hereditary.
BP6 137   PBD6 266

50. **(C)** A malignant neoplasm has a tendency to invade locally. A benign neoplasm is often well circumscribed, although a true capsule is uncommon, and compressed normal surrounding tissue appears to form a discrete border. Such a solitary mucosal lesion is unlikely to represent a metastasis, and the localized lesion is easily resected. Without a family history, a familial cancer with high recurrence risk from multiple polyps is unlikely, and local excision is adequate. Because the lesion is definitely malignant, it must be removed before it increases in size and invades locally or spreads elsewhere.
BP6 138–139   PBD6 267–268

51. **(B)** The condition in this family is xeroderma pigmentosum, an autosomal recessive disorder. Minor damage from sun exposure is not repaired, resulting in mutations that lead to development of skin cancers. Protooncogenes that regulate transcription or encode growth factors or their receptors are associated with other cancers, as are genes that regulate the cell cycle.
BP6 145   PBD6 275–277

52. **(C)** He has HNPCC, which is distinguished from the classic familial polyposis with hundreds of polyps that appear in childhood. HNPCC arises from inheritance of faulty DNA mismatch repair genes.
BP6 156–157   PBD6 295–296

53. **(A)** Estrogen, like many other hormones and drugs, is not by itself carcinogenic, but it is responsible for stimu-

lation of endometrial growth (i.e., hyperplasia), which has a promoting effect when mutations occur to produce carcinoma. Tumor heterogeneity does not refer to two separate kinds of neoplasms; it refers to heterogeneity with a given tumor or metastasis. A paraneoplastic syndrome results from ectopic secretion of a hormone by tumor (e.g., lung cancer cells producing corticotropin). Inherited susceptibility can never be completely excluded when a person has two tumors. This, for example, can occur in patients with inherited mutations in the *p53* gene. However, in this case, there is a clear hormonal basis for the second tumor. Faulty tumor suppressor genes are not involved in hormonal promotion of a neoplasm.
BP6 164–165   PBD6 308

54. **(A)** The M1 designation indicates that distant metastases are present. Elevated corticotropin levels indicate secretion of an ectopic hormone that may produce a paraneoplastic syndrome. A T1 designation means that the overall size of the tumor is not large. The TNM system is used for staging, not grading.
BP6 171   PBD6 321–322

55. **(B)** Primary or secondary immunodeficiency diseases carry an increased risk for neoplasia, particularly lymphomas. B-cell lymphomas of the brain are 1000-fold more common in patients with AIDS than in the general population. Diabetes mellitus can have a variety of complications, although not neoplasia. Hypertension can lead to CNS hemorrhages. Multiple sclerosis is a demyelinating disease without a significant risk for neoplasia. Tuberculosis as a chronic infection may lead to amyloidosis, not neoplasia.
BP6 169   PBD6 315

56. **(D)** The high alkaline phosphatase concentration in a patient with prostate cancer suggests there are metastases to bone. Prostate cancer is not known for paraneoplastic effects. Tumor extension to soft tissues and major organs does not produce an elevated alkaline phosphatase level, except in the liver. The grade of the tumor is not a major factor in this process, although higher-grade lesions are more likely to be metastatic. Angiogenesis does not affect alkaline phosphatase.
BP6 171–172   PBD6 320–321

57. **(C)** Lung cancers increased enormously in the twentieth century because cigarette smoking became so popular. As the number of persons who smoke in a population increases, so do the number of lung cancers. Some cancers of the urinary tract, oral cavity, esophagus, and pancreas are also causally related to smoking.
BP6 142   PBD6 272

58. **(F)** The decrease in the number of gastric cancers may be related to reduced numbers of dietary carcinogens, but the exact reason is obscure.
BP6 142   PBD6 272

59. **(B)** Worldwide, increasing numbers of skin cancers occur because of sun exposure. The ultraviolet light damages the skin and damages cellular DNA, leading to muta-

tions that escape cellular repair mechanisms. Smoking is related to many cancers, but skin cancers are not typically included with this risk factor. Chemotherapeutic agents have carcinogenic potential, particularly the alkylating agents such as cyclophosphamide, but leukemias and lym- phomas are the usual result. Asbestos exposure increases lung carcinoma risk in smokers and can lead to the rare mesotheliomas of pleura. Allergic reactions do not promote cancer.

BP6 165   PBD6 310

Infectious Diseases

BP6 Chapter 9 - General Pathology of
Infectious Diseases
PBD6 Chapter 9 - Infectious Diseases

1. A 35-year-old renal transplant recipient was being treated with cyclosporine, azathioprine, and high doses of corticosteroids. While on this treatment, the patient began to experience headaches and became lethargic. A clinical diagnosis of meningoencephalitis was made. He died 7 days later. Autopsy revealed a gelatinous meningeal exudate, and on sectioning of the brain, multiple small cystlike areas were seen throughout the brain. Under the microscope, these areas contained rounded structures with a prominent capsule that stained brightly with mucicarmine (i.e., histologic stain for mucin). Which of the following tests would have been most useful for diagnosis of this condition during life?

- (A) Examination of cerebrospinal fluid (CSF) with an India ink preparation
- (B) Determination of the CSF glucose and protein content
- (C) A brain biopsy stained for viral inclusions
- (D) Culture of the CSF for *Streptococcus pneumoniae*
- (E) A polymerase chain reaction (PCR) assay to detect Epstein-Barr virus (EBV) genome in the lymphocytes isolated from CSF

2. During a trip to Central America after hurricane Mitch, a 22-year-old female develops a low-volume, bloody diarrhea. This diarrhea resolves in a couple of weeks. At home 8 weeks after the diarrhea is gone, she begins to have some dull right upper quadrant pain. An abdominal CT scan reveals an irregular, 10-cm mass in the right liver lobe that has central necrosis. Which of the following infectious agents is probably implicated in these events?

- (A) *Giardia lamblia*
- (B) *Salmonella typhi*
- (C) *Entamoeba histolytica*
- (D) *Campylobacter jejuni*
- (E) *Yersinia enterocolitica*

3. A male patient comes into a physician's office complaining of a nontender ulcer on the penis that has been present for a week. A scraping of the lesion is performed and a darkfield examination is positive for spirochetes consistent with *Treponema pallidum*. A biopsy of the lesion is most likely to reveal

- (A) Granulomas with suppuration
- (B) Granulomas with caseation
- (C) Acute inflammation with abscess formation
- (D) Obliterative endarteritis with perivascular lymphocytes and plasma cells
- (E) Gummatous inflammation

4. A 24-year-old male has a fever with mainly upper respiratory tract symptoms—runny nose, sneezing, coughing. These symptoms last for a few days, and then he is better, with no sequelae. His infection is promoted by the binding of which of the following organisms to intercellular adhesion molecule-1 (ICAM-1)?

- (A) *Mycoplasma pneumoniae*
- (B) *Haemophilus influenzae*
- (C) Rhinovirus
- (D) Epstein-Barr virus
- (E) *Neisseria meningitidis*

For each of the patient histories in questions 5 through 7, match the most closely associated infectious organism that can cause the clinical findings:

- (A) *Ancylostoma duodenale*
- (B) *Aspergillus fumigatus*
- (C) *Borrelia recurrentis*
- (D) *Brugia malayi*
- (E) *Cryptococcus neoformans*
- (F) Cytomegalovirus (CMV)
- (G) *Leishmania donovani*
- (H) *Listeria monocytogenes*
- (I) *Mycobacterium leprae*
- (J) *Onchocerca volvulus*
- (K) *Plasmodium falciparum*
- (L) Poliovirus
- (M) *Taenia solium*
- (N) *Toxoplasma gondii*
- (O) *Trypanosoma gambiense*

5.   A previously healthy, 21-year-old male presents with a new-onset seizure disorder. A head computed tomography (CT) scan reveals multiple 0.5- to 1.5-cm, cystic, periventricular and meningeal lesions. (   )

6.   A 9-year-old girl has a mild febrile illness with a pharyngitis. She is better in a week. Over the next 2 months, she has increasing right-sided facial drooping with inability to close her right eye. (   )

7.   An American soldier stationed in Saudi Arabia has developed abdominal enlargement over the past 7 weeks, accompanied by a 10-kg weight loss and hyperpigmentation of skin. Physical examination reveals hepatosplenomegaly and lymphadenopathy. With progression of the disease, he develops pancytopenia and succumbs to *Streptococcus pneumoniae* septicemia. (   )

8.   A woman comes to the health center because she has a small vesicle on her right labium majus. She is sexually active. Inguinal lymph nodes are palpable. Because she has a prior history of lymphoma diagnosed 10 years earlier, a biopsy of one of the lymph nodes is done to exclude malignancy. Histologically, the biopsy shows multiple abscesses in which central necrosis is surrounded by palisading histiocytes. This morphology, combined with the clinical picture, is most representative of which of the following conditions?

○ (A) Chlamydial infection (i.e., lymphogranuloma venereum)
○ (B) Herpes simplex virus infection
○ (C) Recurrent non-Hodgkin lymphoma
○ (D) Candidal vaginitis
○ (E) Bacterial vaginosis

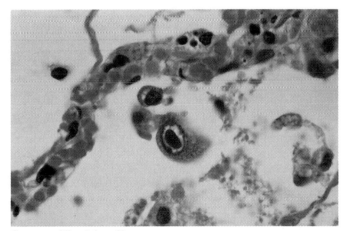

Courtesy of Dr. Arlene Sharpe.

9.   A human immunodeficiency virus (HIV)–positive male has a plasma titer of 26,800 copies of HIV-1 RNA/mL. He presents with increasing respiratory difficulty, and a transbronchial biopsy is performed. On the basis of the clinical and histologic findings shown in the figure, the most causative organism is

○ (A) Epstein-Barr virus (EBV)
○ (B) Cytomegalovirus (CMV)

○ (C) Respiratory syncytial virus
○ (D) Herpes zoster virus
○ (E) Adenovirus

10.   A 60-year-old male presents with bloody diarrhea, abdominal cramps, and fever. He is admitted to the hospital for workup. Sigmoidoscopic examination reveals ulceration in the cecum and ascending colon. Microscopic examination of a colonic biopsy shows flask-shaped mucosal ulcers with extensive necrosis and a modest, nonspecific inflammatory response. The ulcers do not penetrate the muscularis propria. The most likely agent responsible for this patient's diarrhea and mucosal ulceration is

○ (A) *Giardia lamblia*
○ (B) *Entamoeba histolytica*
○ (C) *Shigella* spp.
○ (D) *Salmonella* spp.
○ (E) *Vibrio cholerae*

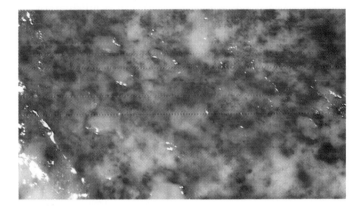

11.   A 24-year-old female has had a bloody diarrhea for the past few days. Colonoscopy reveals the appearance of the rectum and descending colon shown here. She is treated with antibiotics but develops a chronic arthritis after the diarrhea has resolved. HLA typing is done, and she is found to be HLA-B27 positive. Which of the following organisms was most likely to have been identified in her diarrhea stool?

○ (A) *Vibrio cholerae*
○ (B) *Shigella flexneri*
○ (C) *Entamoeba histolytica*
○ (D) *Salmonella typhi*
○ (E) *Helicobacter pylori*

12.   A 23-year-old female is admitted to the hospital with a 2-day history of increasing delirium. On physical examination, she has an acute pharyngitis with an overlying dirty white, tough membrane. She has paresthesias with decreased vibratory sensation. A Gram stain of the pharyngeal membrane reveals numerous small gram-positive rods in a fibrinopurulent exudate. She has an irregular cardiac rhythm. A chest radiograph reveals cardiomegaly. What is the mechanism for development of her cardiac disease?

○ (A) Microabscess formation
○ (B) Endotoxin-mediated hypotension and shock
○ (C) Vasculitis with thrombosis and infarction

○ (D) Granulomatous inflammation
○ (E) Elaboration of an exotoxin

13. A 15-year-old male has a small eschar forming around the site of removal of a tick from his left forearm. A hemorrhagic rash develops over the next few days involving his trunk, extremities, and even his palms and soles. Then, small 0.2- to 0.4-cm foci of skin necrosis develop on his fingers and toes. Which of the following organisms is most likely responsible for the development of these findings?

○ (A) *Rickettsia rickettsii*
○ (B) *Mycobacterium leprae*
○ (C) *Yersinia pestis*
○ (D) *Borrelia burgdorferi*
○ (E) *Leishmania braziliensis*

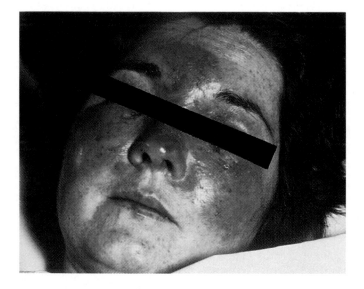

14. The patient shown here has had a high fever for the past 3 days. Which of the following organisms is most likely to produce this finding?

○ (A) *Clostridium botulinum*
○ (B) *Escherichia coli*
○ (C) *Neisseria gonorrhoeae*
○ (D) *Staphylococcus epidermidis*
○ (E) *Streptococcus pyogenes*

15. After World War I, many persons died from an influenza pandemic lasting several years. Which of the following changes in the virus is responsible for such pandemics of influenza?

○ (A) Mutations of the hemagglutinins and neuraminidase
○ (B) Increased ability to bind to ICAM-1 receptor
○ (C) Ability to elaborate exotoxins
○ (D) Recombination with RNA segments from pig viruses
○ (E) Acquisition of antibiotic resistance genes

16. A 52-year-old male has a fever with neutrophilia, and he has a cough that worsens over several days. *Klebsiella pneumoniae* is cultured from his sputum. His condition

improves after a course of therapy with gentamicin. Which of the following complications of this infection is most likely to develop?

○ (A) Gas gangrene
○ (B) Cavitary granulomas
○ (C) Abscess formation
○ (D) Bullous emphysema
○ (E) Adenocarcinoma

17. A bronchopneumonia in a 68-year-old female is complicated by abscess formation and bronchopleural fistula surrounded by a pronounced fibroblastic reaction. At autopsy, within the area of abscess formation are small, grossly visible, 1- to 2-mm, yellowish "sulfur granules." The organism most likely to produce this appearance is

○ (A) *Actinomyces israeli*
○ (B) *Blastomyces dermatitidis*
○ (C) *Chlamydia pneumoniae*
○ (D) *Klebsiella pneumoniae*
○ (E) *Mycobacterium kansasii*

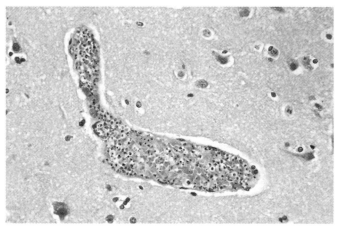

18. An 11-year-old boy had episodic fevers for a week and then developed a severe headache. He became progressively somnolent and died a week later. At autopsy, there is marked cerebral edema with areas of cerebral softening. The microscopic appearance of a cerebral vein is shown in the figure. In which of the following organs does the infectious agent producing his disease proliferate most?

○ (A) Heart
○ (B) Liver
○ (C) Brain
○ (D) Lymph nodes
○ (E) Spleen

19. A 29-year-old male has had hematuria for the past month. An abdominal radiograph reveals a small bladder outlined by a rim of calcification. Cystoscopy is performed, and the entire bladder mucosa is erythematous and granular. Biopsies are taken. Which of the following histologic findings is most likely to be seen?

○ (A) Eggs of *Schistosoma hematobium*
○ (B) Larvae of *Trichinella spiralis*

○ (C) *Taenia solium* cysts
○ (D) Acid-fast bacilli
○ (E) Migrating *Ascaris lumbricoides*

20. A 24-year-old male college student seen by the Health Service complained of 3 weeks of cough, fever, and shortness of breath when walking. The physician found normal cardiac examination results, and a chest radiograph demonstrated mild haziness in the lungs. A presumptive clinical diagnosis of *Mycoplasma pneumoniae* was made after he was found to have an elevated cold agglutinin titer, and he responded to erythromycin therapy. Which set of the following histologic changes is most likely responsible for the pulmonary symptoms in this condition?

○ (A) Neutrophils within bronchioles, extending into alveoli
○ (B) Granulomas with Langhans giant cells
○ (C) Pulmonary infarcts with vascular occlusion by microorganisms
○ (D) Mononuclear (lymphocytes, histiocytes) interstitial infiltrate
○ (E) Collection of neutrophils and fibrin in the pleural space (empyema)

For each of the clinical histories in questions 21 and 22, match the most closely associated lettered host for a parasitic infection:

(A) Cat
(B) Cow
(C) Flea
(D) Louse
(E) Mosquito
(F) Pig
(G) Rat
(H) Sand fly
(I) Snail
(J) Tick
(K) Triatomid bug
(L) Tsetse fly

21. An 18-year-old female gives birth at 33 weeks' gestation to a stillborn boy. Autopsy reveals extensive periventricular cerebral necrosis with calcification and vascular thrombosis in the circle of Willis. Small areas of necrosis also appear in heart and lung. (   )

22. A 6-year-old Mexican girl develops fever with neutropenia, followed by disseminated intravascular coagulation over the course of a week. She dies of an intracerebral hemorrhage. (   )

23. While repairing a fence at his farm, a 40-year-old male cuts the skin over his shin. This wound heals without any complications. Several days later he begins to develop muscle spasms of his face and extremities. These spasms worsen to the point of severe contractions. Which of the following actions by a toxin is responsible for the clinical features in this case?

○ (A) Degradation of muscle cell membranes by phospholipase C

○ (B) Inhibition of acetylcholine release at neuromuscular junctions
○ (C) Stimulation of adenylate cyclase production
○ (D) Cleavage of synaptobrevin in the synaptic vesicles of neurons
○ (E) Cytokine release by T lymphocytes

24. At a convention of veterans, several of the participants begin to develop respiratory difficulty and fever. These men are between 58 and 73 years old, they are all smokers, and many have chronic obstructive lung disease. Chest radiographs of these men demonstrate extensive infiltrates and small abscesses. Sputum specimens reveal as many macrophages as neutrophils on the cytologic smears. Which of the following organisms is most likely to be identified in the sputum?

○ (A) Cytomegalovirus
○ (B) *Pneumocystis carinii*
○ (C) *Legionella pneumophila*
○ (D) *Burkholderia cepacia*
○ (E) *Listeria monocytogenes*

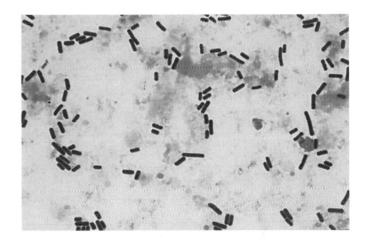

25. A 25-year-old male is involved in a vehicular accident in which he is ejected from the vehicle. He sustains a compound fracture of his right humerus. Several days later, he has marked swelling of his right arm with crepitance. A Gram stain of exudate from the wound site has the appearance as shown here. Which of the following organisms is the causative agent for his infection?

○ (A) *Candida albicans*
○ (B) *Listeria monocytogenes*
○ (C) *Haemophilus influenzae*
○ (D) *Clostridium perfringens*
○ (E) *Bacteroides fragilis*

26. For several weeks, a 52-year-old male has had a chronic cough with low-grade fevers. A chest radiograph shows scattered, upper lobe, 0.3- to 2-cm nodules and hilar adenopathy. A fine-needle aspirate of one of the nodules shows inflammation with mononuclear cells, including macrophages that, with periodic acid–Schiff (PAS) stain, show intracellular, 2- to 5-μm, rounded, yeastlike orga-

nisms. Which of the following infectious diseases is he most likely to have?

- ○ (A) Coccidioidomycosis
- ○ (B) Candidiasis
- ○ (C) Cryptococcosis
- ○ (D) Histoplasmosis
- ○ (E) Blastomycosis

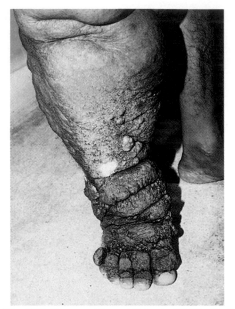

Courtesy of Dr. Willy Pressens, Harvard School of Public Health.

27. The condition shown here in a 40-year-old male has been progressively worsening for years. He also has inguinal lymphadenopathy and scrotal edema. Which of the following infections is this patient most likely to have?

- ○ (A) *Schistosoma mansoni*
- ○ (B) *Echinococcus granulosis*
- ○ (C) *Trichinella spiralis*
- ○ (D) *Leishmania tropica*
- ○ (E) *Wuchereria bancrofti*

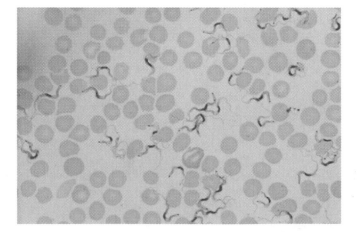

28. A 22-year-old male developed a 1-cm, rubbery, red chancre on his right forearm. After several months, he developed splenomegaly and lymphadenopathy; and 2 months later he succumbed to progressive wasting with cachexia and decreased mentation. At the time of his death, his peripheral blood smear had the appearance depicted in the figure at the bottom of the left column. Where is this disease most likely to have been acquired?

- ○ (A) West Africa
- ○ (B) Central America
- ○ (C) Southeast Asia
- ○ (D) Southern Europe
- ○ (E) Polynesia

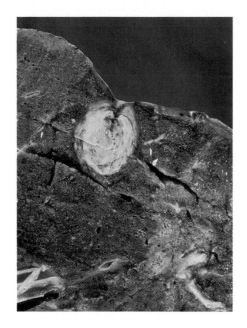

29. A 36-year-old male is singing the blues in Memphis, Tennessee, after a chest radiograph reveals a right lower lobe, peripheral, 2.5-cm mass. He is currently asymptomatic, but he remembers that he had a month-long febrile illness last year. If the gross appearance shown here is representative of the pathologic process in his lung, which of the following mechanisms best explains how he got this infection?

- ○ (A) Mosquito bite on a trip to Africa
- ○ (B) Transfusion of packed red blood cells
- ○ (C) Injection drug use with shared needles
- ○ (D) Ingestion of contaminated milk
- ○ (E) Birds roosting on his air conditioner

30. For which of the following infections is vertical transmission from mother to child a significant cause for rejection as a blood donor later in life?

- ○ (A) *Escherichia coli*
- ○ (B) Hepatitis B virus
- ○ (C) *Plasmodium vivax*
- ○ (D) *Candida albicans*
- ○ (E) *Pneumocystis carinii*

31. A trading ship from the Black Sea docks at an Italian port. The ship's crew has been decimated from an illness marked by a short time course of days from onset of inguinal lymph node enlargement with overlying skin ulceration to prostration and death. A small ulcerated pustule ringed by a rosy rash is seen on the lower extremities of some of the crew. Within days, more than one half of the population of the port city are dead. Which of the following agents is most likely responsible for the rapid spread of this disease?

- (A) Mosquitoes
- (B) Rats
- (C) Sand flies
- (D) Cats
- (E) Ticks

For each of the patient histories in questions 32 through 37, match the most closely associated lettered infectious agent:

(A) Adenovirus
(B) *Aspergillus fumigatus*
(C) *Bacteriodes fragilis*
(D) *Campylobacter jejuni*
(E) *Candida albicans*
(F) *Coccidioides immitis*
(G) Coronavirus
(H) *Corynebacterium diphtheriae*
(I) Coxsackievirus
(J) *Entamoeba histolytica*
(K) Herpes simplex virus
(L) *Histoplasma capsulatum*
(M) *Mucor* species
(N) *Mycobacterium tuberculosis*
(O) *Neisseria gonorrhoeae*
(P) *Pseudomonas aeruginosa*
(Q) *Pneumocystis carinii*
(R) Rotavirus
(S) *Streptococcus pneumoniae*
(T) *Toxoplasma gondii*

32. A 25-year-old female has had pelvic pain, fever, and vaginal discharge for several weeks. On physical examination, she has lower abdominal adnexal tenderness. She also has a painful, swollen knee. (   )

33. A 19-year-old female is admitted with a 2-day history of severe right facial pain. She has right eye proptosis. Laboratory findings include 4+ ketones on urinalysis and a serum glucose concentration of 475 mg/dL. She becomes obtunded. (   )

34. A 6-month-old infant developed diarrhea of 2 days' duration. This resulted from villous atrophy produced by invasion and destruction of the intestinal epithelium and resultant decrease in absorption of sodium and water. (   )

35. A 10-year-old girl with severe neutropenia 1 month after bone marrow transplantation develops fever and difficulty in breathing. A chest radiograph suggests pulmonary

infarcts. At autopsy, pulmonary vessels are occluded by abundant growth of microorganisms. (   )

36. A patient with extensive burns in the surgical intensive care unit develops neutropenia and bilateral pneumonia. At autopsy, the lungs show patchy areas of consolidation. Microscopic examination reveals pulmonary vasculitis and surrounding areas of necrosis with sparse inflammatory exudate. (   )

37. A 50-year-old resident of Phoenix, Arizona, who recently moved to Dallas, Texas, presents with a cough. A chest radiograph reveals a 3.5-cm opacity in the right apical region with central cavitation. An open lung biopsy is done to exclude cancer. Microscopic examination reveals caseating granulomatous inflammation containing large (60-μm) spherules filled with smaller, rounded structures. (   )

38. A watery diarrhea is causing dehydration of a 1-year-old child. Examination of a stool specimen by enzyme immunoassay reveals the presence of rotavirus. The child is given intravenous fluids and makes a complete recovery in a week. Which of the following mechanisms accounts for this diarrhea?

- (A) Decreased absorption of sodium and water
- (B) Increased secretion of sodium and water by epithelial cells
- (C) Presence of Yop virulence plasmid
- (D) Lysis of colonic epithelial cells
- (E) Decreased breakdown of lactose to glucose and galactose

39. A 5-year-old girl developed a blotchy, reddish brown rash on her face, trunk, and proximal extremities over 3 days. On physical examination, she had 0.2- to 0.5-cm ulcerated lesions on the oral cavity mucosa. She also developed generalized lymphadenopathy. A cough with minimal sputum production then progressively worsened over the next 3 days. Which of the following infectious diseases did this child most likely have?

- (A) Mumps
- (B) Varicella zoster virus (VZV) infection
- (C) Rubella
- (D) Mononucleosis
- (E) Rubeola (measles)

40. A chronic abscessing pneumonia of the right middle lobe appears on the chest radiograph of a 42-year-old male known to be HIV positive. A transbronchial biopsy reveals the presence of gram-positive filamentous organisms that are weakly acid fast. His course is further complicated by empyema and acute onset of a headache. A head CT scan reveals a 4-cm discrete lesion of the right hemisphere with ring enhancement characteristic of an abscess. The infectious agent most probably responsible for these findings is

- (A) *Aspergillus fumigatus*
- (B) *Nocardia asteroides*
- (C) *Mycobacterium avium-intracellulare*

○ (D) *Staphylococcus aureus*
○ (E) *Mucor* species

41. A 33-year-old female who is an injection drug user develops a severe headache and neck stiffness. She has no papilledema, and a lumbar puncture is performed. A Gram stain of the CSF obtained reveals many short gram-positive rods. How was this infection most likely to have been acquired?

○ (A) Sharing infected needles
○ (B) Inhalation of droplet nuclei
○ (C) Inoculation through a cut on the skin
○ (D) Eating contaminated dairy products
○ (E) Using a friend's toothbrush

42. A 6-year-old boy developed a rash over his chest that started as 0.5-cm-diameter, reddish macules. In a day or so, the macules became vesicles. A few days later, the vesicles ruptured and crusted over. Crops of these lesions spread to involve the face and the extremities over the next 2 weeks. Decades later, which of the following manifestations of this infection is most likely to appear?

○ (A) Shingles
○ (B) Infertility
○ (C) Paralysis
○ (D) Congestive heart failure
○ (E) Chronic arthritis

43. A 6-year-old child presented with 7 days of diarrhea. A stool culture was positive for *Shigella* spp. What would you expect to see in an endoscopic biopsy of the colon?

○ (A) Epithelial disruption with an overlying exudate of polymorphonuclear leukocytes (neutrophils)
○ (B) Multiple granulomas throughout the wall of the colon
○ (C) Slight increase in the numbers of lymphocytes and plasma cells in the lamina propria
○ (D) Intranuclear inclusions in the enterocytes
○ (E) Extensive scarring of the lamina propria with stricture formation

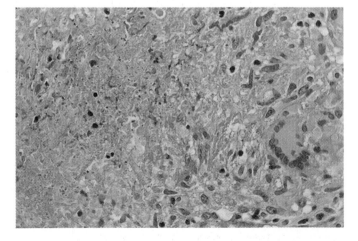

44. A 32-year-old male has had a fever with weight loss over the past 3 months. He has elevated aspartate amino-transferase and alanine aminotransferase concentrations, but his serum bilirubin level is not elevated. A liver biopsy is performed, and the sample has the microscopic appearance as shown in the figure. An acid-fast stain of this tissue is positive. By which of the following mechanisms is the infectious agent being destroyed?

○ (A) Phagocytosis by eosinophils
○ (B) Elaboration of nitric oxide by macrophages
○ (C) Generation of NADPH-dependent oxygen-free radicals
○ (D) Complement-mediated lysis
○ (E) Superoxide formation within phagolysosomes

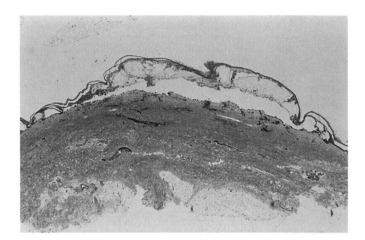

45. A 23-year-old female patient has had recurrent vesicular genital lesions for several years. A genital mucosal lesion is depicted microscopically under low power as shown here. Microscopic examination under higher magnification of this lesion is likely to reveal

○ (A) Dysplastic epithelial cells that contain human papillomavirus sequences
○ (B) Neutrophils containing ingested gram-negative diplococci
○ (C) Multinucleated (syncytial) cells that contain pink-to-purple intranuclear inclusions
○ (D) Perivascular lymphoplasmacytic infiltrate surrounding arterioles, with endothelial proliferation
○ (E) Mononuclear infiltrate with *Trichomonas vaginalis* organisms

For each of the patient histories in questions 46 and 47, match the most closely associated lettered clinical finding resulting from an infectious disease process:

(A) Cerebral abscesses
(B) Chronic arthritis
(C) Dilated cardiomyopathy
(D) Elephantiasis
(E) Hemolysis
(F) Hepatic fibrosis
(G) Leg paralysis
(H) Meningitis
(I) Mucocutaneous ulcers
(J) Myositis

(K) Paranasal bony destruction
(L) Skin anesthesia
(M) Squamous cell carcinoma
(N) Stillbirth
(O) Voluminous watery diarrhea

46. A 45-year-old rice farmer becomes infected by cercaria that penetrate the skin of his feet. The cercaria are released from snails living in the irrigation canals. He develops progressive ascites. (   )

47. A 9-year-old child living in a mud hut in northeastern Brazil is bitten by a reduvid bug, and an erythematous nodule develops at the corner of her mouth. Several years later, she has worsening dyspnea. (   )

For each of the clinical histories in questions 48 through 51, match the most closely associated infectious disease:

(A) African trypanosomiasis
(B) Amebiasis
(C) Aspergillosis
(D) Chagas disease
(E) Cholera
(F) Dengue fever
(G) Filariasis
(H) Hydatid disease
(I) Leishmaniasis
(J) Leprosy
(K) Lyme disease
(L) Malaria
(M) Plague
(N) Schistosomiasis
(O) Syphilis
(P) Tetanus
(Q) Trachoma
(R) Tuberculosis
(S) Typhoid fever

48. A 25-year-old female has a sudden onset of a severe, voluminous, watery diarrhea. She becomes severely dehydrated over the next few days. Microscopic examination of the diarrhea fluid reveals flecks of mucus but no blood and few white blood cells. A blood culture is negative. She recovers in hospital with intravenous fluid therapy over the next week. (   )

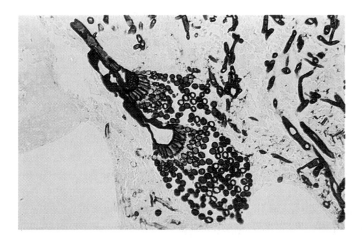

49. A 45-year-old male with a long history of gastrointestinal reflux disease and Barrett esophagus is undergoing chemotherapy for adenocarcinoma of the esophagus. He becomes severely neutropenic, with a white blood cell count of only 50/μL. He then develops a cough and fever. A chest radiograph reveals multiple 0.5- to 2-cm nodules scattered throughout all lung fields. He has a headache and acute-onset seizure disorder. A head CT scan reveals a 1.5-cm, rounded mass in the right parietal lobe. A biopsy of a 1-cm ulcerated mass involving his right nasal septum is shown at the bottom of the left column microscopically with a silver stain. (   )

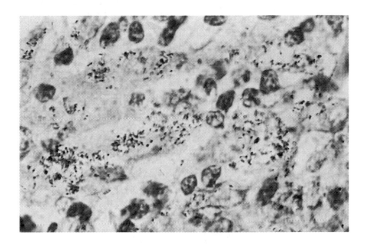

50. A 32-year-old male has developed maculopapular and nodular skin lesions, mainly involving his face, elbows, wrists, and knees. The nodular lesions have slowly enlarged over the past 10 years and are now beginning to cause deformity. However, these lesions are not painful; he has decreased to absent sensation in these areas. A biopsy is taken of a nodular lesion and shown here with acid-fast stain. (   )

51. A 44-year-old female notices an erythematous papule on her left lower leg that becomes a ringlike rash that subsides over several weeks. Over the next 5 months, she has migratory joint and muscle pain. She has substernal chest pain and an irregular heart rhythm. These problems subside, but 2 years after the initial rash appeared, she has a chronic arthritis involving hips, knees, and shoulders. (   )

52. A baby born at term is severely hydropic. There is a diffuse rash with sloughing skin on palms and soles. Within 2 days, the neonate is dead of respiratory distress. Autopsy reveals marked hepatosplenomegaly. There is a periosteitis and osteochondritis. The lungs are pale and poorly aerated, with interstitial mononuclear infiltrates. Serologic tests for which of the following is most likely to be positive in the baby's mother?

○ (A) HIV
○ (B) Herpes simplex, type 2
○ (C) *Toxoplasma gondii*
○ (D) Syphilis
○ (E) Cytomegalovirus

ANSWERS

1. **(A)** He has cryptococcal meningoencephalitis, a complication of his immunocompromised state. *C. neoformans* typically has a thick capsule, making it easily visible with the India ink preparation, a procedure that takes only a few minutes to perform. The CSF glucose and protein levels can aid in determining whether an infection is present and what general type of organism is present, but they do not yield a specific cause. A cryptococcal antigen test would be useful for this patient. Brain biopsies are not commonly done, and other less invasive methods should be pursued first. A bacterial meningitis is possible, and pneumococcus would be a common bacterial cause, but the description here is that of cryptococcosis. PCR probes for EBV are not useful in this case, because an acute viral meningitis does not usually cause a visible exudate, the onset of disease is more insidious, and it is not typically associated with immunocompromised states.
BP6 727   PBD6 379–380

2. **(C)** Amebic liver abscess is an uncommon complication of amebiasis. The colonic lesions are typically gone by the time the liver lesions appear. *E. histolytica* organisms can invade the colonic submucosa, gaining access to venules draining to the portal system. Giardiasis is caused by an intestinal parasite that causes a watery diarrhea. Typhoid fever is a systemic disease that produces splenomegaly more so than hepatomegaly, and abscesses are not common. *Campylobacter* and *Yersinia* can produce various presentations of diarrhea, but abscesses are unexpected.
BP6 269, 496   PBD6 358–359

3. **(D)** Syphilitic chancres occur in the primary stage of syphilis and are characterized by lymphoplasmacytic infiltrates along with an obliterative endarteritis. Similar lesions may also appear with secondary syphilitic mucocutaneous lesions. Caseating granulomatous inflammation is more characteristic for tuberculosis or fungal infections. Acute inflammation with abscess formation is characteristic of bacterial infections such as gonorrhea. Gummatous inflammation can be seen with tertiary syphilis in adults or in congenital syphilis.
BP6 589–592   PBD6 346, 362–364

4. **(C)** Rhinovirus binds to ICAM-1 and accounts for 60% of common colds. *M. pneumoniae* also accounts for some colds, but this agent does not bind to ICAM-1 receptors on host cells. *H. influenzae* can produce sinusitis, otitis media, and bronchopneumonia. EBV infection can produce pharyngitis with infectious mononucleosis, but the course tends to extend over weeks. *N. meningitidis* infections producing meningitis may begin as a mild pharyngitis, but these infections can have a very rapid course over 1 or 2 days.
PBD6 347–348

5. **(M)** He has cysticercosis. Eating uncooked pork can result in the release of larvae that penetrate the gut wall and disseminate hematogenously, often settling in gray and white cerebral tissue, where they develop into cysts.
PBD6 395–396

6. **(L)** Poliomyelitis is an enterovirus spread through fecal-oral contamination. The virus infects the oropharynx first. It then spreads to spinal cord anterior horn cells and bulbar nuclei to produce the paralysis typical of polio. Vaccination has made this disease rare.
PBD6 373

7. **(G)** This is visceral leishmaniasis, or kala-azar. Leishmaniasis is endemic in the Middle East, South Asia, Africa, and Latin America. The organisms proliferate within macrophages in the mononuclear phagocyte system and cause hepatosplenomegaly and lymphadenopathy. Often, there is hyperpigmentation of the skin. Bone marrow involvement and splenic enlargement contribute to reduced production and accelerated destruction of hematopoietic cells, giving rise to pancytopenia.
PBD6 391–392

8. **(A)** Infection with *Chlamydia trachomatis* is one of the more common sexually transmitted diseases, but most cases have only urethritis and cervicitis. However, some strains of *C. trachomatis* can produce lymphogranuloma venereum, a chronic, ulcerative disease that is more endemic in Asia, Africa, and the Caribbean. There is a mixed granulomatous and neutrophilic inflammatory reaction. In contrast, herpes simplex virus produces clear mucocutaneous vesicles with no exudates and is unlikely to involve lymph nodes. Recurrent lymphoma has sheets or nodules of pleomorphic lymphocytes without significant inflammation. Candidiasis can produce superficial inflammation with an exudate but is rarely invasive or disseminated in nonimmunosuppressed individuals. A variety of bacterial infections may involve the vagina.
BP6 595   PBD6 361–362

9. **(B)** This patient has high HIV-1 RNA levels that are consistent with the diagnosis of acquired immunodeficiency syndrome (AIDS). Although patients with AIDS are susceptible to many microbes, infections with CMV are particularly common. This biopsy shows an enlarged cell containing a distinct intranuclear inclusion and ill-defined cytoplasmic inclusions. This is typical of CMV infection. EBV infection is frequently seen in patients with HIV infection, but there are no distinct pulmonary lesions associated with it. Respiratory syncytial virus infections are seen in children and rarely in adults. Herpes zoster infections are most likely to affect the peripheral nervous system and can become disseminated to affect the lungs in immunosuppressed patients. Adenovirus is a common viral pathogen in adults that may produce a clinically significant pneumonia, and intranuclear inclusions may be present, but the cells are not large, and cytoplasmic inclusions are absent.
BP6 429–430   PBD6 726

10. **(B)** Amebiasis is a common cause for dysentery in developing nations. The *E. histolytica* trophozoites can at-

tach to colonic epithelium, invade, and lyse the epithelial cells. In some cases, there can be extensive mucosal involvement with characteristic flask-shaped (i.e., like an Erlenmeyer flask) ulcerations similar to other severe inflammatory bowel diseases. Giardiasis tends to involve the small intestine with variable inflammation but without ulceration. Shigellosis can produce a bloody dysentery with irregular superficial colonic mucosal ulceration, but the organisms typically do not invade beyond the lamina propria. Salmonellosis more typically involves the small intestine and in most cases produces a self-limited enteritis, although more severe disease with dissemination to other organs can occur with *S. typhi* infection. Cholera is characterized by a massive secretory diarrhea without intestinal mucosal invasion or necrosis.
BP6 496　PBD6 358–359

11.　**(B)** The *Shigella* organisms elaborate a shiga toxin that damages colonic epithelial cells. The colonic mucosa is intensely inflamed with ulcerations and pseudomembrane formation (i.e., pale, white patches). *S. flexneri* infections in persons positive for HLA-B27 can lead to Reiter syndrome, with chronic arthritis. *Vibrio* organisms elaborate an exotoxin and do not invade and destroy intestinal epithelium. *E. histolytica* can produce a bloody diarrhea but not Reiter syndrome. Typhoid fever has many systemic problems but not arthritis. *H. pylori* living in gastric mucus drives the processes of chronic gastritis and ulceration of gastric and duodenal mucosal surfaces.
BP6 495　PBD6 355

12.　**(E)** She has diphtheria. The *C. diphtheriae* organisms proliferate in the inflammatory membrane that covers the pharynx and tonsils. These organisms elaborate an exotoxin that produces myocarditis and neuropathy. The organisms do not disseminate to cause inflammation or abscesses or vasculitis elsewhere in the body. Endotoxins tend to be elaborated by gram-negative bacterial organisms. Granulomatous inflammation is more typical for mycobacterial and fungal infections.
BP6 274　PBD6 343,759,1276

13.　**(A)** He has Rocky Mountain spotted fever, which occurs sporadically in the United States in places other than the Rocky Mountains. Rickettsial diseases produce signs and symptoms from damage to vascular endothelium and smooth muscle, similar to a vasculitis. Thrombosis of the affected blood vessels is responsible for foci of skin necrosis. Hansen disease, produced by *M. leprae*, results in skin anesthesia that predisposes to recurrent injury. Plague, caused by *Y. pestis*, can produce focal skin necrosis at the site of a flea bite. Lyme disease, produced by *B. burgdorferi*, can produce an erythema chronicum migrans of skin at the site of a tick bite. Mucocutaneous leishmaniasis mainly involves the nasal and oral regions.
PBD6 384

14.　**(E)** This rash and edema are manifestations of streptococcal erysipelas. Erysipelas is usually caused by types A or C of *Streptococcus*. Streptolysins elaborated by these organisms aid in the spread of the infection. *C. botulinum*

elaborates an exotoxin that when ingested results in paralysis. *E. coli* produces a variety of infections, but skin infections are not common. *N. gonorrhoeae* is best known as a sexually transmitted disease, and a rash is possible, although usually without pronounced swelling. *S. epidermidis* is usually considered a contaminant in cultures.
PBD6 367–368

15.　**(D)** The influenza pandemic in 1918 resulted from an antigenic shift in the influenza A type. This occurs when there is recombination with RNA sequences of influenza viruses found in animals such as pigs. Mutations in the envelope genes are responsible for epidemics. These mutations allow evasion from host antibodies. Influenza viruses do not bind to ICAM-1 receptors; rhinoviruses do. Viruses do not make exotoxins and do not acquire antibiotic resistance. A swine flu virus has been discovered as a cause for the 1918 pandemic.
PBD6 348

16.　**(C)** Bacterial infections are marked by suppurative inflammation, and a virulent organism such as *Klebsiella* can lead to tissue destruction with abscess formation. Gas-forming bacteria, such as *Clostridium* organisms, are unusual respiratory infections. Granulomatous inflammation is characteristic for mycobacterial or fungal infections. Infections of the lung do not result in emphysema. Carcinomas are not sequelae of bacterial infections.
BP6 428–429　PBD6 345

17.　**(A)** Actinomycetes that can produce chronic abscessing pneumonia, particularly in immunocompromised patients, include *A. israeli* and *N. asteroides*. Sulfur granules, formed from masses of the branching, filamentous organisms, are more likely to be seen with *Actinomyces*. *B. dermatitidis* infections tend to produce a granulomatous inflammatory process. Chlamydial infections produce an interstitial pattern, just like most viruses. *Klebsiella* infections, as other bacterial infections, can result in abscess formation, although without distinct sulfur granules. *M. kansasii* infections are similar to *M. tuberculosis* infections in that granulomatous inflammation is prominent.
BP6 420　PBD 335, 722

18.　**(B)** After the infective mosquito bite, *P. falciparum* sporozoites invade liver cells and reproduce asexually. When the hepatocytes rupture, they release thousands of merozoites that infect red blood cells (RBCs). The infected RBCs circulate. These infected RBCs can bind to endothelium in brain, and small cerebral vessels become plugged with the RBCs, resulting in ischemia.
BP6 352–353　PBD6 389–391

19.　**(A)** *S. hematobium* is seen in Africa, particularly the Nile Valley, in areas where irrigation has expanded the range of the host snails. It infects the wall of the urinary bladder, causing severe granulomatous inflammation, fibrosis, and calcification. *T. spiralis* infects striated muscle. Cysticercosis can have a wide tissue distribution, but brain is most often affected. Mycobacterial infections of the urinary tract are uncommon and do not cause bladder fibrosis.

Ascariasis involves the lower gastrointestinal tract, and the worms reside in the lumen.
PBD6 396-397

20. **(D)** *Mycoplasma* infections lead to a primary atypical pneumonia in which there are no alveolar infiltrates, but there is prominent interstitial inflammation. Alveolar and bronchiolar neutrophilic exudates suggest a bacterial agent causing pneumonia. Granulomas with Langhans-type giant cells are typical for tuberculosis. Proliferation of microorganisms with vascular occlusion and infarction is most typical for *Aspergillus* fungal infections. An empyema suggests a bacterial cause for pneumonia with spread to pleura.
BP6 419-420   PBD6 335, 721-722

21. **(A)** Toxoplasmosis is the "T" in the TORCH mnemonic for congenital infections (*t*oxoplasmosis, *o*ther infections, *r*ubella, *c*ytomegalovirus infection, and *h*erpes simplex). The *T. gondii* organisms can cross the placenta to affect the fetus. The mother is typically asymptomatic. The cat is the natural host for *T. gondii*.
PBD6 382-383

22. **(E)** Hemorrhagic fever, or Dengue fever, is caused by an arbovirus of the Flavivirus group. This organism can be devastating because it produces bone marrow suppression and because any antibodies to the virus enhance cellular viral uptake. It is transmitted by the mosquito vector *Aedes aegypti*.
PBD6 383

23. **(D)** He has tetanus. The contamination of a wound with *Clostridium tetani* can result in the elaboration of a potent neurotoxin. This toxin is a protease that cleaves synaptobrevin, a major transmembrane protein of the synaptic vesicles of the inhibitory neurons. The toxin of *S. aureus* produces an enterotoxin that acts as a superantigen and stimulates T-cell cytokine release. Cholera is produced when the toxin elaborated by *V. cholerae* stimulates epithelial cell adenylate cyclase. *C. perfringens* elaborates a variety of toxins, one of which (tetanospasmin) is a phospholipase.
PBD6 368-369

24. **(C)** The original outbreak for which this disease was named occurred at an American Legion convention. *L. pneumophila* is a facultative parasite of macrophages. A high ratio of macrophages to neutrophils is characteristic of the infection. Persons with immunosuppression are at risk for CMV and *Pneumocystis* pneumonia. *B. cepacia* is most often seen in patients with cystic fibrosis who have extensive bronchiectasis. *L. monocytogenes* can produce a disseminated disease with meningitis in immunocompromised adults.
BP6 418   PBD6 377-378

25. **(D)** These large, gram-positive rods are characteristic of *C. perfringens*, which can contaminate open wounds and produce gas gangrene. Candidal infections are typically superficial, and a Gram stain shows gram-positive budding cells with pseudohyphae. Listeriosis can be a congenital or food-borne infection, and the organisms are short, gram-positive rods. *H. influenzae* is a gram-negative rod known best for respiratory and CNS infections. *B. fragilis* can contaminate surgical wounds of the abdomen.
PBD6 369

26. **(D)** The small yeasts of *H. capsulatum* are often intracellular. Infections can be disseminated, involving tissues of the mononuclear phagocyte system. In the lung, histoplasmosis can mimic primary or secondary tuberculosis. The spherules of *C. albicans* are larger and are not intracellular. *C. neoformans* organisms have narrow-based budding and are two to three times larger than *H. capsulatum* organisms. Organisms of *B. dermatitidis* exhibit broad-based budding and are slightly larger than *C. neoformans* organisms.
BP6 425-426   PBD6 352-353

27. (E) This is elephantiasis, which results from lymphatic obstruction when there is an inflammatory reaction to the adult filarial worms *Wuchereria bancrofti*. Schistosomiasis may affect liver or bladder most severely. *Echinococcus* produces hydatid disease of liver, lungs, or bone. *Trichinella* encysts in striated muscle. *Leishmania* can involve the skin with ulceration and enlarge parenchymal organs.
PBD6 397-398

28. **(A)** The findings are consistent with African trypanosomiasis, or sleeping sickness. The eradication of the tsetse fly vector has been a priority for decades. Filarial worms endemic in parts of Central America, Southeast Asia, and Polynesia can also appear in blood but are smaller in size and do not lead to chronic wasting.
PBD6 337, 393

29. **(E)** This is a small "coin lesion" of the lung produced by a granulomatous inflammatory process. One cause for this process is infection with *H. capsulatum*. Bird droppings, especially from pigeons, are a rich source of dusts contaminated with *H. capsulatum*. Fungal and mycobacterial infections are not acquired by transfusion or other parenteral routes, such as sharing intravenous needles. Contaminated milk is a source for *Mycobacterium bovis*, but this is a rare pulmonary infection. Mosquitoes are not generally known as vectors for diseases that cause granulomatous inflammation.
BP6 425-427   PBD6 352-353

30. **(B)** Testing for hepatitis B and C is part of routine screening of blood donors. This form of transmission for hepatitis B is most common in developing nations. *E. coli* can be a congenital infection, but it leaves no major significant lasting sequelae in infants who survive. Malaria, candidal infection, and pneumocystosis are not congenital infections.
BP6 526   PBD6 339

31. **(B)** This incident was the beginning of the Black Death in Europe that persisted through the 14th and 15th centuries. Rodents form the reservoir of infection. Flea bites and aerosols transmit the infection very efficiently. The causative organism, *Y. pestis*, secretes a plasminogen activator that promotes its spread. Plague was endemic in East Asia at the beginning of the 20th century and was carried to San Francisco. Not wanting to produce a panic that could be bad for business or tourism, California's governor at that time did not enforce a quarantine. As a consequence, plague is endemic in wild rodents in the western United States, but it fortunately accounts for only occasional sporadic human infections.
PBD6 387-388

32. **(O)** She has pelvic inflammatory disease, which may be produced by gonococci or *Chlamydia*. *N. gonorrhoeae* and *Chlamydia* are sexually transmitted diseases. Complications of pelvic inflammatory disease include peritonitis, adhesions with bowel obstruction, sepsis with endocarditis, meningitis, arthritis, and infertility.
BP6 593,613   PBD6 362

33. **(M)** Rhinocerebral mucormycosis is a feared complication associated with diabetic ketoacidosis. The broad, nonseptate hyphae invade extensively into paranasal sinuses and orbit and into the central nervous system.
BP6 428   PBD6 380-381

34. **(R)** Rotavirus, an encapsulated RNA virus, is a major cause for diarrhea in infancy. The villous destruction with atrophy leads to decreased absorption of sodium and water. The development of antibodies from secretory immunity in the bowel to rotavirus surface antigens makes older children and adults relatively resistant to rotavirus infection. Such antibodies are present in maternal milk and confer some degree of resistance to babies receiving mother's milk.
BP6 493-494   PBD6 354

35. **(B or M)** *Aspergillus*, *Candida*, and *Mucor* infections may become disseminated in the setting of neutropenia. Vascular invasion can occur with fungal infections, particularly with *Aspergillus* and *Mucor*. After these organisms gain a foothold (hyphae-hold) in tissues, they are very difficult to eradicate.
BP6 428   PBD6 380-381

36. **(P)** *P. aeruginosa* organisms secrete several virulence factors: exotoxin A, which inhibits protein synthesis; exoenzyme S, which interferes with host cell growth; phospholipase C, which degrades pulmonary surfactant; and iron-containing compounds, which are toxic to endothelial cells. These virulence factors result in extensive vasculitis with necrosis. Neutropenic patients are particularly at risk.
BP6 418   PBD6 376-377

37. **(F)** Inhaling the arthrospores of *C. immitis* can lead to coccidioidomycosis. This disease is endemic to the southwestern United States. The infection typically results in granuloma formation, but most persons have subclinical infections. About 10% may be symptomatic with respiratory symptoms, including cough and pleuritic chest pain. Dissemination to extrapulmonary sites occurs in only 1% of cases.
BP6 427   PBD6 353

38. **(A)** Many enteroviruses produce diarrhea by inhibiting the intestinal absorption of intraluminal sodium and water. Most older children and adults have immunity. Cholera is the result of secretion of an exotoxin by the *V. cholerae* organism, which potentiates the epithelial cell production of adenylate cyclase and causes secretory diarrhea. The Yop plasmid confers infectivity to *Yersinia* organisms. Amebae can lyse epithelium, and the diarrhea can be bloody. Decreased breakdown of lactose occurs in disaccharidase deficiency and gives rise to an osmotic diarrhea.
PBD6 354, 815

39. **(E)** The rash and the Koplik spots on the buccal mucosa are characteristic findings for measles, a childhood infection. It occurs only sporadically when immunizations have been administered to a large part of the population. The severity of the illness varies, and a measles pneumonia may complicate the course of this disease, which in some cases can be life threatening. Mumps produces a parotitis and an orchitis. VZV infections in children manifest as chickenpox. Rubella, also called German measles, is a much milder infection than rubeola. Mononucleosis resulting from EBV infection is more likely to occur in adolescence.
PBD6 370

40. **(B)** Although nocardial infections typically start in the lungs, they often become disseminated, particularly to the central nervous system. These infections are most often seen in immunocompromised patients. Aspergillosis can also affect persons with immune compromise, but the fungal hyphae are easily distinguishable on hematoxylin and eosin stains. *Mycobacterium avium-intracellulare* infections are seen in persons with AIDS, but these are short, acid-fast rods that produce poorly formed granulomas. Bacterial pneumonias should also be considered in immunocompromised patients, and septicemia can complicate them, but *S. aureus* organisms form clusters of cocci on Gram stain. Mucor organisms have broad, nonseptate hyphae and are seen most commonly in diabetics and burn patients.
BP6 420   PBD6 334, 722

41. **(D)** The result of the Gram stain is diagnostic for *L. monocytogenes*, an organism more likely to produce disseminated disease in persons who are immunocompromised. These include injection drug users, who are at a high risk for HIV infection. Listeriosis is not known to be

acquired parenterally, although it can be a congenital infection.
BP6 726   PBD6 378

42.   **(A)** The skin lesions are typical for chickenpox, a common childhood infection caused by VZV infection. The infection can remain dormant for years in dorsal root ganglia, only to reactivate when immune status is diminished. Infertility is a complication of mumps orchitis. Paralysis can complicate poliovirus infection. Rheumatic heart disease can appear after group A β-hemolytic streptococcal infection. A chronic arthritis can be seen with Lyme disease after *B. burgdorferi* infection.
PBD6 373-374

43.   **(A)** Shigellosis results in a bloody dysentery because the *Shigella* organisms can invade and destroy the mucosa. There is typically a mononuclear infiltrate extending to the lamina propria with a neutrophilic exudate overlying the ulcerated areas. Granulomatous inflammation may be seen with granulomatous colitis (Crohn disease) and intestinal tuberculosis (rare). An increase in mononuclear inflammatory cells may appear with milder forms of enterocolitis caused by viruses, *Giardia*, and *Salmonella* spp. Intranuclear inclusions in enterocytes point to infection with DNA viruses, such as herpesviruses. Stricture formation may follow intestinal tuberculosis.
BP6 495   PBD6 355

44.   **(B)** This is a granuloma. Activated macrophages are the key cellular component within granulomas. CD4 cells secrete interferon-γ, which activates macrophages to kill organisms with reactive nitrogen intermediates. Eosinophils are not a major component of most granulomas, and they cannot destroy mycobacteria. NADPH-dependent reactive oxygen species are important in the lysis of bacteria by neutrophils. Complement mediated lysis is not involved in the destruction of intracellular bacteria such as *M. tuberculosis*. However, complement activation on the surface of *M. tuberculosis* can opsonize them for uptake by macrophages. *M. tuberculosis* organisms reside in phagosomes, which are not acidified into phagolysosomes. Inhibition of acidification is caused by the urease secreted by mycobacteria.
BP6 421-423   PBD6 349-351

45.   **(C)** This is a vesicle that has resulted from herpes simplex virus (HSV) infection. Most genital infections are caused by HSV-1, and HSV-2 is responsible for most cases of herpetic gingivostomatitis. The viral cytopathic effect results in formation of intranuclear inclusions, multinucleated cells, and cell lysis with vesicle formation in the epithelium. Cervical dysplasias do not produce vesicular lesions and are the result of another sexually transmitted disease—human papillomavirus infection. Gram-negative diplococci are characteristic for *N. gonorrhoeae* infection, another sexually transmitted disease. Lymphoplasmacytic infiltrates may be seen with a chancre caused by *T. pallidum*, the causative agent of syphilis. Trichomoniasis may

produce small blisters or papules, but these are often self-limited and not typically recurrent.
BP6 595-596   PBD6 360-361

46.   **(F)** He is infected with *S. mansoni* or *Schistosoma japonicum*. Female worms in the portal venous system release eggs that incite a granulomatous inflammatory reaction in liver. With time, the portal granulomas undergo fibrosis, compressing the portal veins. This gives rise to severe portal hypertension, splenomegaly, and ascites.
PBD6 396-397

47.   **(C)** She is infected with *Trypanosoma cruzi*, resulting in Chagas disease. The organisms can damage the heart by direct infection or by inducing an autoimmune response that affects the heart because of the existence of cross-reactive antigen. In 20% of infected persons, cardiac failure can occur 5 to 15 years after the initial infection. The affected heart is enlarged, and all four chambers are dilated.
PBD6 393-394

48.   **(E)** The *V. cholerae* organisms are noninvasive. Instead, they produce severe diarrhea by elaboration of an enterotoxin, called cholera toxin. This toxin acts on bowel mucosal cells to cause persistent activation of adenylate cyclase and high levels of intracellular cyclic AMP that drives massive secretion of sodium, chloride, and water. The fluid loss is life threatening because of resultant dehydration.
BP6 495   PBD6 357-358

49.   **(C)** Notice the septate branching hyphae and a fruiting body typical of *Aspergillus* colony. Neutropenia is a risk factor for development of aspergillosis. In immunocompromised patients, the various species of *Aspergillus* can produce sinusitis and pneumonitis most frequently, and dissemination to other sites such as the brain is common.
PBD6 380-381

50.   **(J)** Leprosy, also known as Hansen disease, is caused by the small acid-fast organism *M. leprae*. This organism cannot be cultured in artificial media. Diagnosis is by biopsy of a skin lesion. There are two polar forms of leprosy: tuberculoid and lepromatous. In the tuberculoid form, a delayed hypersensitivity reaction gives rise to granulomatous lesions that resemble tuberculosis. Acid-fast bacilli are rare in such lesions. In contrast, in the lepromatous form, shown in the figure, T-cell immunity is markedly impaired, and granulomas are therefore not formed. Instead, there are large aggregates of lipid-filled macrophages that are stuffed with acid-fast bacilli.
BP6 276   PBD6 385-387

51.   **(K)** The acute stage of Lyme disease is marked by the appearance of erythema chronicum migrans of the skin. As the *B. burgdorferi* organisms proliferate and disseminate, systemic manifestations of carditis, meningitis, and migratory arthralgias and myalgias appear. This is followed

2 to 3 years after initial infection by an arthritis of large joints.
BP6 686–687   PBD6 388–389

52.   **(D)** These are findings of congenital syphilis. Because the spirochetes cross the placenta in the third trimes- ter, early stillbirths do not occur. Most babies born with HIV infection have no initial gross or microscopic patho- logic findings. Herpes infections in the neonate are usually not initially obvious, because most such infections are ac- quired by passage through the birth canal. Congenital toxo- plasmosis and CMV produce severe cerebral disease.
BP6 592   PBD6 362–363

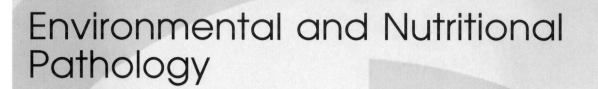

Environmental and Nutritional Pathology

CHAPTER

9

BP6 Chapter 8 - Environmental Diseases
PBD6 Chapter 10 - Environmental and
Nutritional Pathology

1. Since her early twenties, a 55-year-old female has been steadily gaining weight. She is now 164 cm tall and weighs 126 kg. Which of the following complications is she *least* likely to develop?

O (A) Osteoarthritis
O (B) Endometrial carcinoma
O (C) Diabetes mellitus
O (D) Pulmonary emphysema
O (E) Cholelithiasis

2. A 30-year-old male goes on a diving expedition to the Blue Hole off the coast of Belize. Over the course of 30 minutes, he descends to 50 meters, where he begins to feel light-headed and disoriented. He panics and ascends quickly to the surface. He soon experiences difficulty breathing, with dyspnea and substernal chest pain. He then develops a severe headache and vertigo. The best explanation for these findings is

O (A) Hypothermia
O (B) Decompression disease
O (C) Oxygen toxicity
O (D) Multiple contusions
O (E) Hypoxemia

3. A 50-year-old male with a history of chronic alcoholism has had increasing congestive heart failure for the past year. For the past month, he has experienced increasing confusion and disorientation, with difficulty ambulating. He is found on physical examination to have nystagmus and ataxia of gait, along with decreased sensation in his lower extremities. These findings point to a dietary deficiency of

O (A) Folate
O (B) Thiamine

O (C) Pyridoxine
O (D) Niacin
O (E) Riboflavin

4. A 43-year-old female has been taking oral contraceptives for many years and has noticed no side effects. She is at a higher risk than nonusers of developing which of the following tumors?

O (A) Endometrial cancer
O (B) Hepatic adenoma
O (C) Ovarian cancer
O (D) Gallbladder cancer
O (E) Pancreatic adenoma

For each of the clinical histories in questions 5 and 6, match the most closely associated disorder resulting from a nutritional deficiency:

(A) Beriberi
(B) Blindness
(C) Cheilosis
(D) Diabetes mellitus
(E) Goiter
(F) Hematuria
(G) Macrocytic anemia
(H) Marasmus
(I) Microcytic anemia
(J) Pellagra
(K) Rickets
(L) Scurvy

5. A 19-year-old pregnant female receives no prenatal care, eats a diet containing mostly carbohydrates and fats, and takes no prenatal vitamins with iron. The baby is born at term, but the baby is pale and listless in the first week of life. Laboratory tests reveal markedly decreased serum ferritin. (   )

6. A 55-year-old female has dementia worsening over the past year. She also has red, scaling skin in sun-exposed areas. A watery diarrhea has been present for the past month. (   )

7. At a party where a variety of drugs, legal and illicit, are being used, a 29-year-old previously healthy male suddenly collapses. He is taken to the hospital, requiring resuscitation with defibrillation en route to establish a normal cardiac rhythm. On admission, vital signs show his temperature to be 40°C, respirations 36, heart rate 110/min, and blood pressure 175/90 mm Hg. His pupils are dilated. Which of the following drugs is most likely responsible for these findings?

○ (A) Ethanol
○ (B) Heroin
○ (C) Marijuana
○ (D) Phencyclidine
○ (E) Cocaine

8. A suicidal ingestion of 35 g of acetaminophen results in symptoms of nausea and vomiting in a 26-year-old female. Within a day, which of the following laboratory test findings will indicate the most severe organ damage?

○ (A) Hypokalemia
○ (B) Elevated serum creatine kinase level
○ (C) Ketonuria
○ (D) Elevated serum alanine aminotransferase (ALT) level
○ (E) Hyperamylasemia

9. A baby born at term has Apgar scores of 8 and 9 at 1 and 5 minutes. The baby is initially doing well, but at 3 days of life, there is bleeding from the umbilical cord stump, and ecchymoses are observed over the buttocks. This is followed by seizure activity. Which of the following nutrient deficiencies best accounts for these findings?

○ (A) Iron
○ (B) Vitamin E
○ (C) Folic acid
○ (D) Vitamin K
○ (E) Iodine

10. Sir Robert Falcon Scott reaches the South Pole on January 17, 1912, barely a month after Roald Amundsen achieved this goal with his more experienced and prepared expeditionary party. Scott's dejected party must now make the long trip back to their base, but they are weak and running low on supplies. They finally can go no further, ironically only a few kilometers from a cache of supplies. They are found by a rescue team, but too late. Scott and his men are observed to have a hyperkeratotic, papular rash, ecchymoses, and severe gingival swelling with hemorrhages. A contributing cause of death was most likely

○ (A) Rickets
○ (B) Beriberi
○ (C) Scurvy
○ (D) Kwashiorkor
○ (E) Pellagra

11. A basal cell carcinoma is excised from the right lower eyelid of a 72-year-old male. Which of the following

forms of electromagnetic radiation played the greatest role in the development of this neoplasm?

○ (A) Ultraviolet rays
○ (B) Infrared rays
○ (C) Visible rays
○ (D) X-rays
○ (E) Gamma rays

12. Several children between the ages of 3 and 6 have been admitted to a local hospital for encephalopathic crisis. They previously exhibited retarded psychomotor development. Head computed tomography (CT) scans of the children reveal marked cerebral edema. An investigator sent to the housing project where the children live finds a rundown apartment complex with extensive water damage, poor plumbing, lack of ventilation, and peeling, flaking paint. Which of the following toxicities best accounts for the findings in these children?

○ (A) Sodium hypochlorite
○ (B) Ethylene glycol
○ (C) Methanol
○ (D) Kerosene
○ (E) Lead

13. A dull thudding noise followed by the sound of screeching tires is the signal for the emergency department staff to go outside the hospital. At the door to the emergency department, they find the body of a young man who is alive but obtunded. The examining physician notices that the man has a perforated nasal septum, and a prominent callus is present on his right thumb. A head CT scan reveals an acute right frontal lobe hemorrhage. He orders a serum drug screen, expecting to find

○ (A) Cocaine
○ (B) Opiates
○ (C) Cannabinoids
○ (D) Amphetamine
○ (E) Barbiturates

14. While touring the grounds of the Imperial Palace in Kyoto, a 75-year-old female collapses. She is hypotensive with tachycardia. The temperature in the shade is 34°C with 90% humidity. After drinking some cool green tea, she revives and continues on. The best explanation for these findings is

○ (A) Heat cramps
○ (B) Thermal inhalation injury
○ (C) Heat exhaustion
○ (D) Malignant hyperthermia
○ (E) Heat stroke

15. A previously healthy 52-year-old male who is a nonsmoker has an episode of hemoptysis with coughing. A chest radiograph reveals a 6-cm central right upper lobe mass. A sputum cytology shows atypical squamous cells suggestive of lung cancer. Which of the following inhaled pollutants is most likely to lead to these findings?

○ (A) Carbon monoxide
○ (B) Ozone

○ (C) Radon gas
○ (D) Silica
○ (E) Carbonaceous dust

16. Increased numbers of respiratory tract infections are observed among the children living in a community in which most families are at the poverty level. This finding most likely results from a deficiency of

○ (A) Vitamin E
○ (B) Vitamin D
○ (C) Vitamin K
○ (D) Vitamin A
○ (E) Vitamin B_1

For each of the clinical histories in questions 17 and 18, select the most closely associated drug or toxin:

(A) Amphetamine
(B) Barbiturate
(C) Benzodiazepine
(D) Cocaine
(E) Cyanide
(F) Ethanol
(G) Gasoline
(H) Heroin
 (I) Lead arsenate
 (J) Marijuana
(K) Mercuric chloride
(L) Methanol
(M) Organophosphate insecticide
(N) Penicillin
(O) Sulfonamide

17. A 4-year-old child ingests a 100-mL bottle of a clear liquid found under the kitchen sink. He develops central nervous system (CNS) depression over the next few hours. Acidosis is documented on admission to the hospital. Weeks later, it is noticed that the child's visual acuity is markedly decreased. (   )

18. A 20-year-old star football player suddenly collapses during play and suffers an immediate cardiac arrest from which he cannot be resuscitated. The medical examiner is called to investigate this sudden and unexpected death. Autopsy reveals marked coronary atherosclerosis and histologic evidence of hypertension in the renal blood vessels. (   )

19. A 36-year-old male is the owner of the radiator repair shop, where he works cleaning, cutting, polishing, and welding metals. The shop is poorly ventilated. Over several months, he develops worsening malaise with headache, abdominal pains, and difficulty holding on to his tools. A complete blood cell count reveals a microcytic anemia, with basophilic stippling of red blood cells on the peripheral blood smear. Which of the following laboratory tests will support the diagnosis of lead poisoning?

○ (A) Elevated blood levels of ALT and AST in the serum
○ (B) Elevated blood levels of creatine kinase
○ (C) Elevated blood levels of zinc protoporphyrin
○ (D) Hypernatremia
○ (E) Hypocalcemia

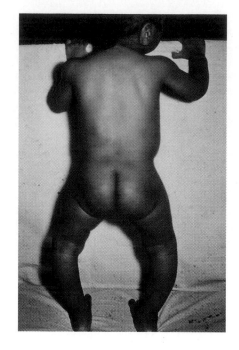

20. The child shown here is most likely to have

○ (A) Papular dermatosis
○ (B) Rickets
○ (C) Pellagra
○ (D) Beriberi
○ (E) Kwashiorkor

21. A boy falls off his bicycle while traveling down the street at 5 km/h. The skin of his right calf and right arm are scraped along the pavement so that the top layer of epidermis is removed. The best term for his injury is

○ (A) Incision
○ (B) Contusion
○ (C) Laceration
○ (D) Burn
○ (E) Abrasion

22. The rate of dental caries and tooth abscesses is high among children in an upper middle class community. This problem could be ameliorated by supplementing the water supply with

○ (A) Zinc
○ (B) Iodine
○ (C) Selenium
○ (D) Fluoride
○ (E) Copper

For each of the clinical histories in questions 23 and 24, match the most closely associated carcinogen:

(A) Acetaldehyde
(B) Arsenic
(C) Asbestos
(D) Benzidine
(E) Chromium
(F) Dioxins
(G) Naphthylamine
(H) Nickel
 (I) Polycyclic aromatic hydrocarbons

(J) Radon gas
(K) Ultraviolet radiation
(L) Vinyl chloride

23.   A 72-year-old male has had increasing dyspnea for the past year. Physical examination reveals decreased breath sounds on auscultating the right chest. A chest radiograph demonstrates a large pleural mass that nearly encases the right lung. A pleural biopsy reveals a malignant mesothelioma. (   )

24.   A 52-year-old male has been a lifeguard at a beach in California for the past 30 years. He has noticed a nodule on the outer helix of his left ear. This nodule is now 0.8 cm in diameter, with a central ulceration. It is excised and histologically determined to be a basal cell carcinoma. (   )

For each of the clinical histories in questions 25 and 26, match the most closely associated pollutant:

(A) Asbestos
(B) Beryllium
(C) Carbon monoxide
(D) Coal dust
(E) Nicotine
(F) Nitrous oxide compounds
(G) Oxygen
(H) Ozone
(I) Polycyclic aromatic hydrocarbons
(J) Silica
(K) Sulfur dioxide

25.   A 60-year-old female has a 90-pack per year history of smoking. She has had an increased cough for several months. In the past week, she had an episode of hemoptysis. A chest radiograph reveals a 7-cm, infiltrative perihilar mass in the right lung. (   )

26.   An older man who lives alone in a poorly ventilated house without central heating uses a small portable kerosene heater to warm the house during the winter months. He is found by a neighbor one morning in an obtunded state. (   )

27.   A 36-month-old male appears chronically ill. He has had a succession of respiratory infections in the past 6 months. The child is underdeveloped, only 50% of ideal body weight, and exhibits marked muscle wasting. Laboratory findings include a normal serum albumin but a decreased hemoglobin. These findings are most characteristic for

O (A) Marasmus
O (B) Leukemia
O (C) Folate deficiency
O (D) Kwashiorkor
O (E) Bulimia

28.   Xerophthalmia leads to erosion of a roughened corneal surface in the eyes of a 3-year-old child. This keratomalacia results in corneal scarring with eventual blindness after several years. The ocular damage could have been prevented by treating a dietary deficiency of

O (A) Protein
O (B) Vitamin K
O (C) Iron
O (D) Niacin
O (E) Vitamin A

29.   A 40-year-old male knows of his family history of colon carcinoma. He is concerned about this and wants to determine how best to reduce his risk. Which of the following dietary practices should he be advised to follow each day?

O (A) Drink a glass of red wine
O (B) Eat a bowl of ice cream
O (C) Reduce intake of chocolate
O (D) Consume more beef
O (E) Eat more vegetables

30.   Sending the children outside to play instead of having them parked for hours in front of the television set is most helpful in developing healthy

O (A) Bones
O (B) Eyes
O (C) Skin
O (D) Lungs
O (E) Kidneys

31.   A 5-year-old child is admitted to the hospital after ingestion of pills he found in a cabinet at home. The child is rapidly becoming obtunded and the major laboratory test findings are a serum AST level of 850 U/L and ALT level of 1052 U/L. The child's respiratory and cardiac status remain stable. Which of the following drugs was probably ingested?

O (A) Acetaminophen
O (B) Penicillin
O (C) Aspirin
O (D) Sulfamethoxazole
O (E) Codeine

32.   A history of heart disease in his mother, father, brother, and uncle prompts a 45-year-old male to consult his physician regarding his risk for coronary artery disease. He has a blood pressure of 125/80 mm Hg. He is 171 cm tall and weighs 91 kg. His blood glucose concentration is 181 mg/dL. What should his physician tell him regarding his diet?

O (A) Reduce your intake of saturated fat.
O (B) Increase your dietary fiber.
O (C) Take vitamin A supplements.
O (D) Do not put salt on your food.
O (E) Drink more water.

33.   A 55-year-old male receives 4000 cGy in divided doses to treat a squamous cell carcinoma of the larynx. A year later, there is no evidence of any residual carcinoma. However, which of the following histologic findings is most likely to be present in this patient?

O (A) Hypocellular bone marrow
O (B) Absent spermatogenesis
O (C) Colonic ulceration

○ (D) Vascular fibrosis
○ (E) Cerebral atrophy

34. During a qualifying match for the World Cup, the goalkeeper is hit in the chest by a football (soccer ball) struck from 10 meters away. He stays in the game. Which of the following injury patterns is most likely to be seen over the chest of the goalkeeper?

○ (A) Contusion
○ (B) Abrasion
○ (C) Laceration
○ (D) Incision
○ (E) Puncture

35. Over the course of 30 minutes, a 19-year-old university student at a fraternity party drinks 2L of mixed alcoholic beverages containing 50% ethanol by volume. He does not ordinarily drink much alcohol. His major use of drugs consists of acetaminophen for headaches. Which of the following complications is he most likely to experience?

○ (A) Hepatic cirrhosis
○ (B) Acute pancreatitis
○ (C) Sudden death
○ (D) Wernicke disease
○ (E) Massive hematemesis

For each of the clinical histories in questions 36 and 37, match the most closely associated nutrient that is deficient in the diet:

(A) Ascorbic acid
(B) Calcium
(C) Fluoride
(D) Folate
(E) Niacin
(F) Pyridoxine
(G) Riboflavin
(H) Selenium
(I) Vitamin A
(J) Vitamin B_{12}
(K) Vitamin K
(L) Zinc

36. A 42-year-old female is found to have a positive tuberculin skin test, and her chest radiograph shows some right upper lobe cavitary lesions. She is placed on isoniazid. However, after 6 months she has developed a peripheral neuropathy. (   )

37. A 75-year-old female lives alone and eats sparingly because of her low fixed retirement income. She has pain in her legs. A radiograph reveals a right tibial subperiosteal hematoma. A cut on her right hand is healing poorly. She has a hyperkeratotic rash. (   )

38. Contact with a frayed electrical cord carrying 120-volt, 10-ampere alternating current through the right hand of a 20-year-old male may result in death through which of the following mechanisms?

○ (A) Bronchoconstriction
○ (B) Cerebral artery thrombosis
○ (C) Heat stroke
○ (D) Gastric hemorrhage
○ (E) Ventricular fibrillation

39. A 5-year-old child exhibits generalized edema, ascites, and areas of desquamating skin over the trunk and extremities. The child has had recurrent upper respiratory infections for the past 2 months. Which of the following laboratory findings is most likely to be present in this child?

○ (A) Hyperglycemia
○ (B) Hypoalbuminemia
○ (C) Abetalipoproteinemia
○ (D) Megaloblastic anemia
○ (E) Hypocalcemia

40. A 48-year-old female has pain in her right wrist after a fall down a flight of stairs. A radiograph of her right hand and arm reveals marked osteopenia, along with a fracture of the radial head. Which of the following underlying diseases is most likely to contribute to her risk for fracture?

○ (A) Coronary atherosclerosis
○ (B) Pulmonary emphysema
○ (C) Primary biliary cirrhosis
○ (D) Chronic lymphocytic leukemia
○ (E) Atrophic gastritis

41. A 61-year-old male with a history of chronic arthritis complains of pronounced tinnitus. He also has some dizziness, with headache. Physical examination reveals some scattered petechiae over the upper extremities. A stool guaiac test result is positive. Which of the following drug toxicities best explains these findings?

○ (A) Penicillin
○ (B) Tetracycline
○ (C) Aspirin
○ (D) Chlorpromazine
○ (E) Quinidine

42. A 26-year-old female has had amenorrhea for the past 8 years. She incurs a right wrist fracture after a minor fall to the ground while getting out of an automobile, and she is found to have decreased bone density on performance of a radiographic densitometry. Laboratory findings include anemia and hypoalbuminemia. The underlying condition that best explains these findings is

○ (A) Kwashiorkor
○ (B) Obesity
○ (C) Anorexia nervosa
○ (D) Scurvy
○ (E) Rickets

43.   The most common worldwide dietary deficiency is

○ (A) Iron
○ (B) Calcium
○ (C) Folate
○ (D) Vitamin C
○ (E) Chocolate

44.   The firemen who initially responded to fight the fires from the Chernobyl nuclear reactor accident were exposed to high radiation levels. Some of them had dosages exceeding 5000 cGy. Within hours, they died from severe damage to

○ (A) Bone marrow
○ (B) Cerebrum
○ (C) Small intestine
○ (D) Heart
○ (E) Lungs

45.   There are no external findings on examination of the body of a 30-year-old female found in her hotel room an hour after firemen extinguish a fire on the floor below. Which of the following injuries best explains her death?

○ (A) Pseudomonas aeruginosa septicemia
○ (B) Inhalation injury
○ (C) Acute myocardial infarction
○ (D) Cerebral edema
○ (E) Malignant hyperthermia

46.   Chronic alcoholics are at increased risk for which of the following disorders?

○ (A) Blindness
○ (B) Carcinoma of the esophagus
○ (C) Carcinoma of the stomach
○ (D) Peripheral vascular disease
○ (E) Acute renal failure

For each of the clinical histories in questions 47 and 48, match the most closely associated drug:

(A) Acetaminophen
(B) Amphetamine
(C) Cannabinoids
(D) Cocaine
(E) Ethanol
(F) Flurazepam
(G) Heroin
(H) Lysergic acid
 (I) Meperidine
(J) Phencyclidine
(K) Phenobarbital
(L) Propoxyphene

47.   A fetus was stillborn at 36 weeks' gestational age to a 23-year-old female. The mother experienced the sudden onset of lower abdominal pain several hours before deliv-ery. An ultrasound scan revealed a large retroplacental hemorrhage. Delivery was accompanied by a 1200-mL blood loss. (   )

48.   A 22-year-old male is brought to the hospital emergency department in a state of respiratory depression. He exhibits convulsions for several minutes before a cardiac arrest ensues. Advanced cardiac life support measures are instituted, and he is stabilized and intubated. While performing a physical examination, the physician notices that he has needle tracks in the left antecubital fossa. He also has a temperature of 39.2°C. A loud diastolic heart murmur is audible. (   )

For each of the clinical histories with accompanying pictures in questions 49 and 50, match the most closely associated environmental insult or nutritional disease state that may be seen involving the skin on physical examination:

(A) Abrasion
(B) Blast injury
(C) Contusion
(D) Electrocution injury
(E) Gunshot wound
(F) Hypothermia
(G) Incision
(H) Kwashiorkor
 (I) Laceration
(J) Pellagra
(K) Scurvy
(L) Sunburn
(M) Therapeutic radiation
(N) Thermal burn
(O) Vitamin A toxicity
(P) Zinc deficiency

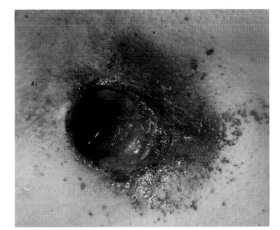

Courtesy of George Katsas, MD. Forensic pathologist, Boston.

49.   A 14-year-old boy was taken to the emergency department of a local hospital, where he died several hours later. His hematocrit was 17%. Figure shows a picture taken at autopsy (   )

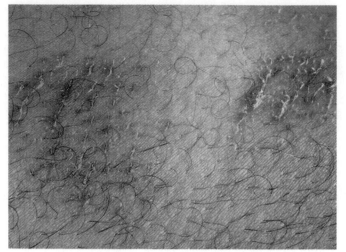

From the teaching collection of the Department of Pathology, Southwestern Medical School, Dallas, TX.

50. A 5-year-old boy is sent to be examined by a physician. This picture was recorded by the physician. A police agency suspects possible child abuse. (   )

ANSWERS

1. **(D)** She is morbidly obese. The extra weight puts strain on joints, particularly on the knees. The relation between endometrial carcinoma and obesity is well established. About 80% of persons with type II diabetes mellitus are obese. There is no association with pulmonary emphysema.
BP6 259-261   PBD6 452-454

2. **(B)** This patient developed decompression sickness on return from diving in the ocean. Too rapid an ascent results in dissolved nitrogen gas coming out of the blood to form bubbles that cause symptoms from occlusion of small arteries and arterioles. This process is called *the bends*. Hypothermia does not have significant symptoms or tissue effects. Oxygen toxicity causes pulmonary diffuse alveolar damage—a process that typically complicates intubation and mechanical ventilation in hospitalized patients. A blast injury may produce contusions, but the water pressure at 50 meters is not great enough to do this. The symptoms he has are not characteristic for hypoxemia.
PBD6 436

3. **(B)** Alcoholics are often deficient in thiamine and other nutrients (ethanol provides "empty calories"). Thiamine deficiency can lead to neuropathy, cardiomyopathy, and Wernicke disease. Alcoholics often have folate deficiency with macrocytic anemia. Pyridoxine or riboflavin deficiency can lead to neuropathy but not cerebral findings. Niacin deficiency leads to pellagra.
BP6 254-255   PBD6 447

4. **(B)** Although hepatic adenomas are rare tumors, there is a well-defined association between these benign liver tumors and prolonged oral contraceptive use. They can regress after cessation of the medication. There is no increase in the risk of endometrial cancer because the presence of progestins in oral contraceptives protects against the effect of estrogens. The incidence of ovarian cancer is actually lower in those who use the pill.
BP6 231   PBD6 414-416

5. **(I)** Iron deficiency gives rise to microcytic anemia. It is common in women of reproductive age, because of menstrual blood loss, and in children with a poor diet. Pregnant women have greatly increased iron needs. Serum ferritin is low in iron deficiency
BP6 258   PBD6 452

6. **(J)** Pellagra is caused by a deficiency of niacin. The classic presentation includes the "3 Ds" of diarrhea, dermatitis, and dementia.
BP6 255-256   PBD6 448

7. **(E)** Cocaine is a powerful vasoconstrictor and has a variety of vascular effects. Many complications result from the cardiovascular effects that include arterial vasoconstriction with ischemic injury and arrhythmias. Hyperthermia is another complication. Acute ethanolism may lead to CNS depression but not serious immediate cardiac effects. Heroin may produce acute pulmonary edema. Marijuana has no serious acute toxicities. Phencyclidine (PCP) produces an acute toxicity that mimics psychosis.
BP6 236   PBD6 412-413

8. **(D)** Acetaminophen toxicity leads to hepatic necrosis, and the ALT and AST levels are elevated. If death is not immediate, hyperbilirubinemia can also be seen. Hypokalemia can be a feature of renal diseases and of glucocorticoid deficiency. The serum creatine kinase level is elevated with injury to skeletal and cardiac muscle. Ketonuria is a feature of absolute insulin deficiency with diabetes mellitus; it is also a feature of starvation. The serum amylase is elevated with pancreatitis.
BP6 231   PBD6 416

9. **(D)** Coagulation factors synthesized by the liver require vitamin K for their production. Hemorrhagic disease of the newborn can occur because endogenous production of vitamin K is limited in neonates. This results from minimal establishment of the intestinal bacterial flora that produce this nutrient. Iron deficiency leads to anemia, not to bleeding. Vitamin E is an antioxidant and is rarely deficient to a degree leading to serious illness. Folic acid helps to prevent a macrocytic anemia. Iodine is needed in small quantities for thyroid hormone synthesis.
BP6 253-254   PBD6 446-447

10. **(C)** Because humans do not generate vitamin C endogenously, they must have a continuous dietary supply. The lack of fresh fruits and vegetables with vitamin C led to scurvy in many explorers in centuries past. Rickets is seen in children deficient in vitamin D. Beriberi leads to heart failure and results from thiamine deficiency. Kwashi-

orkor results from protein deficiency. Pellagra (with diarrhea, dermatitis, and dementia) is seen with niacin deficiency.
BP6 256-257   PBD6 449-451

11. **(A)** Exposure to sunlight is a risk for malignancies involving the skin (i.e., basal cell carcinoma, squamous cell carcinoma, and malignant melanoma). The ultraviolet rays, mainly the UVB component of UV light, are the major causative agent for these malignancies. Infrared radiation causes mainly thermal injury. Visible light has minimal effects. The ambient x-radiation and gamma rays that filter through the earth's atmosphere are very small in quantity.
BP6 711   PBD6 430-431

12. **(E)** Old flaking paint that is lead based has a sweet taste, attracting children to ingest it. The major risk to children from lead ingestion is neurologic damage. Household bleach (sodium hypochlorite) is a local irritant and is not likely to be found in the living conditions of these children. Ethylene glycol is found in antifreeze and can produce acute renal tubular necrosis. Methanol ingestion can cause acute CNS depression, acidosis, and blindness. Kerosene, a hydrocarbon, can cause gastrointestinal and respiratory toxicity when ingested.
BP6 231-233   PBD6 420-422

13. **(A)** Cocaine, as a powerful vasoconstrictive agent, causes ischemic injury to the nasal septum following the route of administration—inhalation. CNS hemorrhages may occur as an acute complication. The callus comes from flicking the lighter for the crack cocaine pipe. Opiates can be CNS and respiratory depressants. Cannabinoids in marijuana do not generally cause serious acute problems. Amphetamines are CNS stimulants. Barbiturates are CNS depressants.
BP6 236-237   PBD6 412-413

14. **(C)** Heat exhaustion results from the failure of the cardiovascular system to compensate for hypovolemia caused by water depletion. It is readily reversible by replacing lost intravascular volume. Vigorous exercise with electrolyte loss can produce muscle cramping typical of heat cramps. Inhalation injury is seen when a fire occurs in an enclosed space, and hot, toxic gases are inhaled. Malignant hyperthermia occurs from a metabolic derangement such as thyroid storm or with drugs such as succinyl choline.
BP6 240   PBD6 434-435

15. **(C)** There is a natural seepage of radon gas from soil, more so in some geographic locations than others. This gas can collect in houses and is a potential cause for lung cancer. The pollutant gases carbon monoxide and ozone are not associated with lung cancer, nor are dusts containing carbon such as coal dust. Silicosis may possibly increase the risk for lung cancer, but there is severe restrictive lung disease with silicosis.
BP6 242-243   PBD6 418

16. **(D)** Vitamin A is important in maintaining epithelial surfaces, and a deficiency can lead to squamous metaplasia of respiratory epithelium, predisposing to infection. Vitamin E deficiency is rare, and when present, it causes neurologic symptoms related to degeneration of the axons in the posterior columns of the spinal cord. Vitamin D deficiency in children leads to rickets, with bone deformities. Vitamin K deficiency can result in a bleeding diathesis. Vitamin B_1 (thiamine) deficiency leads to a variety of problems including Wernicke disease, neuropathy, and cardiomyopathy.
BP6 246-248   PBD6 439-441

17. **(L)** Methanol is metabolized by the same enzymatic pathway as ethanol, but the toxic metabolites formaldehyde and acetaldehyde are produced, which damage the CNS and the retina.
BP6 232   PBD6 412

18. **(D)** Cocaine is a powerful vasoconstrictor, and the cardiac complications include arterial vasoconstriction with ischemic injury and arrhythmias. Atherosclerosis, affecting small peripheral coronary arterial branches, can be marked.
BP6 236-237   PBD6 412-413

19. **(C)** This person has experienced occupational exposure to lead and shows symptoms and signs of lead toxicity. The concentration of zinc protoporphyrin is elevated in chronic lead poisoning, in anemia of chronic disease, and in iron deficiency anemia. Lead interferes with heme biosynthesis and inhibits the incorporation of iron into heme so that zinc is used instead. Hepatic damage with elevation of liver enzymes ALT and AST is not a major feature of lead poisoning. The level of the muscle enzyme creatine kinase is not elevated because muscle is not directly damaged by lead, although a neuropathy can occur. Lead can damage renal tubules and cause renal failure, but specific alterations in electrolytes with elevated sodium or decreased calcium are not specific for lead-induced renal failure.
BP6 232-233   PBD6 420-422

20. **(B)** This skeletal deformity with bowing of the legs results from vitamin D deficiency in children, known as rickets. Hyperkeratosis with follicular plugging from vitamin A deficiency leads to papular dermatosis marked by extensive papular excrescences on the skin. Pellagra from niacin deficiency can lead to dermatitis in sun-exposed areas of skin. Beriberi from thiamine deficiency can result in heart failure with peripheral edema. A diet poor in protein can result in kwashiorkor, with areas of flaking, depigmented skin.
BP6 249-250   PBD6 444-445

21. **(E)** A scraping injury produces an abrasion, but the skin is not broken. An incised wound is made with a sharp instrument such as a knife, leaving clean edges. A contusion is a bruise with extravasation of blood into soft tissues. Lacerations break the skin or other organs in an irregular fashion. A burn injury causes coagulative necrosis without mechanical disruption.
BP6 238   PBD6 432

22. **(D)** Water in some places naturally contains fluoride, and dental problems in children are fewer in these places. Fluoride can be put in the drinking water, but opposition from ignorance or fear is common. Zinc deficiency can produce a hemorrhagic dermatitis. Iodine deficiency can predispose to goiter. Selenium deficiency can result in a myopathy. Copper deficiency can produce neurologic defects. Serious illnesses from trace element deficiencies are rare.
BP6 258   PBD6 452

23. **(C)** Asbestos fibers can cause pulmonary interstitial fibrosis, and there is an increased risk for malignancy. Persons who have had asbestos exposure and who are smokers have a greatly increased incidence of bronchogenic carcinoma. Mesothelioma is uncommon, even in persons with asbestos exposure, but virtually all occurences are in persons who have been exposed to asbestos.
BP6 227-229   PBD6 732-733

24. **(K)** The UVA and UVB portions of the ultraviolet spectrum contribute to an increased incidence of skin cancer in persons with chronic sunlight exposure.
PBD6 430-431

25. **(I)** The infiltrative perihilar mass suggests lung cancer. Polycyclic hydrocarbons and nitrosamines, found in tobacco smoke, are the key contributors to the development of lung cancer.
BP6 223   PBD6 408-409

26. **(C)** Heating devices that burn hydrocarbons such as petroleum products generate carbon dioxide, which can build up to dangerous levels in unventilated or poorly ventilated houses. Chronic carbon monoxide poisoning produces CNS damage. The carbon monoxide binds much more tightly to hemoglobin than does oxygen and leads to hypoxia. Decreased mental functioning generally begins at carboxyhemoglobin levels greater than 20%, with death likely above 60%.
BP6 234   PBD6 418

27. **(A)** Body weight less than 60% of normal with muscle wasting is consistent with marasmus, which results from a marked decrease in total caloric intake. In kwashiorkor, protein intake is reduced more than total caloric intake, and body weight is usually 60% to 80% of normal, with hypoalbuminemia a key laboratory finding. Malignancies can promote wasting, but not to this degree. This child's problems are far more serious then a single vitamin deficiency; a lack of folate could account for the child's anemia, but not wasting. Bulimia is an eating disorder of adolescents and adults that is characterized by binge eating and self-induced vomiting.
BP6 244-245   PBD6 437-439

28. **(E)** Vitamin A is essential to maintain epithelia. The lack of vitamin A affects the function of lacrimal glands and conjunctival epithelium, promoting keratomalacia. Dietary protein is essential for building tissues, particularly muscle, but it has no specific effect in maintaining ocular structures. Vitamin K is beneficial for synthesis of coagulation factors by the liver to prevent bleeding problems. Iron is essential for production of heme to manufacture hemoglobin used in making red blood cells. Niacin deficiency leads to diarrhea, dermatitis, and dementia.
BP6 248   PBD6 439-441

29. **(E)** More fruits and vegetables are recommended in the diet to help prevent colon cancer. Vitamins C and E have an antioxidant and antimutagenic effect. Red wine in moderation may have a beneficial antiatherogenic effect. Ice cream can include animal fat that may promote cancer, as would the animal fat of beef.
BP6 261-262   PBD6 455-456

30. **(A)** Vitamin D can be synthesized endogenously in skin with exposure to ultraviolet light. Vitamin D with calcium helps to build growing bone. The exercise helps build bone mass. Given the increases in air pollution in many cities, pulmonary diseases are increasing, with children being at risk. Renal function is not greatly affected by environment.
BP6 248   PBD6 442-445

31. **(A)** Acetaminophen toxicity produces hepatic necrosis. This effect is enhanced with prior ethanol ingestion. Hepatic necrosis is indicated by extremely high levels of AST and ALT. Penicillin may cause systemic anaphylaxis in a few persons. Aspirin can produce a metabolic acidosis. Sulfa drugs may produce renal failure. Opiates, including codeine, are CNS and respiratory depressants.
BP6 230   PBD6 416

32. **(A)** These findings suggest a diagnosis of diabetes mellitus. He is also obese and most likely has type II diabetes. Type I and type II diabetes greatly increase the risk for early and accelerated atherosclerosis. Decreasing total caloric intake, particularly saturated fat, helps reduce the risk for coronary artery disease. Vegetable and fish oils are better than animal fat in terms of dietary lipid for prevention of atherosclerosis. Dietary fiber helps to reduce the incidence of diverticulosis. Vitamin A has no known effect on atherogenesis. Reducing dietary sodium helps to lower blood pressure. More fluid intake aids renal function.
BP6 261   PBD6 452-454

33. **(D)** Therapeutic doses of radiation can cause acute vascular injury, manifested by endothelial damage and an inflammatory reaction. With time, these vessels undergo fibrosis and suffer severe luminal narrowing. There is ischemia of the surrounding tissue and formation of a scar. The radiation used in therapeutic dosages is carefully delivered in a limited field to promote maximal tumor damage while reducing damage to surrounding tissues. Whole-body irradiation affects marrow, gonads, gastrointestinal tract, and brain.
BP6 242-243   PBD6 428

34. **(A)** A blow with a blunt object produces soft tissue hemorrhage without breaking the skin. An abrasion scrapes away the superficial epidermis. A laceration is an irregular tear in the skin or other organ. An incised wound is made by a sharp object and is longer than a puncture, which has a rounded outline and is deeper than it is wide.
BP6 238   PBD6 432-434

35. (C) The large amount of ethanol ingested over a short time can elevate his blood ethanol to toxic levels, because the alcohol dehydrogenase in liver metabolizes ethanol by first-order kinetics. Cirrhosis is a long-term complication of chronic ethanolism. Likewise, pancreatitis is also a feature of chronic use of ethanol. Wernicke disease is rare, even in alcoholics, and probably occurs from nutritional thiamine deficiency. Hematemesis from gastritis and gastric ulceration are more typically seen with chronic ethanolism, and variceal bleeding is a complication of hepatic cirrhosis. The combination of acetaminophen and ethanol increases the likelihood of hepatic toxicity.
BP6 234-235 PBD6 410-412

36. (F) Isoniazid (INH) is a pyridoxine antagonist. Persons on INH therapy for tuberculosis may need vitamin B₆ supplementation.
BP6 256 PBD6 449

37. (A) Scurvy can be subtle. A diet must contain a constant supply of vitamin C, because none is made endogenously. Older persons with a poor diet are just as much at risk as younger persons.
BP6 256-257 PBD6 449-451

38. (E) Electrical current, especially alternating current, disrupts nerve conduction and electrical impulses, particularly in heart and brain. This can lead to severe arrhythmias, especially ventricular fibrillation. These are immediate effects. The amount of tissue injury from standard (U.S.) household current is generally not great, and there may be just a small thermal injury at the site of entry or exit of the current on the skin.
BP6 240 PBD6 435

39. (B) The findings are consistent with kwashiorkor, a nutritional disorder predominantly of decreased protein in the diet. Hypoalbumenia is characteristic of this condition. The wasting of diabetes mellitus affects adipose tissue and muscle, and edema is not a feature. Abetalipoproteinemia is a rare disorder leading to vitamin E deficiency. Megaloblastic anemia is a feature of specific deficiencies of vitamin B₁₂ or folate. Hypocalcemia can occur as a consequence of vitamin D deficiency.
BP6 244-245 PBD6 437-439

40. (C) The osteopenia can result from osteomalacia, the adult form of vitamin D deficiency. Vitamin D is one of the fat-soluble vitamins, and it requires fat absorption, which can be impaired by chronic cholestatic liver disease, biliary tract disease, and pancreatic disease. Heart disease from atherosclerosis does not affect bone density. Emphysema can result in a hypertrophic osteoarthropathy, but not osteopenia. Leukemias do not tend to erode bone. Atrophic gastritis affects vitamin B₁₂ absorption.
BP6 251 PBD6 444-445

41. (C) Chronic aspirin toxicity (more than 3 g/day) can result in a variety of neurologic problems. Aspirin also inhibits platelet function by suppressing the production of thromboxane A₂, promoting bleeding. The best known complication of penicillin therapy is systemic anaphylaxis.

Tetracycline therapy may be complicated by a fatty liver. Chlorpromazine ingestion may lead to cholestatic jaundice. Quinidine therapy may lead to hemolytic anemia.
BP6 231-232 PBD6 416

42. (C) The decreased food intake from self-imposed dieting in an adult female can lead to changes such as hormonal deficiencies (e.g., follicle-stimulating hormone, luteinizing hormone, thyroxine). The result is diminished estrogen synthesis, which promotes osteoporosis just as in the postmenopausal state. Kwashiorkor is a disease mainly of children who have reduced protein intake. Obesity can be accompanied by specific nutritional deficiencies, even though total caloric intake is increased, but hypogonadism is not a typical feature. Scurvy from vitamin C deficiency does not affect hormonal function. Rickets is a specific deficiency of vitamin D in children resulting in skeletal deformities.
BP6 246 PBD6 439

43. (E) There is never quite enough chocolate, and much of the world's population has to get by without it. Of course, serious dietitians would choose answer A, which is a deficiency most likely to be seen in menstruating women, in pregnant women, and in children. Calcium is most important in growing children for building bones. Folate deficiency leads to macrocytic anemia and is most likely to occur in adults with a poor diet, such as persons with chronic alcoholism. Vitamin C deficiency occurs in persons who do not get enough fresh fruits and vegetables.
BP6 258 PBD6 452

44. (B) The cerebral syndrome occurs within hours with a massive total-body radiation dose. Death can occur with dosages from 200 to 700 cGy but takes days to weeks from injury to radiosensitive marrow and gastrointestinal tract. Muscle tissue is relatively radioresistant. Early findings with radiation lung injury include edema, and interstitial fibrosis develops over years if survival occurs.
BP6 243 PBD6 426-427

45. (B) Fires in enclosed spaces produce hot, toxic gases. The inhalation of these gases can lead to death without any injury from flames. Infections follow a burn injury by days to weeks because of the loss of an epithelial barrier to infectious agents. An acute myocardial infarction is possible but not probable at her age. Cerebral edema is a complication more likely during recovery from a burn injury. The condition of malignant hyperthermia, when core body temperature exceeds 40°C, is produced by metabolic disorders such as hyperthyroidism and drugs such as succinylcholine and cocaine.
BP6 239 PBD6 434

46. (B) Alcohol increases the risk of cancer in the upper aerodigestive tract, including the mouth, pharynx, and esophagus. In the stomach, it can cause acute and chronic gastritis, but there is no reported increase in gastric cancer. Peripheral vascular disease is usually caused by atherosclerosis. Alcohol does not increase atherosclerotic disease incidence. Blindness is an acute toxic effect of methanol

ingestion. Acute renal failure results from ingestion of ethylene glycol.
BP6 234-235 PBD6 412

47. **(D)** Cocaine has powerful vasoactive effects, including vasoconstriction. The effects on the placenta can include decreased blood flow with fetal hypoxia and spontaneous abortion, placentae abruption, and fetal hemorrhages. With chronic maternal cocaine use, the babies demonstrate neurologic impairment.
BP6 236-237 PBD6 412-413

48. **(G)** Heroin is an opiate narcotic that is a derivative of morphine. Opiates are CNS depressants. Overdoses are accompanied by respiratory depression, convulsions, and cardiac arrest. The typical mode of administration is by injection, and there is often an infection, such as an endocarditis, that results from such use.
BP6 237 PBD6 414

49. **(E)** This is the entry site for a gunshot wound made from close range. There is a sharply demarcated skin defect, and the surrounding skin demonstrates some stippling of unburned gunpowder.
BP6 238 PBD6 433

50. **(A)** There are superficial tears in the epidermis, with underlying superficial dermal hemorrhage. Abrasions are made by a scraping type of injury.
BP6 238 PBD6 432

Diseases of Infancy and Childhood

BP6 Chapter 7 - Genetic and Pediatric
           Diseases
PBD6 Chapter 11 - Diseases of Infancy and
           Childhood

1. A baby born at term weighs 1900 g. The head size is normal, but the crown-heel length and foot length are reduced. No external malformations are observed. Through infancy, developmental milestones are delayed. The most likely condition occurring during gestation that could lead to these findings is

○ (A) Pregnancy-induced hypertension
○ (B) Down syndrome
○ (C) Maternal diabetes mellitus
○ (D) Congenital cytomegalovirus
○ (E) Erythroblastosis fetalis

2. An 18-month-old, apparently healthy African-American boy is found dead in his crib one morning. The terrified and distraught parents, both blue-collar workers, are interviewed by the medical examiner and indicate that the child was not ill. The medical examiner finds no gross or microscopic abnormalities at autopsy, and all toxicologic tests are negative. The medical examiner tells the parents that, although she cannot find the cause of death, she feels that sudden infant death syndrome (SIDS) is very unlikely. This conclusion by the medical examiner is based on which of the following factors:

○ (A) Sex of the child
○ (B) Race of the child
○ (C) Age of the child
○ (D) Low socioeconomic background of parents
○ (E) Absence of any abnormality in the respiratory centers

3. A premature male newborn delivered after 28 weeks' gestation develops difficulty in breathing 2 days after birth. A chest radiograph reveals a bilateral ground-glass appearance. He is treated with assisted ventilation and nutritional support. He seems to improve for the first 24 hours but then becomes progressively more cyanotic. He develops terminal seizures and dies 4 days after birth. The most likely histologic finding in the lungs would be

○ (A) Diffuse alveolar septal fibrosis
○ (B) Alveolar hyaline membranes and atelectasis
○ (C) Extensive alveolar transudate
○ (D) Bronchiolar mucus plugging
○ (E) A frothy (bubbly) alveolar exudate

4. Steatorrhea as a consequence of pancreatic acinar atrophy with fibrosis is most likely to be seen in a child with

○ (A) Galactose-1-phosphate uridyl transferase deficiency
○ (B) A low-density lipoprotein (LDL) receptor gene mutation
○ (C) Abnormal fibrillin production by fibroblasts
○ (D) Impaired epithelial cell chloride ion transport
○ (E) Phenylalanine hydroxylase deficiency

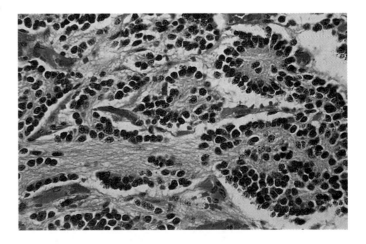

5. An infant is found to have a palpable abdominal mass, along with fever and weight loss. An abdominal CT scan reveals a 5.5-cm mass involving the right adrenal gland. A 24-hour urine homovanillic acid (HVA) is increased. This adrenal is surgically excised, and the histologic appearance

of the mass is shown in the figure. Which of the following clinical or histologic features of this lesion is associated with a poor prognosis?

○ (A) Age younger than 1 year
○ (B) Hyperdiploidy
○ (C) Presence of many ganglion cells
○ (D) N-*myc* gene amplification
○ (E) Malformations of the kidney

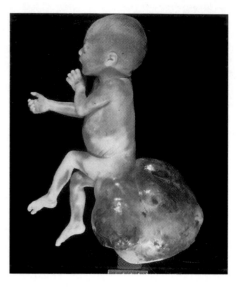

6. A cesarean section must be performed at 27 weeks because of the lesion shown in the figure. The 28-year-old mother began to have preterm labor. The depicted lesion is most likely to be a

○ (A) Teratoma
○ (B) Neuroblastoma
○ (C) Hemangioma
○ (D) Lymphangioma
○ (E) Hamartoma

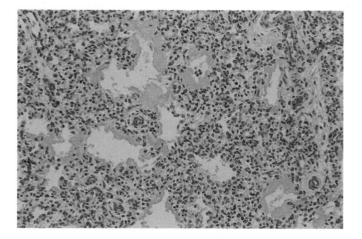

7. A 31-week-gestational-age neonate has initial Apgar scores of 5 and 6 at 1 and 5 minutes; but within an hour, the baby is in severe respiratory distress and dies despite resuscitative measures. Microscopic examination of the baby's lungs at autopsy is shown in the figure. Which of the following conditions best accounts for these findings?

○ (A) Maternal toxemia of pregnancy
○ (B) Marked fetal anemia
○ (C) Congenital toxoplasmosis
○ (D) Immaturity of the lungs
○ (E) Oligohydramnios

8. Soon after birth, a 40-week-gestational-age baby has a heart murmur audible on auscultation of the chest. On echocardiography there is a membranous ventricular septal defect (VSD). Which of the following events is most likely to have resulted in the appearance of this VSD?

○ (A) Dispermy at conception
○ (B) Maternal thalidomide use
○ (C) Maternal rubella infection
○ (D) Erythroblastosis fetalis
○ (E) Folate deficiency

9. The amount of surfactant in the developing lung increases between the 26th and 32nd weeks of gestation. This increase is related to which of the following developmental events?

○ (A) Differentiation of alveoli from embryonic foregut
○ (B) Increased density of pulmonary capillaries
○ (C) Development of ciliated epithelium in airspaces
○ (D) Differentiation of type II alveolar epithelial cells
○ (E) Apoptosis in interlobular mesenchymal cells

10. A 22-year-old primigravida delivers a 38-week-gestational-age male baby that appears normal on physical examination, except for a single midline cleft of the upper lip. This cleft lip interferes with breast-feeding, although the baby gains weight normally. The mother asks you if there is any risk that her other children will be born with a similar malformation. You give the following advice:

○ (A) It is highly unlikely that other offspring will have a similar defect.
○ (B) There is a small but definite risk, in the range of 2% to 7%, that her other children will have a cleft lip.
○ (C) It is likely that one half of her offspring will have cleft lip.
○ (D) The risk of having other children with a similar defect is one in four.
○ (E) Her sons but not daughters are at risk for cleft lip.

11. A 20-year-old female is planning for her first pregnancy, and she is advised by her physician that she must begin a phenylalanine-free diet before conception and must continue with this diet throughout all three trimesters of her pregnancy. Otherwise, her baby could be affected by

○ (A) Mental retardation
○ (B) Muscular weakness
○ (C) Cataracts
○ (D) Anemia
○ (E) Congestive heart failure

12.   Which of the following factors is most likely to increase the risk for neonatal hyaline membrane disease in a 34-week-gestational-age baby?

○ (A) Maternal corticosteroid therapy
○ (B) Chorioamnionitis
○ (C) Gestational diabetes
○ (D) Oligohydramnios
○ (E) Pregnancy induced hypertension

For each of the clinical histories in questions 13 and 14, match the most closely associated infectious agent that may cause infection in the neonatal period:

   (A) *Candida albicans*
   (B) Cytomegalovirus
   (C) Group B streptococcus
   (D) Herpes simplex virus
   (E) Human immunodeficiency virus (HIV)
   (F) *Listeria monocytogenes*
   (G) Parvovirus
   (H) Rubella virus
   (I) *Toxoplasma gondii*
   (J) *Treponema pallidum*

13.   A 33-year-old female is in the 32nd week of pregnancy when she notices lack of fetal movement for 3 days. No fetal heart tones can be auscultated. The fetus is delivered stillborn. Autopsy reveals scattered microabscesses in liver, spleen, brain, and placenta. No congenital anomalies are found. There have been similar fetal losses within the same community over the past 3 months. (   )

14.   A neonate born at 36 weeks' gestation manifests hydrops fetalis and hepatosplenomegaly. The baby is also found to have a hemoglobin concentration of 9.4 g/dL and platelet count of 67,000/μL. The baby has generalized icterus and scattered ecchymoses of the skin. Death occurs at 14 days after birth. Autopsy reveals extensive subependymal necrosis with microscopic evidence for encephalitis. Within the areas of necrosis are large cells containing intranuclear inclusions. (   )

15.   A baby is born prematurely at 32 weeks' gestation. The infant requires 3 weeks of intubation with positive pressure ventilation and dies at 4 months of age. At autopsy the infant's lungs show bronchial squamous metaplasia with peribronchial fibrosis, interstitial fibrosis, and dilation of air spaces. Which of the following conditions best explains these findings?

○ (A) Sudden infant death syndrome
○ (B) Ventricular septal defect
○ (C) Cystic fibrosis
○ (D) Lung injury due to positive pressure ventilation
○ (E) Pulmonary hypoplasia

16.   A baby born at term has become mildly icteric, with a neonatal bilirubin concentration of 4.9 mg/dL over the first few days of life. No morphologic abnormalities are found on physical examination. The pregnancy and the delivery were uncomplicated for the 18-year-old mother. The direct Coombs test on the baby's red blood cells is positive. The baby's blood type is A negative. Based on these findings, which of the following events is most likely to occur?

○ (A) Kernicterus
○ (B) Complete recovery
○ (C) Respiratory distress syndrome
○ (D) Fetal demise in the next pregnancy
○ (E) Hemolytic anemia throughout infancy

17.   A large "port wine stain" involves the left side of the face of a 3-year-old child. This irregular, slightly raised, red-blue area is not painful, but is very disfiguring. Histologically, this lesion is most likely composed of a proliferation of

○ (A) Neuroblasts
○ (B) Lymphatics
○ (C) Fibroblasts
○ (D) Lymphoblasts
○ (E) Capillaries

18.   There is no screening test to detect carriers of mutations in the cystic fibrosis gene (CFTR) because of which of the following limitations?

○ (A) Most mutations in the CFTR cannot be detected by polymerase chain reaction (PCR).
○ (B) Fluorescent in situ hybridization technique for detecting the mutation is very labor intensive and expensive.
○ (C) There are several hundred mutations in the CFTR gene that can give rise to cystic fibrosis.
○ (D) Molecular techniques can detect mutations in CFTR only when both copies of the gene are abnormal.
○ (E) The frequency of heterozygotes in the population is less than 1 in 10,000.

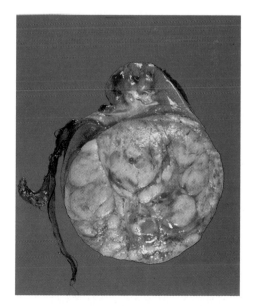

19.   The renal lesion shown here was present in a 3-year-old child who had a palpable abdominal mass. The child later had abdominal distention from bowel obstruction. Which of the following congenital disorders greatly increases the risk of developing this lesion?

○ (A) Edwards syndrome
○ (B) Marfan syndrome
○ (C) Beckwith-Wiedemann syndrome
○ (D) McArdle syndrome
○ (E) Klinefelter syndrome

20. At birth, a male neonate is noticed to be small for 38-weeks' gestational age. Physical examination reveals microcephaly, short palpebral fissures, and maxillary hypoplasia. Which of the following conditions is most likely to lead to these findings?

○ (A) Congenital rubella
○ (B) Placenta previa
○ (C) Maternal diabetes mellitus
○ (D) Trisomy 21
○ (E) Fetal alcohol syndrome

21. At 18 weeks' gestation, ultrasound reveals hydrops fetalis, but no malformations are found. This is the third pregnancy for the 20-year-old mother, whose previous pregnancies all ended in term live births. The baby is liveborn at 36 weeks but has a cord blood hemoglobin level of only 9.2 g/dL, and the total bilirubin concentration is 20.2 mg/dL. Which of the following laboratory test findings best explains the pathogenesis of this baby's disease?

○ (A) Positive Coombs' test result on cord blood
○ (B) Elevated maternal serum α-fetoprotein level
○ (C) Positive maternal hepatitis B surface antigen
○ (D) Diminished glucocerebrosidase activity in fetal cells
○ (E) Placental culture positive for *Listeria monocytogenes*

22. A 3-month-old infant was found dead by his mother late one evening. When she put him in bed only an hour before, he had shown no signs of distress. The baby's term birth had followed an uncomplicated pregnancy, and he had been feeding well and gaining weight normally. What is the medical examiner most likely to find at autopsy?

○ (A) Hyaline membrane disease
○ (B) Cerebral cytomegalovirus
○ (C) Tetralogy of Fallot
○ (D) Adrenal neuroblastoma
○ (E) No abnormalities

23. A 25-year-old gravida 3 para 2 female in her 39th week of pregnancy felt no fetal movement for 1 day. The baby was stillborn on vaginal delivery a day later. Microscopic examination of the placenta revealed marked acute chorioamnionitis. Which of the following infectious agents was most likely responsible for these events?

○ (A) Cytomegalovirus
○ (B) *T. pallidum*
○ (C) Herpes simplex virus
○ (D) *Toxoplasma gondii*
○ (E) Group B *Streptococcus*

24. Soon after birth, a baby of 31 weeks' gestation develops respiratory distress requiring intubation with positive pressure ventilation. Ultrasound at 20 weeks' gestation had revealed no abnormalities. However, premature labor experienced by the 19-year-old mother led to the emergent vaginal delivery. Which of the following prenatal diagnostic tests could have best predicted this baby's respiratory distress?

○ (A) Maternal serum level of α-fetoprotein
○ (B) Amniotic fluid phospholipid analysis
○ (C) Chromosome analysis
○ (D) Coombs test on cord blood
○ (E) Genetic analysis for cystic fibrosis gene

For each of the descriptions of a patient with a genetic disease in questions 25 and 26, select the most closely associated gene product that is likely to be abnormal or absent with that disease?

(A) Adenosine deaminase
(B) Alpha$_1$-antitrypsin
(C) Dystrophin
(D) Factor VIII
(E) Fibrillin
(F) Galactose-1-phosphate uridyl transferase
(G) Globin chains
(H) Glucocerebrosidase
(I) Glucose-6-phosphatase
(J) Hexosaminidase
(K) Lysosomal acid maltase
(L) Muscle phosphorylase
(M) Phenylalanine hydroxylase
(N) Spectrin
(O) Sphingomyelinase

25. A 3-year-old, light-skinned African-American child has developmental delay with mental retardation and inability to walk. The child's urine has a distinctly "mousy" odor. On physical examination, there is no lymphadenopathy or hepatosplenomegaly. The child is not anemic. (   )

26. A term infant develops vomiting with diarrhea a few days after birth. By the end of the first week of life, the neonate is icteric. Cataracts develop a month later. Developmental milestones are not being met at 1 year of age. The baby succumbs to *Escherichia coli* septicemia at age 2. (   )

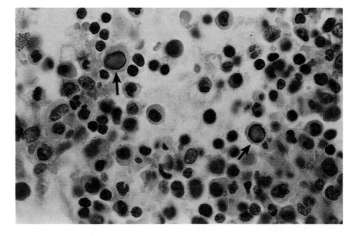

27. A stillborn boy of 33 weeks' gestational age was severely hydropic. The pregnancy was reported by the mother, a 19-year-old primigravida, to be uncomplicated,

and an ultrasound performed at 16 weeks had shown no abnormalities. The mother had only experienced a mild rash involving her face around 18 weeks' gestation. At autopsy, the stillborn is found to have no congenital malformations, although there is cardiomegaly. From the histologic appearance of the bone marrow shown in the figure, the most likely cause for these findings is

○ (A) Maternal IgG crossing the placenta
○ (B) A chromosomal anomaly of the fetus
○ (C) A congenital neuroblastoma
○ (D) Inheritance of two abnormal *CFTR* genes
○ (E) An infection with parvovirus B19

28. A 25-year-old female has had four previous first- and second-trimester spontaneous abortions. She is now in the 16th week of her fifth pregnancy. She has had no prenatal problems so far. Her blood type is A positive, the serologic test for syphilis is negative, and she is rubella immune. Which of the following laboratory tests would be most useful for determining the cause of recurrent fetal loss in this patient?

○ (A) Maternal serum α-fetoprotein determination
○ (B) Genetic analysis for the *CFTR* gene
○ (C) Maternal serologic test for HIV
○ (D) Amniocentesis with chromosome analysis
○ (E) Maternal serum antibody screen

29. Examination of a stillborn fetus delivered at 20 weeks' gestation reveals an abdominal wall defect lateral to the umbilical cord insertion, marked vertebral scoliosis, and a thin, fibrous band constricting the right lower extremity, which lacks fingers. None of the other three pregnancies, which ended in term births for the 31-year-old mother, were similarly affected. These findings are most typical for

○ (A) Trisomy 18
○ (B) Oligohydramnios
○ (C) Maternal fetal Rh incompatibility
○ (D) Amniotic band syndrome
○ (E) Congenital cytomegalovirus infection

30. Synthetic retinoids can be successfully used to treat acne. However, pregnant women are advised against using this medication because retinoic acid can cause congenital malformations. The teratogenic effect of retinoic acid is related to its ability to affect which of the following processes?

○ (A) Increasing the risk of maternal infections
○ (B) Reducing the resistance of fetus to transplacental infections
○ (C) Increasing the likelihood of aneuploidy during cell division
○ (D) Abnormal development of blood vessels in the placenta
○ (E) Disrupting the pattern of expression of homeobox genes

31. Which of the following etiologic factors is the most common cause of congenital malformations?

○ (A) Single-gene mutations of large effect
○ (B) Maternal infections
○ (C) Maternal drug use
○ (D) Interaction of multiple genes with environmental factors
○ (E) Chromosomal aberrations resulting from mitotic errors early during gestation

32. A morphologically normal looking infant born at 37 weeks' gestation weighs 1500 g. This weight is below the 10th percentile for age. Further examination reveals that, although the crown-heel length is below normal for the gestational age, head circumference is normal. Which of the following causes is most likely to be responsible for this condition?

○ (A) Transplacental spread of maternal toxoplasmosis
○ (B) Nondisjunction of chromosomes during maternal oogenesis
○ (C) Nondisjunction of chromosomes within the trophoblast
○ (D) Failure of fetal kidneys to develop
○ (E) Inheritance of mutant alleles at the cystic fibrosis transmembrane conductance regulator (CFTR) from both parents

33. Examination of a 20-week-gestational age stillborn fetus shows amniotic bands that extend from amputated fingers and toes of both feet and another band in a cleft through the right aspect of the skull. How would you classify the underlying abnormality in this case?

○ (A) Disruption
○ (B) Malformation
○ (C) Teratogenesis
○ (D) Inflammation
○ (E) Deformation

34. An 18-month-old male child is not gaining weight normally. His mother notes that the child's abdomen seems larger. There are increased levels of vanillylmandelic acid (VMA) and homovanillic acid (HVA) in the child's urine. An abdominal ultrasound scan is most likely to reveal a mass in the

○ (A) Liver
○ (B) Adrenal
○ (C) Kidney
○ (D) Spleen
○ (E) Colon

35. A baby born at term develops abdominal distention in the first week of life. Meconium ileus is diagnosed. Subsequently, the infant has persistent steatorrhea and fails to develop normally. Which of the following laboratory test findings is most likely related to the infant's underlying disease:

○ (A) Decreased serum thyroxine level
○ (B) Positive HIV serology
○ (C) Elevated sweat chloride
○ (D) Increased urine homovanillic acid level
○ (E) Hyperbilirubinemia

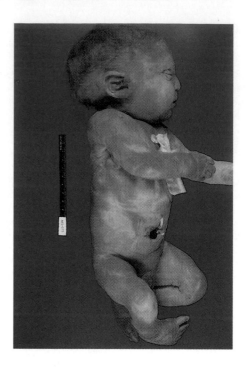

36. A baby born at 36 weeks' gestation shows the facial features and positioning of extremities shown here. The baby soon develops severe respiratory distress. Which of the following conditions best explains these findings?

○ (A) Congenital rubella infection
○ (B) Bilateral renal agenesis
○ (C) Maternal diabetes mellitus
○ (D) Hyaline membrane disease
○ (E) Trisomy 13

ANSWERS

1. **(A)** The baby is small for gestational age because of intrauterine growth retardation. The asymmetric growth suggests a maternal or placental cause. Fetal problems such as chromosomal abnormalities, infections, and erythroblastosis are likely to produce symmetric growth retardation. Babies born to diabetic mothers are likely to be larger than normal for gestational age. Fetal hydrops can accompany congenital infections and erythroblastosis, which may artificially increase fetal weight.
BP6 203   PBD6 461–462

2. **(C)** Although the cause of SIDS is unknown, certain risk factors are well established. Among these is age. SIDS occurs between 1 month and 1 year of age. Ninety per cent of SIDS deaths occur during the first 6 months of life. Although age alone cannot exclude SIDS in this case, all other factors provided increase the risk of SIDS. Male sex, African-American race, low socioeconomic background of parents, and absence of anatomic abnormality all favor the

likelihood of SIDS. The only factor that argues against SIDS in this case is the age of 18 months.
BP6 205   PBD6 481–482

3. **(B)** This premature newborn does not have sufficient type II alveolar cell surfactant production. As a result, the baby has developed hyaline membrane disease. If the baby were to survive but go on to develop bronchopulmonary dysplasia, fibrosis would be apparent. An alveolar transudate or exudate may accompany a variety of conditions but is not the key feature of hyaline membrane disease. Mucus plugging occurs in cystic fibrosis, but this is not a common finding in neonatal lungs.
BP6 204–205   PBD6 471–472

4. **(D)** The abnormal chloride ion transport in cystic fibrosis results in abnormal mucus secretions in pancreatic ducts that cause plugging with subsequent acinar atrophy with fibrosis. Galactose-1-phosphate uridyl transferase deficiency gives rise to galactosemia. Patients with this condition have liver damage but no pancreatic abnormalities. Abnormalities of LDL receptor with familial hypercholesterolemia lead to accelerated atherogenesis. Abnormal fibrillin is a feature of Marfan syndrome. Phenylketonuria results from a deficiency of phenylalanine hydroxylase.
BP6 207–209   PBD6 477–481

5. **(D)** Amplification of the N-*myc* oncogene occurs in about 25% of neuroblastomas, and the greater the number of copies, the worse is the prognosis. Such N-*myc* amplification tends to occur in neuroblastomas with a higher stage or with chromosome 1p deletions. Hyperdiploidy or near triploidy is usually associated with lack of N-*myc* amplification, absence of 1p deletion, and high levels of nerve growth factor receptor Trk A expression. All these bode for good prognosis. The presence of ganglion cells is consistent with a better differentiation and better prognosis; some tumors may differentiate over time and become ganglioneuromas under the influence of Trk A. Renal malformations are not related to neuroblastomas.
BP6 211–212   PBD6 486–487

6. **(A)** Teratomas are benign neoplasms composed of tissues derived from embryonic germ layers (i.e., ectoderm, mesoderm, or endoderm). Teratomas occur in midline locations, and the sacrococcygeal area is the most common. Less common immature or frankly malignant teratomas with neuroblastic elements can occur. Neuroblastomas are malignant childhood tumors most commonly arising in the adrenal. Hemangiomas form irregular red-blue skin lesions that are flat and spreading. Lymphangiomas are most often lateral head and neck lesions in childhood. Hamartomas are masses composed of tissues normally found at a particular site, and they are rare.
BP6 210–211   PBD6 484

7. **(D)** The immaturity of the fetal lungs before 35 to 36 weeks' gestation can be complicated by lack of sufficient surfactant to provide for adequate ventilation after birth. This can result in hyaline membrane disease. Tests on amniotic fluid before birth, including lecithin-sphingomyelin ratio, fluorescence polarization, and lamellar body

counts, are useful to predict the degree of pulmonary immaturity. Maternal toxemia and congenital infections may lead to hyaline membrane disease if the birth occurs prematurely as a consequence of these conditions, but they do not directly affect lung maturity. Oligohydramnios may result in neonatal respiratory distress through the mechanism of pulmonary hypoplasia.
BP6 204-205   PBD6 471-472

8.   **(C)** Rubella infection in the first trimester, when organogenesis is occurring (4 to 9 weeks' gestation), can lead to congenital heart defects. Dispermy leads to triploidy, a condition that rarely results in a live birth. Thalidomide use in the past was an important cause of malformations (almost invariably, prominent limb deformities). The use of thalidomide as an immunosuppressive agent is under consideration. Erythroblastosis fetalis leads to fetal anemia with congestive heart failure and hydrops but not to malformations. Folate deficiency is most likely to be associated with neural tube defects.
BP6 201-202   PBD6 466-467

9.   **(D)** Surfactant is synthesized by type II pneumocytes that line the alveolar sacs. They begin to differentiate after the 26th week of gestation. These cells can be recognized on electron microscopy by the presence of lamellar bodies. Surfactant production increases greatly after 35 weeks' gestation. Other structures in the lung do not synthesize the phosphatidylcholine and phosphatidylglycerol compounds that are important in reducing alveolar surface tension.
BP6 204-205   PBD6 471-472

10.   **(B)** Most malformations, particularly those that are isolated defects, have no readily identifiable cause. They are believed to be caused by the inheritance of a certain number of genes and the interaction of those genes with environmental factors. Their transmission follows the rules for multifactorial inheritance. The rate of recurrence is believed to be in the range of 2% to 7% and is the same for all first-degree relatives, regardless of sex and relationship to the index case.
BP6 201-202   PBD6 466-467

11.   **(A)** Persons with phenylketonuria survive to reproductive age with good mental function when they are treated from infancy with a phenylalanine-free diet. After neurologic development is completed in childhood, the diet is no longer needed. However, a pregnant woman with phenylketonuria has high levels of phenylalanine, which can damage the developing fetus. Going on a phenylalanine-free diet is a major sacrifice, because there are few foods that have no phenylalanine. (Persons without phenylketonuria can find drinking even 100 mL of a liquid phenylalanine-free meal to be difficult.) Phenylketonuria does not affect tissues other than the CNS, and there are no malformations in children with phenylketonuria.
BP6 184   PBD6 475-476

12.   **(C)** The hyperinsulinism in the fetus of a diabetic mother suppresses pulmonary surfactant production. Corticosteroids stimulate surfactant production. Infection may increase the risk for premature birth but does not signifi-

cantly affect surfactant production. Oligohydramnios leads to constriction in utero that culminates in pulmonary hypoplasia, not decreased surfactant. Maternal hypertension may reduce placental function and increase growth retardation but typically does not have a significant effect on the production of surfactant.
BP6 204   PBD6 471-472

13.   **(F)** Listeriosis can be a congenital infection. Pregnant women may have only a mild diarrheal illness themselves, but the organism can prove devastating to the fetus or neonate. Mini-epidemics of listeriosis are often linked to a contaminated food source, such as dairy products, chicken, and hot dogs. Neonatal meningitis can be caused by *L. monocytogenes*.
PBD6 378

14.   **(B)** Although about 90% of cytomegalovirus-infected neonates have no overt disease, infection can be extensive in some cases. The brain is often involved, although the inclusions can be found in many organs. The renal tubular epithelium can be infected, and large cells with inclusions can be seen with urine microscopic examination in some cases. Cytomegalovirus manifested in neonates may have been acquired transplacentally, at birth, or in breast milk.
PBD6 376

15.   **(D)** High-dose oxygen with positive pressure ventilation can cause injury to immature lungs, leading to the chronic lung disease known as bronchopulmonary dysplasia. With SIDS, no anatomic abnormalities are found at autopsy. A VSD could eventually lead to pulmonary hypertension from shunting. Pulmonary manifestations of cystic fibrosis are not manifest at birth or in infancy. Mortality with pulmonary hypoplasia is greatest at birth.
BP6 205   PBD6 472-473

16.   **(B)** This is a mild hemolytic anemia, probably an ABO incompatibility with maternal blood type of O, so that anti-A antibody coats fetal cells. Although most anti-A and anti-B antibodies are IgM, in about 20% to 25% of pregnancies there are also IgG antibodies, which cross the placenta in sufficient titer to produce mild hemolytic disease, at least in most cases. At term, the bilirubin in this case is not high enough to produce kernicterus. At term, respiratory distress is unlikely. ABO incompatibilities are not likely to have as serious consequences for subsequent pregnancies as Rh incompatibility. As the baby matures, the maternal antibody diminishes.
BP6 206   PBD6 473

17.   **(E)** The most common tumor of infancy is a hemangioma, and these benign neoplasms form a large percentage of childhood tumors as well. Though benign, they can be large and disfiguring. A proliferation of neuroblasts occurs in neuroblastoma, a common childhood neoplasm in the abdomen. Lymphangioma is another common benign childhood tumor seen in the neck, mediastinum, and retroperitoneum. Fibromatoses are fibromatous proliferations of soft tissues that form solid masses. Lymphoblasts as part of

leukemic infiltrates or lymphomas are not likely to be seen in skin, but mediastinal masses may be seen.
BP6 210   PBD6 483

18. **(C)** When a genetic disease (e.g., cystic fibrosis) is caused by many different mutations, no simple screening test that can detect all the mutations can be performed. Although 70% of patients with the disease have a 3–base pair deletion that can be readily detected by PCR, the remaining 30% are caused by several hundred allelic forms of CFTR. To detect all would require sequencing of the CFTR genes. This prohibits mass screening.
BP6 207–209   PBD6 478–479

19. **(C)** This uncommon syndrome carries an increased risk for the development of Wilms' tumor, which is a childhood neoplasm arising in the kidney. Renal anomalies such as horseshoe kidney can be seen with Edwards syndrome (trisomy 18) but not neoplasms. Likewise, Marfan syndrome is not associated with an increased risk for malignancy. Children with a deficiency of myophosphorylase in McArdle syndrome can have muscle cramping but are not at risk for neoplasia. The 47,XXY karyotype of Klinefelter syndrome does not carry an increased risk for renal tumors.
BP6 213–214   PBD6 488–489

20. **(E)** Alcohol is perhaps one of the most common environmental teratogens affecting fetuses, although the effects can be subtle. The children so affected tend to continue to be developmentally impaired. Congenital rubella, which has its major effects during organogenesis in the first trimester, results in more pronounced defects, including congenital heart disease. Placenta previa, a low-lying placenta at or near the cervical os, can cause significant hemorrhage at the time of delivery, or uteroplacental insufficiency with growth retardation before delivery. Placental causes of intrauterine growth retardation result in asymmetric growth retardation with sparing of the brain. Maternal diabetes often results in a larger baby, and malformations may be present as well. The findings of trisomy 21 are subtle at birth but typically include brachycephaly, not microcephaly.
BP6 202   PBD6 467

21. **(A)** The baby has erythroblastosis fetalis from maternal antibody coating fetal cells and causing hemolysis. The fetal anemia leads to congestive heart failure and hydrops. Hemolysis results in a very high bilirubin. A high maternal serum level of α-fetoprotein suggests a fetal neural tube defect, and neural tube defects are not associated with hydrops. Viral hepatitis is not a perinatal infection. Diminished glucocerebrosidase activity causes Gaucher disease. This does not lead to perinatal liver failure or anemia. Listeriosis or other congenital infections may produce hydrops and anemia, although not of this severity.
BP6 206–207   PBD6 473–475

22. **(E)** The events suggest SIDS. The cause is unknown, and by definition there are no significant gross or microscopic autopsy findings. Infants with congenital anomalies or infections are unlikely to be doing well. Hyaline membrane disease occurs at birth with prematurity. Congenital neoplasms are a rare cause for sudden death.
BP6 205   PBD6 481–482

23. **(E)** The acute inflammation suggests a bacterial infection, and group B *Streptococcus*, which can colonize the vagina, is a common cause. The infection can develop quickly. Cytomegalovirus, syphilis, and toxoplasmosis are congenital infections that can cause stillbirth, but they are more likely to be chronic. Herpetic infections are most likely to be acquired by passage through the birth canal.
BP6 203   PBD6 470

24. **(B)** The baby most likely had hyaline membrane disease from fetal lung immaturity and lack of surfactant. Surfactant consists predominantly of dipalmitoyl phosphatidylcholine. The adequacy of surfactant production can be gauged by the phospholipid content of amniotic fluid because fetal lung secretions are discharged into the amniotic fluid. The maternal serum alpha-fetoprotein is useful to predict fetal neural tube defects and chromosomal abnormalities. Chromosome analysis may help to predict problems after birth or the possibility of fetal loss. The Coombs test may help to determine presence of erythroblastosis fetalis. Cystic fibrosis does not cause respiratory problems at birth.
BP6 204   PBD6 471–472

25. **(M)** The child has phenylketonuria. The absence of phenylalanine hydroxylase genes give rise to hyperphenylalaninemia, which impairs brain development and can lead to seizures. The block in phenylalanine metabolism results in decreased pigmentation of skin and hair. It also results in the formation of intermediate compounds, such as phenylacetic acid, that are excreted in urine and impart to it a "mousy" odor. Because of the devastating consequences of this inherited disorder and because it can be treated with a phenylalanine-free diet, this is one of the diseases tested for at birth, even though it is rare.
BP6 184–185   PBD6 475–476

26. **(F)** The baby has findings associated with galactosemia, an autosomal recessive condition that can be tested for at birth. Histologically, the liver of affected infants has marked fatty change, and portal fibrosis that increases over time. In addition to hepatic lesions, the patients have diarrhea and develop cataracts. For unknown reasons, they are very susceptible to *E. coli* septicemia.
BP6 185   PBD6 476–477

27. **(E)** The erythroid precursors demonstrate large pink intranuclear inclusions typical for parvovirus. In adults, such an infection typically causes "fifth disease," which is self-limited. However, this is one of the "O" infections in the TORCH mnemonic describing congenital infections (*t*oxoplasmosis, *o*ther infections, *r*ubella, *c*ytomegalovirus infection, and *h*erpes simplex infection). Parvovirus infection in the fetus can lead to a profound fetal anemia with cardiac failure and hydrops fetalis. Erythroblastosis fetalis is unlikely to occur with the first pregnancy, and there is only erythroid expansion, not erythroid inclusions. Al-

though a variety of chromosomal anomalies—monosomy X in particular—may lead to hydrops, malformations are typical. Congenital tumors are an uncommon cause for hydrops, and they should produce a mass lesion. Cystic fibrosis does not affect erythropoiesis.
PBD6 470,474

28. **(D)** Multiple fetal losses earlier in gestation suggest the likelihood of a chromosomal abnormality—the mother or father may be the carrier of a balanced translocation. The maternal serum level of α-fetoprotein can help find cases of fetal neural tube defects, but this is not a cause for early fetal loss. Maternal HIV infection is not a cause for significant fetal loss. Cystic fibrosis produces postnatal problems. Because the mother is blood type A positive, fetal loss with erythroblastosis fetalis is unlikely.
BP6 214-215   PBD6 182

29. **(D)** This is a classic example of an embryonic disruption that leads to the appearance of congenital malformations. Fibrous bands and possible vascular insults may explain such findings, which fall in the spectrum of a "limb-body wall complex" that includes amniotic band syndrome. In trisomy 18 and other chromosomal abnormalities, an omphalocele is the most common abdominal wall defect. Oligohydramnios with diminished amniotic fluid leads to deformations, not disruptions. Rh incompatibility can give rise to erythroblastosis fetalis, which may manifest as hydrops fetalis. Fetuses affected by hydrops present with widespread edema and intense jaundice. A variety of malformations may occur as a result of congenital infections, but not amnionic bands.
BP6 200   PBD6 465

30. **(E)** Retinoic acid embryopathy characterized by cardiac, neural, and craniofacial defects is believed to result from the ability of retinoids to affect the expression of homeobox (HOX) genes. These genes are important in embryonal patterning of limbs, vertebrae, and craniofacial structures.
PBD6 469

31. **(D)** Multifactorial inheritance is the single most common known cause of congenital malformations. This information is useful for advising patients of the likelihood of recurrence. Most cases of congenital anomalies from multifactorial inheritance have recurrence risk that ranges from 2% to 7%. All the other listed causes added together are about equal to multifactorial inheritance.
BP6 201-202   PBD6 466-467

32. **(C)** The infant has asymmetric intrauterine growth retardation that can result from placental causes. Confined placental mosaicism, resulting from genetic errors in dividing trophoblasts, is responsible in 90% of cases. Transplacental spread of infection to the fetus would give rise to proportionate intrauterine growth retardation (IUGR). Nondisjunction of chromosomes during maternal oogenesis

would affect the fetus very early on and would also result in symmetric growth retardation. Failure of kidneys to develop can cause oligohydramnios, and the fetus would be abnormal in appearance. Mutation at both alleles of the CFTR gives rise to cystic fibrosis. This is not associated with intrauterine growth retardation.
BP6 203   PBD6 461-462

33. **(A)** This is amniotic band syndrome, a subset of limb-body wall complex, which results from embryonic disruption with destruction of body regions and formation of fibrous bands. A malformation, such as congenital heart disease, results from an error in morphogenesis. Chromosomal abnormalities can be accompanied by a variety of malformations. Inflammation can produce malformations, as with congenital syphilis, or tissue destruction, as with congenital cytomegalovirus infection. Deformations result from mechanical forces on organs and tissues, an example of which is the facial features seen with oligohydramnios.
BP6 200-201   PBD6 464-465

34. **(B)** The presence of an abdominal mass and metabolites of catecholamines in the urine strongly indicate a neuroblastoma. The adrenal is the most common location for a neuroblastoma. Extra-adrenal paraganglia are other common sites. Hepatoblastomas of the liver and Wilms' tumor of the kidney are childhood tumors but do not secrete catecholamines. Splenic neoplasms are rare at any age. Colon cancers are seen in older persons more commonly but occasionally occur even in teenagers (with an inherited mutation in the APC gene).
BP6 211-212   PBD6 485-487

35. **(C)** The findings are typical for cystic fibrosis, which is an inherited defect in chloride transport. Cretinism from hypothyroidism results in impaired CNS and skeletal development. A baby with congenital HIV infection may have a variety of infections. The increased urine homovanillic acid is a feature of neuroblastoma, a mass lesion that could also cause bowel obstruction but not meconium ileus. Neonatal jaundice has a variety of causes, including the inherited disorder called galactosemia.
BP6 207-209   PBD6 477-481

36. **(B)** The flattened face and deformed feet suggest oligohydramnios resulting from renal agenesis. Fetal kidneys produce urine that becomes the amniotic fluid. Pulmonary hypoplasia is the rate-limiting step to survival. Congenital rubella can lead to a variety of malformations, not deformations. Babies born to diabetic mothers have an increased risk of congenital anomalies. Fetal lung maturity is typically achieved at 34 to 35 weeks' gestation, and hyaline membrane disease is unlikely at 36 weeks. Trisomy 13 is accompanied by a variety of malformations, including those affecting the kidneys. The external features, however, are quite different, and they almost always have midline defects such as cleft lip and palate and microcephaly.
BP6 201   PBD6 465

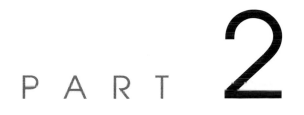

PART 2

DISEASES OF ORGAN SYSTEMS

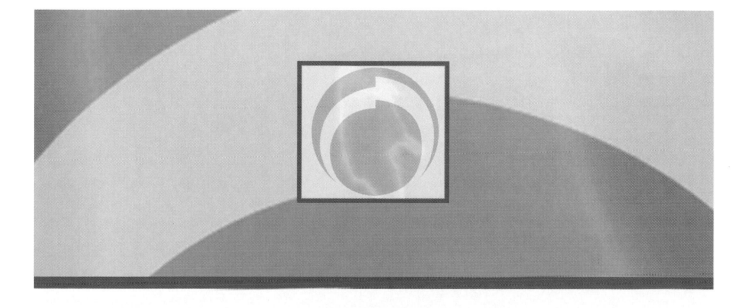

C H A P T E R
11

Blood Vessels

BP6 Chapter 10 - Blood Vessels
PBD6 Chapter 12 - Blood Vessels

1. Atherosclerotic plaques are slowly but constantly changing in ways that promote clinical events. Which of the plaque alterations listed is *least* likely to lead to ischemia in the coronary artery circulation?

- (A) Thinning of the media
- (B) Ulceration of the plaque surface
- (C) Thrombosis
- (D) Hemorrhage into the plaque substance
- (E) Intermittent platelet aggregation

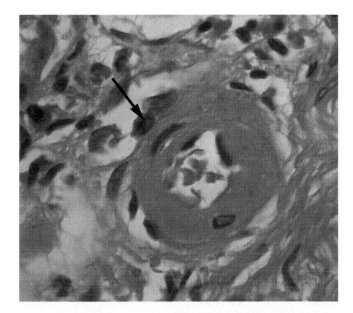

2. The high-magnification microscopic appearance of the kidney shown in the figure is most indicative of which of the following underlying conditions?

- (A) *Escherichia coli* septicemia
- (B) Hypertension
- (C) Colonic adenocarcinoma
- (D) Syphilis
- (E) Polyarteritis nodosa

For each of the patient descriptions in questions 3 through 5, match the associated lettered vascular disease process:

- (A) Angiosarcoma
- (B) Aortic dissection
- (C) Arteriovenous fistula
- (D) Atherosclerotic aneurysm
- (E) Giant cell arteritis
- (F) Glomus tumor
- (G) Granuloma pyogenicum
- (H) Hemangioma
- (I) Henoch-Schönlein purpura
- (J) Kaposi sarcoma
- (K) Polyarteritis nodosa
- (L) Takayasu arteritis
- (M) Telangiectasia
- (N) Thromboangiitis obliterans
- (O) Wegener granulomatosis

3. An 80-year-old male with a long history of smoking survived a small myocardial infarction several years earlier. He has poor pulses peripherally in his lower extremities. His blood pressure is 165/100 mm Hg. Fasting serum glucose measurements are in the range of 170 to 200 mg/dL. He has a 7-cm, pulsating mass in the midline of his lower abdomen. ( )

4. A 7-year-old child presents with abdominal pain, purpuric skin lesions, hematuria, and proteinuria. A skin biopsy shows necrotizing vasculitis of small dermal vessels. A renal biopsy shows immune complex deposition in glo-

meruli with some IgA-rich immune complexes. Serum determinations are negative for antineutrophil cytoplasmic antibodies (p-ANCA and c-ANCA). (   )

5. A 50-year-old male presents with chronic cough, nasopharyngeal ulcers, and a serum urea nitrogen level of 75 mg/dL with a creatinine concentration of 6.7 mg/dL. A nasal biopsy shows necrosis and necrotizing granulomatous inflammation. A transbronchial lung biopsy shows a vasculitis involving the small peripheral pulmonary arteries and arterioles. Granulomatous inflammation is seen within and adjacent to small arterioles. His serologic titers for c-ANCA are high and rising. (   )

6. A 61-year-old male had a myocardial infarction a year ago. This was the first major illness in his life. He now wants to prevent another myocardial infarction, and he is advised to begin a program of exercise and a change in his dietary habits. Which of the following serum laboratory test findings would give the best indication a year later of the success of his diet and exercise regimen?

○ (A) Cholesterol
○ (B) Glucose
○ (C) Potassium
○ (D) Renin
○ (E) Calcium

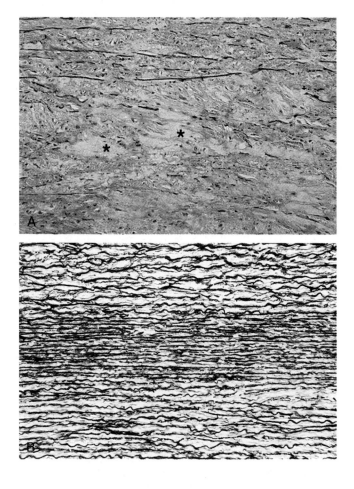

7. A 23-year-old male experiences the sudden onset of severe, sharp chest pain. A chest radiograph reveals a wid-

ened mediastinum. Transesophageal echocardiography shows a dilated aortic root and arch with a tear in the aortic intima 2 cm distal from the great vessels. From the microscopic appearance of the aorta with elastic stain shown in the figure, the most likely underlying disease is

○ (A) Scleroderma
○ (B) Diabetes mellitus
○ (C) Hypertension
○ (D) Marfan syndrome
○ (E) Wegener granulomatosis

8. A pulsatile abdominal mass is palpated in a 40-year-old male who has had worsening abdominal pain for the past week. An abdominal computed tomography (CT) scan reveals a 6-cm fusiform enlargement of the abdominal aorta. He is taken to surgery, and an abdominal aortic graft is placed. The underlying disease process in his case is most likely

○ (A) Polyarteritis nodosa
○ (B) Obesity
○ (C) Diabetes mellitus
○ (D) Systemic lupus erythematosus (SLE)
○ (E) Syphilis

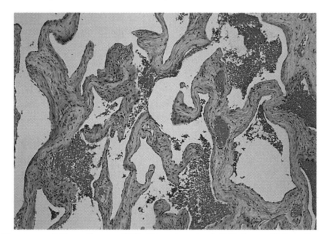

Courtesy of Tom Rogers, MD, Department of Pathology, University of Texas Southwestern Medical School, Dallas, TX.

9. A spongy, 2-cm, dull red, circumscribed lesion has been present since infancy on the upper outer left arm of a 10-year-old male. This lesion is excised, and the microscopic appearance is shown here. This lesion is most likely to be

○ (A) Kaposi sarcoma
○ (B) Angiosarcoma
○ (C) Lymphangioma
○ (D) Telangiectasia
○ (E) Hemangioma

10. A pharmaceutical company is trying to develop an anti-atherosclerosis agent. Which of the following mechanisms of action is likely to have the most effective anti-atherosclerotic effect?

○ (A) Inhibits the release of platelet-derived growth factor (PDGF) and inhibits macrophage-mediated lipoprotein oxidation

(B) Promotes the release of PDGF and inhibits macrophage-mediated lipoprotein oxidation

(C) Inhibits the release of PDGF and promotes macrophage-mediated lipoprotein oxidation

(D) Decreases the level of high-density lipoprotein (HDL) and inhibits macrophage-mediated lipoprotein oxidation

(E) Increases the level of intercellular adhesion molecule-1 (ICAM-1) and vascular cell adhesion molecule-1 (VCAM-1) on endothelial cells and increases endothelial permeability

11. At autopsy, the thoracic aorta of a 73-year-old male has a dilated root and arch, giving the intimal surface a "tree bark" appearance. Microscopically, the aorta shows an obliterative endarteritis of the vasa vasorum. Which of the following laboratory test findings is most likely to be found recorded in this patient's medical record?

(A) High double-stranded DNA titer

(B) p-ANCA positive at 1:1024

(C) Sedimentation rate of 105 mm/h

(D) 4+ ketonuria

(E) Antibodies against *Treponema pallidum*

12. For the past 3 weeks, a 70-year-old female has been recuperating from a bout of viral pneumonia complicated by bacterial pneumonia, during which time she has been bedridden. She now has some swelling and tenderness of her right leg, which is made worse on raising or moving this leg. Her condition is best called

(A) Lymphedema

(B) Disseminated intravascular coagulopathy (DIC)

(C) Thrombophlebitis

(D) Thromboangiitis obliterans

(E) Varicose veins

13. A 49-year-old male is feeling fine when he has his blood pressure checked for the first time in 20 years. He is surprised to find that he has a pressure of 155/95 mm Hg. He has had no serious medical problems and is taking no medications. Which of the following factors is most likely to be important in the initiation of this form of hypertension?

(A) Increased catecholamine secretion

(B) Renal retention of excess sodium

(C) Gene defects in aldosterone metabolism

(D) Renal artery stenosis

(E) Increased production of atrial natriuretic factor

14. A 50-year-old male presents with angina pectoris. Coronary angiography reveals a (fixed) 75% narrowing of the anterior descending branch of the left coronary artery. Which of the following cells is *least* likely to be involved in the pathogenesis of his coronary artery lesion?

(A) Monocytes

(B) Smooth muscle cells

(C) Platelets

(D) Neutrophils

(E) Endothelial cells

15. In the causation of atherosclerosis, which of the following events is considered the most important *direct* biologic consequence of smoking, hypertension, and hypercholesterolemia?

(A) Endothelial injury and its sequelae

(B) Conversion of smooth muscle cells to foam cells

(C) Alterations of hepatic lipoprotein receptors

(D) Inhibition of low-density lipoprotein (LDL) oxidation

(E) Alterations of endogenous factors regulating vasomotor tone

16. For about 5 years, a 55-year-old female has unsightly dilated superficial veins over both lower legs. Which of the following complications is she most likely to suffer as a consequence?

(A) Stasis dermatitis

(B) Gangrenous necrosis of the lower legs

(C) Pulmonary thromboembolism

(D) Disseminated intravascular coagulation

(E) Atrophy of lower leg muscles

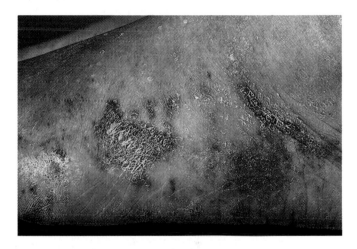

17. The 35-year-old male with the skin lesions shown here is known to have been infected with the human immunodeficiency virus (HIV) for the past 10 years. Which of the following additional infectious agents is most likely to play a role in the development of these skin lesions?

(A) Human herpesvirus 8

(B) Epstein-Barr virus (EBV)

(C) Cytomegalovirus (CMV)

(D) Hepatitis B virus

(E) Adenovirus

18. An 80-year-old male diabetic has a 7-cm, pulsating mass in the midline of his lower abdomen. He has poor pulses in his lower extremities. Which of the following complications of aortic atherosclerosis is responsible for the development of this lesion?

(A) Ulceration of atherosclerotic plaque

(B) Thrombosis overlying atherosclerotic plaque

(C) Hemorrhage into the plaque substance

(D) Atrophy (thinning) of the media

(E) Cystic degeneration of the media along with fragmentation of elastic fibers

19. A 50-year-old male develops the sudden onset of excruciating pain in the chest and back. Physical examination reveals diminished radial pulses bilaterally and normal femoral pulses. The chest radiograph reveals a widened mediastinum. Which of the following underlying conditions is most likely to be etiologically related to this patient's acute problem?

○ (A) A history of diabetes mellitus
○ (B) Myxoid change and fragmentation of elastic lamellae in the aortic media
○ (C) Severe atherosclerosis of proximal aorta
○ (D) A past history of syphilis
○ (E) A congenital cardiac malformation

20. A 40-year-old female has fever and a nonproductive cough of 6 weeks' duration. A transbronchial biopsy reveals necrotizing granulomatous inflammation centered around small peripheral pulmonary artery branches. Laboratory findings include a urinalysis showing the presence of 50 red blood cells per high-power field along with red blood cell casts, a serum creatinine of level of 5.1 mg/dL, and a serum c-ANCA determination positive at a 1:512 titer. Her underlying disease is most likely to be

○ (A) Polyarteritis nodosa
○ (B) Pulmonary hypertension
○ (C) Hyperplastic arteriolosclerosis
○ (D) Giant cell arteritis
○ (E) Wegener granulomatosis

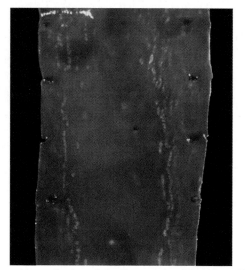

From the teaching collection of the Department of Pathology, University of Texas Southwestern Medical School, Dallas, TX.

21. The gross appearance of the aorta from a 12-year-old male who died of leukemia is shown here. Histologic examination of the linear pale marking is most likely to reveal

○ (A) A core of lipid debris covered by a cap of smooth muscle cells
○ (B) Collection of foam cells, necrotic areas, and calcification
○ (C) A lipid core, granulation tissue, and areas of hemorrhage

○ (D) Lipid-filled foam cells and T lymphocytes
○ (E) Cholesterol clefts surrounded by proliferating smooth muscle cells and foam cells

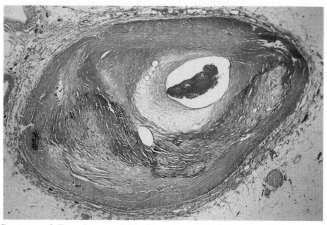

Courtesy of Tom Rogers, MD, Department of Pathology, University of Texas Southwestern Medical School, Dallas, TX.

22. The figure shows the microscopic appearance of the left anterior descending artery found at autopsy of a 59-year-old male. Which of the following laboratory test findings is believed to be etiologically related to the process illustrated here?

○ (A) Low lipoprotein Lp(a)
○ (B) Positive VDRL
○ (C) Low HDL cholesterol
○ (D) Elevated platelet count
○ (E) Low plasma homocysteine

23. After a fall, a 59-year-old female experiences some right hip pain. A radiograph reveals no fractures, but there are calcified, medium-sized arterial branches in the region of the pelvis. What is the significance of this finding?

○ (A) This is a feature of diabetes mellitus.
○ (B) Her blood pressure needs to be checked.
○ (C) This is an incidental finding.
○ (D) She is at risk for gangrenous necrosis.
○ (E) Hyperparathyroidism is likely.

24. For more than a decade, a 45-year-old male has had poorly controlled hypertension in the range of 160/95 mm Hg. For the past 3 months, his blood pressure has increased to 250/125 mm Hg. He now has a serum creatinine level of 3.8 mg/dL. Which of the following vascular lesions is most likely to be found in the kidneys?

○ (A) Hyperplastic arteriolosclerosis
○ (B) Granulomatous arteritis
○ (C) Fibromuscular dysplasia
○ (D) Polyarteritis nodosa
○ (E) Hyaline arteriolosclerosis

25. After a mastectomy with axillary node dissection a year ago, a 47-year-old female has swelling and puffiness of her left arm that persists all the time. The underlying skin appears firm. The arm is not painful or discolored.

She had a bout of cellulitis in this left arm 3 months ago. Her condition is best called

○ (A) Thrombophlebitis
○ (B) Subclavian arterial thrombosis
○ (C) Tumor embolization
○ (D) Lymphedema
○ (E) Vasculitis

For each of the descriptions of patients in questions 26 and 27, match the most closely associated laboratory test finding.

(A) Anti–double stranded-DNA titer of 1:512
(B) c-ANCA titer of 1:256
(C) Cryoglobulinemia
(D) Plasma glucose level of 200 mg/dL
(E) HBsAg positive
(F) Serum HDL cholesterol of 10 mg/dL
(G) HIV positive
(H) Homocystinuria
(I) Serum LDL cholesterol of 210 mg/dL
(J) p-ANCA titer of 1:128
(K) Plasma renin of 15 mg/mL/h
(L) Serologic test for syphilis positive
(M) Total serum cholesterol of 140 mg/dL

26.   A 79-year-old female was diagnosed with a progressive dementia. She was a nonsmoker, and she had a blood pressure of 90/55 mm Hg. She is found at autopsy to have no cerebral atherosclerosis, no coronary atherosclerosis, and only a few lipid streaks in the aorta. Her underlying cause of death is found to be Alzheimer's disease. (   )

27.   A 55-year-old female was found to have a blood pressure of 160/105 mm Hg on several occasions in the past 3 months. She feels fine and has had no major medical conditions during her lifetime. An abdominal ultrasound scan reveals that the left kidney is smaller than the right. An angiogram reveals a focal stenosis of the left renal artery. (   )

28.   In which of the following locations would you *least* expect to find significant atherosclerotic lesions in a patient with risk factors of smoking, hypertension, diabetes mellitus, and serum cholesterol level of 280 mg/dL?

○ (A) Left main coronary artery
○ (B) Aortic bifurcation
○ (C) Circle of Willis
○ (D) Pulmonary artery trunk
○ (E) Common carotid artery

29.   A 75-year-old male has had headaches for several months. On physical examination, he has a prominent palpable right temporal artery that is painful to touch. The biopsied segment of thickened temporal artery shows focal granulomatous inflammation. This condition responds well to corticosteroid therapy. Which of the following complications is most likely in untreated patients?

○ (A) Renal failure
○ (B) Hemoptysis
○ (C) Malignant hypertension

○ (D) Blindness
○ (E) Gangrene of the toes

30.   A 30-year-old female who has smoked cigarettes since she was a teenager has painful thromboses of the superficial veins of her lower legs for a month. Then she experiences episodes when her fingers become blue and cold. Over the next year, she develops chronic, poorly healing ulcerations of her feet. One toe becomes gangrenous and is amputated. Histologically, at the resection margin there is an acute and chronic vasculitis involving medium-sized arteries with segmental involvement. She is best advised that

○ (A) Hemodialysis is necessary
○ (B) She must stop smoking
○ (C) Corticosteroid therapy will be effective
○ (D) Antibiotic therapy for syphilis is required
○ (E) Insulin therapy can control this disease

31.   A 40-year-old male has experienced malaise, fever, and a 4-kg weight loss over the past month. He is found to have a serum urea nitrogen concentration of 58 mg/dL and a serum creatinine level of 6.7 mg/dL. Renal angiography reveals right renal arterial thrombosis, and the left renal artery and branches show segmental luminal narrowing along with focal aneurysmal dilation. While receiving hemodialysis a week later, he is found to have melena in association with abdominal pain and diarrhea. Which of the following laboratory test findings is most likely?

○ (A) Positive c-ANCA
○ (B) Positive antinuclear antibody (ANA)
○ (C) Positive HIV
○ (D) Positive hepatitis B surface antigen
○ (E) Positive Scl-70

32.   A 30-year-old, overweight female is a school teacher who is known to be a strict disciplinarian in the classroom. She presents with angina pectoris, and coronary angiography reveals 75% narrowing of the anterior descending branch of the left coronary artery. Which of the following would be a major risk factor for coronary atherosclerosis in this patient?

○ (A) Obesity
○ (B) Type A personality
○ (C) Diabetes mellitus
○ (D) Sedentary life style
○ (E) Age

33.   Several skin lesions on the upper chest of a 45-year-old male have central pulsatile cores. Pressing on a core causes a radially arranged array of subcutaneous arterioles to blanch. The size of the lesions from core to periphery is 0.5 to 1.5 cm. The underlying disease he is most likely to have in association with these skin lesions is

○ (A) Wegener granulomatosis
○ (B) Micronodular cirrhosis
○ (C) Marfan syndrome
○ (D) Acquired immunodeficiency syndrome
○ (E) Diabetes mellitus

34. Itching with burning pain in the perianal region in a 22-year-old female has been present for several months. Physical examination reveals dilated and thrombosed external hemorrhoids. What underlying process most likely led to her present condition?

○ (A) Rectal adenocarcinoma
○ (B) Pregnancy
○ (C) Polyarteritis nodosa
○ (D) Filariasis
○ (E) Micronodular cirrhosis

ANSWERS

1. **(A)** Atheromatous plaques can be complicated by a variety of pathologic alterations, including hemorrhage, ulceration, thrombosis, and calcification. These processes can increase the size of the plaque and narrow the residual arterial lumen. Although atherosclerosis is a disease of the intima, the media is compressed by the expanding plaque with advanced disease. This causes thinning of the media, which weakens the wall and predisposes to aneurysm formation.
BP6 285-288   PBD6 507-509

2. **(B)** This arteriole shows marked hyaline thickening of the wall, indicative of hyaline arteriolosclerosis. Diabetes mellitus can also lead to this finding. Sepsis can produce DIC with arteriolar hyaline thrombi. The debilitation that accompanies cancer tends to diminish vascular disease due to atherosclerosis. Syphilis can cause a vasculitis involving the vasa vasorum of the aorta. Polyarteritis can involve large to medium-sized arteries in many organs, including kidneys. The affected vessels show fibrinoid necrosis and inflammation of the wall (i.e., vasculitis).
BP6 292-293   PBD6 514-515

3. **(D)** Abdominal aneurysms are most frequently related to underlying atherosclerosis. This patient has multiple risk factors for atherosclerosis, including diabetes mellitus, hypertension, and smoking. When the aneurysm reaches this size, there is a significant risk for rupture.
BP6 299   PBD6 525-526

4. **(I)** Henoch-Schönlein purpura is the multisystemic counterpart in children of IgA nephropathy seen in adults. The immune complexes formed with IgA produce the vasculitis that affects mainly arterioles, capillaries, and venules in skin, gastrointestinal tract, and kidney.
BP6 453   PBD6 517, 961, 965

5. **(O)** Wegener granulomatosis is characterized by necrotizing granulomatous inflammation that typically involves the upper respiratory tract, small to medium-sized vessels, and glomeruli. The lungs are often involved, although other organ sites may also be affected. It is a type of hypersensitivity reaction to an unknown antigen.
BP6 295-296   PBD6 522-523

6. **(A)** The lowering of cholesterol, particularly the LDL cholesterol with the same or increased HDL cholesterol level, indicates a lowered risk for atherosclerotic complications. Atherosclerosis is multifactorial, but modification of diet (i.e., reduction in total dietary fat and cholesterol) with increased exercise is the best way of reducing risk for most persons. Glucose is a measure of control of diabetes mellitus. Potassium, calcium, and renin values may be altered with some forms of hypertension, one of the risk factors for atherosclerosis.
BP6 283-284   PBD6 504-506

7. **(D)** This is cystic medial necrosis, which weakens the aortic media and predisposes to aortic dissection. In a young patient, such as this one, a heritable disorder of connective tissues such as Marfan syndrome must be strongly suspected. Atherosclerosis with diabetes mellitus and hypertension are risk factors for aortic dissection, although at an older age. Scleroderma and Wegener granulomatosis do not typically involve the aorta.
BP6 301   PBD6 526-528

8. **(C)** He has an atherosclerotic abdominal aortic aneurysm. Diabetes mellitus is an important risk factor for atherosclerosis and must be suspected if a young male or premenopausal female presents with severe atherosclerosis. Polyarteritis nodosa does not typically involve the aorta. Obesity is a "soft" risk factor for atherosclerosis. SLE produces small arteriolar vasculitis. Syphilitic aortitis involves the thoracic aorta.
BP6 299   PBD6 525-526

9. **(E)** These dilated, endothelium-lined spaces are filled with red blood cells. The circumscribed nature of this lesion and its long, unchanged course suggest its benign nature. Kaposi sarcoma is uncommon in its endemic form in childhood, and it is best known as a neoplastic complication associated with HIV infection. Angiosarcomas are large, rapidly growing malignancies in adults. Lymphangiomas tend to be more diffuse and are not blood filled, but they are most often seen in children. A telangiectasia is a radial array of subcutaneous dilated arteries or arterioles around a central core, and it may pulsate.
BP6 304-305   PBD6 532-533

10. **(A)** Atherosclerosis is considered a complex reparative response that follows endothelial cell injury. Hypercholesterolemia (i.e., high LDL cholesterol level) is believed to cause subtle endothelial injury. The oxidation of LDL by macrophages or endothelial cells has many deleterious effects. It is chemotactic for circulating monocytes, causes monocytes to adhere to endothelium, stimulates release of growth factors and cytokines, and is cytotoxic to smooth muscle cells and endothelium. Smooth muscle proliferation in response to injury is important in the development of atheromas. This is driven by growth factors, including PDGF. HDL is believed to mobilize cholesterol from developing atheromas and hence high HDL levels are protective. ICAM-1 and VCAM-1 are adhesion molecules on endothelial cells that promote adhesion of monocytes to the site of endothelial injury.
BP6 285-286   PBD6 507-509

11. **(E)** These findings are most suggestive of syphilitic aortitis, a complication of tertiary syphilis, with characteristic involvement of the thoracic aorta. Obliterative endarteritis is not a feature of other forms of vasculitis. High-titer double-stranded DNA antibodies are diagnostic of SLE, and the test result for p-ANCA is positive in various vasculitides, including microscopic polyangiitis. A high sedimentation rate is a nonspecific marker of inflammatory diseases. Ketonuria may occur in persons with diabetic ketoacidosis.
BP6 299–300   PBD6 526

12. **(C)** This is a common problem that results from venous stasis. There is little or no inflammation, but the term is well established. Lymphedema takes longer to develop and is not caused by bed rest alone. DIC more often results in hemorrhage, and edema is not the most prominent manifestation. Thromboangiitis obliterans is a rare form of arteritis that results in pain and ulceration of extremities. Varicose veins are superficial and can thrombose, but they are not related to bed rest.
BP6 302–303   PBD6 530

13. **(B)** This patient has essential hypertension (i.e., no obvious cause for his moderate degree of hypertension). Renal retention of excess sodium is thought to be important in initiating this form of hypertension. This leads to an increased intravascular fluid volume, increase in cardiac output, and peripheral vasoconstriction. Increased catecholamine secretion (as may occur in pheochromocytoma), gene defects in aldosterone metabolism, and renal artery stenosis can all cause secondary hypertension. However, secondary hypertension from all causes is much less common than essential hypertension. Increased production of atrial natriuretic factor reduces sodium retention and therefore reduces blood volume.
BP6 290–291   PBD6 512–513

14. **(D)** Atherogenesis can be considered a chronic inflammatory response of the arterial wall to endothelial injury. The injury promotes participation by monocytes, macrophages, and T lymphocytes. Smooth muscle cells are stimulated to proliferate. Platelets adhere to areas of endothelial injury. However, neutrophils are not a part of atherogenesis, although they may be seen in various forms of vasculitis.
BP6 285–287   PBD6 507–509

15. **(A)** Atherosclerosis is believed to result from some form of endothelial injury and the subsequent chronic inflammation and repair of the intima. All risk factors, including smoking, hyperlipidemia, and hypertension, cause biochemical or mechanical injury to the endothelium. Formation of foam cells occurs after the initial endothelial injury. Lipoprotein receptor alterations may occur in some inherited conditions, but these conditions account for only a fraction of cases of atherosclerosis, and other lifestyle conditions do not affect their action. Inhibition of LDL oxidation should diminish atheroma formation. Vasomotor tone does not play a major role in atherogenesis.
BP6 284–286   PBD6 505–508

16. **(A)** The venous stasis results in hemosiderin deposition and dermal fibrosis with brownish discoloration and skin roughening. Focal ulceration may occur over the varicosities, but extensive gangrene similar to what occurs with arterial atherosclerosis does not occur. The varicosities involve just the superficial set of veins, which may thrombose, but are not the source of thromboemboli, as are the larger deep leg veins. The thromboses in superficial leg veins do not lead to DIC. The varicosities do not affect muscle, although lack of muscular support for veins to "squeeze" blood out for venous return may predispose to formation of varicose veins.
BP6 302   PBD6 529

17. **(A)** Human herpesvirus 8 has been associated with Kaposi sarcoma and can be acquired as a sexually transmitted disease. Kaposi sarcoma is a complication of acquired immunodeficiency syndrome (AIDS). Persons with HIV infection can be infected with a variety of viruses, including EBV and CMV, but these have no etiologic association with Kaposi sarcoma. EBV is a factor in the development of non-Hodgkin lymphoma, and CMV can cause colitis or retinitis or may be disseminated. HBV can be seen in HIV-infected patients as well, particularly those with a risk factor of injection drug use. Adenovirus can be seen in HIV-infected persons, although not frequently; it tends to be a respiratory or gastrointestinal infection.
BP6 305–307   PBD6 535–536

18. **(D)** Aneurysms, including aortic aneurysms, form in areas of weakness of an arterial wall. Abdominal aortic aneurysms are typically atherosclerotic in origin. Atherosclerotic plaques compress the media, and this can cause atrophy of the media. Because the media provides elasticity and support to the vessel wall, weakening of the media predisposes to aneurysmal dilatation. Ulceration, thrombosis, and hemorrhage occur superficially in atheromatous plaques and tend to promote narrowing of arterial lumens, not arterial dilation. Cystic medial necrosis is a feature of Marfan syndrome.
BP6 299   PBD6 525–526

19. **(B)** He has an aortic dissection in which there has been an intimal tear that allows blood to dissect into the aortic media. The dissection in this patient extended to the great vessels to cause tamponade as evidenced by diminished upper extremity pulses. The most frequent preexisting histologically detectable lesion in these cases is cystic medial degeneration (CMD), also known as cystic medial necrosis. Some cases of CMD are associated with Marfan syndrome. Hypertension and atherosclerosis are additional risk factors that can be identified in patients with aortic dissection. Syphilitic aortitis can lead to ischemic aortic medial injury that results in aortic arch dilation with the potential for rupture, but such cases are far less frequent than aortic dissection from CMD.
BP6 300–302   PBD6 526–528

20. **(E)** Pulmonary and renal involvement can be serious and life-threatening with Wegener granulomatosis. Polyarteritis is less likely to involve the lungs, and the inflammation is not typically granulomatous. p-ANCA or c-ANCA

are absent in polyarteritis. Pulmonary vascular hypertensive changes include vascular thickening and tortuosity, although not usually inflammation. Hyperplastic arteriolosclerosis is a lesion most typically seen with malignant hypertension in systemic circulation. Giant cell arteritis is most typical for temporal arteries and branches of the external carotid arteries.
BP6 295-296   PBD6 522-523

21. **(D)** These slightly raised, pale lesions, called fatty streaks, are seen in the aorta of almost all children older than 10 years. They are thought to be precursors of atheromatous plaques. Fatty streaks cause no disturbances in blood flow and are discovered incidentally at autopsy. All the other lesions described are seen in fully developed atheromatous plaques. The histologic features of such plaques include a central core of lipid debris that may have cholesterol clefts and may be calcified. There is usually an overlying cap of smooth muscle cells. Hemorrhage is a complication seen in advanced atherosclerosis. Foam cells, derived from smooth muscle cells or macrophages that have ingested lipid, can be present in all phases of atherogenesis.
BP6 286-289   PBD6 502-503

22. **(C)** The arterial lumen is markedly narrowed by atheromatous plaque complicated by calcification. Hypercholesterolemia with elevated LDL and decreased HDL levels is a key risk factor for atherogenesis. Syphilis (i.e., positive VDRL test result) produces endarteritis obliterans of aortic vasa vasorum. This weakens the wall and predisposes to aneurysms. Although platelets participate in forming atheromatous plaques, their number is not of major importance. Thrombocytosis can result in thrombosis or hemorrhage. Levels of Lp(a) and homocysteine, if elevated, increase the risk for atherosclerosis.
BP6 287-289   PBD6 504-506

23. **(C)** Older adults with calcified arteries often have Mönckeberg medial calcific sclerosis, a benign process that is one form of arteriosclerosis without serious sequelae. Such calcification of arteries is far less likely to be a consequence of atherosclerosis with diabetes or with hypercalcemia. Hypertension is most likely to affect small renal arteries, and calcification is not a major feature, although hypertension is also a risk factor for atherosclerosis.
BP6 283   PBD6 498

24. **(A)** This patient has malignant hypertension superimposed on benign essential hypertension. Malignant hypertension can suddenly complicate hypertension of a lesser severity. The arterioles undergo concentric thickening and luminal narrowing. A granulomatous arteritis is most characteristic for Wegener granulomatosis, which often involves the kidney. Fibromuscular dysplasia involves the main renal arteries and can lead to hypertension but not typically malignant hypertension. Polyarteritis nodosa produces a vasculitis that may involve the kidney. Hyaline arteriolosclerosis is seen with long-standing essential hypertension of moderate degree. These lesions give rise to benign nephrosclerosis. The affected kidneys become symmetrically shrunken and granular because of progressive loss of renal parenchyma and consequent fine scarring.
BP6 292-293   PBD6 514-515

25. **(D)** The mastectomy with axillary lymph node dissection leads to disruption and obstruction of lymphatics in the axilla. Such obstruction to flow of lymph gives rise to lymphedema, a condition that can be complicated by cellulitis. Thrombophlebitis from venous stasis is more commonly a complication seen in the lower extremities. An arterial thrombosis can lead to a cold, blue, painful extremity. Tumor emboli are generally small; they are uncommon. Vasculitis is not a complication of surgery.
BP6 303   PBD6 530-531

26. **(M)** Hypercholesterolemia is a major driving force behind atherogenesis. A total cholesterol level of less than 200 mg/dL carries a low risk for development of complications of atherosclerosis, and clinical events resulting from atherosclerosis are uncommon when the total cholesterol concentration is below 150 mg/dL. It is better to have more HDL cholesterol than more LDL cholesterol.
BP6 284-286   PBD6 504-506

27. **(K)** This is a classic example of a secondary form of hypertension in which a cause can be determined. In this case, the renal artery stenosis reduces glomerular blood flow and reduced pressure in the afferent arteriole, resulting in renin release by juxtaglomerular cells. The renin initiates angiotensin II–induced vasoconstriction, increased peripheral vascular resistance, and increased aldosterone that promotes sodium reabsorption in the kidney, resulting in increased blood volume.
BP6 290-291   PBD6 512-514

28. **(D)** The pulmonary vasculature is under much lower pressure than the systemic arterial circulation and is much less likely to have endothelial damage that promotes atherogenesis. Atherosclerosis is more likely to occur where blood flow is more turbulent, and this occurs at arterial branch points and in the first few centimeters of the coronary arteries.
BP6 284-285   PBD6 507-508

29. **(D)** This patient has clinical features suggesting giant cell (temporal) arteritis. This form of arteritis typically involves large to medium-sized arteries in the head—especially temporal arteries—but also vertebral and ophthalmic arteries. The latter can lead to blindness. Because involvement of the kidney, lung, and peripheral arteries of the extremities is much less common, renal failure, hemoptysis, and gangrene of toes are unusual. There is no association with hypertension.
BP6 297   PBD6 517-518

30. **(B)** She has features of thromboangiitis obliterans (i.e., Buerger disease). This disease, which affects small to medium-sized arteries of the extremities, is strongly associated with smoking. Renal involvement does not occur. Immunosuppressive therapy is not highly effective. Syphilis produces an aortitis. Although peripheral vascular disease

with atherosclerosis is typical for diabetes mellitus, vasculitis is not.

BP6 298–299   PBD6 523

31. **(D)** Segmental involvement of medium-sized arteries with aneurysmal dilation in renal vascular bed and presumed mesenteric vasculitis (e.g., abdominal pain, melena) is most likely caused by polyarteritis nodosa. Polyarteritis can affect many organs at different times. Although the cause of polyarteritis is unknown, about 30% of patients have hepatitis B surface antigen in serum. Presumably, hepatitis B surface antigen–antibody complexes damage the vessel wall. Unlike the situation with microscopic polyangiitis, there is no known association with ANCA. Vasculitis with HIV infection is uncommon. A collagen vascular disease with a positive ANA result, such as SLE, may produce a vasculitis but not in the pattern seen here. The affected vessels are smaller. The Scl-70 autoantibody is indicative of scleroderma, which may produce renal failure.

BP6 293–295   PBD6 520

32. **(C)** Diabetes mellitus is a significant risk factor for early, accelerated, and advanced atherosclerosis. If a premenopausal female or a young male presents with severe coronary atherosclerosis, diabetes must be suspected as a predisposing factor. "Soft" risk factors that play a lesser role in development of atherosclerosis may include obesity, stress, and lack of exercise.

BP6 284   PBD6 504–506

33. **(B)** These lesions are spider telangiectasias, which are a feature of micronodular cirrhosis, typically as a consequence of chronic alcoholism. Spider telangiectasias are thought to be caused by hyperestrinism (i.e., estrogen excess) that results from hepatic damage. Vasculitis tends not to produce skin telangiectasias. The vascular involvement in Marfan syndrome is primarily in the aortic arch with cystic medial necrosis. The most common vascular lesion of skin with AIDS is Kaposi's sarcoma, which is a neoplasm presenting as one or more irregular, red to purple patches, plaques, or nodules. Diabetes mellitus, with accelerated atherosclerosis, is most likely to result in ischemia or gangrene.

BP6 304   PBD6 534

34. **(B)** The hemorrhoidal veins can become dilated from venous congestion. This is most common with chronic constipation, but the pregnant uterus presses on pelvic veins to produce similar congestion that promotes hemorrhoidal vein dilation. Carcinomas are not likely to obstruct venous flow. Polyarteritis does not affect veins. Filarial infections may affect lymphatics, including those in the inguinal region, and produce lymphedema. Portal hypertension with cirrhosis is most likely to dilate submucosal esophageal veins, but hemorrhoidal veins occasionally may be affected. However, cirrhosis would be rare at her age.

BP6 302   PBD6 530

The Heart

BP6 Chapter 11 - The Heart
PBD6 Chapter 13 - The Heart

1. A 50-year-old male experiences episodes of severe substernal chest pain every time he performs any task requiring moderate exercise. These episodes have become more frequent and severe in the past year, but they can be relieved by use of sublingual nitroglycerin. Which of the following cardiac lesions is probably present?

○ (A) Rheumatic mitral stenosis
○ (B) Serous pericarditis
○ (C) Restrictive cardiomyopathy
○ (D) Calcific aortic stenosis
○ (E) Atherosclerotic narrowing of coronary arteries

2. Ten years after receiving an aortic valve bioprosthesis because of infective endocarditis, a 44-year-old female is most likely to suffer which of the following complications?

○ (A) Paravalvular leak
○ (B) Stenosis
○ (C) Hemolysis
○ (D) Embolization
○ (E) Myocardial infarction (MI)

3. The direction of blood flow and the clinical severity of symptoms in tetralogy of Fallot is determined primarily by the

○ (A) Size of the left ventricle
○ (B) Degree of pulmonary stenosis
○ (C) Size of the ventricular septal defect (VSD)
○ (D) Diameter of the tricuspid valve
○ (E) Presence of an atrial septal defect (ASD)

4. A 12-year-old male presented with a sore throat and fever. Throat culture was positive for β-hemolytic *Streptococcus*. Three weeks later, the sore throat had resolved, but the patient developed a reddish rash. On examination, the pediatrician noticed a murmur of mitral regurgitation and

rales over both of the lungs. The patient was admitted to the hospital. During the hospital stay, he had several episodes of atrial fibrillation, and he developed signs of acute left ventricular failure and died of pulmonary edema 2 days after admission. Which of the following changes is *least* likely to be seen in the heart?

○ (A) Fibrinous pericarditis
○ (B) Aschoff nodules in the myocardium
○ (C) Fibrosis of mitral valve with fusion of commissures
○ (D) Foci of fibrinoid necrosis in mitral valve
○ (E) Dilatation of the left ventricle

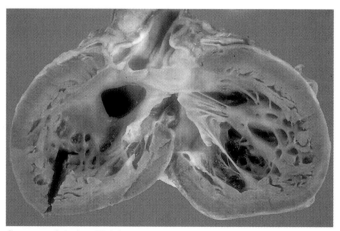

Courtesy of Arthur Weinberg, M.D. Department of Pathology, University of Texas Southwestern Medical School, Dallas, TX.

5. The gross appearance of the heart of a 5-year-old child at autopsy is illustrated here. Which of the following additional pathologic conditions would you most likely find?

○ (A) Chronic renal failure
○ (B) Coronary atherosclerosis
○ (C) Thymic hypoplasia
○ (D) Pulmonary hypertension
○ (E) Dilated cardiomyopathy

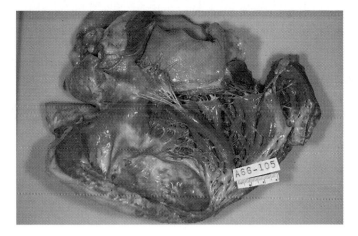

6. The gross appearance of the heart of a 68-year-old male at autopsy is shown here. The most likely complication resulting from this lesion is

○ (A) Cardiac rupture
○ (B) Acute pericarditis
○ (C) Systemic thromboembolism
○ (D) Cardiogenic shock
○ (E) Constrictive pericarditis

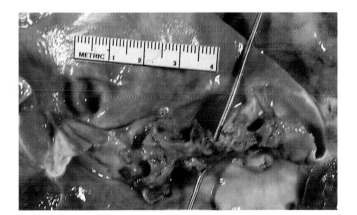

7. The gross appearance of the heart depicted in the figure here was seen at autopsy of a 25-year-old male who died after an illness of less than 3 days' duration. Which of the following laboratory test findings was probably obtained during his hospital course on the day before he died?

○ (A) Elevated anti–streptolysin O titer
○ (B) Positive antineutrophil cytoplasmic autoantibody
○ (C) Increased creatine kinase MB fraction
○ (D) High double-stranded DNA autoantibody titer
○ (E) Positive blood culture for *Staphylococcus aureus*

8. A young patient presents with chronic progressive exercise intolerance. The electrocardiographic results and radiologic evidence suggest severe left ventricular hypertrophy with a prominent septum. The right ventricle is also somewhat thickened. The anterior leaflet of the mitral valve moves into the outflow tract of the left ventricle during systole. Hemodynamic tests reveal an abnormally high ejection fraction but low ventricular volume and low cardiac output. The most likely cause of cardiac abnormalities in this patient is

○ (A) Mutations in β-myosin heavy chain
○ (B) Autoimmunity against myocardial fibers
○ (C) Chronic alcoholism
○ (D) Deposition of amyloid protein
○ (E) Latent enterovirus infection

9. Infection with which of the following organisms is most likely to give rise to a bloody pericardial effusion with a high protein content?

○ (A) *Mycobacterium tuberculosis*
○ (B) Group A *Streptococcus*
○ (C) Coxsackievirus B
○ (D) *Candida albicans*
○ (E) *S. aureus*

10. A young injection drug user presents with fever, a new murmur, and mental status changes. Blood cultures are positive for *S. aureus*, and her white blood cell count is 19,200/μL. An echocardiogram reveals a 1.5-cm vegetation on the mitral valve. Which of the changes listed is *least* likely to be a complication of her disease process?

○ (A) Left atrial dilation
○ (B) Glomerulonephritis
○ (C) Intramyocardial or ring abscesses
○ (D) Central nervous system embolic events
○ (E) Myxomatous degeneration of the mitral valve

11. A 19-year-old male has had a low-grade fever for 3 weeks. On physical examination, he has a temperature of 38.3°C, with a respiration rate of 28, pulse of 104, and blood pressure of 95/60 mm Hg. A tender spleen tip is palpable. Splinter hemorrhages are observed on his fingernails. A heart murmur is auscultated. Which of the following infectious agents best accounts for these findings?

○ (A) *Streptococcus viridans*
○ (B) *Trypanosoma cruzi*
○ (C) Coxsackievirus B
○ (D) *C. albicans*
○ (E) *M. tuberculosis*

12. A thrombotic occlusion of the left circumflex artery occurs in a 50-year-old male with severe coronary atherosclerosis. Within an hour after the thrombus forms, which of the following complications is most likely to occur?

○ (A) Ventricular fibrillation
○ (B) Pericarditis
○ (C) Myocardial rupture
○ (D) Ventricular aneurysm
○ (E) Thromboembolism

For each of the patient histories in questions 13 through 16, match the most closely associated description of a cardiovascular disease process:

(A) Congenitally stenotic pulmonic valve associated with a VSD
(B) Dilation of the aortic valve ring with an aneurysm of the arch of aorta
(C) Fibrinoid necrosis of medium-sized arteries in many organs
(D) Fibrotic mitral valve associated with thickening and fusion of the chordae tendineae
(E) Fragmentation of elastic fibers in the media of the aortic arch
(F) Granulomatous inflammation and fibrosis of the media of the aortic arch with narrowing of aortic lumen
(G) Heavily calcified aortic valve with three cusps
(H) Heavily calcified, congenitally bicuspid aortic valve
(I) "Hooding" deformity and myxomatous degeneration of the mitral valve
(J) Large, destructive vegetations involving the aortic valve
(K) Small, nondestructive vegetations on an otherwise normal mitral valve

13. A 30-year-old African-American male with long-standing essential hypertension collapses after the sudden onset of severe chest pain. On physical examination, his radial pulses are weak but femoral pulses are normal. A chest radiograph reveals widening of the mediastinum. (   )

14. A 35-year-old asymptomatic female is found to have a mid-systolic click heart murmur during a routine physical examination for an insurance policy. (   )

15. A 50-year-old male with a history of a mucin-producing adenocarcinoma of the pancreas dies after a 6-month course complicated by wasting, bronchopneumonia, and stroke. (   )

16. A 35-year-old male with a history of intravenous drug abuse is brought to the hospital emergency room for evaluation of acute onset fever and altered mental status. A head CT scan reveals evidence of a right parietal, 3-cm abscess. (   )

17. A 68-year-old male presents with progressive dyspnea, experienced over the past year. By echocardiography, the left ventricular wall is greatly hypertrophied. His chest radiograph reveals pulmonary edema and a prominent left heart shadow. Which of the following conditions probably led to these findings.

○ (A) Centrilobular emphysema
○ (B) Hypertension
○ (C) Tricuspid valve regurgitation
○ (D) Chronic alcoholism
○ (E) Silicosis

18. At autopsy, the heart of a 73-year-old male shows marked right ventricular and right atrial dilation and hypertrophy. The aorta shows minimal atherosclerosis, and the pulmonary trunk shows moderate atherosclerosis. Which of the following conditions is most likely to have given rise to these findings?

○ (A) Saddle pulmonary thromboembolism
○ (B) Ventricular septal defect (VSD)
○ (C) Chronic obstructive pulmonary disease
○ (D) Rheumatic heart disease (RHD)
○ (E) Hypertrophic cardiomyopathy

19. A 34-year-old female with no history of heart disease has had palpitations, fatigue, and chest pain worsening for the past year. Auscultation of the chest reveals a mid-systolic click. What are the results of an echocardiogram most likely to show?

○ (A) Aortic valvular vegetations
○ (B) Pulmonic stenosis
○ (C) Mitral valve prolapse
○ (D) Patent ductus arteriosus (PDA)
○ (E) Tricuspid valve regurgitation

20. A 15-year-old female jumps up for a block in the third match of a volleyball tournament. She collapses and cannot be revived despite cardiopulmonary resuscitation. She had been healthy all her life and complained only of some limited episodes of chest pain during games in the current school year. Which of the following pathologic findings of the heart is the medical examiner most likely to find?

○ (A) Haphazardly arranged, hypertrophied septal myocytes
○ (B) Extensive myocardial hemosiderin deposition
○ (C) Tachyzoites within foci of myocardial necrosis and inflammation
○ (D) Mitral valvular stenosis with left atrial enlargement
○ (E) Large, friable vegetations with destruction of aortic valve cusps

21. The gross appearance of the heart in the following figure from a 59-year-old male with a history of an increasing renal failure is most characteristic for which of the following underlying conditions?

○ (A) Chronic alcoholism
○ (B) Hypertension
○ (C) Pneumoconiosis
○ (D) Hemochromatosis
○ (E) Diabetes mellitus

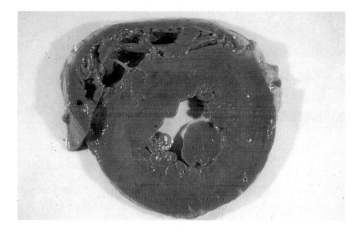

22. A 4-year-old child is less than the 5th percentile for height and weight for age. She is cyanotic and has no exercise tolerance. Arterial blood gas measurement shows decreased oxygen saturation. She now presents with fever and obtundation, and a cerebral CT scan shows a right parietal, ring-enhancing, 3-cm lesion. She is most likely to have which of the following congenital heart diseases?

○ (A) Tetralogy of Fallot
○ (B) Arterial septal defect (ASD)
○ (C) Patent ductus arteriosus (PDA)
○ (D) Coarctation of the aorta
○ (E) Bicuspid aortic valve

23. A 50-year-old male with a history of long-standing diabetes mellitus and hypertension developed pain in the left shoulder and arm. He attributed the pain to arthritis and took some acetaminophen. Over the next several hours, the patient developed shortness of breath, which persisted over the next several days. On the third day, he visited a doctor, who ordered determinations of creatine kinase (CK) and troponin I levels. The total CK activity was within reference range, but the troponin level was elevated. He was admitted to the hospital, where he continued to experience dyspnea over the next 3 days. One day later (7 days after the onset of shoulder pain), the patient suffered from cardiac arrest. Attempted resuscitation was unsuccessful. Postmortem examination reveals a large transmural myocardial infarct (MI) with rupture of the heart and acute hemopericardium. Which of the following statements is supported by the clinical and autopsy data?

○ (A) The patient most probably did not develop MI until day 5 or 6 after the episode of chest pain.
○ (B) The normal CK level obtained on day 3 excludes the possibility of MI in the preceding 72 hours.
○ (C) The normal CK level and elevated troponin level obtained on day 3 are consistent with an acute MI occurring on the day the patient developed shoulder pain.
○ (D) A CK-MB fraction determination would have been a much more sensitive way to detect acute MI than total CK level.

○ (E) A second acute MI most likely occurred on day 6 or 7, because myocardial rupture usually occurs within several hours of the development of a transmural MI.

24. A 45-year-old male experiences crushing substernal chest pain on arriving at work in the morning. Over the next few hours the pain persists and begins to radiate to his left arm. He becomes diaphoretic and short of breath, but he waits until the end of his 8-hour shift to go to the hospital. Which of the following serum laboratory test findings is most useful to diagnose his condition on admission to the hospital?

○ (A) Elevated lipase
○ (B) Elevated aspartate aminotransferase (AST)
○ (C) Elevated CK-MB
○ (D) Elevated alanine aminotransferase (ALT)
○ (E) Elevated lactate dehydrogenase type 1 (LDH-1)

25. A 60-year-old male diabetic has experienced angina on exertion for several years. A previous coronary angiography revealed 75% stenosis of the left anterior descending coronary artery and 50% stenosis of the right coronary artery. His blood pressure is 110/80 mm Hg. In the past few weeks, the frequency and severity of his anginal attacks have increased, and sometimes the pain occurs even when he is lying in bed. The most likely explanation for these changes in his symptoms is

○ (A) Hypertrophy of the ischemic myocardium with increased oxygen demands
○ (B) Increasing stenosis of the right coronary artery
○ (C) Fissuring of the plaque in left coronary artery with superimposed mural (partial) thrombosis
○ (D) Sudden complete thrombotic occlusion of the right and left coronary arteries
○ (E) Reduction in oxygen-carrying capacity from pulmonary congestion

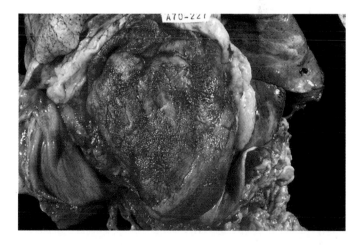

26. A friction rub is audible in a 68-year-old male with the gross appearance of the heart shown here. Which of the following laboratory test findings is most likely present in this patient?

O (A) Positive antinuclear antibody at 1:512
O (B) Elevated anti-streptolysin O titer
O (C) Urea nitrogen level of 98 mg/dL
O (D) Elevated renin level
O (E) Serum creatine kinase (CK) of 500 U/L

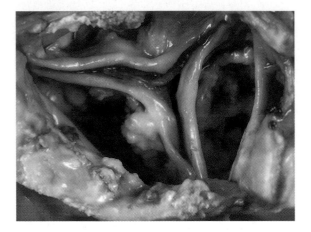

27. From the gross appearance of the aortic valve shown here, which of the following causes most likely contributed to the lesion?

O (A) Chromosomal aneuploidy
O (B) Aging
O (C) Syphilis
O (D) Atherosclerosis
O (E) Systemic lupus erythematosus

28. A 32-year-old North American Caucasian female presents with increasingly severe symptoms of congestive heart failure over 2 weeks. She has no previous history of heart disease. An electrocardiogram shows some runs of ventricular tachycardia, and an endomyocardial biopsy shows focal myocyte necrosis along with a lymphocytic infiltrate. She is most likely to have an infection with which of the following organisms?

O (A) *T. cruzi*
O (B) *S. viridans*
O (C) Coxsackievirus A
O (D) *Toxoplasma gondii*
O (E) *S. aureus*

29. While touring a 17th century European mansion, you notice that the bed in the bedroom was designed so that the occupant slept while sitting up. What cardiac disease in the 40-year-old wife of the mansion's owner at that time would best explain this bed design?

O (A) Libman-Sacks endocarditis
O (B) Giant cell myocarditis
O (C) Rheumatic heart disease
O (D) Atrial myxoma
O (E) Fibrinous pericarditis

30. A harsh, waxing and waning, machinery-like murmur is auscultated in the upper chest of a 2-year-old child with a history of infective endocarditis. Angiography reveals

mild pulmonary hypertension. Echocardiography shows all valves to be normal in configuration. Which of the following lesions did the angiogram most likely show?

O (A) Atrial septal defect (ASD)
O (B) Tetralogy of Fallot
O (C) Aortic coarctation
O (D) Total anomalous pulmonary venous return
O (E) Patent ductus arteriosus (PDA)

31. A 49-year-old previously healthy female reports having had several "fainting spells" in the last 6 months. In each case, she regained consciousness after only a few minutes. Her blood pressure is normal. She has good carotid pulses with no bruits. Which of the following cardiac lesions is most likely to be present?

O (A) Pericardial effusion
O (B) Left atrial myxoma
O (C) Bicuspid aortic valve
O (D) Mitral valve stenosis
O (E) Left anterior descending artery thrombosis

32. A 60-year-old male presents with worsening cough and orthopnea. Echocardiography reveals marked left ventricular hypertrophy and severe aortic stenosis. The remaining cardiac valves are normal. A coronary angiogram demonstrates no significant coronary arterial narrowing. Which of the following conditions best accounts for these findings?

O (A) Diabetes mellitus
O (B) Marfan syndrome
O (C) Bicuspid aortic valve
O (D) Systemic hypertension
O (E) Infective endocarditis

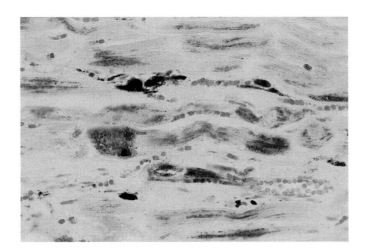

33. The microscopic appearance of the myocardium of a 45-year-old male is seen here with a Prussian blue stain. He had complained of increasing fatigue, exertional dyspnea, and chest pain. Which of the following functional cardiac disturbances was most likely present?

O (A) Dynamic obstruction to left ventricular outflow
O (B) Reduced ventricular compliance resulting in impaired ventricular filling in diastole

○ (C) Mitral and tricuspid valvular insufficiency
○ (D) Lack of ventricular expansion during diastole
○ (E) Reduced ejection fraction from decreased contraction

34.   Physical examination reveals jugular venous distention in the neck of a 50-year-old male, even when he is sitting up. He also has an enlarged and tender liver that can be felt 10 cm below the right costal margin. Pitting edema is observed on his lower extremities. A chest radiograph reveals large pleural effusions. Thoracentesis on the right yields 500 mL of clear fluid with few cells. The most likely cause of this clinical picture is

○ (A) Tricuspid valve stenosis
○ (B) Acute myocardial infarction
○ (C) Pulmonary valve stenosis
○ (D) Chronic obstructive lung disease
○ (E) Primary pulmonary hypertension

35.   Three weeks after a bout of acute pharyngitis, a 10-year-old female develops subcutaneous nodules over the skin of her arms and torso. She also manifests choreiform movements and begins to complain of pain in her knees and hips, particularly with movement. Auscultation of the chest reveals an audible friction rub. Which of the following serum laboratory test findings is most characteristic of the disease affecting this patient?

○ (A) Elevated level of cardiac troponin I
○ (B) Positive antinuclear antibody test
○ (C) Elevated creatinine level
○ (D) Positive rapid plasma reagin test
○ (E) Elevated anti–streptolysin O level

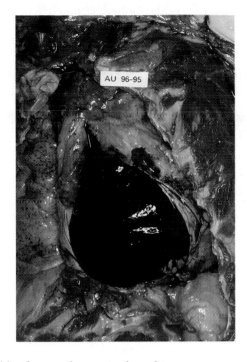

37.   This figure, demonstrating the gross appearance of this heart at autopsy in a 25-year-old male, is most consistent with which of the following underlying causes of death?

○ (A) Diabetes mellitus
○ (B) Disseminated tuberculosis
○ (C) Scleroderma
○ (D) Blunt chest trauma
○ (E) Malignant melanoma

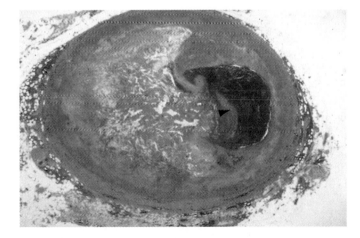

36.   The microscopic appearance of the proximal left anterior descending artery shown in the figure is seen at autopsy of a 37-year-old female. Which of the following conditions is probably the underlying cause of death?

○ (A) Marfan syndrome
○ (B) Acute leukemia
○ (C) Polyarteritis nodosa
○ (D) Diabetes mellitus
○ (E) Chronic alcoholism

38.   A 40-year-old female diagnosed with adenocarcinoma of the stomach with metastases to liver suffers a right cerebral infarction. A few weeks later, she develops severe dyspnea, and a pulmonary ventilation-perfusion scan shows a high probability for pulmonary thromboembolism. Which of the following cardiac lesions is most likely to be present?

○ (A) Cardiac metastases
○ (B) Left ventricular mural thrombosis
○ (C) Constrictive pericarditis
○ (D) Nonbacterial thrombotic endocarditis
○ (E) Calcific aortic valvular stenosis

39.   A month after orthotopic cardiac transplantation for ischemic cardiomyopathy in a 55-year-old male, an endomyocardial biopsy performed. The biopsy shows minimal focal myocyte necrosis with scattered lymphocytes and plasma cells. Which of the following pathologic processes best accounts for the biopsy findings?

○ (A) Autoimmunity
○ (B) Ischemia
○ (C) Infection
○ (D) Rejection
○ (E) Apoptosis

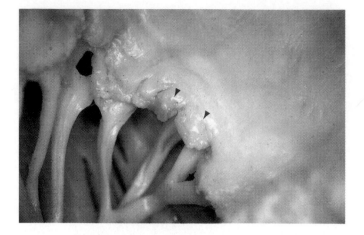

40. A 40-year-old female experiences increasing dyspnea, and the gross appearance of her heart is shown here. These changes in the heart most likely resulted after an infection with

O (A) *Treponema pallidum*
O (B) *Staphylococcus aureus*
O (C) Coxsackievirus B
O (D) Group A *Streptococcus*
O (E) *Toxoplasma gondii*

41. A 15-year-old male complains of pain in his legs when he runs more than 300 m. Physical examination reveals a blood pressure of 165/90 mm Hg along with a temperature of 36.5°C, pulse of 76, and respiration rate of 22 per minute. His radial pulses are 4+, and the dorsalis pedis pulses are 1+. Arterial blood gas measurement reveals normal oxygen saturation. Which of the following lesions is probably present?

O (A) Tricuspid atresia
O (B) Coarctation of the aorta
O (C) Aortic valve stenosis
O (D) Patent ductus arteriosus
O (E) Transposition of the great arteries

42. Physical examination of an asymptomatic 2-year-old child reveals a low-pitched cardiac murmur. An echocardiogram shows presence of the ostium secundum, with a 1-cm diameter defect. Which of the following clinical abnormalities is most likely to be found in this child?

O (A) Pulmonary hypertension
O (B) Pericardial effusion
O (C) Left-to-right shunt
O (D) Mural thrombosis
O (E) Cyanosis

43. A 44-year-old previously healthy male has experienced worsening exercise tolerance accompanied by marked shortness of breath for the past 6 months. A chest radiograph shows an enlarged heart and pulmonary edema. An echocardiogram shows four-chamber cardiac dilation and demonstrates mitral and tricuspid valvular regurgitation. A coronary angiogram demonstrates no more than 10% narrowing of the major coronary arteries. The under-

lying condition that is most likely to be present in this patient is

O (A) Rheumatic heart disease
O (B) Hemochromatosis
O (C) Chagas disease
O (D) Diabetes mellitus
O (E) Idiopathic dilated cardiomyopathy

44. A 19-year-old male suddenly collapses. He is brought to the emergency room, where he is found to be hypotensive. He is found to have an elevated total CK level with CK-MB fraction of 10%. Which of the following underlying conditions is he most likely to have?

O (A) Hereditary hemochromatosis
O (B) Marfan syndrome
O (C) Down syndrome
O (D) DiGeorge syndrome
O (E) Familial hypercholesterolemia

45. Myocarditis in a 14-year-old female is characterized microscopically by focal interstitial inflammation with Aschoff nodules and Anitschkow cells. This is accompanied by the gross appearance of a verrucous endocarditis and a fibrinous pericarditis. This pancarditis resolves over the ensuing weeks. Which of the following complications of this process is most likely to be seen in this patient 20 years later?

O (A) Aortic stenosis
O (B) Right ventricular dilation
O (C) Constrictive pericarditis
O (D) Mitral valve prolapse
O (E) Left ventricular aneurysm

46. The presence of hemorrhage and contraction bands in necrotic myocardial fibers is most likely to be seen in which of the following?

O (A) Subendocardial infarct resulting from diffuse narrowing of coronary arteries
O (B) Transmural infarct caused by complete thrombotic occlusion of a coronary artery
O (C) Transmural infarct complicated by mural thrombosis
O (D) Transmural infarct that is reperfused by thrombolytic therapy
O (E) A healing transmural myocardial infarct

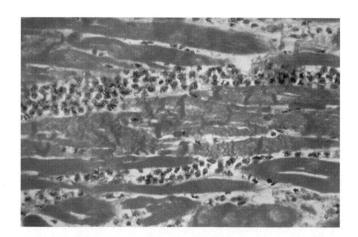

47. The light microscopic appearance of the left ventricular free wall shown on the previous page from a 48-year-old female is most consistent with

O (A) Viral myocarditis
O (B) Two-day-old myocardial infarction (MI)
O (C) Acute rheumatic myocarditis
O (D) Septic embolization
O (E) Restrictive cardiomyopathy

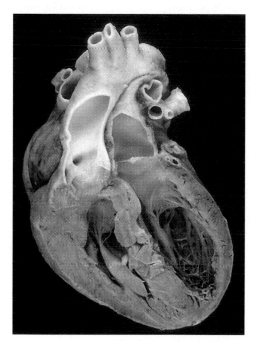

48. A 2-month-old infant has been cyanotic since birth. The baby has worsening congestive heart failure. Based on the gross appearance of the heart shown here, this infant's congenital heart disease is best classified as

O (A) Tetralogy of Fallot
O (B) Pulmonic stenosis
O (C) Truncus arteriosus
O (D) Transposition of the great vessels
O (E) Aortic stenosis

ANSWERS

1. **(E)** His symptoms are typical for angina pectoris when coronary artery narrowing exceeds 75%. Persons with rheumatic heart disease are affected by slowly worsening congestive heart failure (CHF). Pericarditis can produce chest pain, although not in relation to exercise, and it is not relieved by nitroglycerin. Cardiomyopathies result in heart failure but without chest pain. Calcific aortic stenosis leads to left-sided CHF, and the extra workload of the left ventricle may cause angina pectoris. However, calcific aortic stenosis (in the absence of a congenital bicuspid aortic valve) is rarely symptomatic at 50 years of age.
BP6 312   PBD6 554

2. **(B)** Bioprostheses are subject to wear and tear. The leaflets may calcify, resulting in stenosis, or they may perforate or tear, leading to insufficiency. Paravalvular leaks are rare complications of the early postoperative period. Hemolysis is not seen with bioprostheses and is rare with modern mechanical prostheses. Thrombosis with embolization is an uncommon complication of mechanical prostheses, lessened by anticoagulant therapy. Myocardial infarction from embolization or from a poorly positioned valve is rare.
BP6 328   PBD6 578

3. **(B)** The severity of the obstruction to the right ventricular outflow determines the direction of flow. If the pulmonic stenosis is mild, then the abnormality resembles a VSD, and the shunt may be left to right with no cyanosis. With significant pulmonary outflow obstruction, the right ventricular pressure may reach or exceed systemic vascular resistance, and the blood gets shunted from right to left, producing cyanotic heart disease. Even if pulmonic stenosis is mild at birth, the pulmonary orifice does not expand proportionately as the heart grows, and hence cyanotic heart disease supervenes.
BP6 335   PBD6 595

4. **(C)** This patient developed acute left ventricular failure, an uncommon complication of acute rheumatic fever. During the acute phase patients develop pancarditis, and hence pericarditis, valvulitis, myocarditis, and ventricular dilatation are all likely. Fibrosis and fusion of the mitral valve leaflets take several weeks to months to develop.
BP6 322-324   PBD6 570-572

5. **(D)** This is a large VSD. By the age of 5 years, such an uncorrected defect causes marked shunting of blood from left to right, causing pulmonary hypertension. However, the extent of cardiac malfunction is not great enough to produce renal disease, mainly because there is no systemic hypertension. Congenital heart disease is not an antecedent to ischemic heart disease in most cases. The DiGeorge syndrome, with T-cell immune deficiency from thymic hypoplasia, can be accompanied by cardiac defects, but this condition is uncommon and accounts for a very small fraction of all congenital cardiac defects. Dilated cardiomyopathy is an idiopathic condition in most cases. It is characterized by a large, flabby heart with dilation of all four chambers.
BP6 334   PBD6 594

6. **(C)** This enlarged and dilated heart has a large ventricular aneurysm. The aneurysm most likely resulted from a weakening of the ventricular wall at the site of a healed, old MI. Because of the damage to the endocardial lining and stasis and turbulence of blood flow in the region of the aneurysm, mural thrombi are likely to develop. When detached, these thrombi embolize to systemic circulation and can cause infarcts elsewhere. Cardiac rupture and acute pericarditis occur 5 to 7 days after an acute MI. Cardiogenic shock also occurs very early after an acute MI. Constrictive pericarditis follows a previous suppurative or tuberculous pericarditis.
BP6 316   PBD6 563

7. **(E)** This aortic valve has large, destructive vegetations typical for infective endocarditis caused by highly virulent organisms such as *S. aureus*. The verrucous vegetations of acute rheumatic fever are small and nondestructive, and the diagnosis is suggested by an elevated anti–streptolysin O titer. A positive antineutrophil cytoplasmic antibody determination suggests a vasculitis, which is not likely to involve cardiac valves. An elevated CK-MB level suggests myocardial, not endocardial, injury. A positive double-stranded DNA finding suggests a diagnosis of systemic lupus erythematosus, which can produce a nondestructive Libman-Sacks endocarditis.
BP6 326–328 PBD6 573–575

8. **(A)** The clinical and morphologic features are typical of hypertrophic cardiomyopathy. This disease is familial in 50% of cases and is usually transmitted as an autosomal dominant trait. The genetic defects affect the proteins that encode proteins of the cardiac contractile elements. The most common mutation in the inherited forms affects the β-myosin heavy chain. Chronic alcoholism can give rise to dilated cardiomyopathy, and amyloidosis causes restrictive cardiomyopathy.
BP6 331–332 PBD6 581–583

9. **(A)** The most common causes for hemorrhagic pericarditis are metastatic carcinoma and tuberculosis. Group A *Streptococcus* is responsible for rheumatic fever, which acutely can lead to a fibrinous pericarditis and to serous effusions from congestive failure in the chronic form. Coxsackieviruses are known to cause myocarditis. *Candida* is a rare cardiac infection in immunocompromised persons. *S. aureus* is best known as a cause of infective endocarditis.
BP6 337 PBD6 588–589

10. **(E)** This patient is at a high risk for developing complications of infective endocarditis. These findings suggest that she developed staphylococcal septicemia followed by endocarditis of the mitral valve. The impaired functioning of the mitral valve (most likely regurgitation) would give rise to left atrial dilation. The extension of infection from the valve surface to the underlying myocardium produces a ring abscess. Focal or diffuse glomerulonephritis is a complication that develops because antigen-antibody complexes, produced in response to persisting infection, deposit on the glomerular basement membrane. Emboli from the mitral valve would go into systemic circulation and give rise to brain abscesses. Myxomatous degeneration of the mitral valve results from a defect in connective tissues, whether well defined or unknown. The mitral valve leaflets are enlarged, hooded, and redundant.
BP6 326–328 PBD6 569, 574–576

11. **(A)** Prolonged fever, heart murmur, mild splenomegaly, and splinter hemorrhages suggest a diagnosis of infective endocarditis. The valvular vegetations with infective endocarditis are quite friable and can easily break off and embolize. The time course of weeks suggests infection from a less virulent organism, such as *S. viridans*. *T. cruzi* and coxsackievirus B are causes of myocarditis. *Candida* is not a common cause of infective endocarditis but may be

seen in immunocompromised patients. Tuberculosis involving the heart most often manifests as a pericarditis.
BP6 326–328 PBD6 573–575

12. **(A)** In the period immediately after coronary thrombosis, arrhythmias are the most important complication and can lead to sudden cardiac death. It is believed that, even before ischemic injury manifests in the heart, there is greatly increased electrical irritability. Pericarditis and rupture are seen several days later. An aneurysm is a late complication from healing of a large transmural infarction; a mural thrombus may fill an aneurysm and become a source for emboli. If portions of the coronary thrombus break off and embolize, they go into smaller arterial branches in the distribution already affected by ischemia.
BP6 314–316 PBD6 562

13. **(E)** His symptoms suggest aortic dissection. Fragmentation of elastic fibers in the media of the aorta greatly weakens the wall of the aorta and predisposes to aortic dissection. Such cystic medial necrosis can occur in patients with long-standing hypertension or in those with Marfan syndrome.
BP6 301–302, 325–326 PBD6 527–528, 569–570

14. **(I)** She has myxomatous degeneration of the mitral valve (i.e., "floppy mitral valve"), a condition seen in about 3% of the population. There is a potential risk for rupture with acute insufficiency, requiring mitral valve replacement. Other potential complications include infective endocarditis or nonbacterial thrombotic endocarditis with embolization and arrhythmias.
BP6 325–326 PBD6 569–570

15. **(K)** Nonbacterial thrombotic endocarditis often accompanies terminal cancer. This may be a feature of Trousseau syndrome, a paraneoplastic syndrome with a hypercoagulable state. Although the vegetations are bland and nondestructive, they are friable and can easily break off and embolize.
BP6 326 PBD6 567–577

16. **(J)** He probably has an infective endocarditis, and there is evidence of systemic septic embolization to produce the cerebral abscess. Such systemic embolization suggests that the lesions are on the left side of the heart. Although right-sided lesions strongly suggest injection drug use as a cause for infective endocarditis, injection drug users are only slightly more likely to have right-sided lesions. They can have right- and left-sided vegetations.
BP6 326–328 PBD6 574–576

17. **(B)** Hypertension is an important cause of left ventricular hypertrophy and failure. Left-sided heart failure leads to pulmonary edema with dyspnea. Obstructive (e.g., emphysema) and restrictive (e.g., silicosis) lung diseases lead to pulmonary hypertension with right heart failure from cor pulmonale. Likewise, right-sided valvular lesions (i.e., tricuspid or pulmonic valves) predispose to right heart failure. Alcoholism can lead to a dilated cardiomyopathy that affects left and right heart function.
BP6 309 PBD6 549

18. **(C)** This patient has evidence of pulmonary hypertension (pulmonary atherosclerosis) and right-sided heart failure. When this is secondary to lung disease, it is called cor pulmonale, caused most often by pulmonary emphysema and other obstructive lung diseases. Restrictive lung diseases can also lead to cor pulmonale. A VSD predominantly has left ventricular hypertrophy, although after years the left-to-right shunt can cause pulmonary vascular resistance to rise and reverse the shunt; at this stage right ventricular hypertrophy develops. A large pulmonary embolism can produce acute cor pulmonale, mainly with right atrial dilation. RHD affects mainly mitral and aortic valves. A hypertrophic cardiomyopathy affects left ventricular function the most.
BP6 320-321   PBD6 565-566

19. **(C)** She has findings of floppy mitral valve, a condition that is most often asymptomatic. When symptomatic, it can cause fatigue, chest pain, and arrhythmias. Pulmonic stenosis is most often a congenital heart disease. Valvular vegetations suggest an endocarditis, and a murmur is likely to be heard with infective endocarditis causing valvular insufficiency. A PDA causes a shrill systolic murmur. Tricuspid regurgitation is accompanied by a rumbling systolic murmur.
BP6 325-326   PBD6 568-570

20. **(A)** Hypertrophic cardiomyopathy is the most common cause of sudden unexplained death in young athletes. In this condition, there is asymmetric septal hypertrophy that reduces the ejection fraction of the left ventricle, particularly during exercise. Histologically, haphazardly arranged hypertrophic myocardial fibers are seen. Hemochromatosis gives rise to a restrictive cardiomyopathy in middle age. Tachyzoites of *T. gondii* signify myocarditis, a process that may occur in immunocompromised persons. RHD with chronic valvular changes would be unusual at this age, and the course is most often slowly progressive. Valve destruction with vegetations is seen in infective endocarditis. This should be accompanied by signs of sepsis.
BP6 331-332   PBD6 581-583

21. **(B)** The markedly thickened left ventricular wall is characteristic for hypertrophy from increased pressure load from hypertension, which is often associated with chronic renal disease. Chronic alcoholism is associated with a dilated cardiomyopathy. Pneumoconioses produce restrictive lung disease with cor pulmonale and predominantly right ventricular hypertrophy. Hemochromatosis leads to a restrictive cardiomyopathy. Diabetes mellitus accelerates atherosclerosis, leading to ischemic heart disease and MI.
BP6 319-320   PBD6 564-565

22. **(A)** The cyanosis at this early age suggests a right-to-left shunt, and tetralogy of Fallot is the most common cause for cyanotic congenital heart disease. The cerebral lesion suggests an abscess as a consequence of septic embolization from infective endocarditis, which can complicate congenital heart disease. ASDs and PDAs lead to left-to-right shunts. Coarctation is not accompanied by a shunt and cyanosis. A bicuspid valve is asymptomatic until adult life in most cases, and there is no shunt.
BP6 335-336   PBD6 595

23. **(C)** The kinetics of CK, CK-MB, and troponin I elevations after MI are important. Total CK activity begins to rise 2 to 4 hours after an MI, peaks at about 24 hours, and returns to normal by 72 hours. Troponin I levels begin to rise at about the same time as CK and CK-MB but remain elevated for 7 to 10 days. Total CK activity is a sensitive marker for myocardial injury in the first 24 to 48 hours. CK-MB offers more specificity but not more sensitivity. Myocardial rupture occurs 5 to 7 days after myocardial necrosis. This patient developed an MI on the day of the shoulder pain. When he went to the doctor on day 3, the CK levels had returned to normal, but troponin I levels were still elevated. Three days later, he suffered rupture of the infarct.
BP6 317   PBD6 561

24. **(C)** He has symptoms of an acute MI, and of the enzymes listed, CK-MB is the most specific for myocardial injury. The levels of this enzyme begin to rise within 2 to 4 hours of ischemic myocardial injury. Lipase is a marker for pancreatitis. AST is found in a variety of tissues, and therefore elevated levels are not specific for myocardial injury. ALT elevation is more specific for liver injury. The elevation of LDH-1 compared with LDH-2 suggests myocardial injury, but LDH activity peaks at 3 days after an MI.
BP6 317   PBD6 561

25. **(C)** This patient has 75% stenosis of the left anterior descending branch of the coronary artery. This degree of stenosis prevents adequate perfusion of the heart when myocardial demand is increased, as occurs during exertion. Hence, the patient had angina on exertion. In recent weeks, the patient has developed unstable angina which is manifested by increased frequency and severity of the attacks and angina at rest. In most patients, unstable angina is induced by disruption of an atherosclerotic plaque followed by a mural thrombus and, possibly, distal embolization, vasospasm, or both. Hypertrophy of the heart is unlikely in this case because there is neither hypertension nor a valvular lesion. All other possibilities can theoretically give rise to a similar picture, but plaque disruption with mural thrombosis is the most common anatomic finding when the patient develops unstable angina. It is important to recognize this, because unstable angina is a harbinger of MI.
BP6 312   PBD6 554-555

26. **(C)** This is a fibrinous pericarditis. The most common cause is uremia from renal failure. Positive antinuclear antibody suggests a collagen vascular disease, such as systemic lupus erythematosus. Such diseases tend to be accompanied by a serous pericarditis. An elevation of serum CK occurs in MI. An acute MI may be accompanied by a fibrinous exudate over the area of infarction, not the diffuse pericarditis seen here. Elevation of the antistreptolysin titer accompanies rheumatic fever. Acute rheumatic fever may produce a fibrinous pericarditis, but rheumatic fever is not common at this age.
BP6 337   PBD6 588

27. **(B)** This is calcific aortic stenosis, a degenerative change that may occur in a normal aortic valve with aging.

Congenital anomalies with chromosomal aneuploidies (e.g., trisomy 21) are not likely to be associated with aortic stenosis or a bicuspid valve. With syphilis, the aortic root dilates and results in aortic insufficiency. Atherosclerosis does not produce valvular disease from involvement of the valve itself. Systemic lupus erythematosus can sometimes give rise to small sterile vegetations on mitral or tricuspid valves, but these rarely cause valve disease.
BP6 324–325   PBD6 567–568

28.   **(C)** Focal myocardial necrosis with lymphocyte infiltrate is consistent with viral myocarditis. This is not common, and many cases may be asymptomatic. In North America, most cases are caused by coxsackieviruses A and B. This illness may be self-limited, end in sudden death, or progress to chronic heart failure. *T. cruzi* is the causative agent for Chagas disease, seen most often in children. Worldwide, this is probably the most common infectious cause of myocarditis. Septicemia with bacterial infections may involve the heart, but the patient probably is very ill with multiple organ failure. *T. gondii* may cause a myocarditis in immunocompromised patients.
BP6 329–330   PBD6 584–585

29.   **(C)** Paroxysmal nocturnal dyspnea is a feature of left-sided congestive heart failure, and RHD most often involves the mitral, aortic, or both valves. RHD was more common before availability of antibiotic therapy for group A β-hemolytic streptococcal infections. Giant cell myocarditis is a rare cause for cardiac failure that can be right and left sided. Libman-Sacks endocarditis, seen with systemic lupus erythematosus, does not typically impair ventricular function significantly. An atrial myxoma is most often on the left, but the obstruction is often intermittent. Fibrinous pericarditis can produce chest pain, but the amount of accompanying fluid is often not great, and hence cardiac function is not impaired.
BP6 310   PBD6 549

30.   **(E)** Although often not large in size, a PDA can produce a significant murmur and predispose to endocarditis. The left-to-right shunt eventually results in pulmonary hypertension. An ASD is unlikely to produce a loud murmur because of the minimal pressure differential between the atria. Because tetralogy of Fallot has pulmonic stenosis as a component, no pulmonary hypertension results. Aortic coarctations by themselves produce no shunting and no pulmonary hypertension. Total anomalous pulmonary venous return is not accompanied by a murmur because of the low venous pressure.
BP6 335   PBD6 594

31.   **(B)** An atrial myxoma can have a ball-valve effect that intermittently occludes the mitral valve, leading to the syncopal episodes. Most pericardial effusions are not large and do not cause major problems. Large effusions could lead to tamponade, but this is not an intermittent problem. Calcification of a bicuspid valve can lead to stenosis with heart failure, but this condition is progressive. By the time left atrial enlargement with mural thrombosis and risk of embolization occurs from mitral stenosis, she should have

been symptomatic for years. Coronary artery thrombosis results in an acute ischemic event.
BP6 338   PBD6 589–590

32.   **(C)** There is a tendency for bicuspid valves to calcify with aging, which can eventually result in stenosis. In individuals with congenitally bicuspid valves, symptoms appear by 50 to 60 years of age. By contrast, calcific aortic stenosis of tricuspid valves manifests in the seventies or eighties. Ischemic heart disease, expected with diabetes mellitus, does not lead to valvular stenosis. In Marfan syndrome, the aortic root dilates to produce aortic valvular insufficiency. Hypertension accounts for left ventricular hypertrophy, but the aortic valve is not affected. With infective endocarditis, he should be septic, and the valve tends to be destroyed, leading to insufficiency.
BP6 325   PBD6 568

33.   **(B)** The extensive iron deposition signifies hemochromatosis, which reduces ventricular compliance markedly, resulting in a restrictive cardiomyopathy. Dynamic left ventricular outflow obstruction is characteristic for hypertropic cardiomyopathy. Valvular insufficiency of mitral and tricuspid valves can occur with a dilated cardiomyopathy, which also reduces contractility and ejection fraction. Lack of diastolic expansion suggests a constrictive pericarditis.
BP6 332   PBD6 586–587

34.   **(D)** His findings point to a pure right-sided congestive heart failure. This can be caused by right-sided valvular lesions such as tricuspid or pulmonic stenosis, but these are rare. Much more common is pulmonary hypertension resulting from obstructive lung diseases such as emphysema. Primary pulmonary hypertension can also cause right-sided heart failure, but it is a much less common cause than are lung diseases. Because acute MI usually affects the left ventricle, left-sided heart failure is more common in these patients. Chronic left heart failure can eventually lead to right-sided heart failure.
BP6 309–310   PBD6 549–550

35.   **(E)** The findings suggest acute rheumatic fever, which can involve any or all layers of the heart. Because rheumatic fever follows streptococcal infections, the anti–streptolysin O titer is elevated. Cardiac troponins I and T are markers for ischemic myocardial injury. Although their levels may be somewhat elevated because of acute myocarditis that occurs in rheumatic fever, this change is not a characteristic of RHD. Levels of antinuclear antibodies could be elevated with systemic lupus erythematosus, which is most likely to produce a serous pericarditis. The strains of Group A *Streptococcus* that lead to acute rheumatic fever are not likely to cause glomerulonephritis, and an elevated creatinine level is therefore not likely. Positive rapid plasma reagin test suggests syphilis, but the clinical features are not those of syphilis.
BP6 322–324   PBD6 570–572

36.   **(D)** This coronary artery shows marked narrowing from atheromatous plaque, complicated by a recent thrombus. Atherosclerosis is accelerated with diabetes mellitus. When a premenopausal female develops severe atheroscle-

rosis, as in this case, underlying diabetes mellitus must be strongly suspected. The cystic medial necrosis with Marfan syndrome most often involves the ascending aorta and predisposes to dissection that could involve coronaries, although with external compression. Polyarteritis nodosa can involve coronary arteries and give rise to coronary thrombosis. However, in these cases, the vessel wall is necrotic and inflamed. Patients with leukemias can develop hypercoagulable states. When this occurs, there is widespread thrombosis in normal blood vessels. Chronic alcoholics often have less atherosclerosis than do persons of the same age who do not consume large amounts of alcohol.
BP6 311   PBD6 551-552

37.   **(D)** This is a massive hemopericardium with pericardial tamponade. The blunt trauma ruptures the myocardium. Ischemic heart disease with diabetes could lead to a ruptured MI, but that would be unusual at this age. Tuberculosis can cause a hemorrhagic pericarditis, typically without tamponade. Scleroderma is most likely to produce a serous effusion. Melanoma and other metastases can produce a hemorrhagic pericarditis without tamponade.
BP6 337-338   PBD6 587

38.   **(D)** These so-called marantic vegetations may occur on any cardiac valve but tend to be small and do not damage the valves. However, they have a nasty tendency to embolize. They can occur with hypercoagulable states that accompany certain malignancies, especially mucin-secreting adenocarcinomas. This paraneoplastic state is known as Trousseau syndrome. Cardiac metastases are uncommon, and they tend to go to the epicardium. Mural thromboses occur when cardiac blood flow is altered, as in a ventricular aneurysm or dilated atrium. Metastatic tumor can encase the heart to produce constriction, but this is rare. Calcific aortic stenosis occurs at a much older age, usually in the eighth or ninth decade.
BP6 326   PBD6 576

39.   **(D)** Endomyocardial biopsies are routinely performed after cardiac transplantation to monitor rejection. This is not an autoimmune process, because the transplant is "foreign" tissue to the host. Months to years later, the coronary arteriopathy characteristic for cardiac transplants may produce ischemic changes. Infection is a definite possibility, because of the immunosuppressive drugs administered to keep the rejection process under control, although plasma cells are not a key feature of acute infection. Apoptosis is not typically accompanied by inflammation to this degree.
BP6 329   PBD6 579

40.   **(D)** This mitral valve shows shortening and thickening of the chordae typical for chronic rheumatic valvulitis, and the small verrucous vegetations are characteristic of acute rheumatic fever. RHD develops after a streptococcal infection; the immune response against the bacteria damages the heart because streptococcal antigens cross react with the heart. Syphilis leads to aortic root dilation. *S. aureus* most often results in infective endocarditis in the heart. Coxsackievirus B infection can cause viral myocarditis. Toxoplasmosis is a cause for myocarditis in immunocompromised patients.
BP6 321-323   PBD6 570-572

41.   **(B)** In adults, the coarctation is typically postductal, and collateral branches from the proximal aorta supply the lower extremities, leading to the pulse differential from upper to lower extremities. Diminished renal blood flow increases renin production and promotes hypertension. Tricuspid atresia affects the right heart. Aortic valve stenosis causes left heart failure and no pressure differential in the extremities. A PDA produces a left-to-right shunt. Transposition results in a right-to-left shunt with cyanosis.
BP6 336   PBD6 596-597

42.   **(C)** Osteum secundum is the most common form of ASD. Because atrial pressures are low, the amount of shunting from left atrium to right atrium is not great, and this lesion can remain asymptomatic for many years. Eventually, pulmonary hypertension can occur, with reversal of the shunt. Pericardial effusions may occur much later, if congestive heart failure develops. A dilated heart with enlarged atria predisposes to mural thrombosis. Cyanosis is a feature of a right-to-left shunt.
BP6 333-334   PBD6 593-594

43.   **(E)** Congestive heart failure with four-chamber dilation is suggestive of dilated cardiomyopathy. Many cases of dilated cardiomyopathy have no known cause. Dilation is more prominent than hypertrophy, although both are present, and all chambers are involved. RHD should most often produce some degree of valvular stenosis, often with some regurgitation, and the course is usually more prolonged. Hemochromatosis produces a restrictive cardiomyopathy. Chagas disease affects the right ventricle more than the left. With diabetes mellitus and accelerated atherosclerosis, the coronary narrowing should be worse.
BP6 330-331   PBD6 579-581

44.   **(E)** The laboratory findings suggest an acute MI. Persons with familial hypercholesterolemia have accelerated and advanced atherosclerosis, even by the second or third decade. Hereditary hemochromatosis may result in an infiltrative cardiomyopathy with iron overload, more typically in the fifth decade. Marfan syndrome may result in aortic dissection or floppy mitral valve. DiGeorge syndrome can be associated with a variety of congenital heart defects, but survival with this syndrome is usually limited by infections from the cell-mediated immune deficiency.
BP6 317   PBD6 561

45.   **(A)** These findings point to acute rheumatic fever. Chronic rheumatic valvulitis with scarring can follow years later. The mitral and aortic valves are most commonly affected. In almost all cases, the fibrinous pericarditis seen during the acute phase resolves without significant scarring, and constrictive pericarditis does not develop. Mitral valve prolapse can be seen in patients with Marfan syndrome, or more commonly, no antecedent disease can be identified. A left ventricular aneurysm is a complication of ischemic heart disease.
BP6 322-324   PBD6 570-572

46.   **(D)** Reperfusion of an ischemic myocardium by spontaneous or therapeutic thrombolysis changes the morphology of the affected area. Reflow of blood into vascula-

ture injured during the period of ischemia leads to leakage of blood into the tissues (i.e., hemorrhage). Contraction bands are composed of closely packed hypercontracted sarcomeres. They are most likely produced by exaggerated contraction of previously injured myofibrils that are exposed to a high concentration of calcium ions from the plasma. The damaged cell membrane of the injured myocardial fibers allows calcium to penetrate the cells rapidly.

BP6 316–317 PBD6 561

47. **(B)** The picture shows deeply eosinophilic myocardial fibers with loss of nuclei, all indicative of coagulative necrosis. The deeply staining transverse bands are called contraction bands. In between the myocardial fibers are neutrophils. This pattern is most likely caused by an MI that is approximately 24 to 48 hours old. With viral myocarditis, there is minimal focal myocardial necrosis with round cell infiltrates. Rheumatic myocarditis has minimal myocardial necrosis with foci of granulomatous inflamma-

tion (i.e., Aschoff bodies). Septic emboli result in focal abscess formation. There is no significant inflammation with restrictive cardiomyopathies such as amyloidosis or hemochromatosis.

BP6 315   PBD6 560

48. **(D)** There is transposition of the great vessels. The aorta emerges from the right ventricle, and the pulmonic trunk exits the left ventricle. Unless there is another anomalous connection between right and left circulations, this condition is not compatible with extrauterine life. The most common connections include a VSD, PDA, or patent foramen ovale (or ASD). In tetralogy of Fallot, the aorta overrides a VSD but is not transposed. In pulmonic and aortic stenosis, the great arteries are normally positioned but small. In truncus arteriosus, the spiral septum that embryologically separates the great arteries does not develop properly.

BP6 336   PBD6 596

Red Cells and Bleeding Disorders

BP6 Chapter 12 - The Hematopoietic and Lymphoid Systems
PBD6 Chapter 14 - Red Cells and Bleeding Disorders

1. For the past 6 months, a 35-year-old female has had excessively heavy menstrual flow. She has also noticed increasing numbers of pinpoint hemorrhages on her lower extremities in the past month. Physical examination reveals no organomegaly or lymphadenopathy. A complete blood count (CBC) shows a hemoglobin concentration of 14.2 g/dL, hematocrit of 42.5%, mean corpuscular volume (MCV) of 91 fL/red cell, platelet count of 19,000/μL, and white blood cell (WBC) count of 6950/μL. She has melena on admission to the hospital and is given a transfusion of platelets, but her platelet count does not increase. An emergency splenectomy is followed by an increase in platelet count. The most likely basis of her bleeding tendency is

- (A) Abnormalities in production of platelets by mega-karyocytes
- (B) Suppression of pluripotent stem cells
- (C) Destruction of antibody-coated platelets by the spleen
- (D) Excessive loss of platelets in menstrual blood
- (E) Defective platelet-endothelial interactions

2. A 22-year-old female has had malaise with pharyngitis for a couple of weeks. She has Raynaud phenomenon, and she is diagnosed with infectious mononucleosis. Her direct and indirect Coombs tests are positive at 4°C, although not at 37°C. Which of the following substances in her red blood cells (RBCs) can account for these findings?

- (A) Immunoglobulin E (IgE)
- (B) Complement C3b
- (C) Histamine
- (D) Immunoglobin G (IgG)
- (E) Fibronectin

3. A 45-year-old female has chronic hepatitis C infection with serum concentrations of alanine aminotransferase (ALT) of 310 U/L, aspartate aminotransferase (AST) of 275 U/L, total bilirubin of 7.6 mg/dL, direct bilirubin of 5.8 mg/dL, alkaline phosphatase of 75 U/L, and ammonia of 85 μmol/L. She has malaise with nausea and vomiting. Which of the following laboratory test results for hemostatic function is most likely to be abnormal?

- (A) Immunoassay for plasma von Willebrand factor
- (B) Platelet count
- (C) Prothrombin time (PT)
- (D) Fibrin split products
- (E) Bleeding time

4. The peripheral blood smear from a 25-year-old female who has a history of arthralgias for the past 3 years shows hypochromic and microcytic RBCs. Despite a slightly decreased hemoglobin and hematocrit, the total RBC count is normal. Total serum iron and ferritin levels are within the normal range. Hemoglobin electrophoresis demonstrates an elevated hemoglobin A_2 level of about 5.8%. These findings are most typical for

- (A) Autoimmune hemolytic anemia
- (B) β-thalassemia minor
- (C) Infection with *Plasmodium vivax*
- (D) Anemia of chronic disease
- (E) Iron deficiency anemia

5. A 30-year-old female has splenomegaly and anemia with spherocytosis. The circulating RBCs demonstrate an increased osmotic fragility on laboratory testing. An inherited abnormality in which of the following RBC components best accounts for these findings?

- (A) Glucose-6-phosphate dehydrogenase
- (B) A membrane cytoskeletal protein
- (C) α-globin chain
- (D) Heme
- (E) β-globin chain

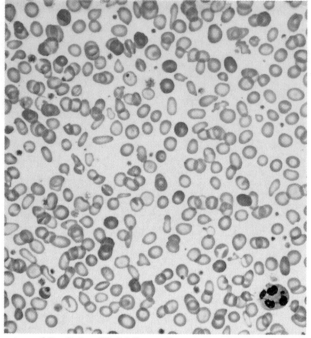

Courtesy of Dr. Robert W. McKenna, Department of Pathology, University of Texas Southwestern Medical School, Dallas, TX.

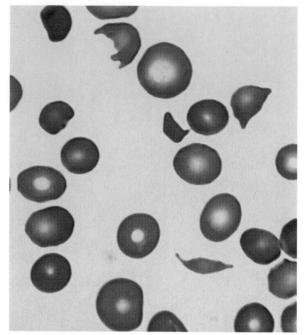

Courtesy of Dr. Robert W. McKenna, Department of Pathology, University of Texas Southwestern Medical School, Dallas, TX.

6. A 69-year-old previously healthy female has been feeling increasingly tired and weak for several months. She is found to be anemic, with a hemoglobin concentration of 9.3 g/dL. The appearance of her peripheral blood smear is shown here. Which of the following conditions should be suspected as the most likely cause for this appearance of the smear depicted here?

O (A) Pernicious anemia
O (B) Gastrointestinal blood loss
O (C) Aplastic anemia
O (D) β-thalassemia major
O (E) Warm autoimmune hemolytic anemia

7. A 76-year-old female notices that small, pinpoint to blotchy areas of superficial hemorrhage have appeared on her gums and on the skin of her arms and legs over several weeks. She is found to have a normal prothrombin time (PT) and partial thromboplastin time (PTT). Her CBC shows a hemoglobin concentration of 12.7 g/dL, hematocrit of 37.2%, MCV of 80 fL/red cell, platelet count of 276,000/μL, and WBC count of 5600/μL. Her template bleeding time is 3 minutes. Her fibrinogen level is normal, and no fibrin split products are detectable. Which of the following conditions best explains these findings?

O (A) Macronodular cirrhosis
O (B) Chronic renal failure
O (C) Meningococcemia
O (D) Vitamin C deficiency
O (E) Metastatic carcinoma

8. Blood culture in a 30-year-old male with hypotension and shock is positive for *Klebsiella pneumoniae*. Scattered ecchymoses are seen over his trunk and extremities. The appearance of his RBCs in a peripheral blood smear is shown in the following figure. These findings are most indicative of which of the following conditions?

O (A) Hereditary spherocytosis
O (B) Autoimmune hemolytic anemia
O (C) Microangiopathic hemolytic anemia
O (D) Iron deficiency anemia
O (E) Megaloblastic anemia

9. A 29-year-old female who has hereditary spherocytosis and mild anemia has developed a low-grade fever with malaise. After a week, she feels very tired and appears pale. Her hematocrit drops from the usual value of 36% to 28%. There is no change in the appearance of red cell morphology. Reticulocytes are absent from the peripheral blood. Her serum bilirubin is within the reference range. Which of the following events has most likely occurred?

O (A) Development of anti–red cell antibodies
O (B) Disseminated intravascular coagulopathy
O (C) Accelerated extravascular hemolysis in the spleen
O (D) Reduced erythropoiesis from parvovirus infection
O (E) Superimposed iron deficiency

10. A 60-year-old male who has terminal carcinoma of the colon develops widespread ecchymoses over his skin surface. The PT is 30 seconds, PTT is 55 seconds, platelet count is 15,200/μL, fibrinogen level is 75 mg/dL, and fibrin split product levels are very elevated. Which of the following morphologic findings would you most expect to find on examination of the peripheral blood smear?

O (A) Howell-Jolly bodies
O (B) Tear-drop cells
O (C) Macro-ovalocytes
O (D) Schistocytes
O (E) Target cells

11. A 30-year-old female has a CBC demonstrating a hemoglobin concentration of 11.8 g/dL and hematocrit of 35.1%. The peripheral blood smear shows that spherocytes and rare nucleated RBCs are present. The direct and

indirect Coombs tests are positive at 37°C, although not at 4°C. She has mild splenomegaly. Which of the following underlying diseases is she most likely to have?

○ (A) Infectious mononucleosis
○ (B) *Mycoplasma pneumoniae* infection
○ (C) Hereditary spherocytosis
○ (D) *Escherichia coli* septicemia
○ (E) Systemic lupus erythematosus (SLE)

12. A young adult patient has just been diagnosed with von Willebrand disease. Which of the following statements should you make to advise the patient of potential consequences of this disease?

○ (A) You may need an allogeneic bone marrow transplant.
○ (B) Expect increasing difficulties with joint mobility.
○ (C) Anticoagulation is needed to prevent deep venous thrombosis.
○ (D) You may have excessive bleeding following tooth extraction.
○ (E) A splenectomy may be necessary to control the disease.

13. Hydroxyurea therapy has been found to be beneficial in patients with sickle cell anemia. The basis for its therapeutic efficacy is

○ (A) An increase in the production of hemoglobin F
○ (B) An increase in the production of hemoglobin A
○ (C) A decrease in overall globin synthesis
○ (D) A stimulation of erythrocyte production
○ (E) An increase in the oxygen affinity of hemoglobin

14. A 73-year-old male who is taking no medications and has been healthy all his life, with no major illnesses or surgeries, is becoming increasingly tired and listless. A CBC indicates a hemoglobin concentration of 9.7 g/dL, hematocrit of 29.9%, MCV of 69.7 fL/red cell, RBC count of $4.28 \times 10^6/\mu L$, platelet count of 331,000/μL, and WBC count of 5500/μL. The most probable explanation for these findings is

○ (A) Iron deficiency
○ (B) Autoimmune hemolytic anemia
○ (C) β-thalassemia major
○ (D) Chronic alcoholism
○ (E) Vitamin B_{12} deficiency

15. Three days after taking an anti-inflammatory medication that includes phenacetin, a 23-year-old African-American male passes dark reddish-brown urine. He is surprised by this, because he has been healthy all his life, with no major illnesses. A CBC demonstrates a mild normocytic anemia, but the peripheral blood smear shows precipitates of denatured globin (i.e., Heinz bodies) with supravital staining and scattered "bite cells" in the population of RBCs. These findings are most typical for

○ (A) α-thalassemia
○ (B) Sickle cell trait
○ (C) Glucose-6-phosphate dehydrogenase deficiency
○ (D) Autoimmune hemolytic anemia
○ (E) β-thalassemia minor

16. A ___ old male who presents with chronic fatigue with weight loss is found to have a hemoglobin concentration of 11.2 g/dL, hematocrit of 33.3%, MCV of 91 fL/red cell, platelet count of 240,000/μL, and WBC count of 7550/μL. He has a serum iron of 80 μg/dL, total iron-binding capacity of 145 μg/dL, and serum ferritin of 565 ng/mL. These findings are most indicative of

○ (A) Iron deficiency anemia
○ (B) Aplastic anemia
○ (C) Anemia of chronic disease
○ (D) Microangiopathic hemolytic anemia
○ (E) Megaloblastic anemia

17. Which of the following infectious agents accounts for the observed distribution of hemoglobin S in human populations?

○ (A) *Cryptococcus neoformans*
○ (B) *Borrelia burgdorferi*
○ (C) *Treponema pallidum*
○ (D) *Plasmodium falciparum*
○ (E) *Clostridium perfringens*

18. A 41-year-old female presents with a 2-week history of multiple ecchymoses on extremities with only minor trauma. She also feels extremely weak. Over the past day she has developed a severe cough productive of yellowish sputum. She has the following CBC findings: hemoglobin concentration of 7.2 g/dL, hematocrit of 21.4%, MCV of 88 fL/red cell, platelet count of 35,000/μL, and WBC count of 1400/μL, with 20 segmented neutrophils, 1 band, 66 lymphocytes, and 13 monocytes. Reticulocytosis is absent. Given these laboratory findings, which of the following points in the history would be most useful in determining the cause of her condition?

○ (A) History of exposure to drugs
○ (B) Dietary history
○ (C) History of recent bacterial infection
○ (D) Menstrual history
○ (E) Family history of anemias

19. A 40-year-old male who suffered from chronic anemia since childhood was admitted to the hospital with fever and pain in the chest. Despite supportive therapy he died a few days later. A small, fibrotic, 5-g spleen filled with deposits of iron and calcium is found at autopsy. Which of the following conditions is most likely to have resulted in this finding?

○ (A) Sickle cell anemia
○ (B) β-thalassemia
○ (C) Malaria
○ (D) Idiopathic thrombocytopenic purpura (ITP)
○ (E) Autoimmune hemolytic anemia

20. A 13-year-old male has less than 1% factor VIII activity measured in plasma. If he does not receive transfusions of factor VIII concentrate, which of the following manifestations of this deficiency is most likely to ensue?

○ (A) Splenomegaly
○ (B) Conjunctival petechiae

○ (C) Hemolysis
○ (D) Hemochromatosis
○ (E) Hemarthroses

21. A 23-year-old female was in her 25th week of pregnancy when she ceased to feel fetal movement. Three weeks later, she has still not delivered, but she suddenly develops dyspnea with cyanosis and is found to be hypotensive. She has large ecchymoses over her skin and melena. She is found to have an elevated PT and PTT. The platelet count is decreased. Her plasma fibrinogen is markedly decreased, and fibrin split products are detected. The most likely cause of her bleeding diathesis is

○ (A) Increased vascular fragility
○ (B) Toxic injury to the endothelium
○ (C) Reduced production of platelets
○ (D) Increased consumption of clotting factors and platelets
○ (E) Defects in platelet adhesion and aggregation

For each of the clinical histories in questions 22 through 24, select the most closely associated lettered mechanism for development of anemia:

○ (A) Mechanical fragmentation of RBCs
○ (B) Increased susceptibility to lysis by complement
○ (C) Nuclear maturation defects due to impaired DNA synthesis
○ (D) Impaired globin synthesis
○ (E) Hemolysis of antibody-coated cells
○ (F) Stem cell defect
○ (G) Oxidative injury to hemoglobin
○ (H) Reduced deformability of the red cell membrane
○ (I) Production of an abnormal hemoglobin
○ (J) Imbalance in the synthesis of α- and β-globin chains

22. A baby is born at 34 weeks' gestation to a gravida 3 para 2 female who is 28 years old. The baby is markedly hydropic and icteric. A cord blood sample is taken, and the direct Coombs test result is positive for the baby's RBCs. (   )

23. A 30-year-old male passes dark brown urine several days after starting the prophylactic antimalarial drug primaquine. His serum haptoglobin concentration is decreased. (   )

24. A 62-year-old male presents to the emergency department in an obvious state of inebriation. He is known in the emergency department because this scenario has repeated itself many times throughout the years. A CBC is ordered, which shows anemia (hemoglobin level of 8.2 g/dL), with a very high MCV (115 fL/red cell), thrombocytopenia, and neutropenia. Microscopic examination of the peripheral blood shows prominent anisocytosis, including very large red cells. Polychromatophilic red cells are difficult to find. A few of the neutrophils demonstrate six to seven nuclear lobes. (   )

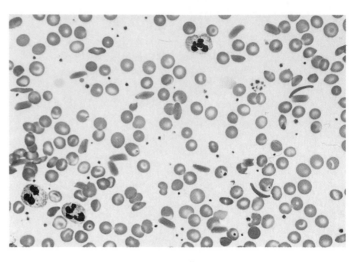

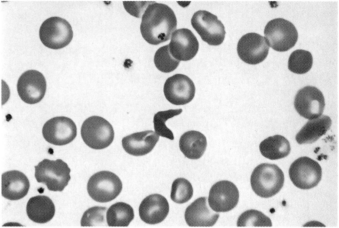

Courtesy of Dr. Robert W. McKenna, Department of Pathology, University of Texas Southwestern School, Dallas, TX.

25. A 12-year-old male experienced the sudden onset of severe abdominal pain and cramping. The peripheral blood smear shown in the figures is most suggestive of which of the following RBC disorders?

○ (A) Hereditary spherocytosis
○ (B) α-thalassemia
○ (C) Paroxysmal nocturnal hemoglobinuria
○ (D) Hemoglobin C disease
○ (E) Sickle cell anemia

26. Patients who inherit mutations that reduce the level of spectrin in the red cell membrane cytoskeleton develop a chronic anemia with splenomegaly. In many such patients, splenectomy reduces the severity of anemia. This beneficial effect of splenectomy is related to which of the following processes?

○ (A) An increase in the synthesis of spectrin in RBC
○ (B) An increase in the deformability of red cells
○ (C) A decrease in the opsonization of red cells
○ (D) A decrease in the trapping of red cells in the spleen
○ (E) A decrease in the production of reactive oxygen species

27. A 39-year-old female presented with a 3-month history of abdominal pain and intermittent diarrhea. Further radiologic examination and colonoscopy established the di-

agnosis of Crohn's disease. Because she failed to respond to medical therapy, part of the colon and terminal ileum were surgically removed. She was transfused with 1 unit of packed RBCs during surgery. Several weeks later, she is apparently healthy but complains of easy fatigability. On investigation, she is found to have the following CBC findings: hemoglobin concentration of 10.6 g/dL, hematocrit of 31.6%, RBC count of 2.69 million/μL, MCV of 118 fL/red cell, platelet count of 378,000/μL, and WBC count of 9800/μL. The most likely condition that explains these findings is

○ (A) Post–blood transfusion hemolytic anemia
○ (B) Iron deficiency
○ (C) Chronic blood loss
○ (D) Vitamin B$_{12}$ deficiency
○ (E) Anemia of chronic disease

28.   A 45-year-old male with *E. coli* septicemia becomes hypotensive and requires increasing pressor support to maintain blood pressure. He develops a guaiac-positive stool and ecchymoses of the skin. A CBC shows that the hemoglobin concentration is 9.2 g/dL and hematocrit is 28.1%. Platelet count is reduced to 70,000/μL. Increased amounts of fibrin split products are identified in the blood. Which of the following conditions is most likely responsible for the low hematocrit?

○ (A) Warm autoimmune hemolytic anemia
○ (B) Paroxysmal nocturnal hemoglobinuria
○ (C) Microangiopathic hemolytic anemia
○ (D) β-thalassemia major
○ (E) Aplastic anemia

29.   A 10-year-old child with homozygous sickle cell anemia had multiple episodes of pneumonia and meningitis with septicemia. The causative organisms cultured included *Streptococcus pneumoniae* and *Haemophilus influenzae*. One final episode of meningitis resulted in the death of the child. The most likely cause of repeated infections in this case is

○ (A) Loss of normal splenic function from recurrent ischemic injury
○ (B) Reduced synthesis of immunoglobulins
○ (C) Impaired neutrophil production
○ (D) Reduced synthesis of complement proteins by the liver
○ (E) Reduced expression of adhesion molecules on endothelial cells

30.   A healthy 19-year-old female suffered blunt abdominal trauma in a motor vehicle accident. On admission to the hospital, her initial hematocrit was 33%, but over the next hour, it dropped to 28%. A paracentesis yielded serosanguineous fluid. She was taken to surgery, where a liver laceration was repaired and a liter of bloody fluid was removed from the peritoneal cavity. Her condition remained stable. A CBC performed 3 days later is most likely to demonstrate which of the following morphologic findings in RBCs in the peripheral blood?

○ (A) Reticulocytosis
○ (B) Leukoerythroblastosis

○ (C) Basophilic stippling
○ (D) Hypochromia
○ (E) Schistocytes

31.   Which of the following parameters reported from a CBC can provide an indication of macrocytosis?

○ (A) Mean corpuscular volume (MCV)
○ (B) Mean corpuscular hemoglobin (MCH)
○ (C) Mean corpuscular hemoglobin concentration (MCHC)
○ (D) Red cell distribution width (RDW)
○ (E) Hematocrit

32.   A 17-year-old male presents with passage of dark urine. He has had multiple bacterial infections over several years and has a history of venous thromboses, including portal vein thrombosis in the previous year. A CBC shows a hemoglobin concentration of 9.8 g/dL, hematocrit of 29.9%, MCV of 92 fL/red cell, platelet count of 150,000/μL, and WBC count of 3800/μL, with a differential count of 24 segmented neutrophils, 1 band, 64 lymphocytes, 10 monocytes, and 1 eosinophil. He has a reticulocytosis. The serum haptoglobin level is very low. A mutation in which of the following gene products could give rise to this clinical condition?

○ (A) Spectrin
○ (B) Glucose-6-phosphate dehydrogenase
○ (C) Phosphatidylinositol glycan A (PIGA)
○ (D) β-globin chain
○ (E) Factor V

33.   A 32-year-old male has had a chronic anemia for many years. Alpha-globin inclusions are present in erythroblasts and erythrocytes, leading to increased phagocytosis by cells of the mononuclear phagocyte system. The result is ineffective hematopoiesis and increased absorption of dietary iron leading to hemochromatosis. These findings are most typical for

○ (A) Autoimmune hemolytic anemia
○ (B) Glucose-6-phosphate dehydrogenase deficiency
○ (C) Megaloblastic anemia
○ (D) β-thalassemia
○ (E) Sickle cell anemia

For each patient described in questions 34 through 37, select the most likely underlying cause of bleeding:

○ (A) Hemophilia A
○ (B) Hemophilia A with inhibitors of factor VIII
○ (C) Vitamin K deficiency
○ (D) von Willebrand disease
○ (E) Heparin therapy
○ (F) Idiopathic thrombocytopenic purpura (ITP)
○ (G) Disseminated intravascular coagulation
○ (H) Thrombotic thrombocytopenic purpura (TTP)
○ (I) Coumadin therapy

34.   A 13-year-old child has a history of bleeding, including severe hemorrhage into the knee joint, requiring multiple transfusions. Other male members of the family have bleeding problems. He has a prolonged PTT and a normal

PT (PT). A 1:1 dilution of patient's plasma with normal pooled plasma does not correct the PTT. (   )

35. A 16-year-old male has a history of easy bruising and hemorrhages into the knee joint that have led to joint deformity. Other male members of the family have also had bleeding problems. He has a prolonged PTT and a normal PT. A 1:1 dilution of this patient's plasma with normal pooled plasma corrects the PTT. (   )

36. A 23-year-old female has had a history of bleeding problems all of her life, primarily heavy menstruation and gum bleeding. A sister and an uncle have similar problems. Bleeding time is prolonged. Her PT is normal, and the PTT is mildly prolonged, but it corrects with a 1:1 dilution with normal pooled plasma. Factor VIII activity is 30% (reference range, 50% to 150%). Her platelet count is within reference range. (   )

37. A 42-year-old female presents with a several-month history of nose bleeds, easy bruising, and increased bleeding with her menstrual periods. There are no other symptoms or signs. Physical examination reveals scattered petechiae over her distal extremities. The peripheral blood smear shows a decrease in platelets and normal red blood cell morphology. Examination of the bone marrow biopsy shows a marked increase in megakaryocytes. Her PT and PTT values are within the reference range. (   )

38. A 3-year-old child of Italian ancestry presents with failure to thrive. Physical examination shows hepatosplenomegaly. His hemoglobin concentration is 6 g/dL, and the peripheral blood smear reveals severely hypochromic microcytic red cells. Total serum iron level is normal. The reticulocyte count is 10%. Hemoglobin electrophoresis reveals very little hemoglobin A. A radiograph of the skull shows maxillofacial deformities. The principal cause of anemia and other abnormalities in this patient is

- O (A) Reduced synthesis of hemoglobin F
- O (B) Reduced red blood cell survival from imbalance in the production of α- and β-globin chains
- O (C) Sequestration of the iron in the reticuloendothelial cells
- O (D) Increased fragility of the erythrocyte membrane
- O (E) Relative deficiency of vitamin B_{12}

39. Worldwide, the most common cause for impaired red blood cell production leading to anemia is

- O (A) Thalassemia
- O (B) Iron deficiency
- O (C) Chronic infection
- O (D) Metastatic carcinoma
- O (E) Toxic marrow injury

40. Your 55-year-old male patient has anemia but no significant past medical or surgical history. He currently feels fine, except for some minor fatigue with exertion. You are asked to determine the adequacy of his total body iron stores. What is the most sensitive and cost-effective test that you should order?

- O (A) Serum iron
- O (B) Serum transferrin

- O (C) Hemoglobin
- O (D) Bone marrow biopsy
- O (E) Serum ferritin

41. A 7-year-old African-American male child known to be suffering from sickle cell anemia presents with severe pain in the bones of the right hand. There is no associated fever or leukocytosis. The most likely pathogenetic factor in the causation of this pain is

- O (A) Defects in the alternative complement pathway
- O (B) Increased adhesion of red blood cells to the endothelium
- O (C) Erosion of bones from stimulation of erythropoiesis
- O (D) Increased red blood cell sickling in the peripheral tissues
- O (E) Increased production of fetal hemoglobin

42. A 78-year-old male presents with worsening malaise and fatigue over the past 5 months. He also has an enlarged spleen. His CBC shows a hemoglobin concentration of 10.6 g/dL, hematocrit of 29.8%, MCV of 92 fL/red cell, platelet count of 95,000/μL, and WBC count of 4900/$\mu\mu$L. The WBC differential count shows 67 segmented neutrophils, 4 bands, 2 metamyelocytes, 22 lymphocytes, 5 monocytes, and 3 nucleated RBCs per 100 WBCs. The peripheral blood smear shows occasional tear-drop cells. An examination of bone marrow biopsy and smear is most likely to show

- O (A) Marrow packed with myeloblasts
- O (B) Marrow fibrosis with greatly reduced hematopoietic islands
- O (C) Replacement of marrow by fat
- O (D) Presence of numerous megaloblasts
- O (E) Marked normoblastic erythroid hyperplasia

43. In your workup of a 50-year-old male with anemia, you are asked to order tests for vitamin B_{12} and folate. What is the most important reason for ordering the tests for these nutrients simultaneously?

- O (A) They are both absorbed similarly.
- O (B) Therapy for one also treats the other.
- O (C) The peripheral blood smear appears the same for both.
- O (D) Aplastic anemia may result from lack of either.
- O (E) Neurologic injury must be avoided.

44. A hemoglobin electrophoresis is performed on the RBCs of a 26-year-old African-American male undergoing a workup of chronic anemia. It shows that almost all of the hemoglobin present is hemoglobin S. In this patient, you would most expect to find which of the following complications of his underlying disease?

- O (A) Micronodular cirrhosis
- O (B) Chronic atrophic gastritis
- O (C) Pigment gallstones
- O (D) A high rate of stillbirths in his family
- O (E) An esophageal web

45. A 42-year-old male hospitalized with *K. pneumoniae* septicemia was observed over the course of 2 days to have decreasing renal and hepatic function. He was bleeding from the endotracheal tube and from his Foley catheter.

His condition continued to worsen, with hypotension and shock, and he died. At autopsy, microthrombi are found in arterioles and capillaries of the kidneys, adrenals, brain, and liver. Which of the following laboratory test results obtained during his terminal course is most characteristic for his condition?

O (A) Increased bleeding time
O (B) Elevated fibrin split products
O (C) Deficiency of von Willebrand factor
O (D) Increased plasma fibrinogen
O (E) Thrombocytosis

46.   A 40-year-old male died from congestive heart failure complicated by arrhythmias. At autopsy, the heart is dark brown and enlarged, with thickened ventricular walls and slight chamber dilation. The liver has a micronodular pattern of cirrhosis and appears dark brown. The myocardium and the liver contain extensive iron deposition as seen with the Prussian blue stain. Which of the following inherited RBC disorders is he most likely to have?

O (A) β-thalassemia major
O (B) Hereditary spherocytosis
O (C) Sickle cell anemia
O (D) Glucose-6-phosphate dehydrogenase deficiency
O (E) β-thalassemia minor

47.   A 31-year-old male has a history of chronic anemia and painful crises with joint and abdominal pain. A head computed tomography scan reveals several small remote infarctions. During one of these acute crises, he is admitted with severe dyspnea. A CBC is performed. Which of the following morphologic findings for RBCs is most likely to be seen on the peripheral blood smear?

O (A) Tear-drop cells
O (B) Sickle cells
O (C) Schistocytosis
O (D) Microcytosis
O (E) Spherocytosis

48.   A diagnosis of systemic lupus erythematosus (SLE) is made in a 61-year-old male who has anemia with a hematocrit of 24%. A urinalysis dipstick examination reveals the presence of blood, but there are no WBCs, RBCs, or casts on the urine microscopic examination. A hemolytic anemia is suspected. Which of the following serum laboratory test findings would best corroborate this diagnosis?

O (A) Elevated d-Dimer
O (B) Negative Coombs antiglobulin test
O (C) Decreased iron
O (D) Elevated antinuclear antibody titer
O (E) Diminished haptoglobin

For each of the patient histories in questions 49 and 50, match the most closely associated hematologic condition that can cause anemia:

O (A) Idiopathic thrombocytopenic purpura (ITP)
O (B) Warm autoimmune hemolytic anemia
O (C) β-thalassemia major
O (D) α-thalassemia major
O (E) Sickle cell anemia
O (F) Hereditary spherocytosis

O (G) Anemia of chronic disease
O (H) Iron deficiency anemia
O (I) Paroxysmal nocturnal hemoglobinuria
O (J) Thrombotic thrombocytopenic purpura (TTP)
O (K) Disseminated intravascular coagulation
O (L) Acute blood loss

49.   A 45-year-old female has a long history of rheumatoid arthritis. A CBC reveals the following: hemoglobin concentration of 11.6 g/dL, hematocrit of 34.8%, MCV of 87 fL/red cell, platelet count of 268,000/μL, and WBC count of 6800/μL. The serum haptoglobin level is normal, and the serum iron concentration is 20 μg/dL; total iron-binding capacity is 195 μg/dL, and the percent saturation is 10.2. The serum ferritin concentration is 317 ng/mL. No fibrin split products are detected. The reticulocyte concentration is 1.1%.

50.   A 54-year-old female presents with the sudden onset of headaches with photophobia worsening for the past 2 days. She has a temperature of 37°C. A CBC shows the following: hemoglobin concentration of 11.2 g/dL, hematocrit of 33.7%, MCV 94 of fL/red cell, platelet count of 32,000/μL, and WBC count of 9900/μL. The peripheral blood smear demonstrates schistocytes. Her serum urea nitrogen level is 38 mg/dL, and the creatinine concentration is 3.9 mg/dL.

51.   A 65-year-old male presents with increasing fatigue, and a CBC shows the following: hemoglobin concentration of 5.9 g/dL, hematocrit of 17.3%, MCV of 96 fL/red cell, platelet count of 150,000/μL, and WBC count of 7800/μL. The reticulocyte concentration is increased at 2.9%. No fibrin split products are detected, and the direct and indirect Coombs test results are negative. Bone marrow demonstrates marked erythroid hyperplasia. Which of the following conditions best explains these findings?

O (A) Blood loss
O (B) Iron deficiency
O (C) Aplastic anemia
O (D) Metastatic carcinoma
O (E) Immunohemolytic anemia

ANSWERS

1.   (C) This patient's bleeding is caused by a low platelet count. She most likely has idiopathic thrombocytopenic purpura (ITP), in which platelets are destroyed in the spleen after being coated with an antiplatelet antibody. The serum contains antiplatelet antibodies that presumably coat the patient's platelets and the transfused platelets. Because spleen is the source of the antibody and the site of destruction, splenectomy can be beneficial. There is no defect in the production of platelets. Suppression of pluripotent stem cells gives rise to aplastic anemia in which there is pancytopenia. Platelet functions are normal with ITP.
BP6 387   PBD6 634-636

2. **(B)** She has cold agglutinin disease with antibody (usually IgM) coating RBCs. The IgM antibodies bind to the red cells at low temperature and fix complement. However, complement is not lytic at this temperature. With a rise in temperature, the IgM is dissociated from the cell, leaving behind C3b. Most of the hemolysis occurs extravascularly in the cells of the mononuclear phagocyte system, such as Kupffer cells in the liver, because of the coating of complement C3b that acts as an opsonin. Raynaud phenomenon occurs in exposed, colder areas of the body such as fingers and toes. She probably has an elevated cold agglutinin titer. IgE is present with allergic conditions, and histamine is released with type I hypersensitivity reactions. IgG is typically involved in warm antibody hemolytic anemia. The anemia is chronic and is not triggered by cold. Fibronectin is an adhesive cell surface glycoprotein that aids in tissue healing.
BP6 351   PBD6 620–621

3. **(C)** Many of the clotting factors that are instrumental in the in vitro measurement of the extrinsic pathway of coagulation, as measured by the PT, are synthesized in the liver. von Willebrand factor is made by endothelial cells, not hepatocytes. The platelet count is not directly affected by liver disease. Increased fibrin split products suggest a consumptive coagulopathy such as disseminated intravascular coagulation (DIC). The bleeding time is a measure of platelet function, which is not significantly affected by liver disease.
BP6 384   PBD6 633

4. **(B)** Although β-thalassemia minor and iron deficiency anemia have hypochromic and microcytic RBCs, there is no increase in hemoglobin A_2 in iron deficiency states. Normal serum ferritin also excludes iron deficiency. Unlike β-thalassemia major, there is usually just a mild anemia without major organ dysfunction. Diseases that produce hemolysis and increase erythropoiesis (e.g., autoimmune hemolytic anemia, malaria) do not alter the composition of β-globin chain production. Anemia of chronic disease may mimic iron deficiency and thalassemia minor with respect to hypochromia and microcytosis. However, it is associated with an increase in the serum concentration of ferritin.
BP6 350   PBD6 617–618

5. **(B)** Spectrin and related proteins (e.g., protein 4.1, ankyrin) are cytoskeletal proteins that are important in maintaining the RBC shape. Hereditary spherocytosis is a condition in which a mutation affects one of several membrane cytoskeletal proteins. These mutations secondarily reduce spectrin synthesis even if the spectrin gene is normal. Spectrin-deficient RBCs are less deformable. The abnormal RBCs appear to lack central pallor on a peripheral blood smear, and they are sequestered and destroyed in the spleen. Glucose-6-phosphate dehydrogenase deficiency is an X-linked condition most commonly affecting black males. Thalassemias with abnormal α- or β-globin chains are associated with hypochromic microcytic anemias.
BP6 343–344   PBD6 607–609

6. **(B)** The RBCs display hypochromia and microcytosis, consistent with iron deficiency. The most common cause for this in older persons is chronic blood loss, and a gas-

trointestinal source (e.g., carcinoma, ulcer disease) should be sought. At age 69 she is not menstruating, and vaginal bleeding is likely to be noticed and is a "red flag" for a gynecologic malignancy. Pernicious anemia from vitamin B_{12} deficiency should result in a macrocytic anemia. The RBCs are generally normocytic with aplastic anemia. Microcytosis may accompany thalassemias, but she would be unlikely to live to age 69 with β-thalassemia major. Autoimmune hemolytic anemias usually produce a normocytic anemia, or the MCV can be slightly elevated with a brisk reticulocytosis.
BP6 353–354   PBD6 629–630

7. **(D)** Platelet number and function in this case are normal, and there is no detectable abnormality in the extrinsic or intrinsic pathways of coagulation as measured by the PT or PTT. Petechia and ecchymoses can result from increased vascular fragility, a consequence of nutritional deficiency (e.g., vitamin C), infection (e.g., meningococcemia), and vasculitic diseases. Meningococcemia is an acute illness. Liver disease should affect the PT. Chronic renal failure may depress platelet function. Metastatic disease does not directly affect hemostasis, although extensive marrow metastases could diminish platelet production.
BP6 384   PBD6 634–635

8. **(C)** The fragmented RBCs, including "helmet cells," are typical for conditions that can produce a microangiopathic hemolytic anemia, such as DIC, TTP, SLE, hemolytic-uremic syndrome (HUS), and malignant hypertension. Such fragmented RBCs can be called schistocytes. Spherocytes may be present with hereditary spherocytosis, but the RBC destruction is extravascular, and fragmented RBCs do not appear in the peripheral blood. In autoimmune hemolytic anemia, the hemolysis is extravascular as well, and spherocytes may be formed. There may be marked anisocytosis and poikilocytosis with iron deficiency and with megaloblastic anemias, but fragmentation of RBCs is not seen.
BP6 352   PBD6 621, 640

9. **(D)** This patient has aplastic crisis, precipitated by a parvovirus infection. In adults who do not have a defect in normal RBC production such as hereditary spherocytosis or sickle cell anemia or who are not immunosuppressed, parvovirus infection is self-limited and often goes unnoticed. When RBC production is shut down with parvovirus, there is no reticulocytosis. Accelerated red cell destruction in the spleen would be expected to cause a rise in serum bilirubin. DIC gives rise to thrombocytopenia, bleeding, and the appearance of fragmented red cells in the blood smear. Iron deficiency does not occur in hemolytic anemias because the iron released from hemolyzed cells is reused.
PBD6 609

10. **(D)** This is an example of a DIC with associated microangiopathic hemolytic anemia. The DIC developed in the setting of a mucin-secreting adenocarcinoma. Howell-Jolly bodies are small, round inclusions in RBCs that appear when the spleen is absent. Tear-drop cells are most characteristic for myelofibrosis and other infiltrative disorders of the marrow. Macro-ovalocytes are seen with megaloblastic anemias, such as vitamin B_{12} deficiency. Tar-

get cells appear when there is hemoglobin C disease or severe liver disease.
BP6 343   PBD6 640–642, 685

11. **(E)** She has a warm autoimmune hemolytic anemia. A positive Coombs test indicates the presence of anti-RBC antibodies in the serum and on the red cell surface. Most cases of warm autoimmune hemolytic anemia are idiopathic, but one fourth occur in persons with an identifiable autoimmune disease such as SLE. Some are caused by drugs such as α-methyldopa. The immunoglobulin coating the RBCs acts as an opsonin to promote splenic phagocytosis. Nucleated RBCs can be seen with active hemolysis, because the marrow compensates by releasing immature RBCs. Infections such as mononucleosis and *Mycoplasma* are associated with cold autoimmune hemolytic anemia (with an elevated cold agglutinin titer). Septicemia is more likely to lead to a microangiopathic hemolytic anemia. The increased RBC destruction with hereditary spherocytosis is extravascular and not immune mediated.
BP6 351   PBD6 620–621

12. **(D)** In most cases of von Willebrand disease, there is a diminished amount of circulating von Willebrand factor, which is necessary for proper platelet adhesion, and affected persons have a mild bleeding tendency. Because the disease is not a disorder of stem cells, transplantation is not helpful. Joint hemorrhages are a feature of hemophilia A and B, not von Willebrand disease. Patients with von Willebrand disease are not prone to thrombosis, as are persons with factor V Leiden mutation or other inherited disorders of anticoagulation. Splenectomy is useful in cases of ITP, but the platelets are not consumed in von Willebrand disease.
BP6 388–389   PBD6 638–639

13. **(A)** In adults with sickle cell anemia, hydroxyurea increases hemoglobin F production, which inhibits the polymerization of hemoglobin S. Because hemoglobin F levels are high for the first 5 to 6 months of life, patients with sickle cell anemia do not manifest the disease during this period. Globin synthesis decreases with the thalassemias. The hemolysis associated with sickling promotes erythropoiesis, but the concentration of hemoglobin S is not changed. Hydroxyurea does not shift the oxygen dissociation curve nor change the oxygen affinity of the various hemoglobins.
PBD6 612

14. **(A)** This man has a microcytic anemia, which is typical for iron deficiency. At his age, bleeding from an occult malignancy should be strongly suspected as the cause of iron deficiency. An autoimmune hemolytic anemia should appear as a normocytic anemia or with a slightly increased MCV with pronounced reticulocytosis. Thalassemias may result in a microcytosis, but β-thalassemia major causes severe anemia soon after birth, and survival to the age of 73 years is unlikely. Macrocytosis should accompany a history of chronic alcoholism, probably because of poor diet and folate deficiency. B$_{12}$ deficiency also results in a macrocytic anemia.
BP6 353   PBD6 627–629

15. **(C)** Glucose-6-phosphate dehydrogenase deficiency is an X-linked disorder that affects about 10% of African-American males. The lack of this enzyme subjects hemoglobin to damage by oxidants, including drugs such as primaquine, sulfonamides, nitrofurantoin, phenacetin, and aspirin (in large doses). Infection can also cause oxidative damage to hemoglobin. Heinz bodies damage the red blood cell membrane, giving rise to intravascular hemolysis. The "bite cells" result from overeager splenic macrophages attempting to pluck out the Heinz bodies, adding an element of extravascular hemolysis. Heterozygotes with α-thalassemia have no major problems, but in cases of α-thalassemia major, perinatal death is the rule. Likewise, β-thalassemia minor and sickle cell trait are conditions with no major problems and no relation to drug usage. Some autoimmune hemolytic anemias can be drug related, but the hemolysis is predominantly extravascular.
BP6 350   PBD6 610–611

16. **(C)** The increased ferritin concentration and reduced total iron-binding capacity are typical for anemia of chronic disease. Increased levels of cytokines such as interleukin-1 and tumor necrosis factor promote sequestration of storage iron with poor utilization for erythropoiesis. Secretion of erythropoietin by the kidney is impaired. A variety of underlying diseases, including cancer, collagen vascular diseases, and chronic infections, may produce this pattern of anemia. Iron deficiency should produce a microcytic anemia with a low serum ferritin. The patient is unlikely to have aplastic anemia, because the platelet count and WBC count are normal. Microangiopathic hemolytic anemias are caused by serious acute conditions such as DIC; these patients have thrombocytopenia caused by widespread thrombosis. Megaloblastic anemias are macrocytic and do not cause a large increase in iron stores.
BP6 354   PBD6 630

17. **(D)** Throughout human history, malaria has been the driving force in increasing the gene frequency for hemoglobin S. Individuals heterozygous for hemoglobin S have the sickle cell trait. They are resistant to malaria because their red blood cells sickle when parasitized and therefore are removed from the circulation by the spleen. Thus, the malarial parasite cannot complete its life cycle. *C. neoformans* can cause granulomatous disease in immunocompromised persons. *B. burgdorferi* is the spirochete that causes Lyme disease. *T. pallidum* is the infectious agent causing syphilis. *C. perfringens* may produce gas gangrene following soft tissue injuries.
BP6 345   PBD6 389–390, 611

18. **(A)** The pancytopenia and absence of a reticulocytosis strongly suggest bone marrow failure. Aplastic anemia has no apparent cause in one half of cases. In other cases, drugs and toxins may be identified. Drugs such as chemotherapeutic agents are best known for this effect. A preceding viral infection may be identified in some cases but bacterial infections do not cause aplastic anemias. Persons with pancytopenia are subject to bleeding disorders from the low platelet count and to infections from the low WBC count. Dietary history would not be helpful because this clinical and laboratory picture is not characteristic of iron

deficiency or vitamin B_{12} deficiency. Menstrual history would be relevant if she had hypochromic microcytic anemia. The only known familial cause of aplastic anemia (i.e., Fanconi's anemia) is rare.
BP6 357 PBD6 630–631

19. (A) This patient has so-called autosplenectomy that results from the multiple infarctions that occur as a consequence of the sickling phenomenon. In childhood, the spleen may initially be enlarged from engorgement of splenic sinusoids with the abnormal masses of sickled cells, but hypoxic tissue damage ensues. Terminally, this patient developed a vaso-occlusive crisis affecting the lung. β-thalassemia major can lead to splenomegaly from extramedullary hematopoiesis. Some of the largest spleens occur because of malaria. With ITP, the spleen is usually of normal size. In autoimmune hemolytic anemias, the spleen may increase in size from extravascular hemolysis and/or extramedullary hematopoiesis.
BP6 346 PBD6 614

20. (E) The severity of hemophilia A depends on the amount of factor VIII activity. With less than 1%, there is severe disease, and joint hemorrhages are common, leading to severe joint deformity with ankylosis. Mild (1% to 5%) and moderate (5% to 75%) activity is often asymptomatic, except with severe trauma. The bleeding tendency is not associated with splenomegaly. Petechiae, seen with thrombocytopenia, are not a feature of hemophilia. Factor VIII deficiency does not affect the lifespan of RBCs. Because persons with factor VIII deficiency are not dependent on RBC transfusions, iron overload is not a usual consequence.
BP6 389 PBD6 638

21. (D) The presence of thrombocytopenia, increased PT and PTT values, fibrin split products, and the low fibrinogen concentration suggest DIC, which was most likely caused by a retained dead fetus, an obstetric complication that can lead to DIC through release of thromboplastins from the fetus. This causes widespread microvascular thrombosis and consumes clotting factors and platelets. There is no damage to the vascular endothelium or vascular wall. Platelet production is normal, but platelets are consumed by widespread thrombosis of small vessels. There is no defect in platelet function.
BP6 385–386 PB 640–642

22. (E) The baby most likely has erythroblastosis fetalis because of maternal antibody coating the fetal cells. A fetal-maternal hemorrhage in utero or at the time of delivery in a previous pregnancy (or with previous transfusion of incompatible blood) can sensitize the mother so that IgG antibodies are made. In subsequent pregnancies, these antibodies (unlike the naturally occurring IgM antibodies) can cross the placenta to attach to fetal cells, leading to hemolysis. Most cases used to be caused by Rh incompatibility (e.g., Rh-negative mother, Rh-positive baby), but the use of RhoGAM administered at birth to Rh-negative mothers has eliminated almost all of such cases. However, other less common blood group antigens can be involved in this process.
BP6 206 PBD6 473–474

23. (G) He has glucose-6-phosphate dehydrogenase deficiency. A drug that leads to oxidative injury to the RBCs, such as primaquine, can induce hemolysis. Oxidant injury to hemoglobin produces inclusion of denatured hemoglobin within RBCs. The inclusions damage the cell membrane directly, giving rise to intravascular hemolysis. These cells have reduced membrane deformability, and they are also removed from the circulation by the spleen.
BP6 350 PBD6 610–611

24. (C) This patient is a chronic alcoholic who has folate deficiency, giving rise to megaloblastic anemia. Folic acid and vitamin B_{12} act as coenzymes in the DNA synthetic pathway. A deficiency of either impairs the normal process of nuclear maturation. The nuclei remain large and primitive looking, giving rise to megaloblasts. The mature red cells are also larger than normal (i.e., macrocytes). The nuclear maturation defect affects all rapidly dividing cells in the body, including other hematopoietic lineages. Patients can have thrombocytopenia and leukopenia. Neutrophils often show defective segmentation, manifested by extra nuclear lobes. Polychromatophilic red cells represent reticulocytes, and they are reduced in number because of the failure of marrow to produce adequate numbers of RBCs despite anemia.
BP6 356 PBD6 622–623

25. (E) The crescent-shaped RBCs (sickled RBCs) are characteristic for hemoglobin SS. This disease is most common in persons of African and eastern Arabian descent. The sickled red cells are susceptible to hemolysis, but they also can cause microvascular occlusions anywhere in the body, including abdominal viscera. These vaso-occlusive episodes cause tissue ischemia and death, resulting in severe pain (i.e., painful crises). α-thalassemia minor is asymptomatic, and α-thalassemia major leads to perinatal death. Paroxysmal nocturnal hemoglobinuria is associated with intravascular hemolysis. Hemoglobin C disease leads to the appearance of target cells.
BP6 345 PBD6 612–614

26. (D) In patients with hereditary spherocytosis, spheroidal cells are trapped and destroyed in the spleen because the abnormal red cells have reduced deformability. Splenectomy is beneficial because the spherocytes are no longer detained by the spleen. Splenectomy has no effect on the synthesis of spectrin; the red cells in spherocytosis are not killed by opsonization. In warm antibody hemolytic anemias, opsonized red cells are removed by the spleen.
BP6 343–344 PBD6 607–609

27. (D) The high MCV is indicative of a marked macrocytosis, greater than would be accounted for by a reticulocytosis alone. The two best known causes for such an anemia, also known as megaloblastic anemia when characteristic megaloblastic precursors are seen in the bone marrow, are vitamin B_{12} and folate deficiency. Because vitamin B_{12} is absorbed in the terminal ileum, its removal can cause B_{12} deficiency. Chronic blood loss and iron deficiency produce a microcytic pattern of anemia, as does iron deficiency. Hemolytic anemia is unlikely several

weeks after blood transfusion. Anemia of chronic disease is generally a normocytic anemia.
BP6 356   PBD6 622-623

28.   **(C)** He has DIC, which can result from gram-negative septicemia. This is a form of microangiopathic hemolytic anemia in which there is deposition of fibrin strands in small vessels. The RBCs are damaged during passage between these strands. Coagulation factors and platelets are consumed, something which does not occur with other forms of hemolytic anemia. Paroxysmal nocturnal hemoglobinuria and the hemolytic anemias do not typically cause a consumptive coagulopathy. Thalassemias produce chronic anemia with ineffective erythropoiesis, and there is also an extravascular hemolytic component without a bleeding complication. Aplastic anemia refers to the loss of marrow stem cell activity and is therefore associated with anemia, leukopenia, and thrombocytopenia. It can follow infections, mostly viral but rarely bacterial.
BP6 343   PBD6 640-642

29.   **(A)** The cumulative damage to the spleen in sickle cell anemia results in autosplenectomy, leaving behind a small fibrotic remnant of this organ. The impaired splenic function with inability to clear bacteria from the bloodstream can occur early in childhood, leading to infection with encapsulated bacterial organisms. There is no impairment in production or function of neutrophils. Levels of serum complement are normal. Adhesion between endothelial cells and red cells is increased in sickle cell anemia.
BP6 346-347   PBD6 613-614

30.   **(A)** The acute blood loss, in this case probably intraperitoneal hemorrhage, results in a reticulocytosis from marrow stimulation by anemia. Leukoerythroblastosis is typical for a myelophthisic process in the marrow. Basophilic stippling of RBCs suggests a marrow injury, such as with a drug or toxin. Hypochromic red cells occur in iron deficiency and thalassemias, both associated with reduced hemoglobin synthesis. Acute blood loss does not give rise to iron deficiency. Schistocytes suggest a microangiopathic hemolytic anemia that may accompany shock or sepsis.
BP6 342   PBD6 605-606

31.   **(A)** The MCV, measured in the obscure unit of femtoliters (fL), provides an indication of the average size of RBCs. The MCV is a directly measured value. The MCH value indicates how much hemoglobin is in each cell, and the MCHC indicates how much hemoglobin is present in a given volume of packed RBCs. The red cell distribution width provides a measure for variation in size of the RBCs and is highest with hemolytic anemias. The hematocrit is calculated by automated instruments from multiplying the RBC count by the MCV; the simple "spun hematocrit" just provides the packed cell volume as a percent of the total volume of the sample of blood.
BP6 342   PBD6 605

32.   **(C)** This patient has paroxysmal nocturnal hemoglobinuria. This disorder results from an acquired myeloid

stem cell membrane defect from a mutation in the PIGA gene. A mutation in this gene prevents the membrane expression of certain proteins that require a glycolipid anchor. These include proteins that protect cells from lysis by spontaneously activated complement. As a result, RBCs, granulocytes, and platelets are exquisitely sensitive to the lytic activity of complement. The red cell lysis is intravascular and hence patients can have hemoglobinuria (i.e., dark urine). Defects in platelet function are believed to be responsible for venous thrombosis. Recurrent infections are possibly caused by impaired leukocyte functions. Patients with paroxysmal nocturnal hemoglobinuria may also have acute leukemia or aplastic anemia as complications. The glucose-6-phosphate dehydrogenase deficiency has an episodic course from exposure to agents such as drugs that induce hemolysis. Spectrin mutations give rise to hereditary spherocytosis. Mutations in β-globin chain can give rise to hemoglobinopathies such as sickle cell anemia. Factor V mutation can present with thromboses, but there is no anemia or leukopenia.
BP6 351   PBD6 619-620

33.   **(D)** The reduced β-globin synthesis results in a relative excess of α-globin chains that precipitate in RBCs and their precursors. These precipitates make the cells more susceptible to damage and removal. This intramedullary loss of red cell precursors is referred to as ineffective erythropoiesis. Unfortunately, it acts as a trigger for greater dietary absorption of iron by unknown mechanisms. Hemolysis of red cells in the periphery (e.g., spleen, liver) releases iron that can be reused for hemoglobin synthesis. In megaloblastic anemias, there is enough iron but not enough vitamin B_{12} or folate. In sickle cell anemia, the β-globin chains are abnormal, leading to sickling of red cells, which are then destroyed in the spleen. However, there is no ineffective erythropoiesis.
BP6 347-348   PBD6 615-616

34.   **(B)** The patient's history is typical of hemophilia A caused by a factor VIII defect or deficiency. The affected patient is male and has male relatives who are affected (i.e., X-linked transmission). There is history of bleeding, especially into joints. PTT is prolonged because factor VIII is required for the intrinsic pathway. PT is normal because the extrinsic pathway does not depend on the function of factor VIII. The inability to correct PTT by mixing with normal plasma is important. If the patient had a deficiency only of factor VIII, the addition of normal plasma, a source of factor VIII, would have corrected the PTT. Failure to correct PTT by normal plasma indicates the presence of an inhibitor of factor VIII in the patient's serum. Such inhibitors are present in about 15% of the patients with hemophilia.
BP6 389   PBD6 639

35.   **(A)** The history in this case is similar to that in question 34. However, the PTT is corrected by normal pooled plasma. The patient has hemophilia A caused by factor VIII deficiency, and inhibitors of factor VIII are absent from patient's serum. An in vitro mixing study of patient and pooled plasma such as this usually corrects an abnormality caused by a deficiency of a procoagulant fac-

tor, but if there is an inhibitor of coagulation in the patient's plasma, the clotting test will show an abnormal result.
BP 389   PBD 639

36. **(D)** This patient has gum bleeding and excessive menstrual bleeding with a normal platelet count. von Willebrand disease is a fairly common bleeding disorder, with an estimated frequency of 1%. In most cases, it is inherited as an autosomal dominant trait. In these cases, a reduction in the quantity of von Willebrand factor impairs platelet adhesion to damaged vessel walls, and hemostasis is compromised. Because von Willebrand factor acts as a carrier for factor VIII, the level of this procoagulant protein (needed for the intrinsic pathway) is diminished, as in this case. However, the levels of factor VIII are rarely reduced enough to be clinically significant. Prolonged PTT corrected by normal plasma is a reflection of factor VIII deficiency.
BP6 388-389   PBD6 638-639

37. **(F)** Reduced platelet number may result from decreased production or increased destruction. Marrow examination in this case reveals plenty of megakaryocytes, excluding decreased production. Accelerated destruction is often immunologically mediated. It may result from well-known autoimmune diseases such as SLE, or it may be idiopathic. When all known causes of thrombocytopenia are excluded, a diagnosis of ITP should be made. This patient seems to have no other symptoms or signs and has no history of drug intake or infections that can cause thrombocytopenia. ITP is most likely. Thrombotic TTP is another entity to be considered. This is typically associated with fever, microangiopathic hemolytic anemia, neurologic symptoms, and renal failure.
BP6 387   PBD6 634-636

38. **(B)** This patient, of Mediterranean origin, has β-thalassemia major. In this condition, there is a severe reduction in the synthesis of β-globin chains without impairment of α-globin synthesis. The free, unpaired α-globin chains form aggregates that precipitate within normoblasts and cause them to undergo apoptosis. The death of red cell precursors in the bone marrow is called ineffective erythropoiesis. Not only does this cause anemia, but it also increases the absorption of dietary iron, giving rise to iron overload. The severe anemia triggers erythropoietin synthesis, which expands the erythropoietic marrow. The marrow expansion encroaches on the bones, causing maxillofacial deformities. Extramedullary hematopoiesis causes hepatosplenomegaly.
BP6 347-348   PBD6 615-617

39. **(B)** Iron deficiency is the most common form of anemia worldwide. The lack of iron impairs heme synthesis. The marrow response is to "downsize" the RBCs, resulting in a microcytic and hypochromic anemia. Thalassemias are uncommon except in certain geographic areas. Likewise, infections and metastases that involve marrow are not common overall, and anemia is probably the easiest problem to treat in a patient with such a problem. Toxic injuries, often from drugs, are uncommon.
BP6 342, 353   PBD6 627-628

40. **(E)** The ferritin is a measure of storage iron, because it is derived from the total body storage pool in liver, spleen, and marrow. About 80% of functional body iron is contained in hemoglobin; the remainder is in muscle myoglobin. Transferrin is a serum transport protein for iron and it is usually about 33% saturated with iron. Persons with severe liver disease may have an elevated serum ferritin level because of release from liver stores. The serum iron concentration by itself gives no indication of iron stores, because in anemia of chronic disease, the iron level may be normal to low, but iron stores are increased. The hemoglobin can be affected by more than just iron stores. A bone marrow biopsy gives a good indication of iron stores, because the iron stain of the marrow demonstrates hemosiderin in macrophages, but such a biopsy is an expensive procedure.
BP6 353   PBD6 627-628

41. **(B)** Patients with sickle cell anemia have painful crises that represent episodes of hypoxic injury and infarction caused by microvascular occlusions. Bones of hands and feet are frequently affected. The vaso-occlusion results from increased adhesiveness of damaged red cell membranes to vascular endothelium. The alternative complement pathway may have defects in sickle cell anemia that impair opsonization of encapsulated bacteria and hence increase susceptibility to infection. The extent of red cell sickling is correlated with the degree of anemia, but it is not correlated with vaso-occlusive episodes.
PBD6 614-615

42. **(B)** Tear-drop RBCs are indicative of a myelophthisic disorder (i.e., something filling the bone marrow such as fibrous connective tissue). The leukoerythroblastosis, including immature RBCs and WBCs, is most indicative of myelofibrosis. Splenomegaly is also typically seen in myelofibrosis. A leukoerythroblastic picture may also be seen with infections and metastases involving the marrow. Marrow packed with myeloblasts is typical of acute myeloid leukemia. In this condition, the peripheral blood would also show myeloblasts and failure of myeloid maturation. Replacement of marrow by fat occurs in aplastic anemia, which is characterized by pancytopenia. Megaloblasts in the marrow would indicate folate or B_{12} deficiency—both causing macrocytic anemia. Hyperplasia of normoblasts occurs in hemolytic anemias. Leukoerythroblastosis is not seen in hemolytic anemias.
BP6 357   PBD6 632-633

43. **(E)** Although both folate and B_{12} deficiency give rise to a macrocytic anemia, a deficiency of vitamin B_{12} can also result in demyelination of the posterior and lateral columns of the spinal cord. The anemia caused by B_{12} deficiency can be ameliorated by increased administration of folate, masking the potential neurologic injury by improving the anemia. Treating B_{12} deficiency does not improve the anemia caused by folate deficiency. Folate has no cofactor for absorption, but B_{12} must be complexed to intrinsic factor, secreted by gastric parietal cells, and then the complex must be absorbed in the terminal ileum, so diseases such as atrophic gastritis and Crohn disease may affect B_{12} absorption more than folate. The peripheral

smear may appear the same, and offers no means for distinguishing these deficiencies. An aplastic anemia is unlikely to result from a nutritional deficiency.
BP6 356   PBD6 625

44. **(C)** The hemolysis that accompanies sickle cell anemia results in an increased indirect hyperbilirubinemia that favors the development of gallstones with bilirubin pigment. Cirrhosis may occur because of hemochromatosis in β-thalassemia major. Chronic atrophic gastritis leads to loss of parietal cells and the resulting vitamin B_{12} malabsorption causes pernicious anemia. Stillbirths suggest thalassemia major. Esophageal webs occur very uncommonly in the setting of chronic iron deficiency anemia.
BP6 347   PBD6 613-614, 893-894

45. **(B)** He has DIC from gram-negative septicemia. Multiple organs are affected, because the microthrombi lead to tissue ischemia and necrosis. Activation of plasmin occurs, leading to fibrinolysis and generation of fibrin split products. DIC is a consumptive coagulopathy in which the PT and the PTT are increased and platelets are reduced (although their function remains normal). A bleeding time should not be ordered if the platelet count is less than 100,000/μL, because it will always be abnormal. The fibrinogen increases in a variety of inflammatory or infectious conditions, but in a consumptive coagulopathy such as DIC, the fibrinogen concentration should be low. Thrombocytosis may lead to thrombosis, hemorrhage, or both, because the platelets are often abnormal and increased in number, but microthrombi are not typical for this condition.
BP6 384-386   PBD6 640-642

46. **(A)** In β-thalassemia major, there is a significant component of ineffective erythropoiesis, leading to expansion of the marrow and a stimulus to absorb more iron from the diet. The excess iron builds up in the tissues, resulting in hemochromatosis with infiltrative cardiomyopathy, hepatic cirrhosis, and "bronze diabetes" from pancreatic islet dysfunction. In comparison, the hemolytic anemia is mild in β-thalassemia minor, and there is very little ineffective erythropoiesis. Hemochromatosis is particularly detrimental to the liver and heart. Chronic anemia may require RBC transfusions that add even more iron to body stores. Other hemoglobinopathies do not have as significant a component of ineffective erythropoiesis, although any condition that leads to transfusion dependency may be complicated by hemochromatosis.
BP6 349   PBD6 616-617

47. **(B)** Such painful crises in an anemic patient are indicative of sickle cell crises with homozygous hemoglobin S. During the crises, the sickled cells form microvascular occlusions that produce tissue hypoxia. Tear-drop cells are indicative of myelofibrosis. Schistocytes, or fragmented red cells, are seen in microangiopathic hemolytic anemias, as may occur in DIC. Microcytosis can be seen with iron deficiency or with thalassemias. Spherocytosis can occur with hereditary spherocytosis or with hemolytic anemias.
BP6 347   PBD6 613-614

48. **(E)** Haptoglobin is a serum protein that binds to free hemoglobin. Ordinarily, circulating hemoglobin is contained within RBCs, but hemolysis can release free hemoglobin. The haptoglobin is used up as the amount of free hemoglobin increases. SLE is an autoimmune disease that can result in hemolysis by means of autoantibodies directed at RBCs, and the direct Coombs test result is often positive. An elevated d-Dimer level suggests a microangiopathic hemolytic anemia. Decreased iron may cause a hypochromic, microcytic anemia, but with hemolysis, the RBCs get recycled, and the iron is not lost. An elevated antinuclear antibody titer may indicate SLE or other autoimmune disease, but it does not predict hemolysis.
BP6 343, 351   PBD6 606

49. **(G)** The iron concentration and iron-binding capacity are both low. However, unlike in anemia of iron deficiency, serum ferritin level is increased. This is typical of anemia of chronic disease. Underlying chronic inflammatory or neoplastic diseases increase the secretion of cytokines such as interleukin-1, tumor necrosis factor, and interferon-γ. These cytokines depress erythropoiesis.
BP6 354   PBD6 630

50. **(J)** The diagnosis of TTP is based on finding transient neurologic problems, fever, thrombocytopenia, microangiopathic hemolytic anemia, and acute renal failure. These abnormalities are produced by small platelet-fibrin thrombi in small vessels in multiple organs. Heart, brain, and kidney are often severely affected.
BP6 387-388   PBD6 636-637

51. **(A)** The marked reticulocytosis and marrow hyperplasia indicate that the marrow is responding to a decrease in RBCs. The reticulocytes are larger RBCs that slightly increase the MCV. Iron deficiency impairs the ability of the marrow to mount a significant and sustained reticulocytosis. Iron deficiency anemia is typically microcytic and hypochromic. Infiltrative disorders such as metastases in marrow would impair the ability to mount a reticulocytosis of this degree. The normal Coombs test results exclude an autoimmune hemolytic anemia. An aplastic marrow is very hypocellular and unable to respond to anemia. It is associated with pancytopenia.
BP6 342-343   PBD6 606-607

White Cells, Lymph Nodes, Spleen, and Thymus

BP6 Chapter 12 - The Hematopoietic and Lymphoid Systems
PBD6 Chapter 15 - White Cells, Lymph Nodes, Spleen, and Thymus

1. A 15-year-old male presents with high fever of 10 days' duration. Physical examination reveals scattered petechial hemorrhages. There is no enlargement of liver or spleen or lymph nodes. Bone marrow examination does not show any abnormal cells. The complete blood count (CBC) demonstrates a hemoglobin concentration of 13.2 g/dL, hematocrit of 38.9%, mean cell volume (MCV) of 93 fL, platelet count of 175,000/μL, and white blood cell (WBC) count of 1850/μL, with the differential count showing 1 segmented neutrophil, 98 lymphocytes, and 1 monocyte per 100 WBCs. These findings are most likely caused by

○ (A) Acute lymphocytic (or lymphoblastic) leukemia (ALL)
○ (B) Acute myeloid leukemia
○ (C) Aplastic anemia
○ (D) Idiopathic thrombocytopenic purpura
○ (E) Overwhelming bacterial infection

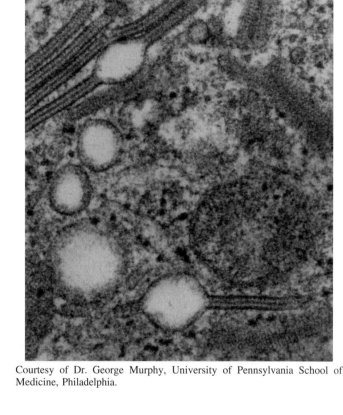

Courtesy of Dr. George Murphy, University of Pennsylvania School of Medicine, Philadelphia.

2. A 9-year-old boy presents with a generalized seborrheic skin eruption and fever. He has been diagnosed and treated for otitis media several times in the past year. He also has mild lymphadenopathy along with hepatomegaly, and splenomegaly. The electron micrograph shown in the figure was taken from a mass lesion involving the mastoid bone. The most likely diagnosis is

○ (A) Acute lymphoblastic leukemia (ALL)
○ (B) Multiple myeloma
○ (C) Hodgkin disease, mixed cellularity type
○ (D) Langerhans cell histiocytosis
○ (E) Disseminated tuberculosis

3. A 67-year-old male has experienced weakness, fatigue, and weight loss worsening over a period of several months. He now has decreasing vision in both eyes, along with headaches and dizziness. His hands are sensitive to cold. On physical examination, he has generalized lymphadenopathy along with hepatosplenomegaly. Laboratory investigations reveal hyperproteinemia, with a serum protein level of 15.5 g/dL and albumin concentration of 3.2 g/dL. A bone marrow biopsy shows infiltration with small plasmacytoid lymphoid cells with Russell bodies in the cytoplasm. Additional investigations are most likely to reveal

○ (A) A monoclonal IgM spike in the serum
○ (B) Punched-out lytic lesions in the skull

○ (C) Hypercalcemia
○ (D) Bence Jones proteinuria
○ (E) t(14;18) translocation

4. A 37-year-old female presents with a fever of a week's duration. A CBC shows a hemoglobin concentration of 13.9 g/dL, hematocrit of 42.0%, MCV of 89 fL, platelet count of 210,000/μL, and WBC count of 56,000/μL. The differential count shows 63 segmented neutrophils, 15 band cells, 6 metamyelocytes, 3 myelocytes, 1 blast, 8 lymphocytes, 2 monocytes, and 2 eosinophils per 100 WBCs. The peripheral blood leukocyte alkaline phosphatase score is increased. The most likely diagnosis is

○ (A) Chronic myelogenous leukemia (CML)
○ (B) Hairy cell leukemia
○ (C) Hodgkin disease, lymphocyte depletion type
○ (D) Leukemoid reaction
○ (E) Acute lymphoblastic leukemia (ALL)

5. A 12-year-old boy presents with bowel obstruction and abdominal distention. Abdominal computed tomography (CT) reveals a 7-cm mass involving the region of the ileocecal valve. Histologic examination of the resected mass shows sheets of intermediate-sized lymphoid cells with nuclei having coarse chromatin and several nucleoli. There are many mitoses. A "starry sky" pattern of macrophages is seen. A bone marrow biopsy is negative for this cell population. Cytogenetic analysis of the lymphoid cells from the mass reveals t(8;14). The most probable diagnosis in this case is

○ (A) Diffuse large B-cell lymphoma
○ (B) Follicular lymphoma
○ (C) Acute lymphoblastic leukemia
○ (D) Plasmacytoma
○ (E) Burkitt lymphoma

6. A 53-year-old male presents with an enlarged supraclavicular lymph node, and physical examination reveals enlargement of the Waldeyer ring of oropharyngeal lymphoid tissue. There is no hepatosplenomegaly. Lymph node biopsy reveals replacement by a monomorphous population of large lymphoid cells with enlarged nuclei and prominent nucleoli. The CBC is normal except for findings of mild anemia. Immunohistochemical staining and flow cytometry of the node reveals that most lymphoid cells are CD19+, CD10+, CD3−, CD15−, and terminal deoxynucleotidyl transferase negative (TdT−). These clinical, histologic, and phenotypic findings are most consistent with a diagnosis of

○ (A) Chronic lymphadenitis
○ (B) Diffuse large B-cell lymphoma
○ (C) Hodgkin disease
○ (D) Lymphoblastic lymphoma
○ (E) Small lymphocytic lymphoma

7. A 50-year-old male presents with headache and dizziness. He has also experienced generalized pruritus of a severe nature. He has had these problems, along with dark stools, for several months. His stool is positive for occult blood, and blood pressure is 165/90 mm Hg. A CBC shows a hemoglobin concentration of 22.3 g/dL, hematocrit

of 67.1%, MCV of 94 fL, platelet count of 453,000/μL, and WBC count of 7800/μL. His problems most likely stem from

○ (A) Myelodysplastic syndrome
○ (B) Essential thrombocytosis
○ (C) Chronic myelogenous leukemia (CML)
○ (D) Erythroleukemia
○ (E) Polycythemia vera

8. A 50-year-old male was diagnosed with a diffuse large cell lymphoma of B cells. He underwent intensive chemotherapy, and a complete remission was achieved that lasted for 7 years. He now presents with fatigue and pulmonary and urinary tract infections. A CBC shows a hemoglobin concentration of 8.7 g/dL, hematocrit of 25.2%, MCV of 88 fL, platelet count of 67,000/μL, and WBC count of 2,300/μL, with a differential count of 15 segmented neutrophils, 5 band cells, 2 metamyelocytes, 2 myelocytes, 6 myeloblasts, 23 lymphocytes, 35 monocytes, and 2 eosinophils per 100 WBCs. A bone marrow biopsy shows 90% cellularity with many immature cells, including ringed sideroblasts, megaloblasts, hypolobated megakaryocytes, and myeloblasts. Karyotypic analysis shows 5q deletions in many cells. His present condition is best characterized as

○ (A) A relapse of his previous lymphoma
○ (B) Transformation of the lymphoma into myeloid leukemia
○ (C) Myelodysplasia related to therapy of his earlier tumor
○ (D) A de novo acute myeloblastic leukemia
○ (E) Myeloid metaplasia with myelofibrosis

9. A 63-year-old female experiences a burning sensation in the hands and feet, and she has had an episode of deep venous thrombosis in the past 2 months. On physical examination, the spleen and liver appear to be enlarged. The peripheral blood smear shows abnormally large platelets. The complete blood count shows a hemoglobin concentration of 13.3 g/dL, hematocrit of 40.1%, MCV of 91 fL, platelet count of 657,000/μL, and WBC of count 17,400/μL. The most likely diagnosis is

○ (A) Essential thrombocythemia
○ (B) Chronic myelogenous leukemia (CML)
○ (C) Myelofibrosis with myeloid metaplasia
○ (D) Acute myelogenous leukemia
○ (E) Polycythemia vera

For each of the clinical histories in questions 10 and 11, match the most closely associated pathologic finding:

(A) Decreased visual acuity
(B) Disseminated intravascular coagulopathy (DIC)
(C) Generalized exfoliative erythroderma
(D) Leukostasis
(E) Mandibular mass
(F) Mediastinal mass
(G) Renal amyloidosis
(H) Scrofula
(I) Seborrheic skin eruptions
(J) Sinus histiocytosis
(K) Small intestinal obstruction
(L) Splenomegaly

10. A 9-year-old boy living in Uganda has a B-cell lymphoma that on chromosome analysis reveals a 46,XY,t(8; 14) karyotype. Histologically, the tumor is formed of intermediate-sized lymphocytes with a high mitotic rate. (   )

11. There is right axillary lymphadenopathy in a 39-year-old female who has a mammogram that demonstrates a 2-cm irregular right upper outer quadrant mass in her right breast. (   )

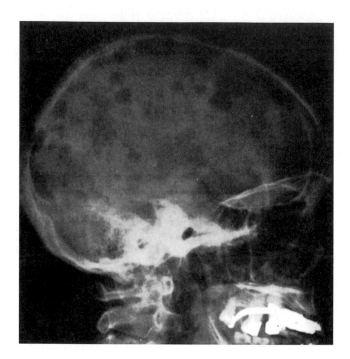

12. A 61-year-old male gives a history of back pain for several months. A skull radiograph is shown here. He has no lymphadenopathy or splenomegaly. His serum blood urea nitrogen level and creatinine concentration are found to be steadily rising. He recently developed a cough productive of yellowish sputum, and a sputum culture grew *Streptococcus pneumoniae*. During the course of his hospitalization, a bone marrow biopsy is performed. The biopsy is most likely to show

○ (A) Scattered small granulomas
○ (B) Numerous plasma cells
○ (C) Nodules of small mature lymphocytes
○ (D) Occasional Reed-Sternberg cells
○ (E) Hypercellularity with many blasts

13. A 26-year-old male has enlarged, nontender cervical lymph nodes. A biopsy of one of the lymph nodes reveals scattered Reed-Sternberg cells along with macrophages, lymphocytes, neutrophils, eosinophils, and a few plasma cells. Which of the following factors elaborated by the Reed-Sternberg cells has led to the appearance of the eosinophils within this lesion?

○ (A) Platelet-derived growth factor (PDGF)
○ (B) Cyclin D1
○ (C) Interleukin-5

○ (D) Trans–retinoic acid
○ (E) Erythropoietin

For each of the clinical histories in questions 14 through 16, match the most closely associated neoplasm:

(A) Acute lymphoblastic leukemia
(B) Acute myeloblastic leukemia
(C) Chronic lymphocytic leukemia
(D) Diffuse large B-cell lymphoma
(E) Follicular lymphoma
(F) Hairy cell leukemia
(G) Hodgkin disease, mixed cellularity type
(H) MALT lymphoma
 (I) Mantle cell lymphoma
 (J) Multiple myeloma
(K) Mycosis fungoides
(L) Thymoma
(M) Waldenström macroglobulinemia

14. A 53-year-old female has had nausea with vomiting and early satiety for several months. An upper endoscopy reveals loss of the rugal folds of the stomach over a 4 × 8 cm area of the fundus. Gastric biopsies reveal the presence of *Helicobacter pylori* organisms in the mucus overlying superficial epithelial cells. There are mucosal and submucosal monomorphous infiltrates of small lymphocytes. When she is treated for the *H. pylori* infection, her condition improves. (   )

15. A 39-year-old male is known to have been infected with the human immunodeficiency virus (HIV) for the past 8 years. Despite antiretroviral therapy with zidovudine, stavudine, and Retrovir, his HIV-1 RNA level has recently been rising and now is 28,000 copies/mL. He is found on physical examination to have stool positive for occult blood. Sigmoidoscopy reveals a 4-cm mucosal mass in the upper rectum. (   )

16. A 50-year-old female presents with fatigue and pallor. Laboratory investigations reveal a hemoglobin concentration of 9 gm/dL, hematocrit of 28%, and reticulocyte count of 0.1%. The MCV, mean corpuscular hemoglobin concentration (MCHC), and serum ferritin level are normal. A bone marrow aspirate shows normal cellularity, but the cells of the erythroid series, such as pronormoblasts, normoblasts, and later stages, are greatly reduced. Other elements are normal in number and differentiation. (   )

17. In which of the following conditions that cause polycythemia is the serum erythropoietin extremely low?

○ (A) Dehydration
○ (B) Renal cell carcinoma
○ (C) Polycythemia vera
○ (D) Cyanotic heart disease
○ (E) High-altitude living

18. A 41-year-old male has a fever, with a temperature of 39.2°C. His CBC shows a hemoglobin concentration of 13.9 g/dL, hematocrit of 40.5%, MCV of 93 fL, WBC of count 13,750/μL, and platelet count of 210,000/μL. The differential count is 75 segmented neutrophils, 10 band

cells, 10 lymphocytes, and 5 monocytes per 100 WBCs. A bone marrow biopsy shows hypercellularity, with a marked increase in myeloid precursors at all stages of maturation and in band neutrophils. Which of the following conditions is most likely to be associated with these clinical and hematologic findings?

- (A) Acute viral hepatitis
- (B) Glucocorticoid therapy
- (C) Lung abscess
- (D) Vigorous exercise
- (E) Acute myeloid leukemia

19. A 37-year-old male known to have been infected with HIV for the past 10 years is admitted with abdominal pain of 3 days' duration. Physical examination reveals abdominal distention with absent bowel sounds. An abdominal CT scan reveals a mass lesion involving the ileum. He is taken to surgery, and an area of bowel obstruction in the ileum is removed. The specimen is examined in the surgical pathology department, and there is a firm, white mass that is 10 cm long and 3 cm in greatest depth. It infiltrates through the wall of the ileum. Histologic studies reveal a mitotically active population of CD19+ lymphoid cells with prominent nuclei and nucleoli. Molecular analysis is most likely to reveal which of the following viral genomes in the lymphoid cells?

- (A) Epstein-Barr virus (EBV)
- (B) Human immunodeficiency virus (HIV)
- (C) Human herpesvirus type 8 (HHV-8)
- (D) Human T-cell leukemia/lymphoma virus type I (HTLV-I)
- (E) Cytomegalovirus (CMV)

20. A 70-year-old male presents with increasing fatigue for the last 6 months. Hematologic workup reveals a CBC with a hemoglobin concentration of 9.5 g/dL, hematocrit of 28%, MCV of 90fL, platelet count of 120,000/μL, and WBC count of 42,000/μL. The peripheral blood smear shows absolute lymphocytosis with a monotonous population of small, round, mature-looking lymphocytes. Flow cytometry shows the cells to be CD19+, CD5+, and TdT−. Cytogenetic and molecular analysis of the cells in the blood is most likely to reveal

- (A) t(9;22) leading to *bcr-abl* rearrangement
- (B) Clonal rearrangement of immunoglobulin (Ig) genes
- (C) Clonal rearrangement of T-cell receptor genes
- (D) t(8;14) leading to c-*myc* overexpression
- (E) t(14;18) leading to *bcl-2* overexpression

21. A 69-year-old woman complains of back pain. A radiograph reveals a partial collapse of T11, along with several 0.5- to 1.5-cm lytic lesions with a rounded "soap bubble" appearance in the thoracic and lumbar vertebrae. A bone marrow biopsy is performed, and a smear of the aspirate is shown in the figure. The most likely laboratory finding in this patient is a (an)

- (A) Monoclonal gammopathy in the serum
- (B) t(9;22) in the karyotype of marrow
- (C) Elevated leukocyte alkaline phosphatase score

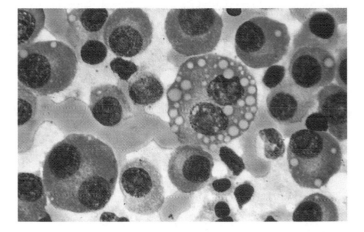

- (D) Decreased serum alkaline phosphatase level
- (E) Platelet count of 750,000/μL

22. A 33-year-old female has had a history of generalized fatigue and night sweats for several months. Physical examination reveals right cervical lymphadenopathy. Biopsy of one lymph node reveals thick bands of fibrous connective tissue with intervening lymphocytes, plasma cells, eosinophils, macrophages, and occasional Reed-Sternberg cells. An abdominal CT scan and bone marrow biopsy show no abnormalities. The subtype and stage of her Hodgkin disease is

- (A) Lymphocyte predominance, stage I
- (B) Mixed cellularity, stage II
- (C) Lymphocyte depletion, stage III
- (D) Lymphocyte predominance, stage II
- (E) Nodular sclerosis, stage I

23. A 7-year-old boy has painful, swollen lymph nodes in his right inguinal region that have worsened over the past week. An inguinal lymph node biopsy is performed. Histologically, the node has large germinal centers containing numerous mitotic figures. There are numerous neutrophils about the follicles and in the sinuses. The most likely cause for these histologic changes is

- (A) Acute lymphoblastic leukemia
- (B) Sarcoidosis
- (C) Follicular lymphoma
- (D) Cat scratch disease
- (E) Acute lymphadenitis

24. A 39-year-old male has subarachnoid and gastrointestinal hemorrhage. The WBC count is 75,000/μL, and most of the WBCs seen on the peripheral blood smear are hypergranular promyelocytes with numerous Auer rods. Schistocytes are seen on the peripheral blood smear as well. The serum D-dimer level is elevated. Cytogenetic analysis of cells from bone marrow biopsy is most likely to yield which of the following karyotypic abnormalities?

- (A) t(8;21)
- (B) t(9;22)
- (C) t(14;18)
- (D) t(15;17)
- (E) t(8;14)

25. A 4-year-old child has appeared listless for about a week. He now complains of pain when he is picked up by his mother, and he demonstrates irritability on touching his arms or legs. In the past couple of days, several large ecchymoses have appeared on his right thigh and left shoulder. A complete blood count reveals a hemoglobin concentration of 10.2 g/dL, hematocrit of 30.5%, MCV of 96 fL, platelet count of 45,000/μL, and WBC count of 13,990/μL. Examination of the peripheral blood smear shows blasts. These blasts lack peroxidase-positive granules but do contain periodic acid–Schiff (PAS)–positive aggregates and stain positively for TdT. Flow cytometry shows the phenotype of blasts to be CD19$^+$, CD3$^-$, and sIg$^-$. He is most likely to have

- ○ (A) Chronic myelogenous leukemia (CML)
- ○ (B) Idiopathic thrombocytopenic purpura
- ○ (C) Acute myelogenous leukemia
- ○ (D) Chronic lymphocytic leukemia
- ○ (E) Acute lymphoblastic leukemia (ALL)

26. Massive splenomegaly is a characteristic clinical feature of all of the following diseases *except*

- ○ (A) Chronic myelogenous leukemia (CML)
- ○ (B) Myelofibrosis with myeloid metaplasia
- ○ (C) Gaucher disease
- ○ (D) Kala-azar
- ○ (E) Infectious mononucleosis

27. A 69-year-old male notices the presence of "lumps" in his right neck that have been enlarging during the past year. Physical examination reveals firm, nontender posterior cervical lymph nodes ranging from 1 to 2 cm in diameter. The overlying skin is intact and not erythematous. One of these cervical lymph nodes is biopsied. Which of the following histologic features provides the best evidence for the presence of malignant lymphoma in this node?

- ○ (A) Presence of lymphoid cells positive for kappa, but not lambda, light chains
- ○ (B) Absence of a follicular pattern
- ○ (C) Proliferation of small capillaries
- ○ (D) Presence of cells that stain with monoclonal antibody to the CD30 antigen
- ○ (E) Absence of plasma cells

28. A 42-year-old male presents with generalized lymphadenopathy along with fever and weight loss. The spleen tip is palpable on physical examination. His peripheral blood WBC count is 24,500/μL, with a differential count of 10 segmented neutrophils, 1 band, 86 lymphocytes, and 3 monocytes per 100 WBCs. A cervical lymph node biopsy reveals a nodular pattern of neoplastic small lymphoid cells. A bone marrow biopsy reveals infiltrates of similar small cells. Cytogenetic analysis reveals t(11;14) in the neoplastic cells. The most likely diagnosis is

- ○ (A) Mantle cell lymphoma
- ○ (B) Follicular lymphoma
- ○ (C) Acute lymphoblastic leukemia
- ○ (D) Burkitt lymphoma
- ○ (E) Small lymphocytic lymphoma

29. A 45-year-old male has fever, weight loss, and lymphadenopathy. The adenopathy becomes very tender after a six-pack of beer. A lymph node biopsy reveals effacement of the nodal architecture by a population of small lymphocytes, plasma cells, eosinophils, and macrophages. Which of the following additional cell types, which stain positively for CD15, is characteristic of this disease?

- ○ (A) Reed-Sternberg cell
- ○ (B) Immunoblast
- ○ (C) Epithelioid cell
- ○ (D) Neutrophils
- ○ (E) Mast cell

30. A 23-year-old female has a positive antinuclear antibody test with a titer of 1:1024 and a "rim" pattern. An anti–double-stranded DNA test is also positive. She has a malar skin rash on physical examination. Her complete blood count demonstrates a hemoglobin concentration of 12.1 g/dL, hematocrit of 35.5%, MCV of 89 fL, WBC count of 4500/μL, and platelet count of 109,000/μL. Which of the following findings is most likely to be demonstrated by a WBC differential count?

- ○ (A) Eosinophilia
- ○ (B) Thrombocytosis
- ○ (C) Monocytosis
- ○ (D) Neutrophilia
- ○ (E) Basophilia

Normal serum

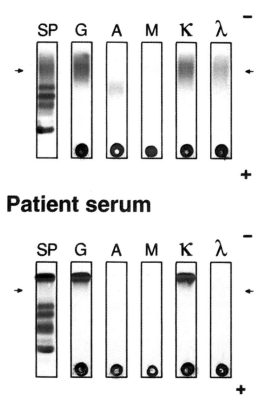

Patient serum

SP, serum protein electrophoresis; G, A, M, κ, and λ are gels with specific stains for IgG, IgA, IgM, kappa light chain, and lambda light chains, respectively. (Courtesy of Dr. David Sacks, Department of Pathology, Brigham and Women's Hospital, Boston, MA.)

31. The finding on serum protein electrophoresis shown in the previous figure from a 58-year-old male with renal failure is most characteristically associated with which of the following laboratory findings?

○ (A) TdT⁺ circulating blasts
○ (B) Bence Jones proteinuria
○ (C) Bone marrow karyotype with t(8;14)
○ (D) Reactive amyloidosis
○ (E) Hematocrit of 62%

32. The *bcr-abl* fusion gene from the reciprocal translocation t(9;22)(q34;q11) results in increased tyrosine kinase activity. This is most characteristic for

○ (A) Follicular lymphoma
○ (B) Chronic myelogenous leukemia (CML)
○ (C) Hodgkin disease, lymphocyte depletion type
○ (D) Acute promyelocytic leukemia
○ (E) Multiple myeloma

33. A 64-year-old male presents with inguinal, axillary, and cervical lymphadenopathy. The nodes are firm and nontender. A biopsy of a cervical node shows a histologic pattern of nodular aggregates of small cleaved lymphoid cells and larger cells with open nuclear chromatin, several nucleoli, and moderate amounts of cytoplasm. A bone marrow biopsy reveals lymphoid aggregates of similar cells. Karyotyping of these lymphoid cells reveals the presence of t(14;18). He is most likely to have

○ (A) Hodgkin disease, nodular sclerosis type
○ (B) Acute lymphadenitis
○ (C) Follicular lymphoma
○ (D) Mantle cell lymphoma
○ (E) Toxoplasmosis

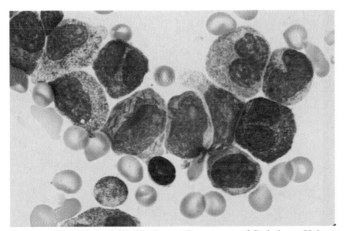

Courtesy of Dr. Robert W. McKenna, Department of Pathology, University of Texas Southwestern Medical School, Dallas, TX.

34. A 35-year-old male has experienced malaise for the past 3 months. A CBC is performed and shows a hemoglobin concentration of 10.8 g/dL, hematocrit of 33.0%, MCV of 90 fL, platelet count of 96,000/μL, and WBC count of 89,600/μL. The peripheral blood smear has the appearance shown here. The most likely complication of this condition is

○ (A) Vertebral compressed fractures
○ (B) Chronic renal failure
○ (C) Disseminated intravascular coagulation (DIC)
○ (D) Small intestinal obstruction
○ (E) Perforated duodenal ulcer

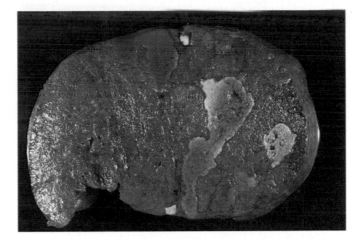

35. The gross appearance of the spleen shown in the figure, from a 27-year-old male with fever and leukocytosis, is most typical for which of the following conditions?

○ (A) Metastatic carcinoma
○ (B) Acute myelogenous leukemia
○ (C) Hodgkin disease
○ (D) Infective endocarditis
○ (E) Disseminated histoplasmosis

For each of the clinical histories in questions 36 and 37, match the most closely associated infectious agent:

(A) *Aspergillus fumigatus*
(B) *Bartonella henselae*
(C) Cytomegalovirus
(D) Epstein-Barr virus
(E) *Escherichia coli*
(F) *Helicobacter pylori*
(G) Hepatitis C virus
(H) Herpes simplex virus
(I) *Strongyloides stercoralis*
(J) *Toxoplasma gondii*
(K) Varicella zoster virus

36. A week after beginning therapy for *Pneumocystis carinii* pneumonia with trimethoprim-sulfamethoxazole, a 29-year-old female has a CBC that shows a hemoglobin concentration of 7.4 g/dL, hematocrit of 22.2%, MCV of 98 fL, platelet count of 47,000/μL, and WBC count of 1870/μL, with a differential count of 2 segmented neutrophils, 2 band cells, 85 lymphocytes, 10 monocytes, and 1 eosinophil per 100 WBCs. A chest radiograph 1 week later demonstrates multiple, 1- to 3-cm nodules in all lung fields. (   )

37. A 23-year-old male undergoing chemotherapy for acute lymphoblastic leukemia has developed a fever and abdominal pain in the past week. He now has a severe

cough. His CBC shows a hemoglobin concentration of 12.8 g/dL, hematocrit of 39.0%, MCV of 90 fL, platelet count of 221,000/μL, and WBC count of 16,475/μL, with differential count of 51 segmented neutrophils, 5 band cells, 18 lymphocytes, 8 monocytes, and 18 eosinophils per 100 WBCs. (   )

38. A 41-year-old male has had several bouts of pneumonia in the past year. He now complains of vague abdominal pain and a dragging sensation. Physical examination reveals marked splenomegaly. A complete blood count shows a hemoglobin concentration of 8.2 g/dL, hematocrit of 24.6%, MCV of 90 fL, WBC count of 2400/μL, and platelet count of 63,000/μL. On the peripheral blood smear are many small leukocytes with reniform nuclei and pale blue cytoplasm with threadlike extensions. Immunohistochemical staining shows that they mark with CD20. Which of the following laboratory test findings is most characteristic of this disease?

○ (A) Tartrate-resistant acid phosphatase in leukocytes
○ (B) Presence of Auer rods in leukocytes
○ (C) Presence of Ph[1] chromosome
○ (D) Presence of toxic granulations in neutrophils
○ (E) Monoclonal IgM in serum

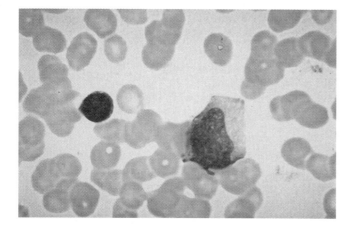

39. The peripheral blood smear shown here is from a previously healthy 26-year-old male who has had a low-grade fever, malaise, pharyngitis, and lymphadenopathy for a couple of weeks. The most likely risk factor for the disease shown here is

○ (A) An inherited disorder of globin chain synthesis
○ (B) Transfusion of packed red blood cells (RBCs)
○ (C) Close personal contact (kissing) with his date
○ (D) Sharing infected needles for intravenous drug use
○ (E) Ingestion of raw oysters

40. A 38-year-old woman presents with bleeding gums. Physical examination reveals hepatosplenomegaly and generalized lymphadenopathy. A complete blood count shows a hemoglobin concentration of 11.2 g/dL, hematocrit of 33.9%, MCV of 89 fL, platelet count of 95,000/μL, and WBC count of 4500/μL. The WBC differential count shows 25 segmented neutrophils, 10 band cells, 2 metamyelocytes, 55 lymphocytes, 8 monocytes, and 1 nucleated

RBC per 100 WBCs. A bone marrow biopsy shows 100% cellularity with many large blasts that are peroxidase negative and nonspecific esterase positive. She is most likely to have

○ (A) Acute lymphoblastic leukemia (ALL)
○ (B) Acute megakaryocytic leukemia
○ (C) Acute promyelocytic leukemia
○ (D) Acute erythroleukemia
○ (E) Acute monocytic leukemia

41. Which of the following combinations of phenotypic-, karyotypic-, and age-related markers predicts the best prognosis in acute lymphoblastic leukemia?

○ (A) Early pre-B (CD19+, CD10+, TdT+); hyperdiploidy; 8 years old
○ (B) T cell (CD3+, CD2+, TdT+); normal karyotype; 2 years old
○ (C) Pre-B (CD19+, CD10+, TdT+, Cμ+); t(9;22); 4 years old
○ (D) Early pre-B (CD19+, CD10+, TdT+); t(9;22); 1 year old
○ (E) Pre-B (CD19+, CD10+, TdT+, Cμ+); normal karyotype; 15 years old

42. A 51-year-old male presents with a generalized exfoliative erythroderma. A skin biopsy reveals the presence of lymphoid cells in the upper dermis and epidermis. These cells have cerebriform nuclei with marked infolding of nuclear membranes. Similar cells are seen on his peripheral blood smear. Which combination of the following phenotypic markers is expressed on the abnormal lymphocytes?

○ (A) CD3+, CD4+, CD8−
○ (B) CD3+, CD4−, CD8+
○ (C) CD19+, sIg+
○ (D) CD19+, CD5+
○ (E) CD33+, CD13+

43. A 65-year-old male presents with a 1-year history that includes fatigue, a 5-kg weight loss, night sweats, and abdominal discomfort. His CBC shows a hemoglobin concentration of 10.1 g/dL, hematocrit of 30.5%, MCV of 89 fL, platelet count of 94,000/μL, and WBC count of 14,750/μL. The WBC differential count shows 55 segmented neutrophils, 9 band cells, 20 lymphocytes, 8 monocytes, 4 metamyelocytes, 3 myelocytes, and 1 eosinophil, with 2 nucleated RBCs per 100 WBCs. The peripheral blood smear also demonstrates tear-drop cells. Serum uric acid level is 12 mg/dL. He has marked splenomegaly on physical examination, although no lymphadenopathy. A bone marrow biopsy shows extensive marrow fibrosis along with clusters of atypical megakaryocytes. Which of the following pathologic findings in his spleen is most likely to account for the enlargement?

○ (A) Reed-Sternberg cells mixed with many more lymphocytes, plasma cells, eosinophils, and macrophages
○ (B) Proliferation of all hematopoietic lineages, with prominence of megakaryocytes
○ (C) Chronic passive venous congestion and fibrosis

○ (D) Multiple caseating granulomas containing macrophages with *Histoplasma capsulatum*

○ (E) Diffuse infiltration by metastatic adenocarcinoma

44. A 60-year-old male presents with vague abdominal discomfort accompanied by some bloating and diarrhea. The stool is positive for occult blood. An abdominal CT scan reveals a 5 × 12 cm mass involving the wall of the distal ileum and adjacent mesentery. A laparotomy is performed, and the mass is resected. Microscopically, the mass is composed of sheets of large lymphoid cells with large nuclei, prominent nucleoli, and frequent mitoses. The neoplastic cells are CD19$^+$ and CD20$^+$ and have the bcl-6 gene rearrangement. Which of the following prognostic features is most applicable to this case?

○ (A) Indolent disease with survival for 7 to 9 years without treatment

○ (B) Aggressive disease that can be cured by aggressive chemotherapy

○ (C) Aggressive disease that does not respond to chemotherapy and transforms to acute leukemia

○ (D) Indolent disease that can be cured by chemotherapy

○ (E) Indolent disease that often undergoes spontaneous remission

45. A 45-year-old male experienced a gradual weight loss for months, along with weakness, anorexia, and easy fatigability. On physical examination, there was marked splenomegaly. A complete blood count showed a hemoglobin concentration of 12.9 g/dL, hematocrit of 38.1%, MCV of 92 fL, platelet count of 410,000/μL, and WBC count of 168,000/μL. The peripheral blood smear is depicted in part *A* of the figure. Karyotypic analysis showed the Ph^1 chromosome. He underwent chemotherapy that reduced the spleen size and the total leukocyte count to the normal range. He remained in remission for 3 years but then began to develop fatigue and experienced a 10-kg weight loss. Physical examination revealed petechial hemorrhages. A complete CBC showed a hemoglobin concentration of 10.5 g/dL, hematocrit of 30%, WBC count of 40,000/μL, and platelet count of 60,000/μL. A peripheral blood smear is depicted in part *B* of the figure. Karyotypic analysis showed 2 Ph^1 chromosomes and aneuploidy. Flow cytometric analysis of the peripheral blood showed CD19$^+$,

CD10$^+$, sIg$^-$, CD3$^-$ cells. Which of the following sequence of events is supported by these findings?

○ (A) This patient had chronic myeloid leukemia (CML) previously and has developed a second malignancy of B cells.

○ (B) This patient had CML and has developed a therapy-associated myelodysplastic syndrome.

○ (C) This patient had CML and acute lymphoblastic leukemia (ALL) at the original presentation. The CML is cured, but has persisted.

○ (D) This patient had transformation of a pluripotent stem cell, manifested initially as CML. With additional mutations, the leukemic stem cells have now emerged as a B-lymphoblastic leukemia.

○ (E) The first and second presentations are completely unrelated; patients' charts should be checked carefully to determine if the two sets of data pertain to different individuals.

46. A 14-year-old boy complains of a feeling of discomfort in his chest. A chest radiograph reveals clear lung fields, but there appears to be widening of the mediastinum. A thoracic CT scan demonstrates a 10-cm mass involving the anterior mediastinum. A biopsy of the mass reveals lymphoid cells with lobulated nuclei showing delicate, finely stippled nuclear chromatin. There is scant cytoplasm. Many mitoses are seen. The cells express TdT, CD1, CD2, and CD5 antigens. The most likely diagnosis is

○ (A) Lymphoblastic lymphoma

○ (B) Burkitt lymphoma

○ (C) Hodgkin disease, nodular sclerosing type

○ (D) Mantle cell lymphoma

○ (E) Follicular lymphoma

47. A 60-year-old female presents with headaches and dizziness. Physical examination reveals a somewhat congested face with a cyanotic appearance. There is mild splenomegaly but no other abnormal finding. Her blood pressure is normal. The patient's history reveals that she has been taking treatment for heartburn with anti-ulcer medications. Laboratory investigations reveal a hemoglobin concentration of 17.5 gm/dL, hematocrit of 65%. The MCV, MCHC, and serum ferritin levels are normal. Total WBC count is 30,000/μL with a differential of polymor-

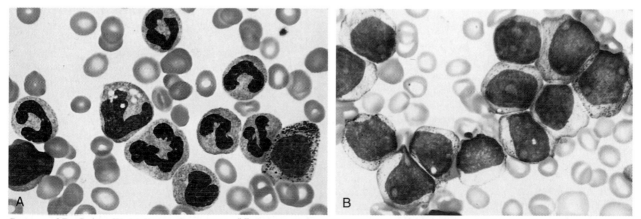

Courtesy of Dr. Robert W. McKenna, Department of Pathology, University of Texas Southwestern Medical School, Dallas, TX.

phonuclear leukocytes 85%, lymphocytes 10%, and mono-cytes 5%. Platelet count is 400,000/μL, and the blood smear shows abnormally large platelets. Her serum erythro-poietin level is undetectable, and the karyotype is normal. Which of the following is a characteristic of the natural history of this disease?

O (A) Death from transformation of the disease into acute B-lymphoblastic leukemia
O (B) Onset of marrow fibrosis with extensive extramed-ullary hematopoiesis in the spleen
O (C) Spontaneous remissions and relapses without any treatment
O (D) Gradual increase in monoclonal serum immuno-globulins
O (E) Development of a gastric lymphoma

48. A 17-year-old female has experienced malaise for several weeks, starting with a mild pharyngitis. Her sclerae are slightly icteric, and she is mildly anemic. The periph-eral blood smear demonstrates atypical lymphocytes. Which of the following laboratory test findings is most likely in this case?

O (A) Basophilia
O (B) Eosinophilia
O (C) Monocytosis
O (D) Monospot test positivity
O (E) 46,XX,t(9;22) karyotype

For each of the clinical histories in questions 49 and 50, match the most closely associated morphologic finding:

(A) Atypical lymphocytes
(B) Auer rods in promyelocytes
(C) Birbeck granules in histiocytes
(D) Döhle bodies in neutrophils
(E) Hairy cells
(F) Hypersegmented neutrophils
(G) Lacunar cells
(H) Lymphoblasts
(I) Megaloblastoid erythroblasts
(J) Myeloblasts
(K) Reticulocytes
(L) Toxic granulations in neutrophils

49. A 38-year-old female has experienced increasing dyspnea. A chest radiograph demonstrates mediastinal wid-ening. A chest CT scan reveals an 8 × 10 cm posterior mediastinal mass that impinges on the trachea and esopha-gus. A mediastinoscopy is performed and the mass is biop-sied. Histologically, there are scattered Reed-Sternberg cells along with lymphocytes and macrophages separated by dense collagenous bands. (   )

50. An 18-month-old child who has developed seborrheic skin eruptions is also found to have hepatosplenomegaly and generalized lymphadenopathy. He has had recurrent upper respiratory and middle ear infections with *S. pneu-moniae* for the past year. A skull radiograph reveals an expansile, 2-cm lytic lesion involving the right parietal bone. (   )

51. A 28-year-old male is admitted with marked hypoten-sion and shock. A CBC shows a hemoglobin concentration of 14.1 g/dL, hematocrit of 42.6%, MCV of 93 fL, WBC count of 12,150/μL, and platelet count of 127,500/μL. The peripheral blood smear demonstrates a differential count of 71 segmented neutrophils, 8 band cells, 14 lymphocytes, and 7 monocytes per 100 WBCs. The neutrophils show cytoplasmic toxic granulations and Döhle bodies. Which of the following conditions is he most likely to have?

O (A) Tuberculosis
O (B) Acute myelogenous leukemia
O (C) Chronic myelogenous leukemia
O (D) Bacterial septicemia
O (E) Infectious mononucleosis

52. A 15-year-old girl has a CBC that demonstrates a hemoglobin concentration of 14.7 g/dL, hematocrit of 43.1%, MCV of 92 fL, platelet count of 233,000/μL, and WBC count of 9750/μL, with the differential count show-ing 58 segmented neutrophils, 4 band cells, 22 lympho-cytes, 4 monocytes, and 12 eosinophils per 100 WBCs. These findings are most likely to be associated with which of the following conditions?

O (A) Bacterial septicemia
O (B) Bronchial asthma
O (C) Chronic myelogenous leukemia (CML)
O (D) Leukemoid reaction
O (E) Viral hepatitis

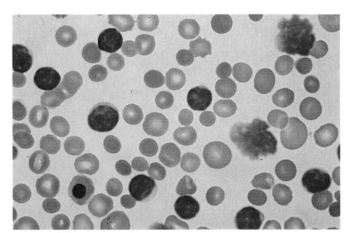

Courtesy of Dr. Jacqueline Mitus.

53. A figure skater who won gold medals at the 1928, 1932, and 1936 Winter Olympic games became progres-sively fatigued in her late fifties, leading to a workup that revealed a CBC with hemoglobin concentration of 10.1 g/dL, hematocrit of 30.5%, MCV of 90 fL, platelet count of 89,000/μL, and WBC count of 31,300/μL. From the pe-

ripheral blood picture shown in the figure, the most likely diagnosis is

O (A) Infectious mononucleosis
O (B) Chronic lymphocytic leukemia (CLL)
O (C) Iron deficiency anemia
O (D) Leukemoid reaction
O (E) Acute lymphoblastic leukemia (ALL)

54. A serum chemistry panel is performed on a healthy 48-year-old male with no complaints other than his worrying about getting older and having cancer. His total serum protein concentration is 7.4 g/dL, and the albumin level is 3.9 g/dL. The serum calcium and phosphorus levels are normal. Urinalysis reveals no Bence Jones proteinuria. A serum protein electrophoresis reveals a small (2.8-g) spike of γ-globulin, which is determined to be IgG kappa by immunoelectrophoresis. A physical examination reveals no hepatosplenomegaly or lymphadenopathy. A bone marrow biopsy reveals normal cellularity with maturation of all cell lines. Plasma cells constitute about 4% of the marrow. A bone scan is normal, with no areas of increased uptake. Which of the following conditions is most likely?

O (A) Solitary plasmacytoma
O (B) Waldenström macroglobulinemia
O (C) Monoclonal gammopathy of undetermined significance
O (D) Heavy-chain disease
O (E) Multiple myeloma

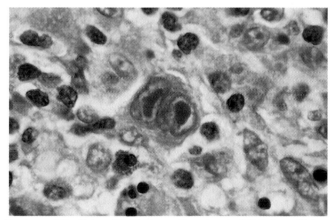

Courtesy of Dr. Robert W. McKenna, Department of Pathology, University of Texas Southwestern Medical School, Dallas, TX.

55. The patient is a 32-year-old female with fatigue, fever, night sweats, and painless right cervical adenopathy. The histologic finding shown here at high power was present in a cervical lymph node that was biopsied. This appearance is most likely to be seen with

O (A) Burkitt lymphoma
O (B) Well-differentiated lymphocytic lymphoma
O (C) Reactive lymphoid hyperplasia
O (D) Hodgkin disease, nodular sclerosis type
O (E) Cytomegalovirus infection

56. A 22-year-old university student presents with easy fatigability. A CBC shows a hemoglobin concentration of

9.5 g/dL, hematocrit of 28.2%, MCV of 94 fL, platelet count of 110,000/μL, and WBC count of 107,000/μL. A bone marrow biopsy shows that the marrow is 100% cellular, with few residual normal hematopoietic cells. Most of the cells in the marrow are large. Their nuclei have delicate chromatin and several nucleoli. The cytoplasm of these cells has azurophilic, peroxidase-positive granules. The most likely diagnosis is

O (A) Chronic lymphocytic leukemia (CLL)
O (B) Acute myelogenous leukemia
O (C) Acute megakaryocytic leukemia
O (D) Chronic myelogenous leukemia (CML)
O (E) Acute lymphoblastic leukemia (ALL)

ANSWERS

1. **(E)** The major finding here is marked granulocytopenia. All that is left on the peripheral smear are mononuclear cells (remember to multiply the percentages in the differential by the total WBC count to get the absolute values; rather than one cell line being overrepresented, another may be nearly missing). Accelerated removal or destruction of neutrophils could account for the selective absence of granulocytes in this case. Overwhelming infections cause increased peripheral use of neutrophils at sites of inflammation. Petechial hemorrhages can also occur in overwhelming bacterial infections, such as those caused by *Neisseria meningitidis*. Bleeding is not likely to be caused by thrombocytopenia, because the platelet count is normal. Normal bone marrow findings exclude acute lymphoid or myeloid leukemia. In aplastic anemia, the marrow is poorly cellular, and there is a reduction in red cells, white cells, and platelet production.
BP6 359   PBD6 646

2. **(D)** Shown here are the famous rodlike tubular Birbeck granules with characteristic periodicity that is seen in Langerhans cell proliferations. In this case, the skin eruptions, organomegaly, and lesion in the mastoid suggest infiltrates in multiple organs. The diagnosis is multifocal Langerhans cell histiocytosis, a disease most often seen in children. In one half of these cases, exophthalmos occurs, and involvement of the hypothalamus and pituitary stalk leads to diabetes insipidus, findings that are then called Hand-Schüller-Christian disease. ALL in childhood can involve the marrow, but does not produce skin or bone lesions. Myeloma is a disease of adults that may produce lytic bone lesions but not skin lesions. Hodgkin disease is seen in young adults and does not produce skin lesions or bone lesions. Tuberculosis may produce granulomatous disease with bony destruction, but the macrophages present in the granulomas are epithelioid macrophages that do not have Birbeck granules.
BP6 383   PBD6 685-686

3. **(A)** This patient has symptoms of hyperviscosity syndrome, such as visual disturbances, dizziness, and head-

aches. He also seems to have Raynaud phenomenon. His bone marrow is full of plasmacytoid lymphocytes that have stored immunoglobulins in the cytoplasm (Russell bodies). All of these suggest that the patient has lymphoplasmacytic lymphoma (i.e., Waldenström macroglobulinemia). In this disorder, neoplastic B cells differentiate to IgM-producing cells, and hence there is a monoclonal IgM spike in the serum. These IgM molecules aggregate and produce hyperviscosity, and some of these agglutinate at low temperatures to produce cold agglutinin disease. Punched-out lytic lesions are typical of multiple myeloma, another monoclonal gammopathy. However, myeloma does not cause liver and spleen enlargement. Hypercalcemia occurs with myeloma because of bone destruction; light chains in urine (Bence Jones proteins) are also a feature of multiple myeloma. A t(14;18) translocation is characteristic of a follicular lymphoma.
BP6 381   PBD6 666-667

4. **(D)** Marked leukocytosis and immature myeloid cells in the peripheral blood can represent an exaggerated response to infection (i.e., leukemoid reaction) or be a manifestation of CML. However, the leukocyte alkaline phosphatase score is high in the more differentiated cell population seen in reactive leukocytosis, whereas in CML, the leukocyte alkaline phosphatase score is low. The Philadelphia chromosome (universally present with CML) is absent with leukemoid reactions. Hairy cell leukemia is accompanied by peripheral blood leukocytes that mark with tartrate-resistant acid phosphatase. Hodgkin disease is not characterized by an increased WBC count. ALL is a disease of children and young adults, and the lymphoid cells do not have leukocyte alkaline phosphatase.
BP6 377   PBD6 681

5. **(E)** Burkitt and Burkitt-like lymphomas can be seen sporadically (in young persons), as an endemic form in Africa (in children), and in association with HIV infection. All forms are highly associated with translocations of the *myc* gene on chromosome 8. In the African form and in HIV-infected patients, the cells are latently infected with EBV, but sporadic cases are EBV negative. Involvement with this form of lymphoma is typically extranodal. Diffuse large cell lymphomas are most common in adults, as are follicular lymphomas. They do not carry the t(8;14) translocation. Acute lymphoblastic lymphomas may be seen in boys at this age, but the mass is in the mediastinum, and the lymphoid cells are T cells. Plasmacytomas appear in older adults and are not likely to produce an abdominal mass.
BP6 368   PBD6 662-663

6. **(B)** Diffuse large B-cell lymphoma occurs in older individuals and frequently presents as localized disease with extranodal involvement, particularly of the Waldeyer ring. The staining pattern indicates a B-cell proliferation (CD19+, CD10+). T-cell (CD3) and monocytic (CD15) markers are absent. TdT can be expressed in B-lineage cells at an earlier stage of maturation. Small lymphocytic lymphoma is also a B-cell neoplasm, but it manifests with widespread lymphadenopathy, liver and spleen enlargement, and lymphocytosis. Lymphoblastic lymphoma is a T-cell neoplasm that occurs typically in the mediastinum of children. Hodgkin disease is characterized by Reed-Sternberg cells. In chronic lymphadenitis, the lymph node has many cell types—macrophages, lymphocytes, and plasma cells. A monomorphous infiltrate is typical of non-Hodgkin lymphomas.
BP6 366-367   PBD6 654-656

7. **(E)** This patient has polycythemia vera. This is a myeloproliferative disorder characterized by an increased RBC mass, with hematocrits typically exceeding 60%. Although the increased RBC mass is responsible for most of the symptoms and signs, these patients have thrombocytosis and granulocytosis as well. This occurs because, like other myeloproliferative disorders, polycythemia vera results from transformation of a multipotent stem cell. The high hematocrit causes an increase in blood volume and distention of blood vessels. Along with abnormal platelet function, this condition predisposes to bleeding. Abnormal platelet function may also predispose to thrombosis. His pruritus and peptic ulceration seem to be the result of the histamine release from basophils. In some patients, the disease "burns out" to myelofibrosis. A few patients "blast out" into acute myelogenous leukemia, and others develop CML. Myelodysplastic syndromes and myeloproliferative disorders, such as essential thrombocytosis, are not accompanied by such an increase in red cell mass. Erythroleukemia is not typically accompanied by such a high hematocrit.
BP6 378-379   PBD6 682-683

8. **(C)** This patient has developed a myelodysplasia, characterized by a cellular marrow in which there are maturation defects in multiple lineages. This diagnosis is supported by the presence of ringed sideroblasts, megaloblasts, abnormal megakaryocytes, and myeloblasts in the marrow. Because the hematopoietic cells fail to mature normally, they are not released into the peripheral blood. The patient has pancytopenia and is susceptible to infections. Myelodysplasias are clonal stem cell disorders that develop de novo or after chemotherapy with alkylating agents, as in this case. The presence of chromosomal deletions such as 5q are markers of post-therapy myelodysplasias. The morphologic abnormalities in the marrow are not seen in any other listed condition.
BP6 376   PBD6 678-679

9. **(A)** Essential thrombocythemia is a myeloproliferative disorder. As with all myeloproliferative diseases, the transformation occurs in a myeloid stem cell. In this form of myeloproliferative disease, the dominant cell type affected is the megakaryocyte, and hence there is thrombocytosis. However, other myeloproliferative disorders can also be accompanied by an increased platelet count. The diagnosis of essential thrombocytosis can be made after other causes for reactive thrombocytosis are excluded and if the bone marrow examination shows increased megakaryocytes without evidence for leukemia. The throbbing, burning pain in the extremities is caused by aggregates of platelets that occlude small arterioles. The major manifestation of this disease is thrombotic or hemorrhagic crises.
PBD6 683

10. **(E)** He has the African variety of Burkitt lymphoma, a B-cell lymphoma that typically appears in the maxilla or mandible of the jaw. This particular neoplasm is related to EBV infection.
BP6 368–369   PBD6 662–663

11. **(J)** Lymph nodes draining from a cancer often demonstrate a reactive pattern, with dilated sinusoids that have endothelial hypertrophy and are filled with histiocytes (i.e., macrophages). Sinus histiocytosis represents an immunologic response to cancer antigens. Not all enlarged nodes are caused by metastatic disease in cancer patients.
BP6 362–363   PBD6 650

12. **(B)** Multiple myeloma produces mass lesions of plasma cells in bone that lead to lysis and pain. The skull radiograph shows typical punched-out lytic lesions, produced by expanding masses of plasma cells. Bence Jones proteinuria can damage the tubules and give rise to renal failure. Multiple myeloma can be complicated by AL amyloid, which can also lead to renal failure. Patients with myeloma often have infections with encapsulated bacteria because of decreased production of IgG, required for opsonization. Granulomatous disease (which is not produced by pneumococcus) may involve the marrow but usually does not produce such sharply demarcated lytic lesions. Nodules of small lymphocytes suggest a small cell lymphocytic leukemia/lymphoma, which is not likely to produce lytic lesions. Reed-Sternberg cells suggest Hodgkin disease. Blasts suggest a leukemic process.
BP6 380–382   PBD6 663–666

13. **(C)** Interleukin-5 acts as an eosinophilic chemotactic factor that makes an eosinophilic cellular component part of the mixed cellularity and nodular sclerosis types of Hodgkin disease. In contrast, the transforming growth factor-β (TGF-β) secreted by eosinophils promotes the fibrosis that is part of nodular sclerosing Hodgkin disease.
PBD6 674

14. **(H)** The mucosa-associated lymphoid tissue (MALT) lesions in the stomach can be associated with the presence of *H. pylori* infection. Although monoclonal (like a neoplasm), these MALT lymphomas can regress with antibiotic therapy for the *H. pylori*.
BP6 368   PBD6 668

15. **(D)** Non-Hodgkin lymphomas of the large diffuse B-cell type can be associated with HIV infection and define the acquired immunodeficiency syndrome (AIDS). AIDS lymphomas tend to be extranodal, and the large cell type can also involve the central nervous system; they have a poor prognosis. In approximately 50% of cases the systemic diffuse large lymphomas contain the EBV genome. Virtually 100% of AIDS-associated central nervous system lymphomas are infected with EBV.
BP6 366–367   PBD6 661–662

16. **(L)** This patient has a rare disorder called pure red cell aplasia, characterized by selective suppression of the erythroid lineage in the bone marrow. This curious entity is

sometimes associated with a thymic tumor. In about one half of such cases, resection of the thymic tumor relieves the red cell aplasia, suggesting some autoimmune mechanisms as the cause of red cell aplasia.
PBD6 632, 693

17. **(C)** Polycythemia vera is a neoplastic disorder of myeloid stem cells that tend to differentiate predominantly along the erythroid lineage, giving rise to polycythemia. The neoplastic erythroid progenitor cells require extremely small amounts of erythropoietin for survival and proliferation, and hence the levels of erythropoietin are virtually undetectable in polycythemia vera. In all other conditions, erythropoietin levels are elevated to produce excess red cells. Erythropoietin secretion is triggered by anoxia in high-altitude dwellers and persons with cyanotic heart disease. Renal tumors produce erythropoietin and trigger a paraneoplastic erythrocytosis. In dehydration, transient polycythemia is caused by hemoconcentration. This does not affect normal erythropoietin secretion.
BP6 378–379   PBD6 682–683

18. **(C)** Chronic infections and chronic inflammatory conditions, such as lung abscess, can lead to an expansion of the myeloid precursor pool in the bone marrow. This is manifested as neutrophilic leukocytosis. Acute viral hepatitis, unlike acute bacterial infections, does not cause neutrophilic leukocytosis. Glucocorticoids may increase the release of marrow storage pool cells and diminish extravasation of neutrophils into tissues. Vigorous exercise can transiently produce neutrophilia from demargination of neutrophils. With acute myelogenous leukemia, the marrow is filled with blasts, not maturing myeloid elements.
BP6 359   PBD6 647–648

19. **(A)** This HIV-positive patient has an extranodal infiltrative mass in the ileum that is made up of B cells (CD19+). This is a diffuse large cell lymphoma of B cells. These tumors contain the EBV genome, and it is thought that immunosuppression allows unregulated proliferation and neoplastic transformation of EBV-infected B cells. HIV is not seen in normal or neoplastic B cells. HHV-8, also called Kaposi sarcoma herpesvirus, is found in the spindle cells of Kaposi sarcoma and in body cavity B-cell lymphomas in AIDS patients. HTLV-1 is related to HIV-1, and it causes adult T-cell leukemia/lymphoma. CMV is not known to cause any tumors.
BP6 367   PBD6 661–662

20. **(B)** The clinical history, the peripheral blood smear, and the phenotypic markers are characteristic of chronic lymphocytic leukemia. This is a clonal B-cell neoplasm in which immunoglobulin genes are rearranged and T-cell receptor genes are in germline configuration. The t(9;22) is a feature of chronic myeloid leukemia. The t(8;14) translocation is typical of Burkitt lymphoma; this occurs in children at extranodal sites. The t(14;18) translocation is a feature of follicular lymphomas. These are distinctive B-cell tumors that involve the nodes and produce a follicular pattern. The lymphoma cells can be present in blood, but they do not look like mature lymphocytes.
BP6 377–378   PBD6 658–659

21. **(A)** The characteristic "punched-out" bone lesions of multiple myeloma seen on radiographs result from areas of bone lysis with plasma cell proliferation. The bone marrow aspirate shows plasma cells. The monoclonal population of plasma cells often produces a monoclonal serum "spike" seen with serum or urine protein electrophoresis. Patients may have hypercalcemia and an increased serum alkaline phosphatase level. The neoplastic cells are generally well differentiated, with features such as a perinuclear "hof," similar to normal plasma cells. The t(9;22) translocation is the Philadelphia chromosome seen with chronic myelogenous leukemia (CML). CML and other myeloproliferative disorders may be accompanied by a thrombocytosis but are unlikely to produce mass lesions or bony destruction.
BP6 380–382   PBD6 663–666

22. **(E)** The bands of fibrosis are typical for the nodular sclerosis type, which is most commonly seen in young adults, particularly females. Involvement of one group of lymph nodes places this in stage I. Mediastinal involvement is common. Most of such cases are stage I or II. The prognosis of such early stage cases is good.
BP6 369–372   PBD6 672–675

23. **(E)** Acute enlargement of nodes that are painful suggests a reactive condition, not a neoplastic process such as a lymphoma or a leukemia. In children, acute lymphadenitis is common. There are many infectious processes that can give rise to this finding, particularly bacterial infections. Sarcoidosis is a chronic granulomatous process characterized by the formation of noncaseating granulomas. Follicular lymphomas are neoplasms of B cells that efface the normal architecture of the lymph nodes. These tumors do not occur in children. Cat scratch disease may produce sarcoid-like granulomas with stellate abscesses.
BP6 361–362   PBD6 649

24. **(D)** This is acute promyelocytic leukemia (M3 class of acute myelogenous leukemia). As in this case, many patients develop disseminated intravascular coagulation. The t(15;17) translocation is characteristic of this disease. It results in the fusion of the retinoic acid receptor gene on chromosome 17 with the promyelocytic leukemia gene on chromosome 15. The fusion gene results in elaboration of an abnormal retinoic acid receptor that blocks myeloid differentiation. Therapy with retinoic acid (vitamin A) can alleviate the block and induce remission in many patients. The t(8;21) abnormality is seen with the M2 variant of acute myelogenous leukemia. The t(9;22) translocation gives rise to the Philadelphia chromosome of chronic myelogenous leukemia. A t(14;18) karyotype suggests a follicular lymphoma. The t(8;14) translocation can be seen with a Burkitt lymphoma.
BP6 375   PBD6 676–678

25. **(E)** This is a childhood ALL of the pre-B cell type. The rapid expansion of the marrow caused by proliferation of blasts can lead to bone pain and tenderness. Features supporting an acute leukemia are anemia, thrombocytopenia, and presence of blasts in the peripheral blood and bone marrow. Anemia and thrombocytopenia result from suppression of normal hematopoiesis by the leukemic clone in the marrow. The phenotype of CD19+, CD3−, sIg− is typical of pre-B cells. TdT is a marker of early T- and B-cell–type lymphoid cells. CML is a disease of adults, and the WBC count is quite high; the peripheral blood contains some myeloblasts, but other stages of myeloid differentiation are also detected. In idiopathic thrombocytopenic purpura, only the platelet count is reduced, because of antibody-mediated destruction of platelets. An acute myelogenous leukemia is a disease of young to middle-aged adults, and there should be peroxidase-positive myeloblasts and phenotypic features of myeloid cells. Chronic lymphocytic leukemia is a disease of older adults, with many small circulating mature B lymphocytes.
BP6 374–375   PBD6 656–658

26. **(E)** Infectious mononucleosis is typically an acute, self-limited EBV-caused disease that gives rise to a mild splenomegaly. Splenic enlargement regresses when the patient recovers. All others are chronic disorders with markedly enlarged spleens. In CML and myelofibrosis, the spleen is the site of proliferation of neoplastic myeloid stem cells. In Gaucher disease, splenic macrophages store glucocerebrosides. Kala-azar is a form of visceral Leishmaniasis caused by *Leishmania donovani* and *L. donovani chagasi*. These parasites lodge in the reticuloendothelial system, including in the spleen, causing massive enlargements.
BP6 390   PBD6 688–689

27. **(A)** All lymphoid neoplasms are derived from a single transformed cell and are therefore monoclonal. Monoclonality in B-cell neoplasms, which comprise 80% to 85% of all lymphoid neoplasms, can often be demonstrated by staining for light chains. Populations of normal or reactive (polyclonal) B cells contain a mixture B cells expressing kappa and lambda light chains. Some lymphoid neoplasms have a follicular pattern, and others do not. A normal pattern of follicles may be absent if the node is involved with some inflammatory conditions or with immune suppression. A proliferation of capillaries is typically a benign, reactive process. The CD30 antigen is a marker for activated T and B cells. Plasma cells are variably present in reactive conditions, but their absence is not indicative of malignancy.
BP6 362–363   PBD6 650–653

28. **(A)** Of the lesions listed here, lymphoblastic lymphoma and Burkitt lymphoma occur in a much younger age group. Burkitt lymphoma has a t(8;14) translocation. The remaining three occur in an older age group. Of these, small lymphocytic lymphoma presents with absolute lymphocytosis and a peripheral blood picture of chronic lymphocytic leukemia. Follicular lymphoma has a distinct and characteristic translocation t(14;18) involving the *bcl-2* gene. In contrast, mantle cell lymphoma has the t(11;14) translocation, which activates cyclin D1 *(bcl-1)* gene. These tumors do not respond well to chemotherapy.
BP6 366   PBD6 667–668

29. **(A)** The features suggest Hodgkin disease, mixed cellularity type, which tends to affect older males. As in all other forms of Hodgkin disease, the Reed-Sternberg cells and variants stain with CD15. These cells also express CD30, an activation marker on T cells, B cells, and monocytes. Clinical symptoms are frequent in the mixed cellularity type of Hodgkin disease, and this histologic type

tends to present in advanced stages. The pain associated with alcohol consumption is a peculiar paraneoplastic phenomenon with Hodgkin disease. The Reed-Sternberg cells make up a relatively small percentage of the tumor mass, with most of the cell population consisting of reactive cells such as lymphocytes, plasma cells, macrophages, and eosinophils. Immunoblasts suggest a B-cell proliferation. Epithelioid cells are seen in granulomatous inflammatory reactions. Neutrophils accumulate at sites of acute inflammation.

BP6 370-371   PBD6 672-676

30. **(C)** She has evidence for an autoimmune disease, most likely systemic lupus erythematosus. This can be accompanied by monocytosis. (Cytopenias can also occur in systemic lupus erythematosus because of autoantibodies against blood elements [a form of type II hypersensitivity].) Eosinophilia is a feature more often seen with allergic conditions, parasitic infestations, and chronic myeloid leukemia (CML). Thrombocytosis usually occurs with neoplastic disorders of myeloid stem cells, such as CML. Basophilia occurs infrequently but may be seen with CML.

PB6 359   PBD6 648

31. **(B)** Multiple myeloma is composed of abnormal plasma cells that tend to retain the ability to secrete immunoglobulins. Heavy and light chain components can be produced. The light chains are excreted in the urine and are known as Bence Jones proteins. Serum protein (SP) electrophoresis is used to screen for the presence of a monoclonal immunoglobulin (M protein). Polyclonal IgG in normal serum (denoted by the arrow in the illustration) appears as a broad band; in contrast, serum from a patient with multiple myeloma contains a single sharp protein band in this region. The suspected monoclonal immunoglobulin is then confirmed and characterized by immunofixation. In this procedure the electrophoresed proteins within the gel are reacted with specific antisera. After extensive washing, only proteins cross-linked by the antisera are retained in the gel, which is then stained for protein. The sharp band in the immunoglobulin region of the patient's SP is recognized by antisera against IgG heavy chain (G) and kappa light chain (κ), indicating that this band is an IgGκ M protein. The levels of polyclonal IgG, IgA (A), and lambda light chain (λ) are also decreased in the patient serum relative to normal serum, a common finding in multiple myeloma. The TdT-positive circulating blasts are seen in lymphoblastic leukemias. The t(8;14) translocation is typical for a Burkitt lymphoma. Amyloidosis, reactive and primary, can give rise to renal failure. In primary amyloidosis, the amyloid is derived from immunoglobulin light chains, and patients may have a monoclonal B-cell proliferation. However, reactive amyloid is made up of nonimmunoglobulin proteins. A markedly increased hematocrit may suggest polycythemia as part of a myeloproliferative process.

BP6 380-382   PBD6 663-666

32. **(B)** This is the Philadelphia chromosome, or Ph[1], that is characteristic for CML. This karyotypic abnormality can be found by cytogenetic techniques, including fluorescence in situ hybridization (FISH). In the few cases that appear negative by karyotyping and by FISH, molecular analysis reveals *bcr-abl* rearrangements. This rearrangement is considered a diagnostic criterion for CML. This is a disease of pluripotent stem cells that affects all lineages, but the granulocytic precursors expand preferentially in the chronic phase. Follicular lymphomas have a t(14;18) karyotypic abnormality involving the *bcl-2* gene. In general, Hodgkin disease and myelomas do not have characteristic karyotypic abnormalities. Acute promyelocytic leukemias often have the t(15;17) abnormality.

BP6 377   PBD6 680-682

33. **(C)** This patient has follicular lymphoma, the most common form of non-Hodgkin lymphoma among adults in the United States. Men and women are equally affected. The neoplastic B cells mimic a population of follicular center cells and hence produce a nodular or follicular pattern. Nodal involvement is often generalized, but extranodal involvement is uncommon. The t(14;18) translocation is characteristic. It causes overexpression of the *bcl-2* gene, and hence the cells are resistant to apoptosis. In keeping with this, follicular lymphomas are indolent tumors that continue to accumulate cells over 7 to 9 years. In Hodgkin disease, there are few Reed-Sternberg cells surrounded by a reactive lymphoid population. The lymphoid population in acute lymphadenitis is reactive, and there is no bone marrow involvement. Mantle cell lymphoma is also a B-cell tumor; it is more aggressive than follicular lymphoma and is typified by the t(11;14) translocation in which the cyclin D1 gene *(bcl-1)* is overexpressed. In toxoplasmosis, there should be a mixed population of inflammatory cells with some necrosis.

BP6 364-366   PBD6 659-661

34. **(C)** This is the M3 variant of acute myelogenous leukemia, with many promyelocytes containing prominent azurophilic granules and short, red, cytoplasmic, rodlike inclusions called Auer rods. Release of the granules can trigger the coagulation cascade, leading to DIC. Leukemias do not tend to produce mass lesions or erode bone, as does multiple myeloma. Chronic renal failure is not a typical feature for leukemias or lymphomas. Small bowel obstruction from lymphoma can occur, typically from B-cell malignancies such as Burkitt lymphoma or diffuse large B-cell lymphoma. *H. pylori* infection, which is a risk factor for peptic ulcer disease, can also be involved in the pathogenesis of gastric B-cell lymphomas.

BP6 374   PBD6 675-677

35. **(D)** The pale, tan to yellow, firm areas are infarcts. These lesions are either wedge-shaped and based on the capsule or more irregularly shaped within the parenchyma. Emboli in the systemic arterial circulation may arise from vegetations on cardiac valves in a patient with infective endocarditis. These can lead to splenic infarction. Emboli exiting the aorta at the celiac axis generally take the straight route to the spleen. Kidneys and brain are other frequent sites for systemic emboli to lodge. Metastases may increase the size of the spleen somewhat but are uncommon in the spleen and are not likely to be accompanied by signs of infection. Although acute myelogenous leukemia and Hodgkin disease can increase the size of the spleen,

there are typically no focal lesions—only uniform infiltration of the parenchyma. Likewise, the congestive splenomegaly with cirrhosis and portal hypertension does not produce focal splenic lesions. There should be scattered granulomas that are rounded and tan with granulomatous diseases of the spleen, such as histoplasmosis.
PBD6 689

36. **(A)** She developed severe neutropenia with pancytopenia from drug toxicity, which predisposed her to sepsis. Aspergillosis is a cause for pulmonary granulomas, and neutropenia is a significant risk factor.
BP6 359   PBD6 646–647

37. **(I)** The eosinophilia suggests a parasitic infestation. Persons who are immunocompromised may have superinfection and dissemination with strongyloidiasis.
BP6 359   PBD6 337, 648

38. **(A)** This patient has hairy cell leukemia, an uncommon neoplastic disorder of B cells (CD20+). These cells infiltrate the spleen and marrow. Pancytopenia results from poor production of hematopoietic cells in the marrow and sequestration of the mature cells in the spleen. There are two characteristic features of this disease: the presence of hairy projections from neoplastic leukocytes in the peripheral blood smear and tartrate-resistant acid phosphatase in the neoplastic cells. Auer rods are seen in myeloblasts in acute myeloblastic leukemia. The Ph[1] chromosome is distinctive for CML. Toxic granulations in neutrophils are most often seen in overwhelming bacterial infections. A monoclonal IgM spike is a feature of lymphoplasmacytic lymphoma (i.e., Waldenström macroglobulinemia).
BP6 378   PBD6 668–669

39. **(C)** The smear shows large, "atypical" lymphocytes that are seen in infectious mononucleosis and other viral infections, such as those caused by CMV. These atypical cells are large lymphocytes with abundant cytoplasm and a large nucleus with fine chromatin. Infectious mononucleosis is caused by EBV and transmitted by close personal contact. Disorders of globin chain synthesis affect red blood cells, as in the thalassemias. Infectious mononucleosis is not known as a transfusion-associated disease. Likewise, injection drug use is typically not a risk factor for infectious mononucleosis but is a risk for bacterial infections, HIV infection, and viral hepatitis. Eating raw oysters is a risk factor for hepatitis A, because the hepatitis A virus is concentrated by the oysters from polluted sea water.
BP6 360   PBD6 371–373

40. **(E)** This patient has an "aleukemic" leukemia, whereby the peripheral blood count of leukocytes is not high, but the leukemic blasts fill the marrow. These blasts show features of monoblasts because they are peroxidase negative and nonspecific esterase positive. This patient has an M5 leukemia, characterized by a high incidence of tissue infiltration and organomegaly. ALL is typically seen in children and young adults. Acute megakaryocytic leukemia is rare and typically accompanied by myelofibrosis, and the blasts react with platelet-specific antibodies. The M3 variant of acute myelogenous leukemia (i.e., promyelocytic leukemia) has many promyelocytes filled with azurophilic granules, making them strongly peroxidase positive. Erythroleukemia is rare and is accompanied by dysplastic erythroid precursors.
BP6 376   PBD6 676–679

41. **(A)** Three markers strongly favor a very good prognosis: early pre-B cell type, hyperdiploidy, and an age between 7 and 10 years. Conversely, poor prognostic markers are T-cell phenotype; an age younger than 2 years; presence of t(9;22); and presentation in adolescence and adulthood.
BP6 374   PBD6 657–658

42. **(A)** The involvement of skin and the presence of lymphocytes with complex cerebriform nuclei in the skin and the blood are features of cutaneous T-cell lymphomas. These are malignancies of CD4+ T cells that may produce a tumor-like infiltration of the skin (i.e., mycosis fungoides) or a leukemic picture without tumefaction in the skin (i.e., Sézary syndrome). Cutaneous T-cell lymphomas are indolent tumors, and patients have a median survival of 8 to 9 years. The other phenotypes provided here are those of mature B cells with CD19+, sIg+; monocytes/granulocytes with CD33+, CD13+; and neoplastic B cells in chronic lymphocytic leukemia with CD19+, CD5+.
PBD6 670

43. **(B)** This patient has classic features of myelofibrosis with myeloid metaplasia. This myeloproliferative disorder is also a stem cell disorder in which neoplastic megakaryocytes secrete fibrogenic factors leading to marrow fibrosis. The neoplastic clone then shifts to the spleen, where it shows trilineage hematopoietic proliferation (i.e., extramedullary hematopoiesis), in which megakaryocytes are prominent. The marrow fibrosis and the extramedullary hematopoiesis in the spleen fail to regulate orderly release of leukocytes into the blood. Therefore, the peripheral blood has immature red cell and white cell precursors (i.e., leukoerythroblastic picture). Tear-drop red cells are misshapen RBCs that are seen when marrow undergoes fibrosis. Marrow injury can have other causes as well (e.g., metastatic tumors, irradiation). These can also give rise to a leukoerythroblastic picture, but splenic enlargement with trilineage proliferation is not usually seen. The other causes mentioned—Hodgkin disease and *H. capsulatum* infection—can cause splenic enlargement but not marrow fibrosis.
BP6 379–380   PBD6 683–685

44. **(B)** This patient has clinical and morphologic features of diffuse large cell lymphoma of B cells. These tumors often involve extranodal sites, show large anaplastic lymphoid cells that involve the tissues diffusely, and contain *bcl-6* gene rearrangements. Their clinical course is aggressive, and they are rapidly fatal if untreated. However, with intensive chemotherapy, 60% to 80% of patients achieve complete remission, and about 50% can be cured.
BP6 366–367   PBD6 661–662

45. **(D)** This patient came with a classic history of CML, confirmed by the presence of different stages of myeloid

differentiation in the blood and by the presence of the Philadelphia chromosome. He went into a remission and then entered a blast crisis involving B cells (CD19⁺). The fact that the B cells carry the original Ph¹ chromosome and some additional abnormalities indicates that the B cells and the myeloid cells belong to the same clone. The best explanation is that the initial transforming event affected a pluripotent stem cell that differentiated along the myeloid lineage to produce a picture of CML. Analysis, even at this stage, reveals that the molecular counterpart of the Ph¹ chromosome — the *bcr-abl* rearrangement — affects all lineages, including B cells, T cells, and myeloid cells. With the evolution of the disease, additional mutations accumulate in the stem cells, which then differentiate mainly along B lineages, giving rise to B-lymphoblastic leukemia.
BP6 377   PBD6 680-682

46.   **(A)** The age and mediastinal location are typical for a lymphoblastic lymphoma involving the thymus. This lesion is in the spectrum of acute lymphoblastic leukemia or lymphoma (ALL). Most ALL cases with lymphomatous presentation are of the pre-T cell type. This is supported by the expression of the T-cell markers CD2, CD5, and CD1. TdT is a marker of pre-T and pre-B cells. A Burkitt lymphoma is a B-cell lymphoma that may also be seen in adolescents but in the region of the jaw or abdomen. Nodular sclerosing Hodgkin disease does occur in the mediastinum, but it involves mediastinal nodes, not thymus. The histologic features of Hodgkin disease include the presence of Reed-Sternberg cells, and this variant has fibrous bands intersecting the lymphoid cells. Mantle cell lymphomas and follicular lymphomas are B-cell tumors usually seen in older patients, and they do not involve the thymus.
BP6 367   PBD6 654-646

47.   **(B)** This patient has polycythemia vera. The symptoms result from the increased hematocrit and blood volume. Undetectable erythropoietin in the face of polycythemia is characteristic of polycythemia vera. Polycythemia vera is a myeloproliferative disorder in which the neoplastic myeloid cells differentiate preferentially along the erythroid lineage. However, other lineages are also affected, and hence there is leukocytosis and thrombocytosis. These patients are Ph¹ chromosome negative. Untreated, these patients die of episodes of bleeding or thrombosis — both related to disordered platelet function and the hemodynamic effects on distended blood vessels. Treatment by phlebotomy reduces the hematocrit. With this treatment, 15% to 20% of the patients characteristically transform into myelofibrosis with myeloid metaplasia. Termination in acute leukemia, unlike in chronic myeloid leukemia, is rare. When it occurs, it is an acute myeloid leukemia, not lymphoblastic leukemia.
BP6 378-379   PBD6 682-683

48.   **(D)** In patients with infectious mononucleosis, multiple clones of B cells are infected by EBV. The EBV genes cause proliferation and activation of B cells, and hence there is polyclonal B-cell expansion. These B cells secrete antibodies with several specificities, including those that cross-react with sheep red blood cells. It is these heterophile antibodies that give a positive monospot test. The

atypical lymphocytes are CD8⁺ T cells that are activated by EBV-infected B cells. There is no increase in basophils, eosinophils, or monocytes in infectious mononucleosis. The t(9;22) gives rise to the Philadelphia chromosome characteristic of chronic myelogenous leukemia.
BP6 360-361   PBD6 371-373

49.   **(G)** The lacunar cells, along with the Reed-Sternberg cells, are indicative of Hodgkin disease, and the fibrous bands suggest the nodular sclerosis type. Lacunar cells have multilobed nuclei containing many small nucleoli. These cells have artifactual retraction of the cytoplasm around the nucleus, giving these cells their distinctive appearance. The nodular sclerosis type of Hodgkin disease is more common in women.
BP6 372   PBD6 670-674

50.   **(C)** The child has Letterer-Siwe disease, a form of Langerhans cell histiocytosis. The Birbeck granules are a distinctive feature identified by electron microscopy that are found in the cytoplasm of the Langerhans cells.
BP6 383   PBD6 685-686

51.   **(D)** Toxic granulations, which are coarse and dark primary granules, and Döhle bodies, which are patches of dilated endoplasmic reticulum, represent reactive changes of neutrophils. These changes are most indicative of overwhelming inflammatory conditions such as bacterial sepsis. Leukemia, granulomatous infections, or viral infections do not cause toxic changes in neutrophils. Infectious mononucleosis is accompanied by an increase in "atypical" lymphocytes.
PBD6 648-649

52.   **(B)** The peripheral eosinophilia seen here is a feature of allergic disorders, including type I hypersensitivity reactions. Extrinsic asthma is a common disorder in which eosinophilia may appear. Infestations with parasites that invade tissues are also known to produce significant eosinophilia. Sepsis most commonly results in a marked neutrophilia and left shift. With CML, the total WBC count is typically high. Although there may be increased eosinophils in CML, the peripheral blood also shows basophils, metamyelocytes, myelocytes, and a few blasts. A leukemoid reaction may appear similar to CML, but the leukocyte alkaline phosphatase level is high in the former, and there is usually no eosinophilia. Viral infections are typically not accompanied by marked increases in the WBC count.
BP6 359   PBD6 648

53.   **(B)** Sonja Henie died from complications of CLL, in which there are increased numbers of circulating small, round, mature lymphocytes with scant cytoplasm. These cells are seen in the blood smear. The cells express the CD5 marker and the pan B-cell markers CD19 and CD20. Most cases have a course of 4 to 6 years before death, and symptoms appear as the leukemic cells begin to fill the marrow. In some patients, the same small lymphocytes appear in tissues, in which case the condition is known as small lymphocytic lymphoma. The lymphocytes seen with infectious mononucleosis are "atypical lymphocytes" that

have abundant, pale blue cytoplasm that seems to be indented by surrounding RBCs. The RBCs in iron deficiency anemia are hypochromic and microcytic, but the WBCs are not affected. Leukemoid reactions are typically of the myeloid type, and the peripheral blood contains immature myeloid cells. The WBC count can be very high, but the platelet count is normal. ALL is a disease of children and young adults, characterized by proliferation of lymphoblasts. These cells are much larger than the cells in CLL and have nucleoli.
BP6 377–378 PBD6 658–659

54. **(C)** Monoclonal gammopathy of uncertain significance (MGUS) is characterized by the presence of an M protein "spike" in the absence of any associated disease of B cells. The diagnosis of MGUS is made when the monoclonal spike is small (>3 g) and the patient has no Bence Jones proteinuria. MGUS may progress to multiple myeloma in about 20% of patients over 10 to 15 years. A plasmacytoma should appear on a bone scan. Waldenström macroglobulinemia should be accompanied by an IgM spike, hepatosplenomegaly, and lymphadenopathy. Heavy chain disease is a rare condition that may be seen with chronic lymphocytic leukemia. In multiple myeloma, the spike is greater than 3 g, and usually the patient has bone lesions.
BP6 381 PBD6 663–666

55. **(D)** This is a Reed-Sternberg cell, which is characteristic for Hodgkin disease. Notice also the nonneoplastic eosinophils, lymphocytes, and macrophages in the background. Reed-Sternberg cells are the neoplastic component in Hodgkin disease, and unlike non-Hodgkin lymphomas, these transformed cells are scattered in a background of a proliferation of nonneoplastic inflammatory cells. As a historical note, the current Rye classification of Hodgkin disease grew out of an international conference held in Rye, Scotland. Nothing much happened at the conference, because everyone wanted to play golf. The meeting's organizer realized that little progress was being made, and he assembled a few of his friends at the bar in the hotel the night before the conference was to end. After a few whiskys, he got them to agree on a simple scheme with four categories, and it has not been revised in more than a quarter of a century since—unlike the many classification schemes for non-Hodgkin lymphomas.
BP6 369–370 PBD6 670–672

56. **(B)** The very high WBC count and the presence of peroxidase-positive blasts (i.e., myeloblasts) filling the marrow are characteristic for acute myeloblastic leukemia. This leukemia is most often seen in persons between the ages of 15 and 39 years. CLL is characterized by the presence of small, mature lymphocytes in peripheral blood and bone marrow of older adults. Megakaryocytic leukemias are rare. CML is also seen in adults, but this is a myeloproliferative process with a range of myeloid differentiation. Most of the myeloid cells are mature, and there are relatively few blasts. ALL occurs in children and young adults. Azurophilic, peroxidase-positive granules distinguish myeloblasts from lymphoblasts.
BP6 374–376 PBD6 657–677

The Lung

BP6 Chapter 13 - Lungs and the Upper
Respiratory Tract
BPD6 Chapter 16 - Diseases of the Lung

1. Over several decades, which of the following inhaled pollutants is most likely to produce extensive pulmonary fibrosis?

- (A) Silica
- (B) Tobacco smoke
- (C) Ozone
- (D) Wood dust
- (E) Carbon monoxide

2. A 50-year-old male has a history of chronic alcoholism. He is found in a stuporous condition after 3 days of binge drinking. His temperature is 39.2°C, and a chest radiograph reveals a 3-cm lesion with an air-fluid level in the right lower lobe. Which of the following organisms are most likely to be detected in bronchoalveolar lavage fluid?

- (A) *Staphylococcus aureus* and *Bacteroides fragilis*
- (B) *Mycobacterium tuberculosis* and *Aspergillus fumigatus*
- (C) *Nocardia asteroides* and *Actinomyces israeli*
- (D) Cytomegalovirus and *Pneumocystis carinii*
- (E) *Cryptococcus neoformans* and *Candida albicans*

3. A 45-year-old male who has smoked two packs of cigarettes for 6 years presents with a 4-year history of chronic cough with copious mucoid expectoration. He also complains that, during several episodes of respiratory tract infections that were diagnosed as "viral flu," he developed difficulty in breathing and tightness of chest, along with audible wheezing. The breathing difficulty was relieved by inhalation of a β-adrenergic agonist and disappeared after the chest infection had resolved. Which of the following pathologic conditions best describes his clinical findings?

- (A) Chronic bronchitis with cor pulmonale
- (B) Chronic bronchitis with asthmatic bronchitis
- (C) Chronic bronchitis with emphysema

- (D) Bronchiectasis
- (E) Hypersensitivity pneumonitis

4. A 75-year-old female has a large (4-cm) atrial septal defect that has never been repaired. The pulmonary condition that is most likely to accompany her congenital heart disease is

- (A) Pulmonary hypertension
- (B) Interstitial fibrosis
- (C) Vasculitis
- (D) Granulomatous inflammation
- (E) Pulmonary infarction

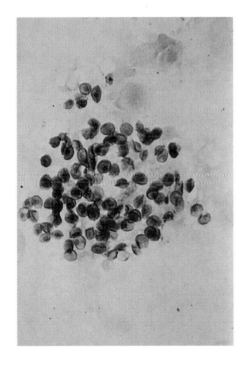

5. Bronchoalveolar lavage fluid from a 40-year-old female who has been ill for 5 years is stained with Gomori methenamine silver (GMS). The high-power microscopic appearance is shown here. The underlying illness in this patient is most probably

- (A) Diabetes mellitus
- (B) Systemic lupus erythematosus (SLE)

○ (C) Acquired immunodeficiency syndrome (AIDS)
○ (D) Sarcoidosis
○ (E) Severe combined immunodeficiency

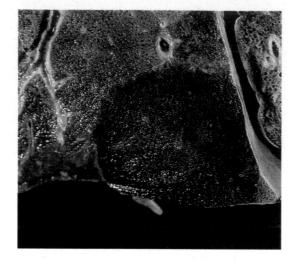

6. The section of right lower lobe shown here from the autopsy of a 60-year-old male. Which of the following clinical scenarios is most likely related to this lesion?

○ (A) A 50-year-old male chronic smoker who has translucent lung fields on radiographs and markedly reduced forced expiratory volume in 1 second (FEV_1)
○ (B) A 60-year-old male with myocardial infarction and congestive heart failure (CHF) who is admitted to the hospital
○ (C) A 55-year-old male chronic smoker who has an infiltrative hilar mass and enlarged, nodular liver
○ (D) An 18-year-old female with cystic fibrosis who has chronic cough with copious sputum production
○ (E) A 60-year-old male sandblaster who has progressive dyspnea

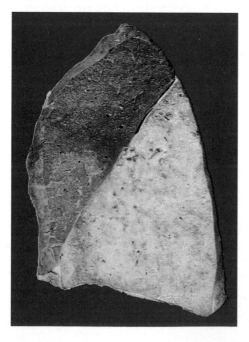

7. For several days, a 52-year-old female has had an increasingly severe cough productive of yellowish sputum. She has a fever of 38.9°C. A chest radiograph demonstrates right lower lung consolidation. The gross appearance of her lung is depicted in the figure. Which of the following pathogens is most likely to be cultured?

○ (A) *Mycoplasma pneumoniae*
○ (B) *Streptococcus pneumoniae*
○ (C) *Cryptococcus neoformans*
○ (D) *Mycobacterium kansasii*
○ (E) *Candida albicans*

8. Which of the following clinical or morphologic features is common to all forms of pneumoconiosis?

○ (A) Marked thickening of the pleura
○ (B) Increased risk of bronchogenic carcinoma
○ (C) Formation of noncaseating granulomas
○ (D) Interstitial pulmonary fibrosis
○ (E) Increased risk of tuberculosis

9. A sputum cytology specimen shows Curschmann spirals, Charcot-Leyden crystals, and acute inflammatory cells in a background of abundant mucus. Many of the inflammatory cells are eosinophils. Which of the following obstructive lung diseases is the patient with such a specimen most likely to have?

○ (A) Bronchiectasis
○ (B) Foreign body aspiration
○ (C) Atopic asthma
○ (D) Centrilobular emphysema
○ (E) Chronic bronchitis

10. A 50-year-old male presents with gradually increasing dyspnea and weight loss. On questioning, the patient admits to smoking two packs of cigarettes per day for 20 years but states that he has not smoked for the past year. Physical examination reveals an increase in the anteroposterior diameter (i.e., "barrel chest"). Auscultation of the chest reveals decreased lung sounds. A chest radiograph shows bilateral hyperlucent lungs; the lucency is especially marked in the upper lobes. The FEV_1 is markedly decreased on spirometry, but the forced vital capacity (FVC) is normal, and FEV_1/FVC is decreased. The pathogenesis of this condition involves all of the following *except*

○ (A) Recruitment of neutrophils and macrophages into the alveoli
○ (B) Release of elastase from neutrophils
○ (C) Inhibition of α_1-antitrypsin activity by neutrophil products
○ (D) Secretion of fibrogenic cytokines by macrophages
○ (E) Damage to the elastic tissue in alveolar septa

11. A 10-year-old female who participated in a screening program developed a 10-mm area of induration on her left forearm 3 days after intracutaneous injection of 0.1 mL of purified protein derivative (PPD). She appears healthy. A chest radiograph is most likely to demonstrate:

○ (A) Marked hilar adenopathy
○ (B) Upper lobe calcifications
○ (C) Extensive opacification

○ (D) Cavitary change
○ (E) No abnormal findings

12. A 63-year-old male worked for 20 years in the sand-blasting business, and he used no respiratory precautions during that time. He now has increasing dyspnea without fever, cough, or chest pain. Which of the following inflammatory cell types is most crucial to the development of his underlying disease?

○ (A) Plasma cell
○ (B) Mast cell
○ (C) Eosinophil
○ (D) Macrophage
○ (E) Natural killer (NK) cell

For each of the clinical histories in questions 13 and 14, match the most closely related pulmonary infectious agent:

○ (A) *Candida albicans*
○ (B) *Coccidioides immitis*
○ (C) Cytomegalovirus
○ (D) Influenza A
○ (E) *Legionella pneumophila*
○ (F) *Mycobacterium tuberculosis*
○ (G) *Mycoplasma pneumoniae*
○ (H) *Nocardia asteroides*
○ (I) *Pneumocystis carinii*
○ (J) *Rickettsia rickettsii*
○ (K) *Staphylococcus aureus*
○ (L) *Streptococcus pneumoniae*

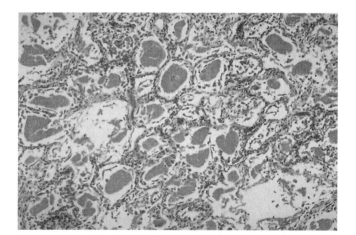

13. A 35-year-old female positive for human immunodeficiency virus (HIV) presents with increasing respiratory difficulty along with fever. A chest radiograph reveals some ill-defined interstitial infiltrates. She develops increasing hypoxemia and dies. At autopsy, the lungs are extensively consolidated and have a pale pink cut surface. The microscopic appearance with routine hematoxylin and eosin staining is shown here. (   )

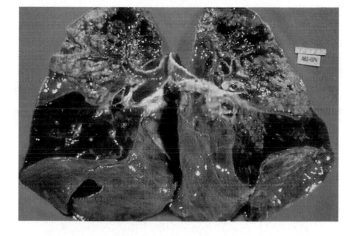

14. A 56-year-old male had a 4-month history of fever, night sweats, and weight loss. In the last month he experienced episodes of hemoptysis. The appearance of the lungs at autopsy is shown here. (   )

15. After a hemicolectomy to remove a colon carcinoma, a 53-year-old male is intubated and receives mechanical ventilation with 100% oxygen. Three days later he has worsening oxygenation, and a chest radiograph demonstrates increasing opacification in all lung fields. A transbronchial lung biopsy shows hyaline membranes that line distended alveolar ducts and sacs. The fundamental mechanism underlying these morphologic changes is

○ (A) Reduced production of surfactant by alveolar type II cells
○ (B) Disseminated intravascular coagulation (DIC)
○ (C) Aspiration of oropharyngeal contents with bacteria
○ (D) Leukocyte-mediated injury to alveolar capillary endothelium
○ (E) Release of fibrogenic cytokines by macrophages

16. A 29-year-old male who was previously healthy, with no major illnesses, experiences the acute onset of hemoptysis. Shortly thereafter, he develops acute renal failure. A chest radiograph shows bilateral fluffy infiltrates. A transbronchial lung biopsy reveals focal necrosis of alveolar walls associated with prominent intra-alveolar hemorrhage. Which of the following laboratory test findings is most likely to be present in serum in this patient?

○ (A) Antineutrophil cytoplasmic antibody
○ (B) Anti-DNA topoisomerase I antibody
○ (C) Antiglomerular basement membrane antibody
○ (D) Antimitochondrial antibody
○ (E) Antinuclear antibody

17. Spirometry performed on a 49-year-old male reveals an increased total lung capacity (TLC) with slightly increased FVC. However, the FEV_1 is decreased, with a decreased FEV_1/FVC ratio. The disease process that should most often be suspected as a cause for these findings is

○ (A) Primary adenocarcinoma
○ (B) Centrilobular emphysema
○ (C) Diffuse alveolar damage
○ (D) Chronic pulmonary embolism
○ (E) Sarcoidosis

18. A 70-year-old female is referred to an ophthalmologist for right eye problems. The findings include enophthalmos, meiosis, anhidrosis, and ptosis. She also has pain in the right upper chest region. A chest radiograph reveals right upper lobe opacification along with bony destruction of the right first rib. Which of the following conditions is she most likely to have?

○ (A) Bronchopneumonia
○ (B) Bronchiectasis
○ (C) Bronchogenic carcinoma
○ (D) Sarcoidosis
○ (E) Tuberculosis

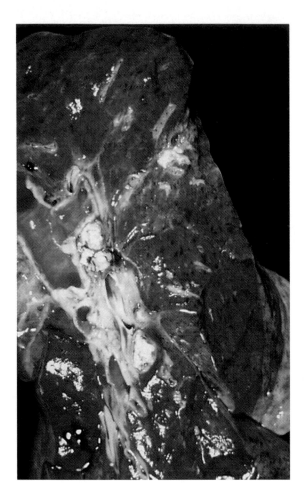

19. The gross appearance of the lung shown in the figure is most likely to be found in which of the following individuals?

○ (A) An HIV-positive patient who has cough, fever, and hepatosplenomegaly
○ (B) An apparently healthy and asymptomatic 15-year-old male who died in an automobile accident
○ (C) An alcoholic who presents with chills, rigors, chest pain, and hemoptysis
○ (D) A patient with cystic fibrosis who presents with history of recurrent lung infections and copious purulent expectoration
○ (E) A 50-year-old male with a 20-year history of heavy smoking who presents with significant weight loss and clubbing of fingers

20. A 60-year-old farmer presents with a 15-year history of increasing dyspnea. The radiograph of the chest shows a bilateral increase in linear markings, and pulmonary function tests reveal reduced FVC with a relatively normal FEV_1 value. A lung biopsy shows interstitial infiltrates of lymphocytes and plasma cells, minimal interstitial fibrosis, and small granulomas. The most likely cause of this clinical and pathologic picture is

○ (A) Chronic inhalation of silica particles
○ (B) Prolonged exposure to asbestos
○ (C) Hypersensitivity to spores of actinomycetes
○ (D) Previous episode of adult respiratory distress syndrome (ARDS)
○ (E) Autoantibodies that react with alveolar basement membranes

21. A local epidemic occurs among children at a summer camp. They all develop upper respiratory tract infections manifested by coryza, pharyngitis, and tracheobronchitis. The children have fever and malaise but minimal sputum production. The total leukocyte count is not markedly elevated. *Mycoplasma pneumoniae* is cultured from the nasopharynx of many of these children. Which of the following histologic patterns is most likely to be found in lung to explain these findings?

○ (A) Alveolar neutrophilic exudates
○ (B) Perivascular granulomatous inflammation
○ (C) Hemorrhagic infarction
○ (D) Hyaline membrane formation
○ (E) Interstitial mononuclear cell infiltrates

22. A 6-year-old child puts the contents of a bag of peanuts in his mouth and then takes a deep breath with the idea of blowing the peanuts out all over his sister. However, he aspirates a peanut during this maneuver. Which of the following complications is this child *least* likely to suffer from this event?

○ (A) Bronchiectasis
○ (B) Resorption atelectasis
○ (C) Bronchopneumonia
○ (D) Pneumothorax
○ (E) Lung abscess

23. A 49-year-old male passes a ureteral calculus that on analysis is found to be composed of calcium oxalate. He is found to have a serum calcium concentration of 6.2 mg/dL, with a serum phosphorus level of 3.9 mg/dL and a serum albumin level of 4.6 g/dL. A chest radiograph reveals a 7-cm right hilar lung mass. A chest computed tomography (CT) scan demonstrates prominent central necrosis in this mass. Which of the following neoplasms is most likely to be associated with these findings?

○ (A) Metastatic colonic adenocarcinoma
○ (B) Small cell anaplastic carcinoma
○ (C) Bronchioloalveolar carcinoma
○ (D) Squamous cell carcinoma
○ (E) Large cell carcinoma

For each of the clinical histories in questions 24 and 25, match the most closely associated pulmonary radiologic finding:

○ (A) Bilateral fluffy infiltrates
○ (B) Bilateral lower lobe cavitation
○ (C) Bilateral pleural effusions
○ (D) Bilateral upper lobe cavitation
○ (E) Diaphragmatic pleural calcified plaques
○ (F) Hyperinflation
○ (G) Left lower lobe, 4-cm solid mass
○ (H) Left main bronchus, 1.5-cm endobronchial mass
○ (I) Marked right pleural thickening
○ (J) Right middle lobe bronchial dilation
○ (K) Right middle lobe, subpleural, 2-cm nodule with hilar adenopathy
○ (L) Right perihilar, 8-cm mass
○ (M) Right pneumothorax
○ (N) Right upper lung, 3-cm nodule with air-fluid level

24.   A 62-year-old male, a smoker for the past 45 years of one pack of cigarettes per day, has developed a cough with hemoptysis during the past month. He has had a 10-kg weight loss over the past year. He is found to have a serum calcium concentration of 12.8 mg/dL, with a phosphorus level of 3.9 mg/dL and an albumin level of 4.2 g/dL. (   )

25.   A 65-year-old male worked in a shipyard for 10 years; he then worked for 5 years in a company that installed home insulation. He experienced increasing dyspnea for several years and eventually died of respiratory failure. At autopsy, there was a firm, tan mass that encased the left lung. Within the lung parenchyma microscopically, many ferruginous bodies were identified. (   )

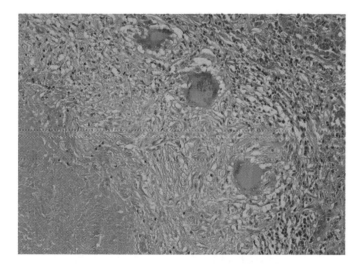

26.   A 46-year-old female has a 3-cm, solitary, left upper lobe mass discovered by chest radiograph. The mass is removed at thoracotomy by wedge resection. The microscopic appearance of this lesion is depicted here. Which of the following conditions does this patient have?

○ (A) Pulmonary hamartoma
○ (B) Pulmonary infarction
○ (C) *Mycobacterium tuberculosis* infection
○ (D) Lung abscess
○ (E) Primary adenocarcinoma

27.   A 3-year-old male has had a cough with headache and a slight fever for 5 days. He is admitted to the hospital after his mother notes that he is having increasing respiratory difficulty. Respiratory syncytial virus is isolated from the child's sputum. Which of the following chest radiographic patterns is most likely to characterize this process?

○ (A) Lobar consolidation
○ (B) Interstitial infiltrates
○ (C) Large pleural effusions
○ (D) Upper lobe cavitation
○ (E) Hyperinflation

28.   A 35-year-old male presents with a 5-year history of episodes of wheezing and coughing. These episodes are more common during the winter months, and he has noticed that they often follow minor respiratory tract infections. In the period between such episodes, he can breathe normally. There is no family history of asthma or other allergies. Results of the complete blood cell count are normal, as is his serum IgE level. The mechanism responsible for the asthmatic attacks in this case is most likely to be

○ (A) Accumulation of mast cells in the airspaces following viral infections
○ (B) Emigration of eosinophils into the bronchi
○ (C) Bronchial hyperreactivity to virus-induced inflammation
○ (D) Secretion of interleukin (IL)-4 and IL-5 by antiviral T cells
○ (E) Hyperresponsiveness to inhaled spores of *Aspergillus*

29.   A 78-year-old male has had increasing dyspnea over the past 4 months. A CT scan shows a dense, bright, right pleural mass encasing most of the left lung, and a pleural biopsy shows spindle and cuboidal cells that invade adipose tissue. Inhalation of which of the following materials is probably an important factor in development of this mass?

○ (A) Asbestos
○ (B) Bird dust
○ (C) Silica
○ (D) Cotton fibers
○ (E) Coal dust

30.   Which of the following morphologic changes can be seen in advanced cases of both obstructive and restrictive lung disease?

○ (A) Marked medial thickening of pulmonary arterioles
○ (B) Destruction of elastic tissue in the alveolar walls
○ (C) Fibrosis of the alveolar walls
○ (D) Hemorrhage in the alveolar lumen
○ (E) Hyaline membranes lining the airspaces

31.   As a child and young adult, a 35-year-old female experienced multiple bouts of severe necrotizing pneumonia. She now suffers for weeks at a time with a cough productive of large amounts of purulent sputum. A chest radiograph reveals areas of right lower lobe consolidation. A bronchogram shows marked dilation of right lower lobe

bronchi. Which of the following mechanisms is the most likely cause of airspace dilation in this patient?

○ (A) Unopposed action of neutrophil-derived elastase
○ (B) Congenital weakness of the supporting structures of the bronchial wall
○ (C) Diffuse alveolar damage (DAD)
○ (D) Destruction of bronchial walls by recurrent inflammation
○ (E) Damage to the bronchial mucosa by major basic protein of eosinophils

32. Two days after surgery with general anesthesia for a coronary artery bypass, a 56-year-old male experiences increasing respiratory difficulty with decreasing arterial oxygen saturations. His heart rate is regular at 78 beats per minute, and his hemoglobin concentration has remained unchanged since surgery at 13.7 g/dL. He is afebrile. After coughing up a large amount of mucoid sputum, his condition improves. The most likely explanation for these findings is

○ (A) Resorption atelectasis
○ (B) Compression atelectasis
○ (C) Microatelectasis
○ (D) Contraction atelectasis
○ (E) Relaxation atelectasis

33. A section of lung from autopsy of a 41-year-old male demonstrates atheroma formation in larger pulmonary arteries, medial thickening of medium-sized arteries, and reduplication of elastic membranes in small tortuous peripheral arteries. The alveoli appear normal. These histologic findings are most likely to be seen in

○ (A) A 30-year-old female with a ventricular septal defect (VSD) who develops cyanosis
○ (B) A 25-year-old male who presents with hemoptysis and renal failure
○ (C) A 30-year-old female with episodes of wheezing for the past 10 years, along with eosinophilia and elevated serum IgE level
○ (D) A 50-year-old male diabetic who develops gangrene of the toes
○ (E) A 30-year-old intravenous drug abuser who develops gram-negative septicemia and shock

34. A 42-year-old male has suffered from chronic sinusitis for several months. He now presents with a mild fever that has persisted for several weeks and with malaise. His serum urea nitrogen concentration is 35 mg/dL, and the serum creatinine level is 4.3 mg/dL. He has a serum alanine aminotransferase (ALT) concentration of 167 U/L and aspartate aminotransferase (AST) of 154 U/L, with a total bilirubin value of 1.1 mg/dL. The cytoplasmic-antineutrophil cytoplasmic antibody (c-ANCA) titer is elevated at 1:256. A transbronchial lung biopsy shows a necrotizing capillaritis with some mild intra-alveolar hemorrhage. A granuloma is seen within the wall of a necrotic small artery. The most likely diagnosis is

○ (A) Goodpasture syndrome
○ (B) Hypersensitivity pneumonitis
○ (C) Systemic lupus erythematosus
○ (D) Wegener granulomatosis
○ (E) Diffuse systemic sclerosis

35. A 45-year-old female who is not a smoker is found to have the PiZZ phenotype of α_1-antitrypsin deficiency. She suffers from increasing respiratory difficulty that limits her activities. What condition is probably present in her lungs?

○ (A) Sarcoidosis
○ (B) Bronchiectasis
○ (C) Interstitial fibrosis
○ (D) Microatelectasis
○ (E) Panacinar emphysema

36. General anesthesia with intubation and mechanical ventilation during surgical procedures increases the risk for postoperative pulmonary infection. By which of the following mechanisms is anesthesia most likely to have this effect?

○ (A) Decreased ciliary function
○ (B) Neutropenia
○ (C) Tracheal erosions
○ (D) Diminished macrophage activity
○ (E) Hypogammaglobulinemia

37. A 45-year-old male has experienced a 5-kg weight loss over the past 3 months after the loss of his job. He recently developed a low-grade fever and cough with mucoid sputum production, and after a week, he noticed blood-streaked sputum. A chest radiograph shows bilateral upper lobe consolidations and focal cavitations. Which of the following diagnostic tests on sputum is most warranted in this situation?

○ (A) Acid-fast stain
○ (B) GMS stain
○ (C) Gram stain
○ (D) Cytologic smear
○ (E) Viral culture

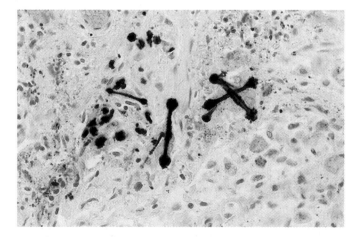

38. A 75-year-old male experienced increasing dyspnea. The microscopic appearance with Prussian blue stain of the lung is shown here. This is most characteristic for

○ (A) Anthracosis
○ (B) Berylliosis
○ (C) Silicosis
○ (D) Calcinosis
○ (E) Asbestosis

39. Which of the following structures in the lung is likely to be affected the most in a patient who smoked a pack and a half of cigarettes per day for 30 years and developed centrilobular emphysema?

○ (A) Alveolar sac
○ (B) Terminal bronchiole
○ (C) Alveolar duct
○ (D) Respiratory bronchiole
○ (E) Capillary

40. A 40-year-old male has had increasing cough with hemoptysis for 2 weeks. He is febrile, and a chest radiograph shows a right upper lobe area of consolidation that improves with antibiotic therapy. However, his cough and the hemoptysis persist. Bronchoscopy reveals an obstructing mass filling the bronchus to the right upper lobe. Which of the following neoplasms is most likely to produce these findings?

○ (A) Hamartoma
○ (B) Adenocarcinoma
○ (C) Large cell carcinoma
○ (D) Kaposi sarcoma
○ (E) Carcinoid tumor

41. A 12-year-old female presents with a history of coughing and wheezing and repeated attacks of difficulty in breathing. Such attacks are particularly common in the spring. Laboratory testing reveals an elevated serum IgE level and peripheral blood eosinophilia. During an episode of acute respiratory difficulty, a sputum sample examined microscopically also has increased numbers of eosinophils. The histologic features that characterize the lung in this condition are

○ (A) Dilation of the respiratory bronchiole and distention of alveoli
○ (B) Dilation of the bronchi with inflammatory destruction of their walls
○ (C) Interstitial and alveolar edema with presence of hyaline membranes that line the alveoli
○ (D) Thickening of the basement membrane of bronchial epithelium, inflammation of the bronchial wall, and hypertrophy of the bronchial wall muscle
○ (E) Patchy areas of consolidation surrounding bronchioles and a neutrophilic exudate in the affected alveoli

42. A 40-year-old male presents with a 6-year history of shortness of breath and weakness. A radiograph of the chest reveals diffuse interstitial markings. Pulmonary function tests reveal diminished FVC, decreased diffusing capacity, and a normal FEV_1/FVC ratio. Which of the following sets of pathologic changes is most likely to be found in his lungs?

○ (A) Voluminous lungs with uniform dilation of air spaces distal to the respiratory bronchioles

○ (B) Chronic inflammatory cells in the bronchi with a marked increase in size of mucous glands
○ (C) Honeycomb lung with widespread alveolar septal fibrosis and hyperplasia of type II pneumocytes
○ (D) Chronic inflammation of the bronchial walls with prominence of eosinophils
○ (E) Edematous, congested lungs with widespread necrosis of alveolar epithelial cells and prominent hyaline membranes

43. The most common outcome of pulmonary thromboembolism is

○ (A) Sudden death
○ (B) Cor pulmonale
○ (C) Hemoptysis
○ (D) Dyspnea
○ (E) No symptoms

44. A 45-year-old male has experienced increasing respiratory difficulty for more than a decade. He can no longer pass the yearly physical examination required to maintain active status as an airline pilot, the only occupation that he has ever had. FEV_1 is normal but FVC is diminished. A chest radiograph shows diffuse interstitial disease but no masses and no hilar adenopathy. An antinuclear antibody test result is negative. The most likely diagnosis is

○ (A) Scleroderma
○ (B) Goodpasture syndrome
○ (C) Silicosis
○ (D) Diffuse alveolar damage
○ (E) Idiopathic pulmonary fibrosis

45. Which of the following features is common to *all* forms of bronchial asthma?

○ (A) Accumulation of eosinophils in the bronchial wall
○ (B) A family history of the disease
○ (C) Preceding viral infection
○ (D) Hyperresponsiveness of the airways
○ (E) Chemical exposure

For each of the clinical histories in questions 46 through 49, match the most closely related pulmonary neoplastic process:

○ (A) Adenocarcinoma
○ (B) Bronchial carcinoid
○ (C) Bronchioloalveolar carcinoma
○ (D) Hamartoma
○ (E) Kaposi sarcoma
○ (F) Large cell carcinoma
○ (G) Mesothelioma
○ (H) Metastatic renal cell carcinoma
○ (I) Non-Hodgkin lymphoma
○ (J) Small cell carcinoma
○ (K) Squamous cell carcinoma

46. A 50-year-old male has developed truncal obesity, hypertension, back pain, and easily bruisable skin during the past 5 months. A chest radiograph reveals a 4-cm mass involving the left hilum of the lung. Cytologic examination

of bronchial washings from bronchoscopy shows round cells that look like lymphocytes but are somewhat larger. The patient is told that, despite the fact that his disease is apparently localized to one side of the chest cavity, surgical treatment is not likely to be curative. (   )

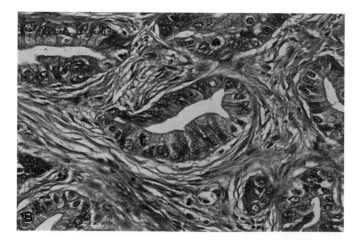

47. A 57-year-old female presents with a 3-week history of cough and pleuritic chest pain. A chest radiograph reveals an ill-defined area of left lower lobe opacification. After a month of antibiotic therapy, she is no better, and the radiographic lesion remains. A left lower lobe lung needle biopsy is performed and shows the histologic appearance seen here. (   )

48. A 64-year-old chain-smoker presents with a 3-month history of cough and loss of weight. Physical examination reveals clubbing of the fingers. Bronchoscopy shows a lesion nearly occluding the right main stem bronchus. A radiograph of the chest shows no hilar adenopathy, but there is cavitation within the 3-cm lesion. The serum chemistry panel results are unremarkable except for a calcium level of 12.3 mg/dL, phosphorus concentration of 2.4 mg/dL, and albumin level of 3.9 g/dL. A bronchoscopic biopsy is performed, and based on the pathologist's report and further testing, the patient is told that a surgical procedure with a curative intent will be attempted. (   )

49. A 37-year-old female nonsmoker presented with cough and loss of weight and appetite. The chest radiograph revealed a subpleural mass. After an open lung biopsy, the patient underwent lobectomy. The microscopic appearance of the lesion is shown in the figure. She remained free of symptoms for the next 10 years. (   )

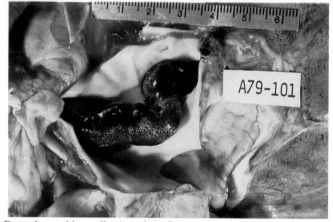

From the teaching collection of the Department of Pathology, University of Texas Southwestern Medical School, Dallas, TX.

50. A 68-year-old female hospitalized for 3 weeks after a cerebral infarction was improving, and she was able to get up and move with assistance. A few minutes after ambulating to the bathroom, she experienced the sudden onset of severe dyspnea. Despite resuscitative measures, she died 30 minutes later. Autopsy findings, shown here, indicate that the most likely mechanism for sudden death in this patient was

○ (A) Atelectasis
○ (B) Hemorrhage
○ (C) Acute right heart failure
○ (D) Bronchoconstriction
○ (E) Edema

51. A 61-year-old female smoked cigarettes for 10 years but stopped smoking 5 years ago. She has experienced increasing dyspnea for months along with a nonproductive cough. A chest radiograph shows prominent hilar lymphadenopathy. A transbronchial biopsy is performed, and the microscopic findings include interstitial fibrosis and small, noncaseating granulomas. One of the granulomas contains an asteroid body in a giant cell. This disease is believed to be caused by

○ (A) Delayed hypersensitivity response to an unknown antigen
○ (B) Immune complexes formed in response to inhaled antigens
○ (C) Diffuse alveolar damage (DAD)
○ (D) Smoke inhalation for many years
○ (E) Infection with atypical mycobacteria

52. A chronic smoker has a 10-year history of cough with mucopurulent sputum. He developed progressive dyspnea over several months, for which he was hospitalized. Physical examination revealed bilateral pedal edema and a soft, enlarged liver. Arterial blood gas determinations

revealed a PO_2 of 58 mm Hg, PCO_2 of 60 mm Hg, pH of 7.19, and HCO_3 level of 31 mmol/L. He was placed on a ventilator and required increasing amounts of oxygen. He died 6 days later, when even 100% oxygen was insufficient to prevent hypoxemia. At autopsy, all of the following are likely to be seen *except*

- (A) Hyaline membranes in alveolar spaces
- (B) Extensive interstitial fibrosis
- (C) Right ventricular hypertrophy and dilation
- (D) Thickening of pulmonary arteriolar walls
- (E) Hypertrophy of bronchial submucosal glands

53. During a cardiac arrest, a 58-year-old male receives cardiopulmonary resuscitative measures and is brought to the hospital, where he is intubated. During the intubation procedure he suffers aspiration of gastric contents (i.e., pasta with mushrooms and peas). Which of the following pulmonary complications is most likely to appear in the week after these events?

- (A) Right lower lobe abscess
- (B) Chronic bronchitis
- (C) Widespread bronchiectasis
- (D) Bronchial asthma
- (E) Left upper lobe infarction

54. After a motor vehicle accident with blunt trauma to the chest, a 30-year-old male is hospitalized. He suffered contusions to the right chest but no lacerations, as determined by physical examination of the chest wall. Within hours of the accident, he develops difficulty breathing and pain on the right. Which of the following radiographic findings is most likely to be present?

- (A) Large bilateral pleural effusions on the chest radiograph
- (B) High probability for pulmonary embolus on the ventilation/perfusion (V/Q) scan
- (C) Extensive centrilobular emphysema on the chest CT scan
- (D) Right rib fractures with pneumothorax
- (E) Bilateral patchy infiltrates on the chest radiograph

55. A pharmaceutical company is designing drugs to treat the recurrent bronchospasms characteristic of bronchial asthma. An antagonist to which of the following mediators do you think will be most effective?

- (A) Complement C3a
- (B) Platelet-activating factor (PAF)
- (C) Interleukin-5 (IL-5)
- (D) Leukotrienes C_4, D_4, and E_4
- (E) Histamine

56. A 59-year-old female presents with shortness of breath. A chest radiograph reveals bilateral pleural effusions, with the right greater than the left. Thoracentesis is performed, and 700 mL of fluid are removed from the right pleural cavity. A cell count shows 5 white blood cells and 10 red blood cells; the fluid is clear and slightly yellow tinged. The most probable cause for this effusion is

- (A) Metastatic adenocarcinoma
- (B) Congestive heart failure (CHF)

- (C) Systemic lupus erythematosus (SLE)
- (D) Chronic renal failure
- (E) Mediastinal malignant lymphoma

57. A 40-year-old female who has been a nonsmoker all her life works as a file clerk at a university that designates all work areas as "nonsmoking." A routine chest radiograph reveals a 3-cm, left upper lobe lung mass. She has no symptoms. The most likely answer to this puzzle is

- (A) Non-Hodgkin lymphoma
- (B) Adenocarcinoma
- (C) Large cell carcinoma
- (D) Mesothelioma
- (E) Squamous cell carcinoma

58. The morning after visiting a friend's farm one summer day, a 25-year-old male experiences the acute onset of fever, cough, and dyspnea. These symptoms are accompanied by headache and malaise. His symptoms subside over several days, at which time a chest radiograph is unremarkable. The most likely cause for these findings is

- (A) *P. carinii* pneumonia
- (B) Hypersensitivity pneumonitis
- (C) Primary atypical pneumonia
- (D) Goodpasture syndrome
- (E) Actinomycosis

ANSWERS

1. (A) Silica crystals incite a fibrogenic response after ingestion by macrophages. The greater the exposure and the longer the time of exposure, the greater is the lung injury. Tobacco smoke leads to loss of lung tissue and emphysema, not fibrosis. Ozone, a component of smog, has no obvious pathologic effects. Particulate matter such as wood dust is mainly screened out by the mucociliary apparatus of upper airways. Carbon monoxide readily crosses the alveolar walls and binds avidly to hemoglobin but does not directly injure lung.
BP6 224   PBD6 731–732

2. (A) He has a lung abscess that most likely resulted from aspiration, something that can occur in persons with a depressed cough reflex or in neurologically impaired persons (e.g., acute alcoholism, anesthesia, Alzheimer disease). The more acutely angled mainstem bronchus to the left lung makes aspiration into the right lung and to the lower lobe more common. Bacterial organisms are most likely to produce abscesses. The most common pathogen is *S. aureus*, along with anaerobes such as *Bacteroides*, *Peptococcus*, and *Fusobacterium* spp. These anaerobes are found normally in the oral cavity and hence are readily aspirated. The purulent, liquefied center of the abscess can produce the radiographic appearance of an air-fluid level. Tuberculosis can produce granulomatous lesions with central cavitation that may be colonized by *Aspergillus*, although not over a few days' time. Nocardial and actinomy-

cotic infections often lead to chronic abscesses without significant liquefaction, and appear in immunocompromised persons. Cytomegalovirus, *Pneumocystis*, and cryptococcal infections are seen in immunocompromised persons and do not typically form abscesses. *Candida* pneumonia is rare.
BP6 428–429   PBD6 722

3. **(B)** This patient meets the clinical definition of chronic bronchitis. He has had persistent cough with sputum production for at least 3 months in 2 consecutive years. This is a disease of smokers and persons living in areas of poor air quality, which explains the chronic cough with mucoid sputum production. However, this patient's episodes of bronchoconstriction set off by viral infections suggest a superimposed element of nonatopic asthma. Cor pulmonale leads to pleural effusions, not bronchoconstriction. Emphysema and chronic bronchitis can overlap in clinical and pathologic findings, but significant bronchoconstriction is not a feature of emphysema. Bronchiectasis results in airway dilation from bronchial wall inflammation with destruction. A hypersensitivity pneumonitis is marked by features of a restrictive lung disease, sometimes with dyspnea, but without mucus production.
BP6 397   PBD6 711–712, 715

4. **(A)** The left-to-right shunt produced by the atrial septal defect leads to increased pulmonary arterial pressure, thickening of the pulmonary arteries, and increasing the pulmonary vascular resistance. Eventually, the shunt may reverse, and this is known as an Eisenmenger complex. Pulmonary fibrosis can be caused by pneumoconioses, collagen vascular diseases, and granulomatous diseases, among others. Pulmonary vasculitis may be seen with immunologically mediated diseases such as Wegener granulomatosis. Granulomatous inflammation does not occur from increased pulmonary arterial pressures. An infarction of the lung can occur with pulmonary embolism.
BP6 413–414   PBD6 705

5. **(C)** Although *P. carinii* pneumonia can be seen with a variety of acquired and congenital immunodeficient states (mainly those affecting cell-mediated immunity), it is most often associated with acquired immunodeficiency syndrome (AIDS) and is diagnostic of AIDS in HIV-infected persons. Diabetics are most prone to get bacterial infections. Persons with autoimmune disease may have cytopenias that predispose to infection, and if they are treated with immunosuppressive drugs, a variety of infections are possible. Likewise, persons with sarcoidosis treated with corticosteroid therapy may have opportunistic infections. A patient with severe combined immunodeficiency is susceptible to *P. carinii* pneumonia, but it is very unlikely that without treatment she would have survived until the age of 40 years.
BP 430–431   PBD6 381–382, 722

6. **(B)** This is a pleural-based "red infarct" typical for pulmonary thromboembolism that affects persons who are immobilized in the hospital such as those with congestive heart failure. The bronchial arterial supply of blood is sufficient to produce hemorrhage but not sufficient to prevent infarction. Persons with underlying cardiac or respiratory diseases that compromise pulmonary circulation are at greater risk for infarction if thromboembolism does occur. Infarction is not a complication of smoking with emphysema. Mass lesions do not obstruct the pulmonary vasculature to cause infarction. Bronchiectasis or bronchopneumonia with cystic fibrosis does not produce infarction; the pneumonia may be hemorrhagic but is not so localized. Pneumoconioses with restrictive lung disease have pulmonary fibrosis but not a compromised vasculature or infarction.
BP6 411–413   PBD6 703–704

7. **(B)** The productive cough suggests an alveolar exudate with neutrophils, and her course is compatible with an acute infection. Bacterial organisms should be suspected. Pneumococcus is the most likely agent to be cultured in persons acquiring a pneumonia outside of the hospital, and particularly when a lobar pneumonic pattern is present, as in this case. The atypical pneumonia of *Mycoplasma* does not result in a purulent sputum, unless there is a secondary bacterial infection, which is a common complication with viral and *Mycoplasma* pneumonias. Cryptococcal and mycobacterial infections typically produce granulomatous disease. *Candida* pneumonia is rare but may occur in immunocompromised patients.
BP6 415–416   PBD6 718–721

8. **(D)** The inhaled inorganic particulate matter is ingested by macrophages and leads to cytokine release that drives fibrogenesis over many years. Diffuse fibrosis with a restrictive pattern of lung disease is the hallmark of pneumoconioses. Pleural thickening in the form of pleural plaques can occur with asbestosis, but pleural thickening may follow any kind of pleuritis, infectious or immunologic. The increased risk for bronchogenic carcinoma is seen mainly in persons with asbestos exposure who smoke. Tuberculosis is not a constant finding with pneumoconioses.
BP6 224–225   BPD6 727–729

9. **(C)** Asthma, particularly extrinsic (atopic) asthma, is driven by a type I hypersensitivity response. The Charcot-Leyden crystals represent the breakdown products of eosinophil granules. The Curschmann spirals represent the whorls of sloughed surface epithelium in the mucin. There can be inflammatory cells in the sputum with bronchiectasis and chronic bronchitis, although without eosinophils as a major component. Foreign body aspiration may result in inflammation but without eosinophils. Inflammation is not a component of emphysema.
BP6 397   PBD6 715

10. **(D)** His findings are predominantly those of an obstructive lung disease—emphysema. Smoking is a major cause for this disease. The inflammation that can accompany smoking leads to increased neutrophil elaboration of elastase, along with elaboration of macrophage elastase not inhibited by the antiprotease action of α_1-antitrypsin. This results in a loss of lung tissue, not fibrogenesis. Fibrogenesis is typical for restrictive lung diseases, such as pneumoconioses that follow inhalation of dusts.
BP6 400   PBD6 710

11. **(E)** Most *M. tuberculosis* infections are asymptomatic and subclinical. Active disease is uncommon, although a preceding illness or poor living conditions increase the risk. Calcifications and cavitation are complications most often seen following reinfection or reactivation of tuberculosis infections in adults. Lymphadenopathy is more frequent with primary tuberculosis infections.
BP6 420-421   PBD6 722-725

12. **(D)** Silica is a major component of sand, which contains the mineral quartz. The small silica crystals are inhaled, and their buoyancy allows them to be carried to alveoli. There they are ingested by macrophages, which then secrete cytokines that recruit other inflammatory cells and promote fibrogenesis. Plasma cells secrete immunoglobulins, which are not a major component of this process. Mast cells and eosinophils are prominent in type I hypersensitivity response. NK lymphocytes are more likely to be a prominent component of inflammatory processes directed against infectious agents.
BP6 226-227   PBD6 731-732

13. **(I)** *P. carinii* pneumonia is one of the most common opportunistic infections in patients with HIV infection who develop AIDS. The pneumonia is typically a diffuse process, accounting for the extensive pink alveolar exudate, but there is minimal inflammation. GMS stain can demonstrate that the exudate consists of numerous *P. carinii* cysts.
BP6 430-431   PBD6 376

14. **(F)** There is prominent upper lobe cavitation in the tan-to-white caseating granulomas, typical for reactivation-reinfection tuberculosis in adults.
BP6 424   PBD6 725

15. **(D)** The clinical and morphologic picture is of (ARDS) adult respiratory distress syndrome. This is characterized by diffuse alveolar damage, which is initiated in most cases by the injury to capillary endothelium by neutrophils and macrophages. Leukocytes aggregate in alveolar capillaries and release toxic oxygen metabolites, cytokines, and eicosanoids. The damage to the capillary endothelium allows leakage of protein-rich fluids. Eventually, the overlying alveolar epithelium is also damaged. Reduced surfactant production causes respiratory distress syndrome with hyaline membrane disease in newborns. ARDS and DIC can complicate septic shock, but DIC is not the cause of ARDS. Aspiration of bacteria causes bronchopneumonia. Release of fibrogenic cytokines is important in the causation of chronic diffuse pulmonary fibrosis.
BP 405-406   PBD6 700-703

16. **(C)** He has Goodpasture syndrome. Renal and pulmonary lesions are produced by an antibody directed against an antigen common to basement membrane in glomerulus and alveolus. This leads to a form of type II hypersensitivity reaction. Antineutrophil cytoplasmic autoantibodies (c-ANCA or p-ANCA) are best known as markers for various forms of systemic vasculitis. The anti-DNA topoisomerase I antibody is a marker for scleroderma. The antinuclear antibody is a general screening test for a variety of autoimmune conditions, typically collagen vascular diseases such as SLE.
BP6 411   PBD6 739

17. **(B)** These findings point to an obstructive lung disease, such as emphysema, that occurs from airway narrowing or from loss of elastic recoil. Adenocarcinomas, similar to other primary lung tumors, typically involve one lung and do not produce small airway disease. Diffuse alveolar damage is an acute restrictive lung disease. Chronic pulmonary embolism does not affect FVC, because the airways are not affected, but there is a ventilation/perfusion mismatch. Sarcoidosis is a form of chronic restrictive lung disease.
BP6 395   PBD6 706-708

18. **(C)** She has Horner syndrome as a result of cervical sympathetic ganglion involvement by invasive carcinoma. Such a tumor in this location with these associated findings is called a Pancoast tumor. Infectious processes such as a pneumonia are not likely to impinge on structures outside of the lung. Bronchiectasis is a process destructive of bronchi within the lung. Sarcoidosis can result in marked hilar adenopathy with a mass effect, but involvement of the superior cervical ganglion is unlikely. Likewise, tuberculosis is a granulomatous disease that can lead to hilar adenopathy, although usually without destruction of extrapulmonary tissues.
BP6 434   PBD6 745-746

19. **(B)** This is the so-called Ghon complex, consisting of a small subpleural granuloma with extensive hilar nodal caseating granulomas. The Ghon complex is a feature of primary tuberculosis, which is most often a subclinical disease of younger persons. Persons who are immunocompromised, such as persons with HIV infection, do not mount a good granulomatous response and have more extensive poorly formed granulomas, dissemination of tuberculosis, or both. Persons with chronic alcoholism are at greater risk for reactivation or reinfection, secondary tuberculosis. Hemoptysis also suggests secondary tuberculosis, which is a more extensive upper lobe granulomatous disease. Persons with cystic fibrosis develop widespread bronchiectasis, with infection by bacterial agents, particularly *Pseudomonas aeruginosa* and *Burkholderia cepacia*. A heavy smoker with weight loss and clubbing of fingers is likely to have a lung cancer. The depicted subpleural lesion is not typical of an infiltrative neoplasm; it is instead very well circumscribed.
BP6 422-423   PBD6 723-724

20. **(C)** He has "farmer's lung," which is a form of hypersensitivity pneumonitis caused by inhalation of actinomycete spores. These spores contain the antigen that incites the hypersensitivity reaction. Because type III (early) and type IV immune hypersensitivity reactions are involved, granuloma formation can occur. The disease abates when the patient is no longer exposed to the antigen. Chronic exposure can lead to more extensive interstitial lung disease. Silicosis can produce a restrictive lung disease with fibrosis, but there are nodules of fibrosis that develop over years with minimal inflammation. Asbestosis is another pneumoconiosis that can also produce interstitial fibrosis over many years, and the risk for neoplasia is increased.

Persons who have resolution of ARDS tend not to have progressive interstitial disease. If resolution fails to occur, there is interstitial fibrosis, but no granulomas are formed. Antibodies directed against pulmonary basement membrane are a feature of Goodpasture syndrome, which mainly produces pulmonary hemorrhage.
BP6 410–411 PBD6 737

21. **(E)** Primary atypical pneumonias may result from a variety of infectious agents, including viruses, chlamydiae, and rickettsiae, although mycoplasmal infections are most common in children and young adults. About one half of cases of *Mycoplasma* infection are accompanied by an increased cold agglutinin titer. Neutrophilic exudates are typical for bacterial pneumonias. Granulomatous inflammation can appear with vasculitides and infections such as tuberculosis. A hemorrhagic infarction is most often the result of a pulmonary thromboembolus, although infection with *Aspergillus* may lead to vascular invasion and thrombosis. Hyaline membranes are seen with acute lung injuries (diffuse alveolar damage).
BP6 419–420 PBD6 721–722

22. **(D)** Pneumothorax is unlikely because local obstruction does not produce enough air trapping to cause an air leak, particularly in a normal child's lung. The obstruction by a foreign body can lead to localized bronchiectasis. Complete obstruction of a bronchus can result in resorption of air and localized atelectasis. Distal to an obstruction, a bronchopneumonia can develop, which can lead to a lung abscess.
BP6 394 PBD6 699, 751

23. **(D)** Most paraneoplastic syndromes involving lung carcinomas are associated with small cell anaplastic (oat cell) carcinomas, but hypercalcemia is one exception. Most commonly, it is caused by squamous cell carcinoma. Metastatic disease can also lead to hypercalcemia when bone metastases are present, but metastases to the lung usually present as multiple masses, not one large mass. Bronchioloalveolar carcinomas are not common and are not often associated with hormone-like factor production. Large cell carcinomas are not commonly the cause for a paraneoplastic syndrome.
BP6 434 PBD6 746–747

24. **(L)** He probably has a squamous cell carcinoma of lung, which is most likely to produce a paraneoplastic syndrome with hypercalcemia. Squamous cell cancers tend to be large, central masses, and they are strongly associated with smoking.
BP6 433–434 PBD6 746

25. **(E)** This patient is at occupational risk for asbestos exposure. The inhaled asbestos fibers become encrusted with iron, and they appear as the characteristic ferruginous bodies with iron stain. The firm, tan mass encasing the pleura is most likely a mesothelioma. Asbestosis more commonly gives rise to pleural fibrosis. This is seen grossly as a dense pleural plaque, which is often calcified. In addition, asbestosis can give rise to interstitial fibrosis and lung cancer; the latter especially occurring in smokers.
BP6 227–229 PBD6 732–733

26. **(C)** There is pink, amorphous tissue at the lower left representing caseous necrosis. The rim of the granuloma has epithelioid cells and Langhans giant cells. Caseating granulomatous inflammation is most typical for *M. tuberculosis* infection. A hamartoma is a benign neoplastic process, with the mass composed of pulmonary tissue elements, including cartilage and bronchial epithelium. A pulmonary infarct should have extensive hemorrhage. A lung abscess would have an area of liquefactive necrosis filled with tissue debris and neutrophils. A carcinoma may have central necrosis, not caseation, and there should be atypical, pleomorphic cells forming the mass.
BP6 423–424 PBD6 723–726

27. **(B)** Respiratory syncytial virus pneumonia is most common in children, and it can occur in epidemics. Viral, chlamydial, and mycoplasmal pneumonias are most often interstitial, without neutrophilic alveolar exudates. The diagnosis is often presumptive, because culture is difficult and expensive. Lobar consolidation is more typical for a bacterial process, such as can be seen with *S. pneumoniae* infection. Pleural effusions can be seen with pulmonary inflammatory processes but are most pronounced with heart failure. Cavitation is most likely to complicate secondary tuberculosis in adults. Hyperinflation can accompany bronchoconstriction with asthma.
BP6 419–420 PBD6 340–341, 721–722

28. **(C)** This history is typical of nonatopic, or intrinsic, asthma. There is no family history, no eosinophilia, and a normal serum IgE level. The fundamental abnormality in such cases is bronchial hyperresponsiveness (i.e., the threshold of bronchial spasm is intrinsically low). When airway inflammation occurs after viral infections, the bronchial muscles go into spasm, and an asthmatic attack occurs. Such bronchial hyperreactivity may also be triggered by inhalation of air pollutants such as ozone, sulfur dioxide, and nitrogen dioxide. Accumulation of mast cells and eosinophils is typical of atopic asthma. Secretion of IL-4 and IL-5 by type 2 helper T cells (T_H2 cells) also occurs in cases of allergic asthma. Bronchopulmonary aspergillosis refers to colonization of asthmatic airways by *Aspergillus*, followed by development of additional IgE antibodies.
BP6 397 PBD6 712–714

29. **(A)** He has a malignant mesothelioma. This is a rare tumor even in persons with a history of asbestos exposure. These tumors appear decades after exposure. More common in persons with asbestos exposure is bronchogenic carcinoma, particularly when there is a history of smoking. Bird dust can lead to hypersensitivity pneumonitis. Silicosis is typified by interstitial fibrosis with a slight increase in the risk for bronchogenic carcinoma. Inhalation of cotton fibers (i.e., byssinosis) leads to symptoms related to bronchoconstriction. Coal dust inhalation can lead to marked anthracosis but without a significant risk for lung cancer.
BP6 435–436 PBD6 151–153, 732–733

30. **(A)** Changes of pulmonary hypertension are characteristic for restrictive and obstructive lung diseases. This explains, for example, the occurrence of cor pulmonale and right-sided CHF in persons with chronic obstructive pulmonary disease or with pneumoconiosis. Destruction of elastic tissue in alveolar walls is a process seen with emphysema. Fibrosis of alveolar walls occurs with restrictive lung

diseases. Alveolar hemorrhage is not a feature of restrictive or obstructive lung disease. Hyaline membranes are seen with diffuse alveolar damage (adult respiratory distress syndrome), which acts more like an acute restrictive lung disease.
BP6 413–414   PBD6 705–706

31.   **(D)** This patient has a typical history of bronchiectasis. In this condition, irreversible dilation of bronchi results from inflammation and destruction of bronchial walls after prolonged infections or obstruction. Serious past bouts of pneumonia can predispose to bronchiectasis. Unopposed action of elastases damages the elastic tissue of alveoli, giving rise to emphysema. DAD is an acute condition that gives rise to adult respiratory distress syndrome. Bronchial mucosal damage by eosinophils occurs in bronchial asthma. It does not cause destruction of the bronchial wall.
BP6 403–404   PBD6 716–717

32.   **(A)** Resorption atelectasis is most often the result of a mucous or mucopurulent plug obstructing a bronchus. It can occur postoperatively, or it may complicate bronchial asthma. Compression atelectasis results from accumulation of air or fluid in the pleural cavity, as can happen with a pneumothorax, hemothorax, or pleural effusion. Microatelectasis can occur postoperatively, in DAD, and in respiratory distress of the newborn from loss of surfactant. Contraction atelectasis occurs when fibrous scar tissue surrounds the lung. Relaxation atelectasis is a synonym for compression atelectasis.
BP6 394   PBD6 699–700

33.   **(A)** These pulmonary vascular changes are typical for pulmonary hypertension that can occur with right heart failure. Initially, a VSD produces a left-to-right shunt, because left ventricular pressures are higher than the right. Over time, the shunt results in pulmonary vascular alterations from this hypertension. With increasing pulmonary hypertension, the right ventricular pressure rises, and there is a right-to-left shunt accompanied by cyanosis from mixing of deoxygenated blood with oxygenated blood. The hemoptysis with renal failure suggests Goodpasture syndrome, an acute cause for pulmonary hemorrhage mediated by antibody directed against glomerular and pulmonary basement membranes. The wheezing with eosinophilia suggests atopic asthma, an episodic condition affecting mainly the bronchi, not the vasculature, of the lungs. Diabetics develop systemic arterial atherosclerosis but not pulmonary atherosclerosis. Infection with septicemia may lead to diffuse alveolar damage with hyaline membranes, an acute event without chronic vascular changes.
BP6 413–414   PBD6 705–706

34.   **(D)** Vasculitis is a key feature of Wegener granulomatosis. Although multiple organs can be affected, the lung and kidney are most often involved. The c-ANCA test result is often positive, whereas a positive p-ANCA result suggests microscopic polyangiitis. Renal and pulmonary disease may be present with Goodpasture syndrome, with a positive result for anti–glomerular basement membrane antibody but no c-ANCA or p-ANCA positivity. With hypersensitivity pneumonitis, an initial type III hypersensitivity response is followed by a type IV response, and renal disease is not expected. With SLE, renal disease is far

more likely than pulmonary disease, and c-ANCA or p-ANCA positivity is not expected. Of the collagen vascular diseases, systemic sclerosis is more likely to produce significant pulmonary disease, but hemoptysis is not a prominent feature, and the c-ANCA result is not likely to be positive.
BP6 411   PBD6 522–523, 738–739

35.   **(E)** The lack of the anti-elastase activity of α_1-antitrypsin promotes damage to the pulmonary elastic tissue, resulting in loss of structures throughout lung acini and causing panacinar emphysema. There is irreversible dilation of respiratory bronchioles to terminal alveoli. This is more pronounced in the lower lung lobes, where greater perfusion occurs. Sarcoidosis is a granulomatous, mainly interstitial disease. Bronchiectasis results from chronic and destructive inflammation of bronchi. Interstitial fibrosis results from inhalation of injurious dusts (e.g., silica, asbestos) or lung injury in collagen vascular diseases. Microatelectasis can occur postoperatively or with loss of surfactant in diffuse alveolar damage.
BP6 399–400   PBD6 709–710

36.   **(A)** The anesthetic gases tend to reduce the ciliary function of the respiratory epithelium that lines the bronchi. The mucociliary apparatus helps to clear organisms that are inhaled into the respiratory tree. The anesthetic gases and drugs do not typically result in marrow failure with neutropenia. The subglottic tracheal region, where the cuff of the endotracheal tube is located, can become eroded, but this is more likely to occur when intubation is prolonged for weeks. Macrophage function is not significantly affected by anesthesia. The levels of γ-globulins in serum are not reduced by the effects of anesthesia.
BP6 414   PBD6 718–719

37.   **(A)** Upper lobe cavitation suggests reactivation or reinfection tuberculosis in adults, and hence, acid-fast stain should be done. The GMS stain is helpful for finding fungi and for finding cysts of *P. carinii*. A Gram stain is most useful for determining what bacterial organisms may be present. The cytologic smear can be most helpful in screening for malignant cells. A viral illness, which typically produces an interstitial pneumonia, should not account for upper lobe cavitation.
BP6 423–425   PBD6 722–725

38.   **(E)** The ferruginous bodies shown here are long, thin crystals of asbestos that have become encrusted with iron and calcium. The inflammatory reaction incited by these crystals promotes fibrogenesis and resultant pneumoconiosis. Berylliosis is marked by noncaseating granulomas. Anthracosis is a benign process seen in all city dwellers as a consequence of inhaled carbonaceous dust. Silica crystals are not covered by iron and tend to result in formation of fibrous nodules (i.e., silicotic nodules). Calcium deposition may occur along alveolar walls with a high serum calcium (i.e., metastatic calcification).
BP6 227–228   PBD6 732–734

39.   **(D)** Centrilobular emphysema results from damage to the central or proximal part of the lung acinus, with relative sparing of the distal acinar structures (i.e., alveolar ducts and alveolar sacs). With panacinar emphysema, the lung lobule is involved from the respiratory bronchiole to

the terminal alveoli. In paraseptal emphysema, the distal acinus is involved.
BP6 398-399   PBD6 707-709

40. **(E)** Most pulmonary carcinoids are central, obstructing masses involving a bronchus. They are neuroendocrine tumors with a somewhat unpredictable behavior, although many are resectable and follow a benign course. They typically present with hemoptysis and consequences of bronchial obstruction. In this case, the pneumonia in the right upper lobe probably resulted from obstruction to drainage caused by the tumor. Adenocarcinomas are common lung tumors but are typically peripheral. A hamartoma is an uncommon but benign pulmonary lesion that is also located peripherally. Large cell carcinomas are typically large, bulky, peripheral masses. Kaposi sarcoma can be seen involving the lung in some patients with AIDS, and the tumor often has a bronchovascular distribution, but obstruction is uncommon.
BP6 435   PBD6 747-748

41. **(D)** This child has atopic asthma, a form of type I hypersensitivity reaction in which there are presensitized, IgE-coated mast cells in mucosal surfaces and submucosa of airways. Contact with an allergen results in degranulation of the mast cells, with release of mediators, such as leukotrienes, histamine, and prostaglandins, that attract leukocytes, particularly eosinophils, and promote bronchoconstriction. The characteristic histologic changes in the bronchi follow from the inflammation. Dilation of the respiratory bronchiole is a feature of centrilobular emphysema. Bronchial dilation with inflammatory destruction is a feature of bronchiectasis. Hyaline membranes are seen with acute diffuse alveolar damage. Neutrophilic exudates with consolidation are seen with pneumonic processes, typically from bacterial infections.
BP6 395-397   PBD6 713-715

42. **(C)** The spirometric data suggest a restrictive lung disease process. The progressive pulmonary interstitial fibrosis of a restrictive lung disease such as a pneumoconiosis can eventually lead to dilation of remaining airspaces, giving a "honeycomb" appearance. The loss of lung tissue with emphysema also leads to airspace dilation but without alveolar wall fibrogenesis. The increase in mucus glands with chronic bronchitis leads to copious sputum production but not fibrogenesis. Eosinophilic infiltrates suggest atopic asthma, an episodic disease without fibrogenesis. Hyaline membranes along with edema, inflammation, and focal necrosis are features of diffuse alveolar damage (i.e., adult respiratory distress syndrome) in the acute phase; if patients survive for weeks, diffuse alveolar damage may resolve to honeycomb change.
BP6 395, 404   PBD6 726-727

43. **(E)** Most pulmonary emboli are small and clinically silent. Sudden death may occur with large emboli that occlude the main pulmonary arteries. Cor pulmonale can result from repeated embolization with reduction in the pulmonary vascular bed. Hemoptysis with pulmonary embolism is uncommon, although it may occur when a hemorrhagic infarction results from thromboembolism. Dyspnea can occur with medium to large emboli.
BP6 412-413   PBD6 703-704

44. **(E)** This patient has chronic restrictive lung disease. The exact cause for many slowly progressive cases of restrictive lung disease is unknown. These cases must be distinguished from identifiable causes such as infections, collagen vascular diseases, drugs, and pneumoconioses. Scleroderma may produce a progressive restrictive lung disease, but there are usually other manifestations affecting the skin, and the antinuclear antibody test result is typically positive. Goodpasture syndrome is a rare cause for sudden onset of severe hemoptysis. Silicosis is a progressive interstitial disease, but his occupation as a pilot would tend to exclude exposure to dusts. Diffuse alveolar damage is an acute form of interstitial disease.
BP6 407-408   PBD6 735-736

45. **(D)** The key feature of asthma (regardless of cause) is the hyperreactivity of the airways to various stimuli leading to episodic, reversible bronchoconstriction. Eosinophils are a feature of atopic asthma, which may run in families. Viral infections tend to produce the inflammation that predisposes to nonatopic asthma. A variety of chemical fumes and dusts are predisposing factors in occupational asthma.
BP6 395-397   BPD6 712-715

46. **(J)** This patient has features of Cushing syndrome, a paraneoplastic syndrome resulting from ectopic corticotropin production (most often from a pulmonary small cell carcinoma), which drives the adrenal cortices to produce an excess of cortisol. Small cell carcinomas are aggressive tumors that tend to metastasize early. Even when they appear to be small and localized, they are not or will not remain so. Surgery therefore is not an option for these patients. They are treated as if they have systemic disease.
BP6 434   PBD6 746-747

47. **(C)** Bronchioloalveolar carcinoma is a peripheral tumor that can mimic a pneumonia. Most are well differentiated. Large cell carcinomas are also peripheral, but the cells are large and pleomorphic and form sheets. Squamous cell carcinomas can be peripheral on occasion (although most are central) and are composed of pink, polygonal cells that have intercellular bridges. If well-differentiated, squamous cell carcinomas show keratin pearls. Most small cell carcinomas are also central in location and are composed of cells that resemble lymphocytes. The tumor cells, however, are about twice the size of lymphocytes.
BP6 433   PBD6 742-745

48. **(K)** This chain smoker has a carcinoma of the lung in the right bronchus. Of all lung cancers, the one most likely to produce paraneoplastic hypercalcemia is squamous cell carcinoma. These tumors can also undergo central necrosis, and hence a cavity may form. Localized squamous cell carcinomas, unlike small cell carcinomas, may be cured by surgery.
BP6 433-434   PBD6 743-746

49. **(A)** The most common primary lung malignancy in women and in nonsmokers is adenocarcinoma. Overall, lung cancers in nonsmokers are far less frequent than in smokers. Adenocarcinomas primary in lung tend to be small, peripheral masses that are amenable to surgical excision and have a better overall prognosis than other forms of lung cancer.
BP6 433   PBD6 744

50. **(C)** This is a saddle pulmonary thromboembolus. Sudden death occurs from hypoxemia or from acute cor pulmonale with right heart failure. Because the airways are not obstructed, the lungs do not collapse, and there is no bronchoconstriction. Such an acute course does not leave time for a hemorrhagic pulmonary infarction to occur. Edema is not a feature of thromboembolism.
BP6 412   PBD6 703

51. **(A)** The clinical and morphologic features strongly suggest sarcoidosis. This granulomatous disease has an unknown cause, but the presence of granulomas and activated T cells in the lungs indicates a delayed hypersensitivity response to some inhaled antigen. Lung involvement, occurring in about one third of cases, may be asymptomatic or may lead to restrictive lung disease. Hypersensitivity pneumonitis is an immune-complex disease that is triggered by inhaled allergens. This form of lung disease is characterized by acute dyspneic episodes. There can be granulomas in the lung, but lymph node enlargement is not seen. Diffuse alveolar damage is an acute lung injury seen in ARDS. Smoking causes chronic bronchitis and emphysema. Atypical mycobacteria cause caseating granulomas, as does *M. tuberculosis*.
BP 409–410   PBD6 734–735

52. **(B)** This patient had chronic bronchitis with terminal adult respiratory distress syndrome (ARDS) and diffuse alveolar damage. Answers C, D, and E are features of chronic bronchitis complicated by pulmonary hypertension and cor pulmonale. Hyaline membranes are caused by ARDS and are seen early in the course of this disorder. Patients who survive ARDS can develop diffuse pulmonary fibrosis as the damaged alveoli heal. However, 6 days is not sufficient time for the development of fibrosis.
BP 405–406   PBD6 700–703

53. **(A)** Lung abscesses can result from aspiration of oropharyngeal or nasopharyngeal contents, and bacterial organisms that are part of normal flora can be picked up and transported to the lungs. The straighter bronchus to the right lung is more likely to conduct aspirated material. Chronic bronchitis is a clinical diagnosis made when a patient has a chronic productive cough. Bronchiectasis can occur from bronchial inflammation and destruction after obstruction or infection; cystic fibrosis is the best known disease to produce a widespread pattern of bronchiectasis. Asthma, which can lead to bronchoconstriction, is not a

complication of aspiration. Pulmonary infarcts are a complication of pulmonary thromboembolism.
BP6 428–429   PBD6 722

54. **(D)** Blunt trauma to the chest can lead to rib fracture. The sharp bone can penetrate the pleura and produce an air leak, resulting in a pneumothorax. Although pulmonary embolus and pneumonia are possible complications in hospitalized patients, they would not occur this quickly. Edema and hydrothorax are unlikely from trauma alone; hemorrhage is more likely. Although a pneumothorax can complicate rupture of a bulla with emphysema, this is most likely with paraseptal emphysema, not centrilobular emphysema.
BP6 436   PBD6 751

55. **(D)** The leukotrienes C_4, D_4, and E_4 promote intense bronchoconstriction and mucin production. Prostaglandin D_2 is also a bronchoconstrictor, but its role is less well defined than that of leukotrienes. PAF increases vascular permeability and aids in histamine release from platelet granules. IL-5, along with PAF, is chemotactic for neutrophils. C3a increases vascular permeability. Histamine acts only during the early acute phase of type I hypersensitivity reactions. It plays very little role in chronic bronchial asthma, when the late-phase reaction takes over.
BP6 396   PBD6 713

56. **(B)** Congestive heart failure is common compared with the other listed conditions. The cell count and appearance indicate that this is a transudate. The lymphoma may lead to a chylothorax, and carcinomas involving the pleura tend to produce blood-tinged fluid. SLE and renal failure tend to produce effusions with more protein or cells.
BP6 436   PBD6 750–751

57. **(B)** Adenocarcinoma is the most common primary lung malignancy in nonsmokers. It tends to be peripheral, making surgical resection an option in many cases. Large cell carcinomas are also more likely to be peripheral, but they tend to be larger masses. Primary lymphomas of the lung are uncommon. A mesothelioma is a rare neoplasm, even in persons with asbestos exposure, and it arises on the pleura. Some squamous cell carcinomas can be peripheral, but they are most likely to occur in persons who smoke.
BP6 433   PBD6 744–745

58. **(B)** He has acute symptoms after exposure to an antigen, often actinomycetes or fungi (molds). The symptoms improve when the person leaves the environment where the antigen was. The pulmonary pathologic changes are usually minimal, with interstitial mononuclear infiltrates. *P. carinii* pneumonia is most likely to occur in immunocompromised patients. Atypical pneumonia, as can be seen with *Mycoplasma* infection, tends to have symptoms that persist longer, and a chest radiograph demonstrates bilateral infiltrates. Goodpasture syndrome is a rare cause of acute-onset hemoptysis. Actinomycosis tends to produce a more chronic pneumonitis.
BP6 410–411   PBD6 737

Head and Neck

PBD6 Chapter 17 - Head and Neck
BP6 Chapter 13 - The Lungs and Upper
          Respiratory Tract
BP6 Chapter 15 - The Oral Cavity and
          Gastrointestinal Tract

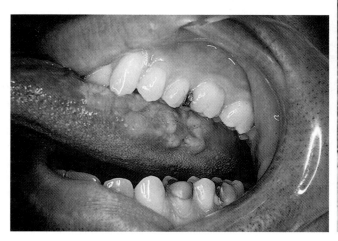

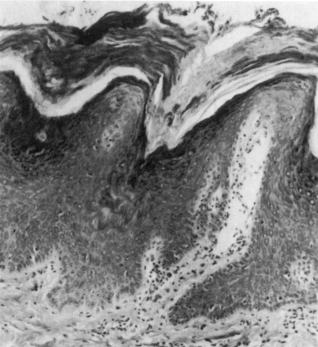

1. A 55-year-old male noticed for more than a year the presence of the lesions seen in the figures. The etiologic factor that probably contributed the most to the appearance of these lesions is

- (A) Dental caries
- (B) Herpes simplex virus type 1 (HSV-1)
- (C) Smoked and pickled foods
- (D) Chronic sialadenitis
- (E) Smoking

2. After a bout of the "flu," a 25-year-old male notices the appearance of several clear vesicles on his upper lip. These 0.3-cm vesicles rupture, leaving shallow, painful ulcers that heal during the next 4 weeks. Several months later, after a skiing trip, this scenario is repeated. The most likely finding associated with these lesions is

- (A) Biopsy demonstrating squamous epithelial hyperkeratosis
- (B) Positive serology for herpes simplex virus type 1 (HSV-1)
- (C) Atypical lymphocytes seen on the peripheral blood smear
- (D) Cytologic scraping showing budding cells with pseudohyphae
- (E) A mononuclear inflammatory infiltrate on biopsy

3. A 50-year-old male has had difficulty breathing through his nose for several months. He also has some dull facial pain. A head computed tomography (CT) scan reveals a 4-cm mass involving the nasopharynx on the right that erodes adjacent bone. The mass is excised, and microscopically, it is composed of large epithelial cells having

indistinct cell borders and prominent nuclei. There are mature lymphocytes scattered through this undifferentiated neoplasm. Which of the following factors most likely played the greatest role in the development of this lesion?

○ (A) Epstein-Barr virus (EBV) infection
○ (B) Sjögren syndrome
○ (C) Smoking
○ (D) Allergic rhinitis
○ (E) Wegener granulomatosis

4. Over the past 10 years, a 50-year-old male has had progressive difficulty hearing, particularly on the left side. Audiometry testing reveals that he has a bone conduction type of deafness. He has a brother and a mother who are similarly affected. Which of the following conditions is he most likely to have?

○ (A) Otosclerosis
○ (B) Schwannoma
○ (C) Cholesteatoma
○ (D) Otitis media
○ (E) Chondrosarcoma

For each of the clinical histories in questions 5 and 6, match the most closely associated neoplastic and nonneoplastic process that may produce a mass lesion in the head and neck region:

○ (A) Angiofibroma
○ (B) Cholesteatoma
○ (C) Malignant lymphoma
○ (D) Mucoepidermoid carcinoma
○ (E) Olfactory neuroblastoma
○ (F) Papilloma
○ (G) Paraganglioma
○ (H) Plasmacytoma
○ (I) Pleomorphic adenoma
○ (J) Pyogenic granuloma
○ (K) Squamous cell carcinoma
○ (L) Warthin tumor

5. A 60-year-old female has a mass arising in a minor salivary gland located on the buccal mucosa beneath the tongue on the right. The mass is 2.5 cm in diameter and movable. It is excised, and histologically, it is malignant and locally invasive. The tumor recurs within a year. (   )

6. A 3-cm, nontender, mobile, discrete mass is palpable on the left side of the face of a 60-year-old female. The mass is anterior to the ear and just superior to the mandible and has been slowly enlarging for several years. Histologic examination of the excised lesion demonstrates ductal epithelial cells in a myxoid stroma containing islands of chondroid and bone formation. (   )

7. A 23-year-old male has difficulty breathing through his nose that has become progressively worse for the last 2 months. Physical examination reveals glistening, translucent, polypoid masses filling the nasal cavity bilaterally. When these masses are excised, they are seen histologically to have respiratory mucosa overlying an edematous stroma with scattered plasma cells and eosinophils. Which of the following laboratory test findings is most likely?

○ (A) Elevated hemoglobin A_{1C} level in serum
○ (B) Increased serum IgE level
○ (C) Nuclear staining for EBV antigens
○ (D) Tissue culture positive for *Staphylococcus aureus*
○ (E) Positive antinuclear antibody test result

8. A 65-year-old female notices a lump on the right side of her face that has been enlarging for the past year. On physical examination, there is a 3- to 4-cm, firm, mobile, painless mass palpable in the region of the right parotid gland. The oral mucosa appears normal. She does not complain of difficulty chewing food or talking. Which of the following conditions is most likely to account for these findings?

○ (A) Sialolithiasis
○ (B) Pleomorphic adenoma
○ (C) Sjögren syndrome
○ (D) Mucoepidermoid carcinoma
○ (E) Malignant lymphoma

9. A 6-year-old male has had increasing difficulty breathing, and the character of his voice has also changed over the past 3 months. Endoscopic examination reveals three soft, pink excrescences on the true vocal cords and in the subglottic region. These masses range from 0.6 to 1.0 cm in diameter. They are excised and microscopically show finger-like projections of orderly squamous epithelium overlying fibrovascular cores. Immunostaining for human papillomavirus 6 (HPV-6) antigens is positive. What advice would you give the parents of this boy, based on these findings?

○ (A) A total laryngectomy is necessary
○ (B) Therapy with acyclovir is indicated
○ (C) The boy should not overuse his voice
○ (D) These lesions are likely to recur many times
○ (E) Congenital heart disease may be present

10. On physical examination of the oral cavity, the right buccal mucosa of a 68-year-old male reveals some discrete white patches with a leathery surface. The lesions are spread over a 0.7 × 2.5 cm area. A biopsy of one of the lesions shows squamous epithelial acanthosis with marked hyperkeratosis. These lesions are most likely to have resulted as a consequence of

○ (A) Eating chili peppers
○ (B) Chewing spearmint gum
○ (C) French kissing
○ (D) Chewing tobacco
○ (E) Human immunodeficiency virus (HIV) infection

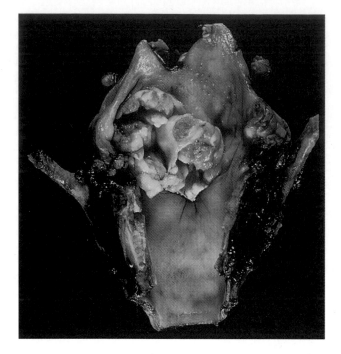

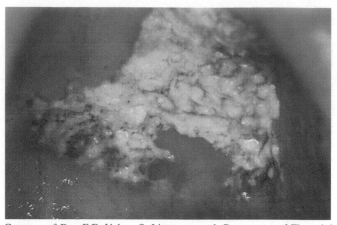

Courtesy of Drs. E.E. Vokes, S. Lippman, et al, Department of Thoracic/Head and Neck Oncology, Texas Medical Center, Houston, TX. Reprinted with permission from The New England Journal of Medicine 328:184, 1993.

11. A 70-year-old male has experienced increasing hoarseness for almost 6 months. He recently had an episode of hemoptysis. The lesion depicted here was identified by endoscopy. He underwent biopsy, followed by laryngectomy and neck dissection. Which of the following etiologic factors probably played the greatest role in the development of this lesion?

○ (A) Human papillomavirus infection
○ (B) Type I hypersensitivity
○ (C) Smoking
○ (D) Repeated bouts of aspiration
○ (E) EBV infection

For each of the clinical histories in questions 12 and 13, match the most closely associated inflammatory process involving the head and neck region:

○ (A) Aphthous ulcer
○ (B) Oral thrush
○ (C) Hairy leukoplakia
○ (D) Lichen planus
○ (E) Leukoplakia
○ (F) Allergic rhinitis
○ (G) Pharyngitis
○ (H) Tonsillitis
○ (I) Singer nodule
○ (J) Otitis media
○ (K) Sialadenitis
○ (L) Xerostomia

12. A 49-year-old male has used chewing tobacco and snuff for many years. The lesion shown here is on the hard palate and cannot be removed by scraping. Biopsy of this lesion shows a thickened squamous mucosa. Several years later, biopsy of a similar lesion is found to have carcinoma in situ. (   )

13. A 35-year-old male who is known to be HIV positive is found on physical examination to have areas of adherent, yellow-tan, circumscribed plaque on the lateral aspects of his tongue. This plaque is lifted off as a pseudomembrane to reveal an underlying granular, erythematous base. (   )

14. A 17-year-old female notices a sensitive, small, gray-white area along the lateral border of her tongue during final examination week. On examination, this is a 0.3-cm, shallow, ulcerated lesion with an erythematous rim. It disappears in a couple of weeks. What is the most probable cause for this finding?

○ (A) Aphthous ulcer
○ (B) Oral thrush
○ (C) Herpes simplex stomatitis
○ (D) Leukoplakia
○ (E) Sialadenitis

15. A 5-year-old male has had repeated bouts of otitis media. S. aureus and Pseudomonas aeruginosa have been cultured, and the right tympanic membrane has perforated. Which of the following complications is he most likely to suffer as a consequence of these events?

○ (A) Otosclerosis
○ (B) Labyrinthitis
○ (C) Squamous cell carcinoma
○ (D) Eosinophilic granuloma
○ (E) Cholesteatoma

16. A 17-year-old female is concerned about a "bump" on her neck that she has noticed for several months. It does not seem to have increased in size appreciably during

that time. On physical examination, there is a discrete, slightly movable nodule located in the midline just above the thyroid. The lesion is excised. Microscopic examination reveals a cystic mass lined by squamous and respiratory epithelium. Which of the following additional histologic elements would you expect to be found adjacent to the cyst?

○ (A) Malignant lymphoma
○ (B) Thyroid follicles
○ (C) Serous salivary glands
○ (D) Squamous cell carcinoma
○ (E) Noncaseating granulomas

ANSWERS

1. **(E)** The lesion is a whitish, well-defined mucosal patch on the tongue. This is the appearance of leukoplakia, a premalignant lesion that can give rise to squamous cell carcinoma. Pipe smoking and chewing tobacco are implicated in the appearance of leukoplakia. Chronic alcoholism is also implicated, but the association is less strong than with tobacco. Ill-fitting dentures may lead to leukoplakia but far less commonly than with smoking. Dental caries are not a risk for leukoplakia, unless the affected tooth becomes eroded and misshapen. Infections and inflammation are not a recognized risk factor for oral leukoplakia or squamous oral cancers. The type of food eaten has less of a correlation with cancer of the oral cavity than with cancer of the esophagus.
BP6 473-474   PBD6 760-761

2. **(B)** Also known as "cold sores" or "fever blisters," the lesions of HSV-1 are common. Many people have HSV-1, and the oral and perianal lesions appear during periods of stress. Recurrence is the norm. Leukoplakia is marked by hyperkeratosis. Atypical lymphocytes are seen with infectious mononucleosis, which may be accompanied by a rash but does not produce vesicular lesions of the skin. Budding cells with pseudohyphae suggest a candidal infection with oral thrush. A mononuclear infiltrate is quite nonspecific and can be seen with aphthous ulcers.
BP6 471-472   PBD6 757

3. **(A)** This is a nasopharyngeal carcinoma. There is a strong association with EBV infection, which contributes to transformation of squamous epithelial cells. Sjögren syndrome is associated with malignant lymphomas, but these typically arise in the salivary gland, not the nasal cavity. Smoking is not associated with nasopharyngeal carcinoma, although smoking contributes to oral and esophageal cancers. Allergic rhinitis is associated with development of nasal polyps, but these do not become malignant. Wegener granulomatosis can involve the respiratory tract with granulomatous inflammation and vasculitis, but the nasopharyngeal region is not commonly affected, and there is no risk of malignancy.
BP6 437   PBD6 764

4. **(A)** Otosclerosis can be familial, particularly when it is severe. It results from fibrous ankylosis followed by bony overgrowth of the little ossicles of the middle ear. A schwannoma typically involves the eighth cranial nerve and results in a nerve conduction form of deafness. Schwannomas are usually unilateral, although familial neurofibromatosis could result in the appearance of multiple schwannomas. A cholesteatoma is typically a unilateral process that complicates chronic otitis media in a child or young adult. Otitis media by itself is usually self-limited and uncommon in an adult. Chondrosarcomas may involve the skull in older adults but are rare and are solitary, bulky masses in the region of the jaw.
PBD6 767

5. **(E)** Mucoepidermoid carcinomas can arise in salivary glands. They account for most neoplasms, particularly those that are malignant, within minor salivary glands. Low-grade mucoepidermoid carcinomas may invade but their prognosis is still good, with a 90% 5-year survival rate. High-grade mucoepidermoid carcinomas can metastasize and have a 5-year survival rate of only 50%.
PBD6 772

6. **(I)** Pleomorphic adenoma is the most common tumor of the parotid gland. They are rarely malignant, although they can be locally invasive.
BP6 475   PBD6 770-771

7. **(B)** These are nasal polyps, which can be associated with allergic rhinitis, a form of type I hypersensitivity often called hay fever. In some patients, this inflammation results in the formation of polyps in the nasal cavity. Type I hypersensitivity is associated with high IgE levels in the serum. The elevated hemoglobin A_{1C} level is indicative of diabetes mellitus, which is not a risk for polyp formation, but ketoacidosis can predispose to nasopharyngeal mucormycosis. EBV infection can be found in nasopharyngeal carcinomas. *S. aureus* is often found colonizing the nasal cavity, but it does not often cause problems. Autoimmune diseases are not associated with nasal polyp formation.
PBD6 762

8. **(B)** Pleomorphic adenoma is the most common benign salivary gland tumor and the most common tumor of the parotid gland. They tend to be slow growing and most act in a benign fashion, although local invasion and recurrence are potential problems. Sialolithiasis is usually accompanied by sialadenitis and is therefore quite painful. It may produce some gland enlargement but not usually a mass effect. Sjögren syndrome can produce some salivary gland enlargement, but the process is typically bilateral. A mucoepidermoid tumor can occur in salivary glands, but this tumor is much less common than a pleomorphic adenoma. Malignant lymphomas of the salivary gland are uncommon.
BP6 475   PBD6 769-771

9. **(D)** He has juvenile laryngeal papillomatosis, which is caused by HPV types 6 and 11. These lesions frequently recur after excision but may regress after puberty. If laryngeal papillomas arise in adulthood, they are usually solitary

and do not recur. There is no effective antiviral therapy for HPV. Although these lesions can be found throughout the airways, they are benign and do not become malignant. The appearance of these lesions is not related to the use of the voice. This is not a congenital condition and is not syndromic.
BP6 537   PBD6 766

10. **(D)** The clinical and histologic features indicate leukoplakia. Oral leukoplakia can appear in a variety of intraoral sites and the lower lip border. Pipe smoking and tobacco chewing are good ways to generate these white patches. Irritation from misaligned teeth or dentures is another way to produce leukoplakia. Transformation to dysplasia and carcinoma is possible. The type of food or chewing gum is not a risk factor, although the chewing of betel nut in some parts of the world is a risk factor for oral cancer. One's social behavior might be a risk factor for infections such as herpes simplex. HIV infection is most often associated with oral thrush (i.e., candidiasis) and with HSV infections.
BP6 472–473   PBD6 759–760

11. **(C)** This is a large, fungating neoplasm that is typical in appearance for a laryngeal squamous cell carcinoma. The most common risk factor is smoking, although alcoholism also plays a role. About 5% of cases harbor HPV sequences. The etiologic significance of this is not clear. Allergies with type I hypersensitivity may result in transient laryngeal edema but not neoplasia. Aspiration may result in acute inflammation but not neoplasia. EBV infection is associated with nasopharyngeal carcinomas.
BP6 437–438   PBD6 765–766

12. **(E)** The raised white patches suggest leukoplakia. This is a premalignant condition. Risk factors include tobacco use, particularly chewing tobacco, and chronic irritation. HPV has been implicated in some lesions.
BP6 472–473   PBD6 759–760

13. **(B)** He has oral thrush, a lesion resulting from oral candidiasis in persons who are immunocompromised. The lesion is typically superficial. Multinucleated cells suggest a herpesvirus infection, which typically has vesicles that ulcerate. Atypical squamous epithelial cells usually come from areas of oral leukoplakia. Leukocytes can be present with a variety of oral lesions, and a variety of bacterial organisms live in the oral cavity.
BP6 472   PBD6 757

14. **(A)** This common lesion is also known as a canker sore. Such lesions are never large, but they are annoying and tend to occur during periods of stress. The lesion is not infectious, but it probably has an autoimmune origin. Oral thrush is a superficial infection with *Candida* that occurs in diabetic, neutropenic, and immunocompromised patients. Herpetic lesions are typically vesicles that can rupture. Leukoplakia represents white patches of thicker mucosa from hyperkeratosis and may be a precursor to squamous cell carcinoma in a few cases. Inflammation of a salivary gland (i.e., sialadenitis), typically a minor salivary gland in the oral cavity, may produce a localized, tender nodule.
BP6 471   PBD6 757

15. **(E)** Cholesteatomas are not true neoplasms but are cystic masses lined by squamous epithelium. The desquamated epithelium and keratin degenerates, resulting in cholesterol formation and giant cell reaction. Although histologically benign, cholesteatomas can gradually enlarge, eroding and destroying the middle ear and surrounding structures. They occur as a complication of chronic otitis media. Otosclerosis is abnormal bone deposition in the ossicles of the middle ear that results in bone deafness in adults. Labyrinthitis is typically caused by a viral infection and is self-limited. Although cholesteatomas have a squamous epithelial lining, malignant transformation does not occur. An eosinophilic granuloma of bone occasionally may be seen in the region of the skull in young children, but it is characterized by the presence of Langerhans cells.
PBD6 767

16. **(B)** The location is classic for a thyroglossal duct (tract) cyst, which is a developmental abnormality that arises from elements of the embryonic thyroglossal duct extending from the foramen cecum of the tongue down to the thyroid gland. One or more remnants of this tract may enlarge to produce a cystic mass. Although lymphoid tissue often surrounds these cysts, malignant transformation does not occur. The cysts may contain squamous epithelium, but squamous cell carcinoma does not arise from such a cyst. If there is a cystic lesion with lymphoid tissue and squamous carcinoma in the neck, it is probably a metastasis from an occult head and neck primary. Salivary gland choristomas are unlikely at this site. Granulomatous disease is more likely to involve lymph nodes in the typical locations in the lateral neck regions.
PBD6 767–768

The Gastrointestinal Tract

BP6 Chapter 15 - The Oral Cavity and
Gastrointestinal Tract
PBD6 Chapter 18 - The Gastrointestinal Tract

1. A 30-year-old female presents with diarrhea, weight loss, fatigue, and malabsorption. After a biopsy is taken from the upper jejunum, the patient is placed on a special diet, producing dramatic improvement. Which of the following microscopic features would the biopsy most likely reveal?

○ (A) Lymphatic obstruction
○ (B) Noncaseating granulomas
○ (C) Flat mucosa with increased intraepithelial lymphocytes
○ (D) Foamy macrophages within the lamina propria
○ (E) Crypt abscesses

2. A 35-year-old male enjoys eating a chicken salad sandwich. However, 2 days later, he experiences cramping abdominal pain with fever and a watery diarrhea. He recovers completely in a few days. The most likely cause for these findings is infection with

○ (A) *Yersinia enterocolitica*
○ (B) *Escherichia coli*
○ (C) *Entamoeba histolytica*
○ (D) *Salmonella enteritidis*
○ (E) Rotavirus

3. In which of the following conditions is a biopsy most likely to demonstrate histologic evidence for granulomatous inflammation?

○ (A) Celiac sprue
○ (B) Crohn disease
○ (C) Ulcerative colitis
○ (D) Autoimmune gastritis
○ (E) Reflux esophagitis

4. A 55-year-old male who had an acute myocardial infarction presented a year later with severe abdominal pain and bloody diarrhea. Physical examination revealed a diffusely tender abdomen with absence of bowel sounds. Ab-

dominal radiographs (plain films) showed no free air. Laboratory investigations revealed a normal complete blood count (CBC) and normal levels of serum amylase, lipase, and bilirubin. His condition deteriorated, with the development of irreversible shock. At autopsy, which of the following lesions is most likely to be found?

○ (A) Acute appendicitis
○ (B) Acute pancreatitis
○ (C) Transmural infarction of the small bowel
○ (D) Acute cholecystitis
○ (E) Pseudomembranous colitis

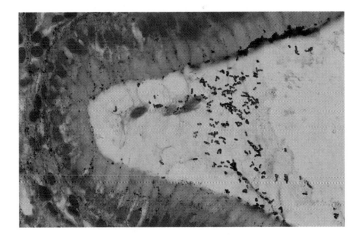

5. A 59-year-old male has been bothered by nausea and vomiting for several months. He has experienced no hematemesis. On physical examination, there is no abdominal tenderness, and bowel sounds are present. An upper endoscopy is performed, and there are erythematous areas of mucosa with thickening of the rugal folds in the gastric antrum. Gastric biopsies are performed. The microscopic appearance of one of these biopsies with a Steiner silver stain is depicted in the figure. The organisms on the luminal surface are most likely to be

○ (A) *Candida albicans*
○ (B) *Helicobacter pylori*
○ (C) *Salmonella typhi*
○ (D) *Tropheryma whippleii*
○ (E) *Clostridium difficile*

For each of the clinical histories in questions 6 and 7, match the most closely associated neoplastic condition involving the gastrointestinal tract:

(A) Adenocarcinoma
(B) Burkitt lymphoma
(C) Carcinoid tumor
(D) Kaposi sarcoma
(E) Leiomyoma
(F) Leiomyosarcoma
(G) Lipoma
(H) Mucinous cystadenoma
(I) Neuroendocrine carcinoma
(J) Neurofibroma
(K) Peutz-Jeghers polyp
(L) Squamous cell carcinoma
(M) Tubular adenoma
(N) Villous adenoma

6. A 38-year-old male has been seropositive for human immunodeficiency virus (HIV) for the past 10 years. He has developed oral thrush, and his CD4 lymphocyte count is 118/μL. He has severe nausea and vomiting. An upper endoscopy reveals a dozen gastric mucosal nodules. These nodules are 0.6 to 1.8 cm in diameter and are reddish purple. (   )

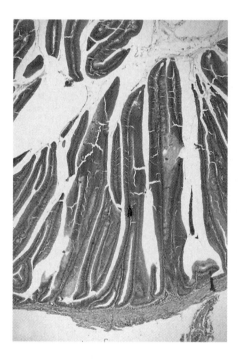

7. On a routine physical examination, a 70-year-old male is found to have stool positive for occult blood. A colonoscopy is performed and reveals a 5-cm-diameter, sessile mass located in the upper portion of the descending colon at 50 cm. The low-power histologic appearance of this lesion is shown here. Because of unexpected hypotension during the procedure, the lesion is not removed. After recovery, the patient is so scared that he refuses any intervention. Five years later, he presents with constipation, anemia, and weight loss. On surgical exploration, a 7-cm

annular lesion encircling the colon is seen. What is the diagnosis of the lesion that he has now developed? (   )

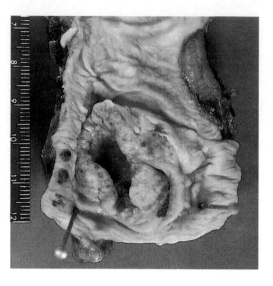

8. A 70-year-old male with a long history of chronic alcoholism has had increasing difficulty with swallowing for the past 2 months. Upper endoscopy reveals an ulcerative mid-esophageal, 3-cm mass that partially occludes the esophageal lumen. He undergoes esophagectomy, and the gross appearance of the lesion is shown here. A microscopic section of this mass is most likely to show

○ (A) Multinucleated cells with intranuclear inclusions
○ (B) Squamous cell carcinoma
○ (C) Dense collagenous scar
○ (D) Adenocarcinoma
○ (E) Thrombosed vascular channels

9. A 33-year-old male living in New York is bothered by a low-volume, mostly watery diarrhea associated with flatulence. These symptoms occur episodically, but they have been persistent for the past year, and he has lost 5 kg. He has no fever, nausea, vomiting, or abdominal pain. Stool examination results for ova and parasites are negative, and the stool is negative for occult blood. A stool culture yields no pathogens. A biopsy of the upper part of the small bowel shows severe diffuse blunting of villi and a chronic inflammatory infiltrate in the lamina propria. Which of the following therapeutic options is most likely to benefit this patient?

○ (A) Parenteral vitamin B_{12}
○ (B) Antibiotic therapy
○ (C) Gluten-free diet
○ (D) Supplementation with fat-soluble vitamins
○ (E) Corticosteroid therapy

10. An office potluck lunch party is held at noon on Thursday. A variety of meats, salads, breads, and desserts brought in earlier that morning are served. Everyone has a good time, and most of the food is consumed. At mid-afternoon, the single office restroom is overwhelmed by multiple employees suffering from an acute, explosive diar-

rheal illness. Which of the following infectious agents is probably responsible for this turn of events?

○ (A) *Escherichia coli*
○ (B) *Staphylococcus aureus*
○ (C) *Vibrio parahaemolyticus*
○ (D) *Clostridium difficile*
○ (E) *Salmonella enteritidis*

11. During July "Black and White Days," a week-long local community celebration of the dairy industry (Holstein cows are black and white), a 40-year-old male suffers from episodic abdominal bloating with flatulence and explosive diarrhea. During the rest of the year, he does not consume milk shakes or ice cream sodas and is not symptomatic. Which of the following conditions best accounts for these findings?

○ (A) Celiac sprue
○ (B) Autoimmune gastritis
○ (C) Cholelithiasis
○ (D) Disaccharidase deficiency
○ (E) Cystic fibrosis

12. For the past year, a 20-year-old male has had increasingly voluminous, bulky, and foul-smelling stools. He has also lost about 10 kg during that time. There is no history of hematemesis or melena. He has some bloating but no abdominal pain. Which of the following laboratory findings is most likely present on examination of the stool?

○ (A) Increased quantitative stool fat
○ (B) *Giardia lamblia* cysts
○ (C) Positive result for occult blood
○ (D) Positive stool culture for *Vibrio cholerae*
○ (E) *E. histolytica* trophozoites

13. A 68-year-old female has suffered from burning substernal pain for many years. This pain occurs after meals. She now has difficulty swallowing. Endoscopy reveals a lower esophageal mass that nearly occludes the lumen of the esophagus. Biopsy of the mass is most likely to reveal the presence of which of the following neoplasms?

○ (A) Adenocarcinoma
○ (B) Leiomyosarcoma
○ (C) Squamous cell carcinoma
○ (D) Non-Hodgkin lymphoma
○ (E) Carcinoid tumor

14. A 6-week-old infant has been feeding poorly for a week, and his mother notices that much of the milk that the baby ingests is forcefully vomited within an hour. The baby was delivered at term and had been doing well up until that time. Which of the following conditions is most likely to explain these findings?

○ (A) Pyloric stenosis
○ (B) Tracheo-esophageal fistula
○ (C) Diaphragmatic hernia
○ (D) Duodenal atresia
○ (E) Annular pancreas

15. An upper gastrointestinal radiographic series reveals gastric outlet obstruction in a 53-year-old female who has had nausea, vomiting, and mid-epigastric pain for several months. Upper endoscopy reveals an ulcerated, 2 × 4 cm mass at the pylorus. Which of the following neoplasms is most likely to be seen on biopsy of this mass?

○ (A) Non-Hodgkin lymphoma
○ (B) Neuroendocrine carcinoma
○ (C) Squamous cell carcinoma
○ (D) Adenocarcinoma
○ (E) Leiomyosarcoma

16. A 60-year-old male is severely anemic, and on rectal examination, his stool occult blood test result is found to be positive. However, no mucosal lesion is palpable. On physical examination of the abdomen, he has active bowel sounds with no masses or areas of tenderness. A colonoscopy reveals no identifiable source for his bleeding. Angiography reveals a 1-cm focus of dilated and tortuous vascular channels in the mucosa and submucosa of the cecum. The condition most likely to be present is

○ (A) Mesenteric vein thrombosis
○ (B) Internal hemorrhoids
○ (C) Angiodysplasia of the colon
○ (D) Collagenous colitis
○ (E) Colonic diverticulosis

17. A 73-year-old female is found to have iron deficiency anemia. She has no vaginal bleeding, hematemesis, hemoptysis, or melena. However, a stool guaiac test result is positive. A colonoscopy reveals a lesion whose gross appearance is shown here after partial colectomy. The lesion depicted here is most likely to be a (an)

○ (A) Malignant lymphoma
○ (B) Adenocarcinoma
○ (C) Leiomyosarcoma
○ (D) Tubular adenoma
○ (E) Carcinoid tumor

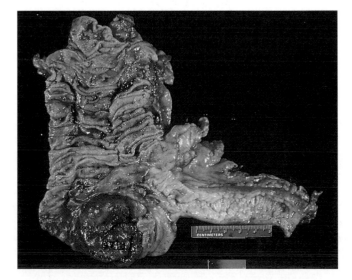

18. A 23-year-old female has had a bloody, mucoid diarrhea for the past week. A stool specimen is negative for ova and parasites. A sigmoidoscopy is performed, and there is friable, erythematous mucosa extending from the rectum to the mid-descending colon. A rectal biopsy shows acute mucosal inflammation with crypt abscesses and epithelial cell necrosis. Which of the following diseases is she most likely to have?

○ (A) Shigellosis
○ (B) Ulcerative colitis
○ (C) Crohn disease
○ (D) Diverticulitis
○ (E) Ischemic colitis

19. A 52-year-old male has experienced weight loss and nausea for the past 6 months. He does not have vomiting or diarrhea. Upper endoscopy reveals a 6-cm-diameter area of irregular pale fundic mucosa with loss of the rugal folds. A biopsy reveals a monomorphous infiltrate of lymphoid cells. *H. pylori* organisms are identified in mucus overlying adjacent mucosa. He receives antibiotic therapy for *H. pylori*, and the repeat biopsy shows a resolution of the infiltrate. The condition that best explains these findings is

○ (A) Chronic gastritis
○ (B) Burkitt type malignant lymphoma
○ (C) Autoimmune gastritis
○ (D) Mucosa-associated lymphoid tissue (MALT) tumor
○ (E) Crohn disease

20. A 70-year-old man ingests large quantities of nonsteroidal anti-inflammatory drugs (NSAIDS) for his chronic degenerative arthritis of the hips and knees. He has observed some recent epigastric pain along with nausea and vomiting. He then has an episode of hematemesis. Which of the following lesions will gastric biopsies most probably show?

○ (A) Epithelial dysplasia
○ (B) Hyperplastic polyp
○ (C) Acute gastritis
○ (D) Adenocarcinoma
○ (E) *H. pylori* infection

21. A barium swallow is performed in a 44-year-old female who has had difficulty swallowing for months. Radiographically, there is marked dilation of the esophagus with "beaking" in the distal portion where marked luminal narrowing exists. A biopsy of the lower esophagus shows prominent submucosal fibrosis without much inflammation. The most likely cause for these findings is

○ (A) Portal hypertension
○ (B) Iron deficiency
○ (C) Barrett esophagus
○ (D) CREST syndrome
○ (E) Hiatal hernia

22. A 35-year-old man presents with epigastric pain that tends to occur 2 to 3 hours after a meal and is relieved by antacids or food. There is no history of weight loss. He is a nonsmoker and not an alcoholic. A urea breath test result is positive, and a gastric biopsy result is positive for ure-

ase. He is asked to take a 2-week course of antibiotics. Four days after starting the treatment, he begins to feel well, and he discontinues the antibiotic treatment. Several weeks later, epigastric pain similar to the one he experienced earlier returns. If he does not seek further treatment, which of the following complications could develop?

○ (A) Hematemesis
○ (B) Fat malabsorption
○ (C) Hepatic metastases
○ (D) Carcinoid syndrome
○ (E) Vitamin B$_{12}$ deficiency

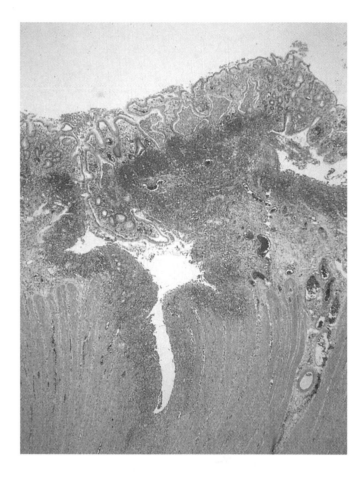

23. A 27-year-old male experiences the sudden onset of marked abdominal pain. His abdomen is diffusely tender and distended, with absent bowel sounds. He is taken to surgery, and a 27-cm segment of terminal ileum with a firm, erythematous serosal surface is removed. The microscopic appearance of a section through the ileum is shown here. Which of the following additional complications is most likely to develop as a result of this disease process?

○ (A) Metastatic adenocarcinoma
○ (B) Mesenteric artery thrombosis
○ (C) Intussusception
○ (D) Hepatic abscess
○ (E) Enterocutaneous fistula

For each of the clinical histories in questions 24 and 25, match the most closely associated condition producing inflammation in the gastrointestinal tract.

(A) Appendicitis
(B) Autoimmune gastritis
(C) Barrett esophagus
(D) Celiac disease
(E) Collagenous colitis
(F) Crohn's disease
(G) Diverticulitis
(H) Ischemic colitis
(I) Peptic ulcer
(J) Pseudomembranous colitis
(K) Spontaneous bacterial peritonitis
(L) Typhlitis
(M) Ulcerative colitis
(N) Whipple disease

24. A 59-year-old male with a long history of chronic alcoholism has noticed increasing abdominal girth for the past 6 months. He has had increasing abdominal pain for the past 2 days. Physical examination reveals a fluid wave, along with prominent caput medusae over the abdomen. There is diffuse abdominal tenderness. An abdominal radiograph reveals no free air. Paracentesis removes 500 mL of cloudy yellow fluid. A Gram stain of the fluid reveals gram-negative rods. (   )

25. A 62-year-old male with acute pyelonephritis has been receiving antibiotic therapy with cefotaxime, clindamycin, and nafcillin for the past 16 days. He now develops lower abdominal pain along with a severe diarrhea. *C. difficile* toxin is identified in a stool specimen. (   )

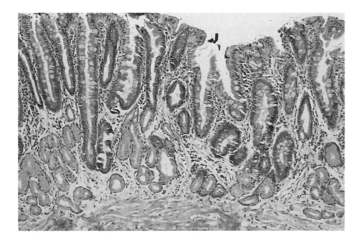

26. A 59-year-old male has had increasing difficulty with swallowing during the past 6 months. An endoscopy is performed, and biopsy of the lower esophagus yields the microscopic appearance shown here. Which of the following complications is most likely to occur with this lesion?

○ (A) Hematemesis
○ (B) Squamous cell carcinoma
○ (C) Adenocarcinoma
○ (D) Achalasia
○ (E) Lacerations (Mallory-Weiss syndrome)

27. One day after a meal of raw oysters, a healthy, 21-year-old woman develops watery diarrhea. Her stool is negative for occult blood. She has no abdominal distention or tenderness, and bowel sounds are present. The diarrhea subsides over the next couple of days. Which of the following organisms is most likely responsible for this case of food poisoning?

○ (A) *Y. enterocolitica*
○ (B) *S. aureus*
○ (C) *Cryptosporidium parvum*
○ (D) *E. histolytica*
○ (E) *V. parahaemolyticus*

28. A 57-year-old female noticed burning epigastric pain after meals for more than 1 year. An endoscopy reveals an erythematous patch in the lower esophageal mucosa. A biopsy of this lesion shows basal squamous epithelial hyperplasia, elongation of lamina propria papillae, and scattered intraepithelial neutrophils with some eosinophils. These findings are most typical for

○ (A) Barrett esophagus
○ (B) Esophageal varices
○ (C) Reflux esophagitis
○ (D) Scleroderma
○ (E) Iron deficiency

29. A 49-year-old woman presents with abdominal cramps and diarrhea. The stool specimen shows blood and mucus but no ova or parasites. These symptoms continue for 2 weeks, and the patient then begins to feel better without any treatment. The history reveals that similar episodes of self-limited pain and diarrhea have occurred several times during the past 20 years. Colonoscopy during one such episode revealed diffuse and uninterrupted mucosal inflammations and superficial ulceration extending from the rectum to the ascending colon. Colonic biopsies from this area showed a diffuse, predominantly mononuclear, infiltrate in the lamina propria. This patient is at a high risk for developing which of the following complications?

○ (A) Carcinoma of the colon
○ (B) Carcinoid of the rectum
○ (C) Primary biliary cirrhosis
○ (D) Fat malabsorption
○ (E) Pseudomembranous colitis

30. A 41-year-old male has been HIV positive for the past 8 years. His CD4 lymphocyte count is now 285/μL. For the past 2 weeks, he has experienced pain on swallowing. There is no hematemesis. He has no nausea or vomiting. Which of the following lesions best accounts for these findings?

○ (A) Esophageal squamous cell carcinoma
○ (B) Achalasia
○ (C) Lower esophageal fibrosis with stenosis
○ (D) Herpes simplex esophagitis
○ (E) Gastroesophageal reflux disease

31. A 67-year-old female has experienced a 9-kg weight loss with severe nausea, vomiting, and early satiety over the past 4 months. Upper endoscopy reveals that the entire

gastric mucosa is eroded and has an erythematous, cobble-stone appearance. An upper gastrointestinal radiographic series shows that the stomach is small and shrunken. Which of the following histologic findings is the gastric biopsy most likely to demonstrate?

- (A) Early gastric carcinoma
- (B) Leiomyosarcoma
- (C) Granulomatous inflammation
- (D) Chronic atrophic gastritis
- (E) Signet-ring cell adenocarcinoma

32. A 51-year-old male experiences the sudden onset of massive emesis of bright red blood. There have been no prior episodes of hematemesis. He is known to be hepatitis B surface antigen positive. His hematemesis is most likely a consequence of which of the following abnormalities of the esophagus?

- (A) Varices
- (B) Barrett esophagus
- (C) Candidiasis
- (D) Reflux esophagitis
- (E) Squamous cell carcinoma

33. A 16-year-old male who is receiving chemotherapy for acute lymphocytic leukemia presents with pain during swallowing food. Upper endoscopy reveals 0.5- to 0.8-cm mucosal ulcers in middle to lower esophageal region. These shallow ulcers are round and sharply demarcated with an erythematous base. The most probable cause for these findings is

- (A) Aphthous ulcerations
- (B) Herpes simplex esophagitis
- (C) Gastroesophageal reflux
- (D) *Candida* esophagitis
- (E) Mallory-Weiss syndrome

34. An 11-month-old, previously healthy infant is found by his mother to have no stool on inspection of the diaper. She notices also that the baby's abdomen is distended. On examination by the physician, the abdomen is very tender. Which of the following lesions best accounts for these findings?

- (A) Meckel diverticulum
- (B) Duodenal atresia
- (C) Hirschsprung disease
- (D) Pyloric stenosis
- (E) Intussusception

35. A 22-year-old female has had several episodes of aspiration of food associated with difficulty in swallowing. A barium swallow shows marked esophageal dilation above the level of the lower esophageal sphincter. A biopsy of the lower esophagus reveals absence of the myenteric ganglia. The condition that best accounts for these findings is

- (A) Hiatal hernia
- (B) Plummer-Vinson syndrome
- (C) Barrett esophagus
- (D) Systemic sclerosis
- (E) Achalasia

36. During a routine physical examination in a 53-year-old female, a rectal examination reveals stool positive for occult blood. A colonoscopy is performed and reveals a solitary 1.5-cm, rounded, erythematous polyp on a 0.5-cm stalk located at the splenic flexure. The polyp is removed. Histologically, it has the appearance shown in the following figures at low and high magnifications. When discussing these findings with the patient, which of the following statements is most appropriate?

- (A) You have inherited one defective copy of the APC gene.

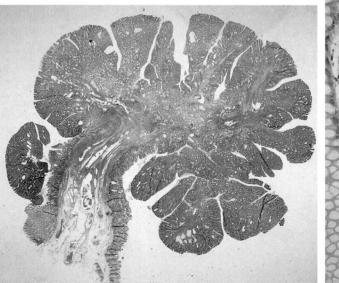

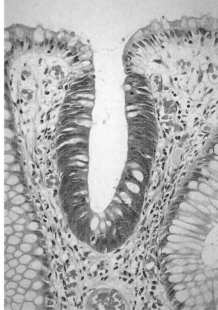

○ (B) Other family members probably have colonic polyps.

○ (C) Many more polyps will appear in the next few
years.

○ (D) There is a high probability that you will develop
endometrial cancer.

○ (E) A detailed workup to detect metastases from this
lesion is not warranted.

37. In her ninth month of pregnancy, a 20-year-old female has increasing pain on defecation and notices some
bright red blood on the toilet paper. She has had no previous gastrointestinal problems. After delivery of the baby,
her rectal pain subsides, and there is no more bleeding.
The most likely cause for these findings is

○ (A) Angiodysplasia
○ (B) Ischemic colitis
○ (C) Intussusception
○ (D) Hemorrhoids
○ (E) Volvulus

38. A neonate born at 32 weeks' gestational age was in
stable condition 3 days after birth and was feeding well.
There was no respiratory distress. However, the next day
the baby's abdomen appears distended and is tender. The
stool is positive for occult blood. Bacteremia and death
from septic shock ensues. What is the pathologist most
likely to find at autopsy that can account for the baby's
course?

○ (A) Dark red necrotic ileum and cecum
○ (B) Markedly dilated colon above the sigmoid
○ (C) Purulent ascitic fluid
○ (D) Markedly enlarged mesenteric lymph nodes
○ (E) A 5-cm mass in the retroperitoneum

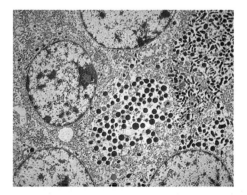

39. A 26-year-old male is brought to the emergency room
after sustaining abdominal gunshot injuries. While repairing
the small intestine at laparotomy, the surgeon notices a 2-
cm mass near the site of bowel perforation. This yellow-
tan and submucosal ileal mass is resected. The electron
micrograph shown in the figure depicts a neoplastic cell
from the mass. The cell of origin of this tumor is most
likely to be a

○ (A) Lipoblast
○ (B) Ganglion cell

○ (C) Neuroendocrine cell
○ (D) Smooth muscle cell
○ (E) Mucin-secreting epithelial cell

40. A 20-year-old female has experienced some nausea
and vague lower abdominal pain for the past 24 hours, but
now the pain has become more severe. On physical examination, the pain is worse in the right lower quadrant, with
rebound tenderness. Her stool is negative for occult blood.
Abdominal radiographs (plain films) reveal no free air. A
serum pregnancy test is negative. Which of the following
laboratory test findings is most useful to aid in the diagnosis of her condition?

○ (A) Hyperamylasemia
○ (B) Hypernatremia
○ (C) Increased serum carcinoembryonic antigen
○ (D) Increased serum alkaline phosphatase
○ (E) Leukocytosis

41. A 45-year-old female has a total serum bilirubin concentration of 8.9 mg/dL and a direct bilirubin level of 6.8
mg/dL. The serum alanine aminotransferase (ALT) level is
125 U/L, and the aspartate aminotransferase (AST) level is
108 U/L. A liver biopsy shows histologic findings characteristic for sclerosing cholangitis. Which of the following
gastrointestinal tract diseases is most likely to coexist in
this patient?

○ (A) Chronic pancreatitis
○ (B) Diverticulosis
○ (C) Ulcerative colitis
○ (D) Celiac sprue
○ (E) Peptic ulceration

42. One week after a trip to Central America, a 31-year-
old woman has an increasingly severe diarrhea. Gross examination of the stools reveals some mucus and blood
streaking. This diarrheal illness subsides in a couple of
weeks, but then she becomes febrile, with abdominal pain
in the right upper quadrant. An abdominal ultrasound reveals a 10-cm, irregular, partially cystic mass in the right
hepatic lobe. These findings are most suggestive of infection with

○ (A) *Giardia lamblia*
○ (B) *Cryptosporidium parvum*
○ (C) *Entamoeba histolytica*
○ (D) *Clostridium difficile*
○ (E) *Strongyloides stercoralis*

43. A 51-year-old female has been feeling tired for
months. A CBC demonstrates a hemoglobin concentration
of 9.5 g/dL, hematocrit of 29.1%, mean cell volume
(MCV) of 124 fL, platelet count of 268,000/μL, and WBC
count of 8350/μL. The reticulocyte index is low. Hypersegmented polymorphonuclear lymphocytes (PMNs) are
seen on the peripheral blood smear. Which of the following conditions involving the gastrointestinal tract is she
most likely to have?

○ (A) Ulcerative colitis of the rectum
○ (B) Adenocarcinoma of the cecum
○ (C) Barrett esophagus

○ (D) Chronic atrophic gastritis
○ (E) Chronic pancreatitis

44. Significant passage of meconium fails to occur after a normal birth at term. Three days postpartum, the baby vomits all oral feedings. An abdominal ultrasound shows marked colonic dilation above a narrow segment in the sigmoid region. A biopsy of this narrowed region shows an absence of ganglion cells in the muscle wall and submucosa. The most likely cause for these findings is

○ (A) Hirschsprung disease
○ (B) Trisomy 21
○ (C) Volvulus
○ (D) Colonic atresia
○ (E) Necrotizing enterocolitis

45. Gastric defense mechanisms against peptic ulcer disease include all of the following *except*

○ (A) Bicarbonate secretion into surface mucus
○ (B) Rapid gastric epithelial regeneration
○ (C) Surface epithelial cell mucus secretion
○ (D) Delayed emptying of gastric contents
○ (E) Robust mucosal blood flow

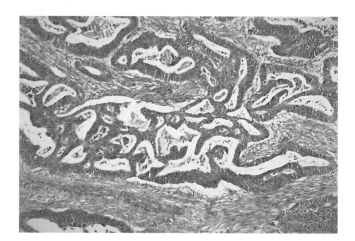

46. A microscopic section from an ulcerative lesion projecting into the cecum of a 30-year-old male is depicted here. This patient was found to have a stool positive for occult blood on routine physical examination. Which of the following molecular biologic events is believed to be critical in the development of such lesions?

○ (A) Overexpression of E-cadherin gene
○ (B) Amplification of *Erb-B2* gene
○ (C) Germ-line transmission of a defective *Rb* gene
○ (D) Germ-line transmission of a defective DNA mismatch repair gene
○ (E) Translocation of retinoic acid receptor-α gene

47. A 19-year-old male has a stool positive for occult blood on rectal examination. A colonoscopy is then performed, followed by a colectomy. The gross appearance of

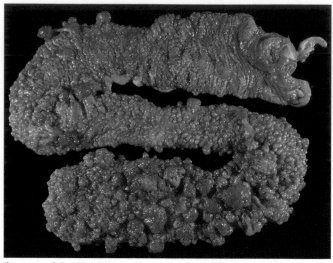

Courtesy of Dr. Tad Wicczorck, Brigham and Women's Hospital, Boston, MA.

the mucosal surface of this specimen is shown here. Molecular analysis of this patient's normal fibroblasts is likely to show a mutation in which of the following genes?

○ (A) APC
○ (B) *p53*
○ (C) *K-ras*
○ (D) HNPCC
○ (E) DCC

For each of the clinical histories in questions 48 and 49, match the most closely associated infectious agent:

(A) *Campylobacter jejuni*
(B) *Candida albicans*
(C) *Clostridium perfringens*
(D) *Cryptosporidium parvum*
(E) *Entamoeba histolytica*
(F) *Giardia lamblia*
(G) *Helicobacter pylori*
(H) *Mycobacterium tuberculosis*
(I) *Rotavirus*
(J) *Salmonella typhi*
(K) *Shigella flexneri*
(L) *Tropheryma whippleii*
(M) *Vibrio cholerae*
(N) *Yersenia enterocolitica*

48. A 46-year-old female with a long history of heartburn and dyspepsia experiences the sudden onset of severe mid-epigastric pain. An abdominal radiograph reveals free air under the diaphragm. She is immediately taken to surgery, and a perforated duodenal ulcer is repaired. (   )

49. An 8-month-old infant has a watery diarrhea that lasts for a week. There is no occult blood in the stool, and no ova or parasites are identified in a stool specimen. The child has a mild fever during her illness but no abdominal pain or swelling. Her parents give her plenty of fluids, and the infant recovers with no sequelae. (   )

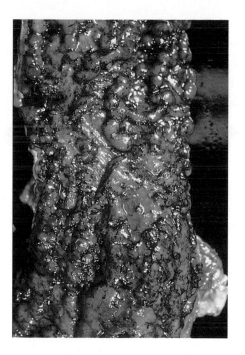

50. The gross appearance of the colectomy specimen shown in the figure from a 35-year-old female with migratory polyarthritis and ankylosing spondylitis is most characteristic for

○ (A) Ulcerative colitis
○ (B) Diverticulitis
○ (C) Pseudomembranous colitis
○ (D) Adenocarcinoma
○ (E) Familial adenomatous polyposis coli

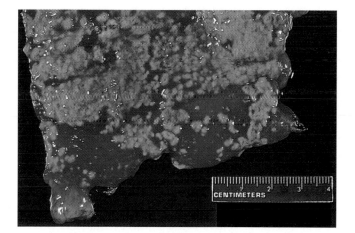

51. A 45-year-old woman is being treated for pneumonia complicated by septicemia in the hospital. She has required multiple antibiotics and was intubated and mechanically ventilated earlier in the course. On the 20th hospital day, she is observed to have abdominal distention. Bowel sounds are absent, and an abdominal radiograph reveals dilated loops of small bowel suggestive of ileus. She now has a low volume of bloody stool that is positive for *C. difficile* toxin. She is taken to surgery, and at laparotomy, a portion of distal ileum and cecum is resected. From the gross appearance of the mucosal surface shown here, the complication she has suffered is most likely to be

○ (A) Mesenteric arterial thrombosis
○ (B) Pseudomembranous enterocolitis
○ (C) Intussusception
○ (D) Cecal volvulus
○ (E) Toxic megacolon

52. After an extensive thermal burn injury involving 70% of his total body skin surface area, a 52-year-old previously healthy male was hospitalized in stable condition. However, 3 weeks after the initial burn injury, he was found to have melanotic stools. All attempts to resuscitate him failed. At autopsy the most likely finding will be

○ (A) Multiple small (2- to 5-mm in diameter) ulcers throughout the gastric mucosa that penetrate the submucosa and the muscularis propria
○ (B) Prominent and tortuous veins at the gastroesophageal junction with overlying irregular 0.5- to 1-cm ulcerations penetrating to submucosa
○ (C) A single, 1-cm, punched-out ulcer in the gastric antrum that penetrates the submucosa, with the ulcer base filled with granulation tissue
○ (D) Multiple small (2- to 5-mm in diameter) ulcers throughout the gastric mucosa that are confined to the mucosa
○ (E) Multiple small (2- to 5-mm in diameter) ulcers in metaplastic columnar epithelium at the lower end of the esophagus

53. A 68-year-old woman with a history of rheumatic heart disease is hospitalized with severe congestive heart failure. Several days after admission, she develops abdominal distention. An abdominal radiograph reveals no free air. There is absence of bowel sounds. Her stool is positive for occult blood. Colonoscopy reveals patchy areas of mucosal erythema with some overlying tan exudate in the ascending and descending colon. No polyps or masses are identified. The best explanation for these findings is

○ (A) Ulcerative colitis
○ (B) Volvulus
○ (C) Shigellosis
○ (D) Mesenteric vasculitis
○ (E) Ischemic colitis

54. A 27-year-old male had intermittent cramping abdominal pain for several weeks. He had some diarrhea with stools that were found to be positive for occult blood. These symptoms subsided in several days. However, the abdominal pain recurs 6 months later, along with perianal pain and formation of a perirectal fistula. Colonoscopic examination reveals many areas of mucosal edema and ulceration and some areas that appear quite normal. Microscopic examination of a biopsy shows patchy acute and chronic inflammatory infiltrate, crypt abscesses, and several noncaseating granulomas. The underlying disease process that best explains these findings is

○ (A) Crohn disease
○ (B) Amebiasis

○ (C) Shigellosis
○ (D) Sarcoidosis
○ (E) Ulcerative colitis

55. A 49-year-old male has complained of "heartburn" after meals for the past decade. Upper endoscopy is performed, and an esophageal biopsy is taken from an erythematous area of velvety mucosa just above the gastroesophageal junction. Microscopically, the mucosa demonstrates columnar metaplasia with goblet cells. The most probable cause for these findings is

○ (A) Esophageal varices
○ (B) Radiation therapy
○ (C) Achalasia
○ (D) Gastroesophageal reflux disease
○ (E) Iron deficiency anemia

56. A 65-year-old female has a positive stool occult blood test on a routine physical examination. A barium enema reveals numerous 1-cm outpouchings of the sigmoid and descending colon. Which of the following complications is most likely to occur from her colonic disease?

○ (A) Adenocarcinoma
○ (B) Pericolic abscess
○ (C) Bowel obstruction
○ (D) Malabsorption
○ (E) Toxic megacolon

57. A 54-year-old female has had increasing abdominal distention for the past 2 weeks. Paracentesis yields 1000 mL of slightly cloudy serous fluid. Cytologic examination of the fluid reveals malignant cells consistent with adenocarcinoma. Which of the following primary sites for this neoplasm is *least* likely to be the source of the metastases?

○ (A) Stomach
○ (B) Pancreas
○ (C) Ovary
○ (D) Jejunum
○ (E) Colon

For the clinical history in question 58, match the most closely associated description of a gastrointestinal mucosal histopathologic finding:

(A) Blunting and flattening of villi containing increased numbers of lymphocytes and plasma cells
(B) Crypt distortion with crypt abscess formation and superficial ulceration
(C) Densely packed tubular glands lined by dysplastic cells with hyperchromatic nuclei
(D) Extensive diffuse hemorrhage and necrosis
(E) Infiltrates of large monoclonal B lymphocytes
(F) Intact epithelium with overlying mucus containing *H. pylori* organisms
(G) Irregular ulceration with chronic inflammation and granuloma formation
(H) Saclike protrusion of the mucosa through the muscularis

(I) Sharply demarcated ulceration with epithelial cells containing intranuclear inclusions
(J) Tearing of an intact mucosa with resultant extensive hemorrhage

58. A 32-year-old male presents with a 1-week history of nausea and vomiting. He has cachexia, having lost 15 kg in the past 2 months. A 10-cm, nontender mass is palpable in the mid-abdominal region. An abdominal computed tomography (CT) scan reveals that this mass involves the small intestine. He is found to be HIV positive. (   )

ANSWERS

1. **(C)** This patient has malabsorption that responded to dietary treatment. She probably has celiac disease (i.e., gluten sensitivity). The histologic features of celiac disease are flattening of the mucosa, diffuse and severe atrophy of the villi, and chronic inflammation of the lamina propria. There is an increase in intraepithelial lymphocytes. Lymphatic obstruction occurs in Whipple disease. In addition foamy macrophages accumulate in the lamina propria. They contain periodic acid—Schiff (PAS)-positive granules that under the electron microscope reveal an actinomycete called *T. whippleii*. Noncaseating granulomas are found in the intestinal wall in Crohn disease. Crypt abscesses are nonspecific and can be seen in inflammatory bowel disease.
BP6 498   PBD6 813

2. **(D)** Infection by one of several *Salmonella* species (not typhi) leads to a self-limited diarrhea. This is a form of food poisoning, typically from contaminated poultry products. *Y. enterocolitica* is most often found in contaminated milk or pork products and may disseminate to produce lymphadenitis and further extraintestinal infection. A variety of diseases result from contamination with various strains of *E. coli*, based on the characteristics of the organisms and whether they invade or produce an enterotoxin. Poultry products are usually not contaminated with *E. coli*. Amebiasis from *E. histolytica* can be an invasive, exudative infection. The stools contain blood and mucus. Rotavirus is most often seen in children; in adults, a self-limited watery diarrhea is the rule; there is no particular association of this infection with a specific food product.
BP6 495   PBD6 806–808

3. **(B)** Granulomas are a feature of Crohn disease, although they are present in only about one half of cases. They can be located anywhere from the mucosa to the serosa and are typically small and noncaseating. The inflammation of celiac sprue consists predominantly of mononuclear cells. Ulcerative colitis can be difficult to distinguish from Crohn disease, although the inflammation of ulcerative colitis is typically mucosal, and granulomas are absent. With autoimmune gastritis, there is mucosal atrophy and minimal chronic inflammation. The esophageal inflammation seen with gastroesophageal reflux

disease shows a mixture of acute and chronic inflammatory cells.
BP6 502   PBD6 821

4. **(C)** The history of myocardial infarction suggests that this patient had severe coronary atherosclerosis. Atheromatous disease most likely involved the mesenteric vessels as well, giving rise to thrombosis of the blood vessels that perfuse the bowel. The symptoms and signs suggest infarction of the gut. Acute appendicitis rarely leads to such a catastrophic illness, unless there is perforation. (The absence of free air in the radiograph argues against perforation of any viscus). Acute pancreatitis can also be a serious abdominal emergency, but normal levels of amylase and lipase tend to exclude this. Acute cholecystitis can present with severe abdominal pain, but bloody diarrhea and absence of bowel sounds (i.e., paralytic ileus) are unlikely. Pseudomembranous colitis develops in the setting of antibiotic therapy.
BP6 491–492   PBD6 820–822

5. **(B)** *H. pylori* lives in the gastric mucus and is associated with a variety of gastric disorders from chronic gastritis to peptic ulcers to adenocarcinoma. Erythema and thickened rugal folds in this patient indicate chronic gastritis. *Candida* produces mucosal plaques in immunocompromised patients, typically in the oral cavity, sometimes in the esophagus, and rarely in the stomach. *S. typhi* is the causative agent of typhoid fever, and pathologic lesions are most often observed in the small bowel. *T. whippleii* is the infectious agent associated with the malabsorption seen in Whipple disease. *C. difficile* is associated with a pseudomembranous enterocolitis.
BP6 482–484   PBD6 790–792

6. **(D)** Kaposi sarcoma, along with non-Hodgkin lymphoma and anorectal squamous carcinoma, can be associated with AIDS. It can be found anywhere in the body, including gastrointestinal tract. Kaposi sarcoma is a vascular lesion—hence the color. These lesions are rarely large enough to cause obstruction.
BP6 125   PBD6 535–537

7. **(A)** This patient had a large villous adenoma (depicted). There is a high probability (>40%) that large villous adenomas (>4 cm in diameter) will progress to invasive adenocarcinoma. These lesions, when they occur in the descending colon, are annular and cause obstruction.
BP6 506–507   PBD6 830

8. **(B)** This large, ulcerated lesion with heaped up margins is a malignant tumor of the esophageal mucosa. There are two main histologic types of esophageal carcinomas—squamous cell carcinoma and adenocarcinoma—with distinct risk factors. Smoking and alcoholism are the most frequent risk factors for esophageal squamous cell carcinoma in the Western world. Adenocarcinoma is most likely to arise in the lower third of the esophagus and be associated with Barrett esophagus. Intranuclear inclusions suggest infection with herpes simplex virus or cytomegalovirus, both of which are more likely to produce ulceration without a mass, and both are seen in immunocompromised

patients. Chronic inflammation may lead to stricture and not to a localized mass. Thrombosed veins occur with sclerotherapy for esophageal varices; they do not produce an ulcerated mass.
BP6 480   PBD6 783–786

9. **(C)** The clinical and histologic features are most suggestive of celiac sprue. This rare chronic disease may be manifested in childhood, but in some persons, it may not be bothersome until young adulthood. Celiac sprue results from gluten sensitivity. Exposure to the gliadin protein in wheat, oats, barley, and rye (but not rice) results in intestinal inflammation. Hence, a trial of gluten-free diet is the most logical therapeutic option. This usually cures the symptoms and restores normal mucosal histology. Antibiotic therapy can be beneficial if the malabsorption is caused by tropical sprue or Whipple disease. The histologic features of Whipple disease are distinct. The mucosa is laden with distended macrophages containing PAS-positive granules and a gram-positive actinomycete called *T. whippleii*. Tropical sprue is very unlikely in a resident of North America. Supplemental fat-soluble vitamins can reduce vitamin deficiency but cannot resolve malabsorption. Vitamin B_{12} is indicated in pernicious anemia, characterized by the presence of atrophic gastritis. Corticosteroid therapy is nonspecific and is sometimes used to treat inflammatory bowel disease.
BP6 498   PBD6 813

10. **(B)** The clinical features suggest food poisoning caused by the ingestion of a preformed enterotoxin. *S. aureus* grows in the food (milk products and fatty foods are favorites) and elaborates an enterotoxin that, when ingested, produces diarrhea within hours. Some strains of *E. coli* can produce a variety of diarrheal illnesses but without a preformed toxin. *V. parahaemolyticus* is found in shellfish. *C. difficile* can produce a pseudomembranous colitis in patients treated with broad spectrum antibiotics. *Salmonella enteritidis* is most often found in poultry products, but the diarrheal illnesses takes a couple of days to develop.
BP6 494–495   PBD6 809

11. **(D)** Disaccharidase (lactase) deficiency is an uncommon congenital condition (or a rare acquired condition) in which the lactose in milk products is not broken down into glucose and galactose, resulting in an osmotic diarrhea and gas production from gut flora. Affected persons do not always make the connection between diet and symptoms, or they do not consume enough milk products to become symptomatic. Celiac sprue is also diet related and results from a sensitivity to gluten in some grains. An autoimmune gastritis is most likely to result in vitamin B_{12} malabsorption. Cholelithiasis could result in biliary tract obstruction with malabsorption of fats or with right upper quadrant abdominal pain. Cystic fibrosis affects the pancreas to produce mainly fat malabsorption.
BP6 497   PBD6 815

12. **(A)** This patient is most likely to have fat malabsorption. Smelly, bulky stools containing increased amounts of fat (steatorrhea) are characteristic for malabsorption of fats. Pancreatic or biliary tract diseases are important causes of

fat malabsorption. Giardiasis produces mainly a watery diarrhea. Malabsorption with steatorrhea is unlikely to be associated with any bleeding. Cholera results in a massive watery diarrhea. Amebiasis can produce findings ranging from a watery diarrhea to dysentery with mucus and blood in the stool.

BP6 493   PBD6 806

13. **(A)** Adenocarcinomas of the esophagus are typically located in the lower esophagus, where the Barrett esophagus arises in the setting of long-standing gastroesophageal reflux disease. Barrett esophagus is associated with a greatly increased risk of developing adenocarcinoma. Leiomyosarcoma of the esophagus is rare and unrelated to a history of "heartburn." Squamous cell carcinomas of the esophagus are most often associated with a history of chronic alcoholism and smoking. Malignant lymphomas of the gastrointestinal tract do not commonly occur in the esophagus and are not related to reflux esophagitis. Carcinoid tumors occur in different parts of the gut, including the appendix, ileum, rectum, stomach, and colon.

BP6 480-481   PBD6 786-787

14. **(A)** This condition occurs several weeks after birth because of hypertrophy of pyloric smooth muscle. A tracheoesophageal fistula, diaphragmatic hernia, and duodenal atresia are serious conditions manifested at birth and often associated with multiple anomalies. Pyloric stenosis is a sporadic condition that occurs typically without other associated anomalies. Annular pancreas is an anomaly that is rare.

BP6 482   PBD6 789

15. **(D)** The most likely cause for a large mass lesion in the stomach is a gastric carcinoma, and these lesions are adenocarcinomas. Squamous cell carcinomas appear in the esophagus. Malignant lymphomas and leiomyosarcomas are less common but do occur, and they tend to form bulky masses in the fundus. Neuroendocrine carcinomas are rare.

BP6 489   PBD6 800-801

16. **(C)** Angiodysplasia refers to tortuous dilations of mucosal and submucosal vessels, seen most often in the cecum in individuals older than 50 years of age. These lesions, although not common, account for 20% of significant lower intestinal bleeding. Bleeding is usually not massive but can occur intermittently over months to years. This lesion is very difficult to diagnose and is often found radiographically. The focus (or foci) of abnormal vessels can be excised. Mesenteric venous thrombosis is rare and may result in bowel infarction with severe abdominal pain. Hemorrhoids at the anorectal junction can account for bright red rectal bleeding, but they can be seen or palpated on rectal examination. Collagenous colitis is a rare cause for a watery diarrhea that is typically not bloody. Colonic diverticulosis can be associated with hemorrhage, but the outpouchings should be seen with colonoscopy.

BP6 493   PBD6 823

17. **(B)** This large, fungating mass is a typical adenocarcinoma of the right colon. Such cancers are unlikely to obstruct, but they can bleed a small amount over months to years and give rise to iron deficiency anemia. Adenomas and carcinoid tumors average 1 cm or less in diameter. They are not ulcerated masses. A leiomyosarcoma produces a bulky mass but is not common and does not project as a fungating mass in the cecum. Malignant lymphomas can also be bulky masses, but they are not exophytic and are rare except in persons with immunocompromised states such as AIDS.

BP6 510   PBD6 834

18. **(B)** The continuous mucosal involvement to a demarcated end point is more typical of ulcerative colitis than Crohn disease, both of which are idiopathic inflammatory bowel diseases. Infections with *Shigella* species should involve most of the colon. Diverticular disease is unusual at this age, as is ischemic bowel disease.

BP6 501-502   PBD6 818-820

19. **(D)** Gastrointestinal lymphomas of a special type that arise from mucosa-associated lymphoid tissue (MALT) are called MALT lymphomas. Gastric lymphomas that occur in association with *H. pylori* infection are made up of monoclonal B cells, whose growth and proliferation remains dependent on cytokines derived from T cells that are sensitized to *H. pylori* antigens. Treatment with antibiotics eliminates *H. pylori* and therefore the stimulus for B-cell growth. MALT lesions can occur anywhere in the gastrointestinal tract, although they are rare in esophagus and appendix. *H. pylori* infection may be seen in chronic gastritis, and this may precede lymphoma development. Burkitt lymphoma and other non-Hodgkin lymphomas that are not MALT lymphomas do not regress with antibiotic therapy. Crohn disease is rare in the stomach and is not related to *H. pylori* infection.

BP6 513   PBD6 837-838

20. **(C)** Prolonged use of NSAIDs is an important cause of acute gastritis. Excessive alcohol consumption and smoking are also possible causes. Acute gastritis tends to be diffuse and, when severe, can lead to significant hemorrhage that is difficult to control. Epithelial dysplasia may occur in the setting of chronic gastritis. It is a forerunner of gastric cancer. Hyperplastic polyps of the stomach do not result from acute gastritis but may arise in the setting of chronic gastritis. Acute gastritis does not increase the risk for gastric adenocarcinoma. *H. pylori* infection is not associated with acute gastritis.

BP6 483-484   PBD6 789-790

21. **(D)** Esophageal dysmotility is the "E" in CREST syndrome, the limited form of systemic sclerosis (i.e., scleroderma). Although this disease is autoimmune in nature, little inflammation is seen by the time the patients come to clinical attention. There is increased collagen deposition in submucosa and muscularis. Fibrosis may affect any part of the gastrointestinal tract, but the esophagus is the site most often involved. Portal hypertension gives rise to esophageal varices, not fibrosis. For a diagnosis of Barrett esophagus, columnar metaplasia must be seen histologically, and there is often a history of gastroesophageal reflux disease. An upper esophageal web associated with iron deficiency ane-

mia might produce difficulty in swallowing, but this is a rare condition. Hiatal hernia is frequently diagnosed in persons with reflux esophagitis, and this can lead to inflammation, ulceration, and bleeding, but formation of a stricture is uncommon.
BP6 476, 112–113   PBD6 778–779

22. **(A)** The clinical symptoms suggest peptic ulcer. In most cases, peptic ulcers are associated with *H. pylori* infection. These bacteria secrete urease that can be detected by oral administration of ^{14}C-labeled urea. After drinking the labeled urea solution, the patient blows into a tube. If *H. pylori* urease is present in the stomach, the urea is hydrolyzed, and labeled CO_2 is detected in the breath sample. Detection of urease in a gastric biopsy specimen is also used for diagnosis of *H. pylori* infection. If not properly treated, peptic ulcers can develop many complications, including massive bleeding that may be fatal. There is no fat malabsorption because no step in fat absorption occurs in the stomach. Peptic ulcers rarely progress to gastric carcinoma, and hence metastases are unlikely. Carcinoid tumors can occur in the stomach, but they are rare and are not related to peptic ulcer disease, which this patient has. Vitamin B_{12} deficiency can occur with autoimmune atrophic gastritis, because intrinsic factor, required for vitamin B_{12} absorption, is produced in gastric parietal cells.
BP6 484–486   PBD6 793–796

23. **(E)** The ileum shows chronic inflammation with lymphoid aggregates. The inflammation is transmural, affecting the mucosa, submucosa, and muscularis. A deep fissure extending into the muscularis is also seen. These histologic features are highly suggestive of Crohn disease. Extension of fissures into the overlying skin can produce enterocutaneous fistulas, although enteroenteric fistulas between loops of bowel are more common. Mesenteric artery thrombosis, typically a complication of atherosclerosis, is unlikely in a 27-year-old man. Intussusception may occur when there is a congenital or acquired obstruction in the bowel. Hepatic abscess can follow amebic colitis.
BP6 499–500;   PBD6 816–818

24. **(K)** Spontaneous bacterial peritonitis is an uncommon complication seen in about 10% of adult patients with cirrhosis of the liver who have ascites. The ascitic fluid provides an excellent culture medium for bacteria, which can invade the bowel wall or spread hematogenously to the serosa. Spontaneous bacterial peritonitis can also appear in children, particularly those with nephrotic syndrome and ascites. The most common organism cultured is *E. coli*.
PBD6 841

25. **(J)** Pseudomembranous colitis, caused by overgrowth of *C. difficile*, occurs when the normal gut flora is altered by broad spectrum antibiotic therapy.
BP6 495–496   PBD6 809–810

26. **(C)** The biopsy shows columnar metaplasia, typical for Barrett esophagus. Patients with a greater than 2-cm focus of Barrett esophagus are at 30-fold to 40-fold higher risk of developing adenocarcinoma than the general popu-

lation. Squamous cell carcinomas do occur in the esophagus, but they do not arise in the setting of Barrett esophagus. Their occurrence is related to smoking and alcohol consumption. Hematemesis is a complication of esophageal varices and other conditions such as peptic ulcers. Achalasia refers to failure of relaxation of the lower esophageal sphincter that gives rise to dilatation of the proximal portion of esophagus. Mallory-Weiss syndrome is associated with vertical lacerations in the esophagus that may occur with severe vomiting and retching.
BP6 479   PBD6 781–782

27. **(E)** Raw or poorly cooked shellfish can be the source for *V. parahaemolyticus*, which, unlike *V. cholerae*, tends to produce a milder diarrhea. *Y. enterocolitica* is invasive and can produce extraintestinal infection. *S. aureus* can produce food poisoning through elaboration of an enterotoxin that causes an explosive diarrhea in a couple of hours after being ingested. *Cryptosporidium* as a cause for a watery diarrhea is most often seen in immunocompromised persons. *E. histolytica* produces colonic mucosal invasion with exudation and ulceration. Therefore, stools contain blood and mucus.
BP6 495   PBD6 808

28. **(C)** These are changes of an ongoing inflammatory process resulting from reflux of acid gastric contents into the lower esophagus. Gastroesophageal reflux disease (GERD) is a common problem that stems from a variety of causes, including sliding hiatal hernia, decreased tone of the lower esophageal sphincter, and delayed gastric emptying. Patients may give a history of "heartburn" after eating. Barrett esophagus is a complication of long-standing GERD and is characterized by columnar metaplasia of the squamous epithelium that normally lines the esophagus. There may be inflammation and mucosal ulceration overlying varices, but this condition does not usually have heartburn as the major feature. Progressive fibrosis with stenosis is seen with scleroderma. A rare complication of iron deficiency is the appearance of an upper esophageal web (i.e., Plummer-Vinson syndrome).
BP6 478–479   PBD6 780–781

29. **(A)** This patient has clinical and histologic features of ulcerative colitis. Particularly important are relapsing and remitting episodes of diarrhea with blood and mucus and diffuse inflammation and ulceration of the rectal and colonic mucosa. One of the most dreaded complications of ulcerative colitis is the development of colonic adenocarcinoma. The risk is 20-fold to 30-fold higher, compared with control populations, in patients who have had the disease for 10 years or longer. Carcinoid tumors can occur in the rectum, but there is no association with ulcerative colitis. Ulcerative colitis is associated with several extraintestinal manifestations, including sclerosing cholangitis, but it has no relationship to primary biliary cirrhosis. Fat malabsorption does not occur in ulcerative colitis because the ileum is not involved. Pseudomembranous colitis is caused by *C. difficile* infections in the setting of antibiotic treatment.
BP6 502   PBD6 818–820

30. **(D)** A person infected with HIV with low CD4$^+$ cell counts is at great risk for developing infections. Herpes

simplex and *Candida* are the most likely upper gastrointestinal infections involving esophagus. Squamous cell carcinoma of the esophagus is not related to HIV infection. Achalasia, caused by a failure of relaxation of the lower esophageal sphincter, is not a feature of HIV infection or immunosuppression. Fibrosis with stenosis is a feature of reflux and of scleroderma.
BP6 125   PBD6 782

31.   **(E)** This is the linitis plastica (leather bottle) appearance of diffuse gastric carcinoma. Histologically, these carcinomas are composed of gastric-type mucus cells that infiltrate the stomach wall diffusely. The individual tumor cells have a signet-ring appearance, because the cytoplasmic mucin pushes the nucleus to one side. Early gastric carcinoma, by definition, is confined to the mucosa and submucosa. Leiomyosarcomas tend to be bulky masses. Granulomas are rare at this site. The rugal folds are lost with chronic atrophic gastritis, but there is no significant scarring or shrinkage.
BP6 489   PBD6 800–801

32.   **(A)** Variceal bleeding is a common complication of hepatic cirrhosis, which can be an outcome of chronic hepatitis B infection. The resultant portal hypertension leads to dilated submucosal esophageal veins that can erode and bleed profusely. Barrett esophagus is a columnar metaplasia that results from gastroesophageal reflux disease. Bleeding is not a key feature of this disease. Esophageal candidiasis may be seen in immunocompromised patients, but it most often produces raised mucosal plaques. Esophageal reflux may produce acute and chronic inflammation and rarely produce massive hemorrhage. Esophageal carcinomas may bleed, but not enough to cause massive hematemesis.
BP6 478   PBD6 783

33.   **(B)** These "punched-out" ulcers result from rupture of the herpetic vesicles. Herpesvirus and *Candida* infections typically occur in immunocompromised patients, and both can involve the esophagus. However, with candidiasis the gross appearance is that of tan to yellow plaques. Aphthous ulcers (i.e., canker sores) can also be seen in immunocompromised persons, but these shallow ulcers are seen most frequently in the oral cavity. GERD can produce acute and chronic inflammation with some erosion, although not typically in a sharply demarcated pattern; GERD has no relation to immune status. Mallory-Weiss syndrome results from mucosal tears of the esophagus. Such laceration of the esophagus can occur with severe vomiting and retching.
BP6 478   PBD6 782

34.   **(E)** Intussusception occurs when one small segment of small bowel becomes telescoped into the immediately distal segment. This disorder can have a sudden onset in infants and may occur in the absence of an anatomic abnormality. Almost all cases of Meckel diverticulum are asymptomatic, although in some cases functional gastric mucosa is present that can lead to ulceration with bleeding. Duodenal atresia (which typically occurs with other anomalies) and Hirschsprung disease should have clinical

manifestations soon after birth. Pyloric stenosis is seen much earlier in life and is characterized by projectile vomiting.
BP6 490, 504   PBD6 826

35.   **(E)** In achalasia, there is incomplete relaxation of the lower esophageal sphincter. Most cases are "primary," or of unknown origin. They are believed to be caused by degenerative changes in neural innervation, and hence the myenteric ganglia are usually absent from the body of the esophagus. There is a long-term risk for development of squamous cell carcinoma. Reflux esophagitis may be associated with hiatal hernia, but myenteric ganglia remain intact. The Plummer-Vinson syndrome is a rare condition caused by iron deficiency anemia, and it is accompanied by an upper esophageal web. In Barrett esophagus, there is columnar epithelial metaplasia, but the myenteric plexuses remain intact. Systemic sclerosis (i.e., scleroderma) is marked by fibrosis with stricture.
BP6 477   PBD6 778–779

36.   **(E)** This is a solitary pedunculated adenoma of the colon with no evidence of malignancy. Under high magnification, a small focus of dysplastic, non–mucin-secreting epithelial cells is seen lining a colonic crypt, giving rise to "tubular" architecture. Such a small (<2 cm) solitary tubular adenoma is unlikely to harbor a focus of malignancy, and hence a search for metastases is unwarranted. Those who inherit a mutant APC gene usually develop hundreds of polyps at a young age, therefore, this patient does not need genetic testing for a somatic mutation in the *APC* gene. Patients with hereditary nonpolyposis colorectal cancer have an increased risk for endometrial cancer and develop colon cancer at a young age.
BP6 508–509   PBD6 829–830

37.   **(D)** This patient has hemorrhoids. This is a common problem that can stem from any condition that increases venous pressure and causes dilation of internal or external hemorrhoidal veins above and below the anorectal junction. Angiodysplasia of the colon leads to intermittent hemorrhage, typically in older persons. Ischemic colitis is rare in young persons, because the most common underlying cause (severe atherosclerotic disease involving mesenteric vessels) is seen at an older age. Intussusception and volvulus are rare causes for mechanical bowel obstruction that occur suddenly in adults and are surgical emergencies.
BP6 493   PBD6 823

38.   **(A)** This baby has neonatal necrotizing enterocolitis, a complication of prematurity. Necrotizing enterocolitis is believed to result from immaturity of the gut immune system and is often precipitated by oral feeding. The necrotic bowel can perforate. Hirschsprung disease with colonic dilation above an aganglionic segment has a lack of stools but no necrosis. A bacterial peritonitis could be seen with ascites as a consequence of necrotizing enterocolitis. However, this is a complication, not the cause. Mesenteric lymphadenitis can likewise accompany infection and on occasion cause bowel obstruction but is not the cause for necrotizing enterocolitis. A retroperitoneal mass such as a neuroblastoma could be present at birth and can sometimes

cause bowel obstruction from a mass effect but not necrotizing enterocolitis.
BP6 497   PBD6 809

39.   **(C)** This is a carcinoid tumor. The cytoplasm of the tumor cell contains small, dark, round dense core (neurosecretory) granules that are characteristic of neuroendocrine cells. The gross appearance of this tumor and its location are also characteristic of carcinoid tumors. Many small carcinoids and other small, benign bowel tumors are discovered incidentally. Most are 2 cm in diameter or smaller.
BP6 512   PBD6 836

40.   **(E)** These findings point to acute appendicitis. The elevated WBC count with neutrophilia is helpful but not decisive, and the choice to operate must be made with clinical judgment. Hyperamylasemia occurs in acute pancreatitis. Diarrhea with fluid loss and dehydration can lead to hypernatremia. The serum carcinoembryonic antigen level can be increased in patients with colonic cancers. However, this test is not specific for colon cancer. The alkaline phosphatase level can be increased with biliary tract obstruction.
BP6 514   PBD6 839-840

41.   **(C)** Sclerosing cholangitis is a serious extraintestinal manifestation of idiopathic inflammatory bowel disease, most often ulcerative colitis or, to a lesser extent, Crohn disease. Pancreatitis and cholangitis may be complications of biliary tract lithiasis, but they have no association with sclerosing cholangitis. Diverticulosis may be complicated by diverticulitis, but the liver is not involved. Peptic ulcer disease does not lead to hepatic complications.
BP6 503, 543-545   PBD6 818-820

42.   **(C)** Diarrhea with mucus and blood in the stools can be caused by several enteroinvasive microorganisms, including *Shigella dysenteriae* and *E. histolytica*. In most cases, the diarrhea is self-limited. The initial episode of diarrhea could have been caused by one of several organisms. However, the occurrence of a liver abscess after an episode of diarrhea most likely results from *E. histolytica* infection. Colonic mucosal and submucosal invasion *by E. histolytica* allows the organisms to gain access to submucosal veins draining to the portal system and to the liver. *Giardia* produces a self-limited, watery diarrhea. Dissemination of *Cryptosporidium* and *Strongyloides* may occur in immunocompromised patients. *C. difficile* causes pseudomembranous colitis after antibiotic therapy.
BP6 496   PBD6 811

43.   **(D)** She has a megaloblastic anemia, with a high mean cell volume. Delayed maturation of the myeloid cells leads to hypersegmentation of PMNs. She most likely has pernicious anemia, resulting from autoimmune atrophic gastritis. Loss of gastric parietal cells from autoimmune injury causes a deficiency of intrinsic factor. In the absence of this factor, vitamin B_{12} cannot be absorbed in the distal ileum. Rectal ulcerative colitis does not affect gastrointestinal absorptive function significantly. The focal nature of a carcinoma is also unlikely to affect absorption of nutrients, and the cecum is not involved with B_{12} absorption. The

gastroesophageal reflux leading to Barrett esophagus does not affect gastric production of intrinsic factor. Pancreatitis may affect absorption of fats, but the B vitamins are water soluble and not affected, and B_{12} has its own mechanism for absorption.
BP6 356, 482   PBD6 622-625, 791

44.   **(A)** This patient has Hirschsprung disease. The aganglionic segment of the bowel wall produces a functional obstruction with proximal distention. Atresias are congenitally narrowed segments of bowel—usually small intestine—that occur with other anomalies. Patients with trisomy 21 may have intestinal (usually duodenal) atresias. Volvulus is a form of mechanical obstruction that occurs from twisting of the small bowel on the mesentery or twisting of a segment of the colon (sigmoid or cecal regions). Necrotizing enterocolitis is a complication of prematurity.
BP6 490-491   PBD6 805

45.   **(D)** Delayed emptying promotes ulceration by keeping the stimulus to acid secretion active. The bicarbonate acts as a buffer to prevent damage from acid. The epithelium of the gastrointestinal tract regenerates quickly to repair injury. The mucus covering the surface epithelium guards against injury. Robust mucosal blood flow, aided by prostaglandin secretion, helps to diminish the amount of acid back-diffused into the mucosa.
BP6 484-485   PBD6 788

46.   **(D)** The lesion is an adenocarcinoma, showing irregular glands infiltrating the muscle layer. Such a lesion in a 30-year-old male strongly indicates a hereditary predisposition. One form of hereditary colon carcinoma results from inheritance of a defective copy of the DNA mismatch repair genes. A second mutation at the same locus inactivates both copies of such genes and cripples the ability to repair certain forms of DNA damage. The resultant genomic instability predisposes to early onset colon carcinoma. This type of cancer is called hereditary nonpolyposis colorectal carcinoma (HNPCC). Unlike familial adenomatous polyposis (FAP) syndrome, HNPCC does not lead to the development of hundreds of polyps in the colon. E-cadherin is required for intercellular adhesion. Its levels are reduced, not increased, in carcinoma cells. Detection of c-Erb-B2 (HER2-neu) expression is important in breast cancers. Germ-line inheritance of the tumor suppressor gene Rb predisposes to retinoblastoma and osteosarcoma, not colon carcinoma. Translocation of the retinoic acid receptor gene is characteristic of acute promyelocytic leukemia.
BP6 507-508   PBD6 832-833

47.   **(A)** This young patient's colon shows hundreds of polyps. This is most likely a case of familial adenomatous polyposis syndrome (FAP), which results from having inherited one mutant copy of the APC tumor suppressor gene. Every somatic cell of this individual will most likely have one defective copy of the APC gene. Polyps are formed when the second copy of the APC gene is lost in many colonic epithelial cells. Without treatment, colonic cancers arise in 100% of these patients because of accumulation of additional mutations in one or more polyps, typi-

cally by the third decade. Patients with the hereditary non-polyposis colorectal carcinoma also have an inherited susceptibility to develop colon cancer, but, unlike in FAP, they do not develop numerous polyps. The other three genes, *p53*, *K-ras*, and DCC, can all be mutated in sporadic colon cancers, but the somatic cells of these patients do not show abnormalities of these genes.
BP6 508–509   PBD6 831–833

48.   **(G)** Although not found in the duodenum, the *H. pylori* organisms result in an altered microenvironment in the stomach that favors peptic ulcer disease in stomach and duodenum. Virtually all duodenal peptic ulcers are associated with *H. pylori*. Ulceration can extend through the muscularis and result in perforation, as occurred in this case.
BP6 484–485   PBD6 793–796

49.   **(I)** Rotavirus is the most common cause for viral gastroenteritis in children. It is a self-limited disease that affects mostly infants and young children, who can lose a significant amount of fluid. The death rate is less than 1%.
BP6 494   PBD6 806

50.   **(A)** This segment of the colon shows diffuse and severe ulceration characteristic of ulcerative colitis. The inflammation from ulcerative colitis shown here is so severe that areas of mucosal ulceration have left pseudopolyps, or islands of residual mucosa. Ulcerative colitis is a systemic disease and is associated in some patients with migratory polyarthritis, ankylosing spondylitis, and primary sclerosing cholangitis. Diverticulitis can have severe inflammation, although without extensive mucosal necrosis. The tan-green pseudomembrane of pseudomembranous colitis lies above the mucosa, which remains largely intact. The carpet of polyps seen with familial polyposis is not accompanied by significant inflammation or necrosis.
BP6 502   PBD6 818–820

51.   **(B)** The opened colon shows fibrinopurulent debris attached to the mucosa. These patches are called pseudomembranes. Pseudomembranous enterocolitis is a complication of broad-spectrum antibiotic therapy, which alters gut flora to allow overgrowth of *C. difficile* or other organisms capable of inflicting mucosal injury. This gross pattern can also appear from ischemic injury that is vascular or mechanical, but the time course for and history of this patient support an iatrogenic cause. A dilated, thinned toxic megacolon is an uncommon complication of ulcerative colitis.
BP6 495–496   BD6 809–810

52.   **(D)** These are so-called stress ulcers, known also as Curling ulcers with burn injuries. The ulcers are small (< 1 cm) and shallow, never penetrating the muscularis propria, but they can bleed profusely. Similar lesions can occur after traumatic or surgical injury to the central nervous system (i.e., Cushing ulcers). Esophageal varices can cause massive hematemesis, but they are seen in the setting of portal hypertension, caused most commonly by cirrhosis. Metaplastic columnar epithelium at the lower end of the esophagus is seen in Barrett esophagus, resulting from chronic gastroesophageal reflux disease.
BP6 487   PBD6 796

53.   **(E)** Hypotension with hypoperfusion from heart failure is a common cause for ischemic bowel in hospitalized patients. The ischemic changes begin in the mucosa in scattered areas, becoming confluent and transmural over time. This can give rise to paralytic ileus and bleeding from the affected regions of the bowel mucosa. Ulcerative colitis usually gives rise to marked mucosal inflammation with necrosis, usually in a continuous distribution from the rectum upward. Volvulus is a form of mechanical obstruction from twisting of the small intestine on its mesentery or twisting of the cecum or sigmoid colon, resulting in compromised blood supply that can lead to infarction of the twisted segment. Shigellosis is an infectious diarrhea that gives rise to diffuse colonic mucosal erosion with hemorrhage. A mesenteric vasculitis is uncommon but could lead to bowel infarction.
BP6 492   PBD6 822

54.   **(A)** The clinical and histologic features are consistent with Crohn disease. This is one of the idiopathic inflammatory bowel diseases. It is marked by segmental bowel involvement and transmural inflammation that leads to strictures, adhesions, and fistula. Ulcerative colitis has mucosal involvement extending variable distances from the rectum. Unlike Crohn disease, the mucosal involvement is diffuse and does not show "skip areas." Fissures and fistulas are not frequently seen in ulcerative colitis. Shigellosis and amebiasis are infectious processes that can cause mucosal ulceration, but they do not produce granulomas or fissures. Sarcoidosis can involve many organs and give rise to noncaseating granulomas. However, involvement of the intestines is uncommon, and it does not give rise to an ulcerative disease.
BP6 499–500   PBD6 816–218

55.   **(D)** Columnar metaplasia of the lower esophageal mucosa, also called Barrett esophagus, is a consequence of chronic gastroesophageal reflux disease. The metaplasia may be accompanied by inflammation. Varices result from long-standing portal hypertension; although there may be some associated inflammation, columnar metaplasia is not present. Irradiation may produce inflammation and eventual fibrosis, but there is no columnar metaplasia. Achalasia refers to failure of relaxation of the lower esophageal sphincter (LES). This gives rise to progressive dilation of the esophagus above the level of LES. Upper esophageal webbing may rarely accompany iron deficiency.
BP6 479   PBD6 781–782

56.   **(B)** She has colonic diverticulosis, which may be accompanied by intermittent minimal bleeding and rarely by severe bleeding. One or more diverticula may become inflamed (i.e., diverticulitis) or, less commonly, perforate to produce an abscess, peritonitis, or both. Diverticular disease is not a premalignant condition. The diverticula project outward, and even with inflammation, luminal obstruction is unlikely. Malabsorption is not a feature of diverticular disease. Toxic megacolon is an uncommon complication of inflammatory bowel disease.
BP6 503–504   PBD6 823–824

57.   **(D)** Carcinomas of the small intestine are rare, and most of them are periampullary in location. Carcinomas of the stomach, pancreas, ovary, and colon are more common and hence much more likely to be the source of peritoneal metastases. Ascites can occur when the peritoneum is seeded with secondary tumors. Ovarian carcinomas are the most likely to do this.
BP6 511   PBD6 826–827

58.   **(E)** He has a non-Hodgkin lymphoma associated with AIDS. These are high-grade B-cell neoplasms that have a poor prognosis. Kaposi sarcoma, non-Hodgkin lymphoma, and anorectal squamous cell carcinoma are the malignancies seen in the gastrointestinal tract that are associated with HIV infection. Besides AIDS, lymphomas of the gastrointestinal tract may be seen in patients with sprue. Sporadic MALT lymphomas are associated with *H. pylori* infection.
BP6 125   PBD6 837

The Liver and the Biliary Tract

PBD6 Chapter 19 - The Liver and Biliary Tract
BP6 Chapter 16 - Pathology of the Liver
and Biliary Tract

1. Three weeks after a meal at the Trucker's Cafe, a 28-year-old male develops malaise. He has a mild scleral icterus, fatigue, and loss of appetite. His symptoms abate over the next 3 weeks. On returning to the cafe, he finds that it has been closed by the city's health department. Which of the following laboratory test findings is he most likely to have?

○ (A) Hepatitis B surface antibody
○ (B) Hepatitis D IgM antibody
○ (C) Hepatitis C antibody
○ (D) Hepatitis A IgM antibody
○ (E) Hepatitis B core antibody

2. Chronic hepatitis is most likely to occur after acute infection with which of the following viruses?

○ (A) Hepatitis A virus
○ (B) Hepatitis B virus
○ (C) Hepatitis C virus
○ (D) Hepatitis E virus (HEV)
○ (E) Coinfection with hepatitis B and D viruses

3. Six weeks after a trip to Central America, a 33-year-old female develops fever with right upper quadrant pain. She had a blood-tinged watery diarrhea for about a week at the end of her trip, but that subsided several weeks ago. She now has a total bilirubin level of 5.4 mg/dL, with a direct bilirubin concentration of 4.9 mg/dL and alkaline phosphatase level of 175 U/L. Abdominal computed tomography (CT) reveals a 7-cm right hepatic mass with central necrosis and discrete borders. Which of the following organisms is the most likely etiologic agent for these findings?

○ (A) *Mycobacterium bovis*
○ (B) *Escherichia coli*
○ (C) *Candida albicans*
○ (D) *Echinococcus granulosus*
○ (E) *Entamoeba histolytica*

4. A 48-year-old man has increasing abdominal girth and icterus. Serum laboratory findings include a total bilirubin concentration of 5.2 mg/dL, direct bilirubin of 4.2 mg/dL, alkaline phosphatase of 95 U/L, aspartate aminotransferase (AST) of 300 U/L, alanine aminotransferase (ALT) of 158 U/L, total protein concentration of 6.4 g/dL, and albumin concentration of 2.2 g/dL. The prothrombin time is 18 seconds (control, 12 seconds). The blood ammonia level is 105 micromol/L. The most likely cause for these findings is

○ (A) Choledocholithiasis
○ (B) Acute hepatitis A infection
○ (C) Metastatic adenocarcinoma
○ (D) Primary biliary cirrhosis
○ (E) Alcoholic liver disease

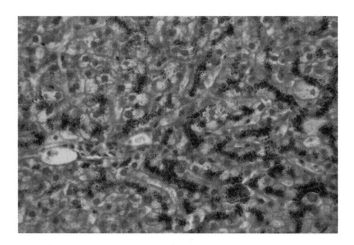

5. A 44-year-old male with diabetes mellitus, congestive heart failure, and chronic polyarthritis is found to have a markedly increased serum ferritin concentration. He has smoked cigarettes for 20 years. He undergoes a liver biopsy, and the microscopic appearance of the liver is seen here with Prussian blue stain. Based on these findings, what is the advice you would give?

○ (A) You need to markedly reduce your alcohol consumption.
○ (B) A cholecystectomy should be performed.
○ (C) Your siblings may be at risk for developing the same condition.

○ (D) You will most likely develop acute fulminant hepatitis.

○ (E) Smoking for many years led to this condition.

For each of the case histories in questions 6 and 7, select the most appropriate diagnosis:

(A) Acute hepatitis A virus (HAV) infection
(B) Acute hepatitis B virus (HBV) infection
(C) Acute hepatitis C virus (HCV) infection
(D) Chronic HAV infection
(E) Chronic HBV infection
(F) Chronic HCV infection
(G) Coinfection with HBV and hepatitis delta virus (HDV)
(H) Extrahepatic biliary atresia
(I) Gilbert syndrome
(J) Primary biliary cirrhosis
(K) Primary hemochromatosis
(L) Primary sclerosing cholangitis
(M) Reye syndrome
(N) Superinfection of chronic hepatitis B by HDV
(O) Wilson disease

6.   A 12-year-old boy with Down syndrome who lives in a residential care facility with other mentally retarded children presents with a history of listlessness, malaise, and mild fever for 2 or 3 days. Scleral icterus and dark urine are observed by one of the caregivers. The child is brought to the clinic, where physical examination reveals mild scleral icterus and mild right upper quadrant tenderness. Based on the history and laboratory results below, what is the most likely diagnosis? (   )

AST	437 U/L	HBsAg	−
ALT	553 U/L	Anti-HBc, total	+
Total bilirubin	6.0 mg/dL	Anti-HBc, IgM fraction	−
Direct bilirubin	3.5 mg/dL	Anti-HAV, total	+
Albumin	4.8 g/dL	Anti-HAV, IgM fraction	+
Urine urobilinogen	Increased	Anti-HCV	−
Alkaline phosphatase	178 U/L	Anti HDV	−

7.   A 27-year-old male intravenous drug user presents to the emergency room with a history of nausea, vomiting, and passage of dark urine. Examination reveals scleral icterus and mild jaundice, and fresh and healed track marks on the arms and legs. Neurologic examination shows a confused, somnolent young man oriented only to person. Based on the history and laboratory data below, what is the most likely explanation for these findings? (   )

AST	2342 U/L	HBsAg	+
ALT	2150 U/L	Anti-HBc, total	+
Total bilirubin	8.3 mg/dL	Anti-HBc, IgM	−
Direct bilirubin	4.5 mg/dL	Anti-HAV, total	+
Albumin	2.7 g/dL	Anti-HAV, IgM	−
Urine urobilinogen	Increased	Anti-HCV	−
Alkaline phosphatase	233 U/L	Anti-HDV, total	+
		Anti-HDV IgM	+

8.   A 36-year-old female has become increasingly icteric for the past month. In the past, she has had several bouts of colicky, mid-abdominal pain. A liver biopsy shows bile duct proliferation and intracanalicular bile stasis, but there is no inflammation or necrosis. Which of the following serum laboratory test findings is most likely to be present?

○ (A) Markedly increased antimitochondrial antibody
○ (B) Hepatitis C antibody
○ (C) Markedly elevated indirect bilirubin
○ (D) Elevated alkaline phosphatase
○ (E) Increased ammonia

9.   A 56-year-old man from Shanghai, China has had a 10-kg weight loss over the past 3 months and has felt tired. An abdominal CT scan reveals a 10-cm, solid mass in the left lobe of a nodular liver. Laboratory testing reveals that he is hepatitis B surface antigen (HBsAg) positive, hepatitis C antibody negative, and hepatitis A antibody negative. A liver biopsy of the lesion reveals a hepatocellular carcinoma. The mechanism that is most likely responsible for development of liver cancer in this patient is

○ (A) Insertion of HBV DNA in the vicinity of the *c-myc* oncogene
○ (B) Inherited mutation in the DNA mismatch repair genes
○ (C) Repeated cycles of liver cell necrosis and regeneration caused by HBV infection
○ (D) Development of a hepatic adenoma that accumulates mutations
○ (E) Coinfection with *Clonorchis sinensis*

10.   A 42-year-old female had bouts of colicky right upper quadrant abdominal pain for a week, along with fever and chills. She then developed icterus, with total bilirubin level of 7.1 mg/dL and direct bilirubin concentration of 6.7 mg/dL. Abdominal ultrasound revealed cholelithiasis and dilation of the common bile duct, along with two cystic lesions in the right lobe of liver 0.8 and 1.5 cm, respectively. Which of the following infectious agents is most likely to produce these findings?

○ (A) *Clonorchis sinensis*
○ (B) *Cryptosporidium parvum*
○ (C) Cytomegalovirus
○ (D) *Entamoeba histolytica*
○ (E) *Escherichia coli*

11.   A 30-year-old intravenous drug user presented with a history of malaise, fever, and jaundice. Serologic testing revealed the presence of HBsAg, hepatitis B DNA, and anti-hepatitis B core IgG antibodies. He was lost to follow-up but returned 2 years later in an emergency room with hematemesis and ascites. Serologic testing revealed the same findings as before. Sclerotherapy was done to treat esophageal varices, and he was discharged. Again, he failed to return. Five years after this last episode, he presents with weight loss, abdominal pain, and rapid enlargement of the abdomen. Which of the following laboratory

tests is most likely to be diagnostic of *this phase* of his disease?

○ (A) Prolonged prothrombin time
○ (B) Elevated serum α-fetoprotein (AFP) level
○ (C) Elevated ALT level
○ (D) Elevated serum alkaline phosphatase level
○ (E) Elevated serum ferritin level

12. Over the past 4 days, a previously healthy 38-year-old woman has become increasingly obtunded. She has scleral icterus. She is afebrile and has a blood pressure of 110/55 mm Hg. Laboratory investigations reveal a prothrombin time of 38 seconds (with a control of 13), an ALT level of 1854 U/L, AST level of 1621 U/L, and serum albumin concentration of 1.8 g/dL. Which of the following additional serum laboratory test findings would you most likely expect to be present?

○ (A) Increased alkaline phosphatase level
○ (B) Hepatitis C virus antibody
○ (C) Increased amylase level
○ (D) Positive antinuclear antibody
○ (E) Increased ammonia level

13. A 58-year-old female has experienced gradually increasing malaise, icterus, and loss of appetite for the last 6 months. She has a total bilirubin concentration of 7.8 mg/dL, AST of 190 U/L, ALT of 220 U/L, and alkaline phosphatase of 26 U/L. A liver biopsy shows piecemeal necrosis of hepatocytes at the limiting plate with portal fibrosis and a mononuclear infiltrate in the portal tracts. These findings are most typical for

○ (A) HAV infection
○ (B) Congestive heart failure
○ (C) Choledocholithiasis
○ (D) Hemochromatosis
○ (E) HCV infection

14. A 53-year-old male comes to the emergency room with marked hematemesis. On physical examination, he has a temperature of 35.9°C, pulse of 112/min, respiration rate of 26/min, and blood pressure of 90/45 mm Hg. He has a distended abdomen with a fluid wave, and the spleen tip is palpable. Which of the following liver diseases is most likely to be present?

○ (A) Cirrhosis
○ (B) Cholangiocarcinoma
○ (C) Massive hepatic necrosis
○ (D) Fatty change
○ (E) HAV infection

15. A 40-year-old female donates blood because she cares about helping to alleviate the chronic shortage of blood. Unfortunately, she is found to be positive for HBsAg and is therefore excluded as a blood donor. She feels fine, and liver function test results, including those for total bilirubin, AST, ALT, alkaline phosphatase, and albumin, are normal. Further serologic testing produces negative results for HAV IgM, hepatitis B core antibody, and HCV antibody. Repeat testing 6 months later yields the same results.

There are no physical examination findings of significance. What should you tell this patient?

○ (A) You acquired this infection through injection drug use.
○ (B) You will develop clinical overt hepatitis within a year.
○ (C) You probably have a chronic carrier state from vertical transmission.
○ (D) These test results are probably erroneous and need to be repeated.
○ (E) You should get a hepatitis B vaccination series.

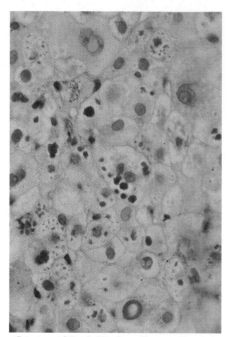

Courtesy of Dr. I. Wanless, Toronto Hospital.

16. A 28-year-old male experiences shortness of breath. As a neonate, he developed marked icterus, but he has felt well since then. A family history of liver disease leads to performance of a liver biopsy. The microscopic appearance of the liver biopsy is seen here with periodic acid–Schiff (PAS) stain. This patient is at a very high risk for development of

○ (A) Diabetes mellitus
○ (B) Congestive heart failure
○ (C) Emphysema
○ (D) Ulcerative colitis
○ (E) Systemic lupus erythematosus

17. The cut surface of the liver at autopsy from a 70-year-old woman is shown in the following figure. The liver is enlarged and tense with a blunted edge. Which of the following underlying conditions did she most likely have?

○ (A) Polyarteritis nodosa
○ (B) Chronic alcoholism
○ (C) Polycythemia vera
○ (D) Cor pulmonale
○ (E) Chronic hepatitis C

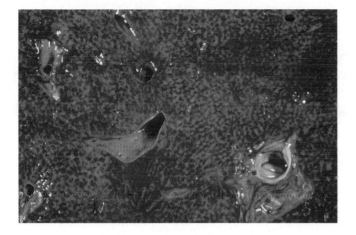

18.   Which of the following is the most important predictor of whether a patient with viral hepatitis will develop chronic liver disease with progression to cirrhosis?

O (A) The presence of chronic inflammatory cells in the portal tract

O (B) The degree to which hepatic transaminase enzymes are elevated

O (C) The length of time that hepatic enzymes remain elevated

O (D) The specific form of hepatitis virus responsible for the infection

O (E) The presence of inflammatory cells in the sinusoids on a liver biopsy

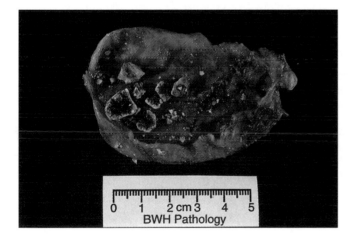

19.   A patient presents with colicky right upper quadrant abdominal pain for a week. There is also some nausea, but no vomiting or diarrhea. The patient's gallbladder, shown here, is removed by laparoscopic cholecystectomy. Which of the following patients is most likely to develop this condition?

O (A) A 16-year-old, black female with sickle cell anemia
O (B) A 50-year-old male with Crohn disease
O (C) A 40-year-old female with jaundice, pruritus, and ulcerative colitis
O (D) A 50-year-old, obese, Native-American female
O (E) A 19-year-old, male intravenous drug abuser

Questions 20 through 22 relate to the same patient with the following history:

A 60-year-old male with a 30-year history of excessive drinking presented with hematemesis. On examination, he was found to have ascites, mild jaundice, and an enlarged spleen. He also had gynecomastia, spider telangiectasias of the skin, and testicular atrophy. Rectal examination revealed prominent hemorrhoids and a normal-sized prostate. Emergency upper endoscopy revealed dilated, bleeding blood vessels in the esophagus. Sclerotherapy was used to control the bleeding.

20.   In this patient, which of the following symptoms or signs is *not* caused by portal hypertension?

O (A) Hematemesis
O (B) Ascites
O (C) Spider telangiectasias of skin
O (D) Splenomegaly
O (E) Hemorrhoids

21.   Laboratory examination revealed the following results:

Hematocrit	25%	Total bilirubin	5.4 mg/dL
Prothrombin time	20 sec	Direct bilirubin	3.0 mg/dL
Total WBC count	$12 \times 10^3/\mu L$	Sodium	136 mEq/L
AST	270 U/L	Potassium	6.0 mEq/L
ALT	95 U/L	Albumin	2.8 g/dL
Alkaline phosphatase	180 U/L	Urinalysis:	positive bilirubin

Which of the following laboratory findings seen in this patient best indicates a defect in the *synthetic* functions of liver?

O (A) Bilirubinuria
O (B) Prothrombin time
O (C) AST level
O (D) Total and direct bilirubin levels
O (E) Alkaline phosphatase level

22.   Despite supportive therapy, the patient went into a coma and died. Which of the following morphologic changes in the liver is most likely to be found?

O (A) A shrunken liver with a wrinkled capsular surface that microscopically shows massive irregular areas of necrosis without any obvious pattern

O (B) Diffusely nodular liver with small, uniform nodules that microscopically shows diffuse fibrosis encircling nodules of regenerative hepatocytes; liver cells contain fat globules

O (C) Diffusely nodular liver with small, uniform nodules that microscopically shows diffuse fibrosis encircling regenerative nodules; liver cells contain PAS-positive, globular cytoplasmic inclusions

O (D) Markedly enlarged, yellow, greasy liver that microscopically shows preservation of the architecture and marked fatty change

○ (E) Diffusely nodular, intensely green liver with small, uniform nodules that microscopically shows prominent bile stasis and fibrous bridging between portal areas

23. Which of the following conditions is *least* likely to be seen in association with cholelithiasis in a 38-year-old female?

○ (A) Adenocarcinoma of the gallbladder
○ (B) Obesity
○ (C) Hemolytic anemia
○ (D) Crohn disease
○ (E) Chronic hepatitis B

24. A 61-year-old male has had ascites for the past year. After a paracentesis with removal of 1 L of slightly cloudy, serosanguinous fluid, physical examination reveals a firm, nodular liver. Laboratory findings include positive serum HBsAg and presence of hepatitis B core antibody. He has a markedly elevated serum α-fetoprotein (AFP) level. Which of the following hepatic lesions is he most likely to have?

○ (A) Hepatocellular carcinoma
○ (B) Massive hepatocyte necrosis
○ (C) Marked steatosis
○ (D) Wilson disease
○ (E) Autoimmune hepatitis

For each of the patient histories in questions 25 through 27, match the most closely associated gross or histologic finding in the liver:

(A) Adenocarcinoma
(B) Cirrhosis
(C) Concentric "onion skin" bile duct fibrosis
(D) Copper deposition
(E) Extrahepatic biliary fibrosis and stricture
(F) Granulomatous bile duct destruction
(G) Hepatic venous thrombosis
(H) Massive hepatocellular necrosis
(I) Microvesicular steatosis
(J) PAS-positive periportal globules
(K) Piecemeal hepatocellular necrosis at interface of portal tracts
(L) Subcapsular hematoma

25. A 50-year-old male presents with massive hematemesis. He has a history of chronic alcoholism, but he quit drinking ethanol 10 years ago. He has been taking no medications. Serologic test results for hepatitis A, B, and C are negative. (   )

26. A 52-year-old female has experienced malaise that has worsened for the past year. She now has mild scleral icterus. There is no ascites or splenomegaly. Her serum serologic test results show positive hepatitis C IgG antibody, positive HCV RNA, negative hepatitis A antibody, negative HBsAg, negative antinuclear antibody, and negative antimitochondrial antibody. Her condition remains stable for months. (   )

27. A 41-year-old man has experienced progressive fatigue, pruritus, and icterus for several months. A

colectomy was performed 5 years ago for treatment of ulcerative colitis, and now cholangiography reveals widespread obliteration of intrahepatic bile ducts, with a beaded appearance in remaining ducts. (   )

28. A 19-year-old woman is bothered by a tremor at rest. This becomes progressively worse over the next 6 months. She then begins to act strangely, leading to a diagnosis of an acute psychosis. On physical examination, she has slight scleral icterus. A slit-lamp examination shows corneal Kayser-Fleischer rings. Laboratory findings for serum include a total protein concentration of 5.9 g/dL, albumin of 3.1 g/dL, total bilirubin of 4.9 mg/dL, direct bilirubin of 3.1 mg/dL, AST of 128 U/L, ALT of 157 U/L, and alkaline phosphatase of 56 U/L. Which of the following additional serum laboratory test findings is most likely in this case?

○ (A) Decreased serum ceruloplasmin level
○ (B) Positive HBsAg
○ (C) Decreased α_1-antitrypsin level
○ (D) Increased serum ferritin level
○ (E) Positive antimitochondrial antibody

29. A 55-year-old male has developed abdominal pain and jaundice over several weeks' time. An abdominal CT scan demonstrates a markedly thickened gallbladder wall. A cholecystectomy is performed, and the slightly enlarged gallbladder on sectioning contains a fungating, 4×7 cm, firm, lobulated, tan mass. Which of the following findings was most likely associated with this mass?

○ (A) Amebic dysentery
○ (B) Ulcerative colitis
○ (C) *C. sinensis* infection
○ (D) Cholelithiasis
○ (E) Primary sclerosing cholangitis

30. A 47-year-old male has experienced intermittent upper abdominal pain for several weeks. A liver biopsy shows intracanalicular cholestasis in the centrilobular regions, along with swollen liver cells and portal tract edema. There is no necrosis and no fibrosis. There is no increase in stainable iron. Liver function test results show that he has a total protein level of 7.3 g/dL, albumin of 5.2 g/dL, total bilirubin of 7.5 mg/dL, direct bilirubin of 6.8 mg/dL, AST of 35 U/L, ALT of 40 U/L, and alkaline phosphatase of 207 U/L. The most probable cause for these findings is

○ (A) Chronic passive congestion
○ (B) HBV infection
○ (C) Choledocholithiasis
○ (D) Extrahepatic biliary atresia
○ (E) Veno-occlusive disease

31. A 42-year-old woman has noticed generalized pruritus for several months. This pruritus is not relieved by application of topical corticosteroid-containing creams. Laboratory findings include a total bilirubin level of 1.8 mg/dL, direct bilirubin of 1.2 mg/dL, AST of 55 U/L, ALT of 58 U/L, alkaline phosphatase of 289 U/L, total protein of 6.8 g/dL, albumin of 3.4 g/dL, and total cholesterol of 344 mg/dL.

Which of the following serologic laboratory test findings is most likely to be positive in this patient?

○ (A) Anti-parietal cell antibody
○ (B) Anti-centromere antibody
○ (C) Anti-ribonucleoprotein
○ (D) Antimitochondrial antibody
○ (E) Anti–double-stranded DNA

32.   A 35-year-old female consults her physician because she has noticed an increasing yellowish hue to her skin for the past week. She has no abdominal pain or tenderness on physical examination, and the liver span is not increased. Laboratory findings on a serum specimen include a hemoglobin concentration of 11.7 g/dL, albumin of 3.5 g/dL, total protein of 5.5 g/dL, total bilirubin of 8.7 mg/dL, direct bilirubin of 0.6 mg/dL, alkaline phosphatase of 35 U/L, AST of 39 U/L, and ALT of 24 U/L. Which of the following conditions is she most likely to have?

○ (A) Cholelithiasis
○ (B) Hemolytic anemia
○ (C) Viral hepatitis A
○ (D) Micronodular cirrhosis
○ (E) Oral contraceptive use

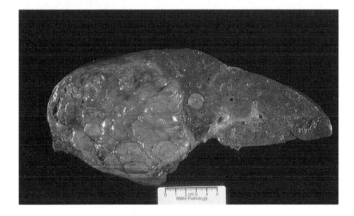

33.   At autopsy, the liver of a 41-year-old female has the gross appearance shown here. Ingestion of which of the following substances is most likely to have played a role in the development of this condition?

○ (A) Aflatoxins
○ (B) Raw oysters
○ (C) Aspirin
○ (D) Iron pills
○ (E) Nitrites

34.   The liver shown in the following figure at autopsy is from a 56-year-old male. The immediate cause of death was bacterial peritonitis with *E. coli* septicemia. What underlying disease most commonly accounts for these findings?

○ (A) Alpha₁-antitrypsin deficiency
○ (B) HEV infection
○ (C) Hereditary hemochromatosis
○ (D) Primary sclerosing cholangitis
○ (E) Chronic alcoholism

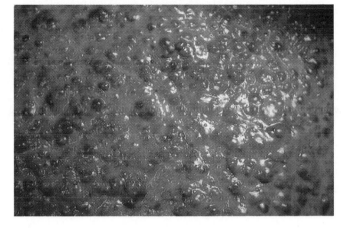

For each of the clinical histories in questions 35 and 36, match the most closely associated condition associated with liver disease:

(A) Alcoholic hepatitis
(B) Alpha₁-antitrypsin deficiency
(C) Autoimmune hepatitis
(D) Budd-Chiari syndrome
(E) Choledocholithiasis
(F) Extrahepatic biliary atresia
(G) Hepatic adenoma
(H) HAV infection
(I) HBV infection
(J) HDV infection
(K) Hepatorenal syndrome
(L) Hereditary hemochromatosis
(M) Primary biliary cirrhosis
(N) Primary sclerosing cholangitis
(O) Wilson disease

35.   A 36-year-old woman is in her sixth month of pregnancy, but she is unsure of her dates because she was taking oral contraceptives at the time she became pregnant. She experiences the sudden onset of severe abdominal pain. An ultrasound of the abdomen reveals a 7-cm, subcapsular, well-circumscribed hepatic mass. Paracentesis yields bloody fluid. At laparotomy, the right lower lobe mass, which has ruptured through the liver capsule, is resected. (   )

36.   A 44-year-old female has noticed increasingly severe generalized pruritus for the past 8 months. Serum levels of alkaline phosphatase and cholesterol are elevated. She has an elevated antimitochondrial antibody titer, but antinuclear antibodies are not present. When her serum total bilirubin concentration increases, a liver biopsy is performed that reveals nonsuppurative, granulomatous destruction of medium-sized bile ducts. (   )

37.   Which of the following modes of transmission of HBV is most likely to give rise to a carrier state?

○ (A) Blood transfusion
○ (B) Heterosexual transmission
○ (C) Vertical transmission during childbirth

○ (D) Oral transmission
○ (E) Needle-stick injury

38. The day of a final examination in anatomy, a 26-year-old medical student notices that she has a mild degree of scleral icterus. She has never had a major illness. Liver function tests show total protein level of 7.9 g/dL, albumin of 4.8 g/dL, alkaline phosphatase of 32 U/L, AST of 48 U/L, ALT of 19 U/L, total bilirubin of 4.9 mg/dL, and direct bilirubin of 0.8 mg/dL. The scleral icterus is gone in 2 days. The condition most likely to produce these findings is

○ (A) Choledochal cyst
○ (B) Primary biliary cirrhosis
○ (C) Gilbert syndrome
○ (D) Hepatitis A
○ (E) Dubin-Johnson syndrome

39. A 48-year-old male presents with colicky right upper quadrant pain. He has had nausea for the past 2 days. His temperature is now 38.8°C. His white blood cell (WBC) count is 11,200/μL, with a differential count of 71 segmented neutrophils, 9 band cells, 13 lymphocytes, and 7 monocytes per 100 WBCs. These findings are most typical for

○ (A) Acute hepatitis A
○ (B) Extrahepatic biliary atresia
○ (C) Acute cholecystitis
○ (D) Primary sclerosing cholangitis
○ (E) Adenocarcinoma of the gallbladder

40. A 49-year-old male experiences increasing ascites, and a liver biopsy demonstrates diffuse portal tract bridging fibrosis and nodular regeneration of liver cells. There is no hepatocyte necrosis and no cholestasis. Within the areas of fibrosis, bile duct proliferation and mononuclear cell inflammatory infiltrates can be seen. These findings are most characteristic for

○ (A) Alcoholic hepatitis
○ (B) Cirrhosis
○ (C) Acute viral hepatitis
○ (D) Acetaminophen toxicity
○ (E) Chronic passive congestion

41. Four days after a previously healthy 4-year-old child appears to be recovering from a bout of the "flu," he develops severe vomiting and irritability. He is admitted to a hospital, where he becomes increasingly icteric and lethargic. Laboratory testing reveals a total bilirubin level of 7.8 mg/dL, direct bilirubin of 6.1 mg/dL, alkaline phosphatase of 125 U/L, AST of 622 U/L, and ALT of 705 U/L in serum. The blood ammonia concentration is 119 μmol/L. The child dies of cerebral edema. Which of the following histologic features do you most expect to find in the liver at autopsy?

○ (A) Atresia of extrahepatic bile ducts
○ (B) PAS-positive 2- to 6-μm hepatic globules in periportal hepatocytes
○ (C) Marked microvesicular steatosis

○ (D) Extensive intrahepatic hemosiderin deposition
○ (E) Inflammation with loss of intrahepatic bile ducts

42. Antibodies to which of the following forms of viral hepatitis do not confer immunity from reinfection?

○ (A) HAV
○ (B) HBV
○ (C) HCV
○ (D) HDV
○ (E) HEV

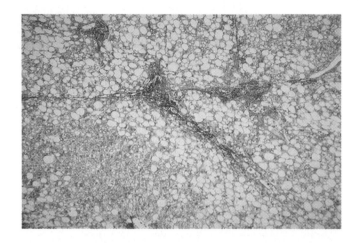

43. This is the microscopic appearance of a liver biopsy. Collagen is stained blue by a trichrome stain. Which of the following clinical scenarios is most likely related to this histology?

○ (A) A 65-year-old, obese woman with a history of chronic cholelithiasis
○ (B) A 50-year-old male with a history of alcoholism
○ (C) A 56-year-old male with skin pigmentation, diabetes, and ascites
○ (D) A 40-year-old female with intense pruritus, jaundice, and xanthomas of the skin
○ (E) A 45-year-old male with pruritus, jaundice, and a history of chronic ulcerative colitis

44. After experiencing malaise and increasing icterus for 6 weeks, a 42-year-old male comes to you for care. You find that he has the following serum serologic test results: negative HAV IgM, positive HBsAg, positive hepatitis core IgM antibody, negative HCV antibody. You are most confident to advise him that

○ (A) Donating blood a month before is the source of his infection.
○ (B) Complete recovery without sequelae is most probable.
○ (C) There is a significant risk for development of fulminant hepatitis.
○ (D) There is significant risk for development of hepatocellular carcinoma.
○ (E) All serologic test results will become negative in a year.

45. A 51-year-old male with a long history of chronic alcoholism has a firm nodular liver on physical examina-

tion. Laboratory findings include a serum albumin level of 2.5 g/dL and a prothrombin time of 28 seconds (control, 13 seconds). He was hospitalized last year with upper gastrointestinal hemorrhage. Which of the following additional physical examination findings is he most likely to have?

○ (A) Splinter hemorrhages
○ (B) Diminished deep tendon reflexes
○ (C) Caput medusae
○ (D) Papilledema
○ (E) Distended jugular veins

46. A 45-year-old female has had increasing pruritus and icterus for several months. Liver function tests show total protein level of 6.3 g/dL, albumin of 2.7 g/dL, total bilirubin of 5.7 mg/dL, direct bilirubin of 4.6 mg/dL, AST of 77 U/L, ALT of 81 U/L, and alkaline phosphatase of 221 U/L in serum. A liver biopsy reveals destruction of portal tracts and loss of bile ducts along with lymphocytic infiltrates. Which of the following laboratory test findings is most likely?

○ (A) Positive hepatitis C antibody
○ (B) Positive antimitochondrial antibody
○ (C) Elevated sweat chloride level
○ (D) Increased serum ferritin level
○ (E) Decreased α_1-antitrypsin

For each of the clinical histories in questions 47 through 49, match the most closely associated morphologic finding associated with liver disease:

(A) Adenocarcinoma
(B) Apoptosis
(C) Centrilobular congestion
(D) Cholestasis
(E) Extrahepatic biliary fibrosis
(F) Granulomatous bile duct destruction
(G) Cirrhosis with hemosiderin deposition
(H) Lymphoid aggregates
(I) Macrovesicular steatosis
(J) Mallory bodies
(K) Periportal PAS-positive globules
(L) Portal fibrosis

47. A 50-year-old male has increasing dyspnea as a consequence of idiopathic pulmonary fibrosis. Physical exami-

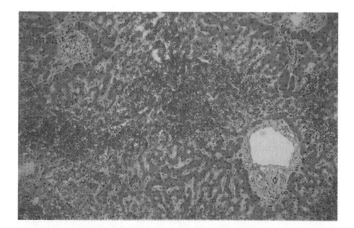

nation reveals elevated jugular venous pressure and pedal edema. He has an AST level of 221 U/L, ALT of 234 U/L, lactate dehydrogenase of 710 U/L, total bilirubin of 1.2 mg/dL, alkaline phosphatase of 48 U/L, albumin of 3.5 g/dL, and total protein of 5.4 g/dL. The representative microscopic appearance of this process is depicted in the figure. (   )

48. Two siblings, both in their forties, have developed insulin-dependent diabetes mellitus. They have exhibited darker skin pigmentation over the past few years. On physical examination, the liver edge is firm. There is pain and limited mobility of elbow and knee joints. (   )

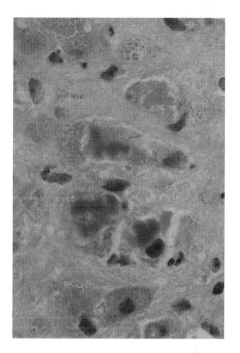

49. After a heavy bout of drinking, a chronic alcoholic feels acutely ill. He develops nausea, upper abdominal pain, and jaundice. The complete blood count reveals a total WBC count of 16,120/μL, with differential count of 82 segmented neutrophils, 8 band cells, 8 lymphocytes, and 2 monocytes per 100 WBCs. A liver biopsy is depicted in the figure. (   )

ANSWERS

1. (D) This person developed a mild, self-limited liver disease after a meal at a restaurant. He most likely developed hepatitis A by consumption of contaminated food or water. The presence of hepatitis A IgM antibody indicates recent infection. The IgM antibody is replaced in a few months by IgG antibodies. The latter give lifelong immunity from reinfection. The incubation period for HAV infection is short, and the illness is short and mild, with no

significant tendency for development of chronic hepatitis. The most common mode of infection for hepatitis A is through the fecal-oral route. Hepatitis B and C infections have a longer incubation period and are most often acquired parenterally. Hepatitis D is caused by coinfection with HBV or by superinfection in a hepatitis B carrier.
BP6 525–529   PBD6 856–857

2.   (C) The incidence of chronic hepatitis is highest with HCV infection. More than 50% of those infected with this virus develop chronic hepatitis, and many progress to cirrhosis. This is in part related to the fact that IgG antibodies against HCV that develop after acute infection are not protective.
BP6 528   PBD6 860–861

3.   (E) Amebic abscesses are an uncommon complication seen after amebic dysentery. From the colonic mucosa, amebae gain access to submucosal veins and are carried through the portal venous system to the liver. The colonic lesions are typically healed when patients present with the amebic liver abscess. *M. bovis* can infect the gastrointestinal tract and may spread to lymph nodes, but usually no further. *E. coli* hepatic abscesses are most likely the result of an ascending biliary tract infection. Disseminated candidiasis in immunocompromised persons may produce multiple, small hepatic abscesses. Echinococcal liver abscesses are generally not necrotic and do not follow a diarrheal illness.
BP6 534   PBD6 358, 867

4.   (E) This patient has liver cell injury (indicated by elevated transaminase levels), some loss of liver function (indicated by the abnormal prothrombin time), and cholestasis. All of these are not specific for a given type of liver injury. However, the AST level that is higher than the ALT level is characteristic for liver cell injury associated with chronic alcoholism. His disease is decompensating, as evidenced by elevated blood ammonia. Choledocholithiasis results in a conjugated hyperbilirubinemia, although without a high ammonia level as evidence of liver failure. Hepatitis A is typically a mild disease, without a preponderance of direct bilirubin. Metastases are not likely to obstruct all biliary tract drainage or lead to liver failure severe enough to cause elevations of blood ammonia. Primary biliary cirrhosis is rare, particularly in males, and the alkaline phosphatase should be much higher.
BP6 522, 535, 538   PBD6 852–853, 872–873

5.   (C) This patient has clinical, histologic, and laboratory features of genetic hemochromatosis. In this condition, iron overload occurs because of excessive absorption of dietary iron. The absorbed iron is deposited in many tissues, including heart, pancreas, and liver, giving rise to heart failure, diabetes, and cirrhosis. The Prussian blue stain stains the iron blue, as seen in this biopsy. High serum ferritin concentration is an indicator of a vast increase in body iron. Genetic hemochromatosis is an autosomal recessive condition, and hence siblings are at risk for developing the same disease.
BP6 538–540   PBD6 873–874

6.   (A) This patient has a short history of jaundice, with evidence of acute hepatitis and significant transaminase elevations. The serologic findings are supportive of acute hepatitis A because he has anti-HAV IgM antibodies. This indicates recent infection, because anti-HAV IgG antibodies form during recovery. In contrast, the patient has antibodies against hepatitis B core antigen that do not type as IgM. By inference, he has IgG antibodies against hepatitis B core antigen. This is indicative of past HBV infection. Absence of HBsAg supports this. Hepatitis A infections are acquired by the fecal-oral route and are likely to occur in institutions such as those for mentally retarded children.
BP6 525–526   PBD6 856–857

7.   (N) This patient has serologic evidence for superinfection of HDV on chronic hepatitis caused by HBV. The evidence for chronic hepatitis B is the presence of HBsAg and anti-hepatitis B core IgG antibody. (Note that the presence of anti-hepatitis B core (anti-HBc) total with absence of anti-hepatitis B core IgM (anti-HBcIgM) antibody indicates that an anti-hepatitis B core antibody other than IgM is present. It is usually IgG.) The evidence of recent HDV infection is the presence of anti-HDV IgM antibodies. HBV and HDV infections are likely to occur in injection drug users by the parenteral route. HDV cannot replicate in the absence of HBV, hence, isolated HDV infection does not occur. When HDV infection is superimposed on chronic HBV, three outcomes are possible: mild HBV hepatitis may be converted to fulminant disease, acute hepatitis may occur in an asymptomatic HBV carrier, or chronic progressive disease may develop, culminating in cirrhosis.
BP6 528–529   PBD6 861–862

8.   (D) The findings suggest obstructive jaundice from biliary tract disease (e.g., gallstones). Elevation of the serum alkaline phosphatase level is characteristic of cholestasis. The alkaline phosphatase comes from bile duct epithelium and hepatocyte canalicular membrane. Primary biliary cirrhosis with an increased antimitochondrial antibody titer should eventually lead to bile duct destruction. Most cases of active HCV infection are accompanied by some degree of inflammation with fibrosis. With obstructive biliary tract disease, the direct bilirubin should be elevated, not the indirect bilirubin. The blood ammonia concentration increases with worsening liver failure. When hepatic failure is sufficient to cause hyperammonemia, mental obtundation is seen. In this case, the patient only has jaundice.
BP6 521   PBD6 850

9.   (C) There is a long-term risk for hepatocellular carcinoma in persons infected with HBV. This infection is more common (often from vertical transmission) in Asia than in North America and Europe, and it accounts for more cases of primary liver cancer worldwide than other causes such as chronic alcoholism. HBV does not encode any oncogene, nor does it integrate next to a known oncogene, such as c-*myc*. Most likely, neoplastic transformation occurs because HBV induces repeated cycles of liver cell death and regeneration. This increases the risk of accumulating mutations during several rounds of cell division. Unlike colon carcinomas, hepatic carcinomas are not known to proceed from a stage of adenoma. The hereditary nonpolyposis co-

lon carcinoma syndrome (HNPCC) is associated with inherited DNA mismatch repair genes. Infection with the liver fluke *C. sinensis* predisposes to bile duct carcinoma.
BP6 548–550   PBD6 888–889

10. **(E)** This patient has a history of gallstones and has developed an ascending cholangitis caused by *E. coli*. These bacteria reach the liver by ascending the biliary tree. Obstruction from lithiasis is the most common risk factor. Development of cystic lesions in the right lobe of the liver suggests that the patient has developed liver abscess. *C. sinensis* is a liver fluke that is a risk factor for biliary tract cancer. Cryptosporidiosis in immunocompromised patients can occasionally occur in the biliary tract and elsewhere. Cytomegalovirus infection can also be seen in immunocompromised patients, but it produces a picture more like hepatitis, without biliary tract disease. Amebiasis involving the liver is most likely to present with a history of diarrhea with blood and mucus.
BP6 553   PBD6 898

11. **(B)** This intravenous drug user developed chronic hepatitis B, as evidenced by persistence of HBsAg, HBV DNA, and anti-hepatitis B core IgG antibodies. Up to 80% or 90% of persons with a history of injection drug use are found to have serologic evidence for HBV or HCV infection. Ruptured varices and ascites suggest that he went on to develop cirrhosis with portal hypertension. His final presentation, with weight loss and rapid enlargement of abdomen, suggests that a hepatocellular cancer has developed. This can be confirmed by an elevated AFP level in most cases.
BP6 548–550   PBD6 888–890

12. **(E)** The history points to an acute fulminant hepatitis with massive hepatic necrosis. The loss of hepatic function from destruction of 80% to 90% of the liver results in hyperammonemia from the defective hepatocyte urea cycle. An elevated alkaline phosphatase concentration suggests extrahepatic or intrahepatic biliary obstruction. Fulminant hepatitis from HCV is rare. An elevated amylase level suggests pancreatitis. An autoimmune hepatitis with a positive antinuclear antibody finding is not likely to produce a fulminant hepatitis.
BP6 522   PBD6 852

13. **(E)** This patient has clinical evidence of liver disease persisting for 6 months, and histologic evidence of hepatic necrosis with portal inflammation and fibrosis. These are features of chronic hepatitis. Of all the hepatitis viruses, HCV is most likely to cause chronic hepatitis, and HAV is the least likely to produce chronic disease. Hepatic congestion with right heart failure produces centrilobular necrosis but not portal fibrosis. Choledocholithiasis leads to extrahepatic biliary obstruction and an elevated alkaline phosphatase level but is not likely to produce hepatocellular necrosis. Hemochromatosis can produce portal fibrosis and cirrhosis, but the liver cells have prominent accumulation of golden-brown hemosiderin pigment.
BP6 525–528   PBD6 856, 860–861

14. **(A)** The findings point to portal hypertension with bleeding esophageal varices. Cirrhosis alters hepatic blood flow to produce portal hypertension. A mass lesion, such as a cholangiocarcinoma, is not likely to obstruct blood flow in this manner, nor does massive necrosis. Fatty change can increase liver size and can be seen in association with alcoholic cirrhosis, but steatosis alone does not elevate portal venous pressure. HAV infection rarely results in significant chronic liver disease.
BP6 523–524   PBD6 853–856

15. **(C)** Persistence of HBsAg in serum for 6 months or more after initial detection denotes a carrier state. Worldwide, most persons with a chronic carrier state for HBV acquired this infection in utero or at birth. Only 1% to 10% of adult HBV infections yield a chronic carrier state. The carrier state is stable in most persons, although they become a reservoir for infection of others.
BP6 530   PBD6 864

16. **(C)** The PAS-positive globules in the liver seen here are characteristic for α_1-antitrypsin (AAT) deficiency. AAT deficiency can lead to chronic hepatitis and to cirrhosis. Deficiency of AAT also allows unchecked action of elastases in the lung that destroy the elastic tissue and cause emphysema. Diabetes mellitus and heart failure are features of hemochromatosis, a condition of iron overload. Iron deposition in liver is detected by the Prussian blue stain. Ulcerative colitis is strongly associated with primary sclerosing cholangitis, a condition in which there is inflammation and obliterative fibrosis of bile ducts. Systemic lupus erythematosus is a systemic immune complex disease that may affect many organs. Liver involvement, however, is uncommon.
BP6 541   PBD6 875–876

17. **(D)** This is the classic "nutmeg" appearance of the liver with chronic passive congestion from right-sided heart failure. Several forms of obstructive and restrictive lung diseases can cause cor pulmonale. Polyarteritis nodosa can lead to focal hepatic infarction. Chronic alcoholism results in hepatic steatosis, cirrhosis, or both. Polycythemia vera is the most common cause for Budd-Chiari syndrome. In this disease, hepatic vein thrombosis is followed by rapid hepatic congestion. This is a rare condition—far less common than cor pulmonale. Chronic HCV infection can lead to portal fibrosis and cirrhosis.
BP6 546–547   PBD6 882–883

18. **(D)** The most important predictor of whether a patient with viral hepatitis will develop chronic liver disease is the etiologic agent that caused the hepatitis. Of all the hepatotropic viruses, infection by HCV is the most likely to progress to chronicity and ultimately to cirrhosis. HAV, HEV, and hepatitis G virus (HGV) almost never cause chronic hepatitis. The pattern of histologic change, the degree of transaminase elevation, and the duration of transaminase elevation are relatively poor predictors of chronicity.
BP6 525   PBD6 856

19. **(D)** These are cholesterol gallstones. They are pale yellow but acquire a variegated appearance by trapping bile pigments. By comparison, pigment stones are uniformly dark. Risk factors for such stones include Native-American

descent, female sex, obesity, and increasing age. These factors cause secretion of bile that is supersaturated in cholesterol. Patients with sickle cell anemia develop pigment stones. Severe ileal dysfunction, as occurs in Crohn disease, can also predispose to pigment stones. Jaundice, pruritus, and ulcerative colitis are associated with primary sclerosing cholangitis, not gallstones. Intravenous drug abusers are at risk for viral hepatitis, not gallbladder disease.
BP6 550–552   PBD6 893–895

20.   **(C)** Spider telangiectasias (i.e., angiomas) refer to vascular lesions in the skin characterized by a central, pulsating, dilated arteriole from which small vessels radiate. This lesion results from hyperestrogenism (which also contributes to the testicular atrophy). The failing liver is unable to metabolize estrogens normally. Therefore, spider angiomas are a manifestation of hepatic failure. Ascites, splenomegaly, hemorrhoids, and esophageal varices are all related to portal hypertension, with resultant collateral venous congestion and dilation.
BP6 304, 522   PBD6 534

21.   **(B)** Prothrombin time depends on the synthesis of prothrombin along with other vitamin K–dependent clotting factors by the liver. Albumin is also manufactured in the liver, and hypoalbuminemia occurs with hepatic failure. Bilirubinuria occurs when there is conjugated bilirubin in the blood, as occurs in obstructive jaundice. AST is an hepatic enzyme whose levels are elevated when liver cells are injured. Total and direct bilirubin levels reflect the balance between bilirubin production from red cell turnover and the ability of the liver to excrete this pigment. The alkaline phosphatase level is elevated when there is obstruction to the flow of bile.
BP6 522   PBD6 852–853

22.   **(B)** This patient had chronic alcoholism, giving rise to cirrhosis. The liver is diffusely nodular, with small uniform, regenerative nodules separated by fibrous bands. Alcohol ingestion also causes fatty liver. PAS-positive inclusions are found in cirrhosis due to α_1-antitrypsin deficiency. A cirrhotic liver that is intensely green is most likely a late sequela of biliary obstruction.
BP6 523, 535   PBD6 853, 869–871

23.   **(E)** Viral hepatitis is not a risk factor for development of biliary tract lithiasis. Most gallbladder carcinomas occur in the setting of cholelithiasis. Obesity in middle-aged women is a risk factor for cholesterol gallstones. Chronic hemolysis and the disturbance of the enterohepatic circulation of bile salts with Crohn disease predispose to the formation of pigment gallstones.
BP6 551–554   PBD6 893–895

24.   **(A)** The elevated AFP level is most suggestive of hepatocellular carcinoma, which arises in the background of cirrhosis. The presence of HBsAg and anti-hepatitis B core antibody indicates chronic infection with HBV, which gave rise to cirrhosis and, ultimately, liver cell cancer. Massive hepatocyte necrosis is not likely late in the course of chronic hepatitis and cirrhosis. Massive liver cell necrosis gives rise to a shrunken, not enlarged or nodular liver. Steatosis is a nonspecific change seen in several forms of

hepatocyte injury. It can be seen in alcoholic liver disease and some forms of hepatitis. It does not cause an elevation of the AFP level. With Wilson disease or autoimmune hepatitis, cirrhosis can occur, but the incidence of these diseases is much less frequent than HBV infection.
BP6 548–549   PBD6 888–890

25.   **(B)** The massive upper gastrointestinal bleeding suggests esophageal varices as a consequence of portal hypertension from cirrhosis. If he is not currently drinking, no fatty change exists. The architectural changes of cirrhosis persist for decades after cirrhosis develops.
BP6 535–538   PBD6 869–872

26.   **(K)** She has evidence of HCV infection and has had symptoms of liver disease for 1 year. Clinically, she has chronic hepatitis (>6 months) that may have followed an asymptomatic acute hepatitis C. The anti-HCV IgG is not protective. This is supported by continued HCV viremia. One half of cases of hepatitis C go on to chronic hepatitis, but a fulminant hepatitis is not common. Chronic hepatitis is characterized by necrosis of hepatocytes at the interface between portal tracts and the liver lobule. This eventually leads to bridging necrosis and, finally, cirrhosis. At this time, however, the patient has no signs and symptoms of cirrhosis.
BP6 528   PBD6 860–861

27.   **(C)** This patient has primary sclerosing cholangitis; ulcerative colitis coexists in 70% of these patients. The major targets in primary sclerosing cholangitis are intrahepatic bile ducts. They undergo a destructive cholangitis that leads eventually to periductal fibrosis and cholestatic jaundice. Eventually, cirrhosis and liver failure can occur. Granulomatous bile duct destruction is seen in primary biliary cirrhosis.
BP6 543–544   PBD6 879–880

28.   **(A)** She has Wilson disease, an inherited disorder in which toxic levels of copper accumulate in tissues, particularly brain, eye, and liver. The gene for Wilson disease encodes a copper-transporting ATPase in the hepatocytes. With mutations in this gene, copper cannot be secreted into plasma. Ceruloplasmin is an α_2-globulin that carries copper in plasma. Because copper cannot be secreted into plasma, ceruloplasmin levels are low. A positive HBsAg result is indicative of HBV, which infects only the liver. Chronic liver disease and panlobular emphysema may occur with α_1-antitrypsin deficiency. An increased serum ferritin may indicate hereditary hemochromatosis. A positive antimitochondrial antibody finding can be seen with primary biliary cirrhosis.
BP6 540–541   PBD6 875

29.   **(D)** Almost all gallbladder carcinomas are adenocarcinomas, and most are found in gallbladders that also contain gallstones. Amebic dysentery can be complicated by amebic liver abscess; the amebae do not cause gallbladder infection. Ulcerative colitis is associated with primary sclerosing cholangitis. Infection with the biliary tree fluke *C. sinensis* is a risk factor for biliary tract cancer, not gallbladder cancer. Similarly, primary sclerosing cholangitis increases the risk of developing cholangiocarcinoma.
BP6 554–555   PBD6 899–900

30. **(C)** The intermittent upper abdominal pain is a nonspecific symptom that is often seen in patients with gallstones. When a stone slips into the common bile duct, intrahepatic cholestasis occurs. This explains the conjugated hyperbilirubinemia and the increased alkaline phosphatase. Chronic passive congestion from heart failure does not typically produce hyperbilirubinemia. Active viral hepatitis should be accompanied by some hepatocellular necrosis. Extrahepatic biliary atresia is a rare neonatal condition. Veno-occlusive disease is rare and is accompanied by hyperbilirubinemia and cholestasis but without evidence for biliary tract obstruction.
BP6 520–521, 553   PBD6 848–851, 898

31. **(D)** She has findings characteristic for primary biliary cirrhosis, which has a peak incidence in middle-aged females. Later in the disease, jaundice may increase with progressive destruction of intrahepatic bile ducts. The positivity for antimitochondrial antibody is a characteristic finding seen in most cases. Anti-parietal cell antibody is seen in chronic atrophic gastritis that gives rise to pernicious anemia. Anticentromere antibody typically occurs in systemic sclerosis. Anti-ribonucleoprotein antibodies can occur in a variety of connective tissue diseases, including mixed connective tissue disease. Anti–double-stranded DNA antibodies are diagnostic of systemic lupus erythematosus.
BP6 543   PBD6 878–879

32. **(B)** She has an unconjugated hyperbilirubinemia, which can result from hemolysis. With increased red blood cell destruction, there is more bilirubin than can be conjugated by the hepatocytes. Obstructive jaundice with biliary tract lithiasis results in mostly conjugated hyperbilirubinemia. The total bilirubin concentration may be increased with viral hepatitis, cirrhosis, and with drugs. Although direct and indirect hyperbilirubinemia may occur in these conditions, conjugated hyperbilirubinemia predominates.
BP6 518–521   PBD6 848–851

33. **(A)** Aflatoxin is a hepatotoxin and is the product of the fungus *Aspergillus flavus* growing on moldy peanuts. Aflatoxin can be carcinogenic, leading to development of hepatocellular carcinoma, as shown here. Oysters can concentrate HAV from sea water contaminated with sewage, and eating raw oysters can result in HAV infection. Aspirin has been implicated in causing Reye syndrome, in which there is extensive microvesicular steatosis. Prolonged and excessive intake of oral iron, rarely, can cause secondary hemochromatosis. Nitrites have been causally linked with cancers in the upper gastrointestinal tract.
BP6 548–550   PBD6 888–890

34. **(E)** The diffuse nodularity with depressed scars between the nodules is characteristic of cirrhosis. The most common cause for cirrhosis in the Western world is alcohol abuse. Alpha$_1$-antitrypsin deficiency and hereditary hemochromatosis can result in a cirrhosis, but both of these diseases are uncommon. With hereditary hemochromatosis, the liver should have a dark brown gross appearance from the extensive iron deposition. Of the various forms of viral hepatitis, those caused by HBV and HCV are the most likely to be followed by cirrhosis. This complication is rare to nonexistent with HAV, HGV, and HEV infection. With sclerosing cholangitis, there is portal fibrosis but not much nodular regeneration, so the liver is green and hard and has a finely granular surface.
BP6 523, 535–536   PBD6 870–871

35. **(G)** This patient has a circumscribed mass in the liver, suggesting a benign tumor such as hepatic adenoma. These tumors, which develop in young women who have used oral contraceptives, can enlarge and rupture from estrogenic stimulation during pregnancy.
BP6 548   PBD6 887–888

36. **(M)** The presence of obstructive jaundice, granulomatous destruction of bile ducts, and elevated titers of antimitochondrial antibodies is characteristic of primary biliary cirrhosis. This is an autoimmune condition that may be associated with other autoimmune phenomena (e.g., scleroderma, thyroiditis, glomerulonephritis). Cirrhosis is a late complication of this disease that can persist for 20 years or more.
BP6 543,   PBD6 878–879

37. **(C)** Vertical transmission, in endemic regions, produces a carrier rate of 90% to 95%. Development of viral hepatitis requires an immune response against virus-infected cells. In immunocompetent individuals, HBV causes development of HBsAg–specific T cells that cause apoptosis of infected liver cells. During the neonatal period, immune responses are not fully developed, and hence hepatitis does not occur. The high carrier rate is medically significant because it increases the risk of hepatocellular carcinomas 200-fold. In these populations, coexistent cirrhosis may be absent in up to 50% of patients. By contrast, in Western countries, where HBV is not endemic, cirrhosis is present in 80% to 90% of patients who develop liver cancer.
BP6 526, 530   PBD6 857, 864

38. **(C)** She has Gilbert syndrome, resulting from decreased levels of uridine diphosphate glucuronosyltransferese (UGT). Up to 7% of persons may have decreased levels of this enzyme, and this condition is often never diagnosed. Stress may cause transient unconjugated hyperbilirubinemia to a point that scleral icterus is detectable when the serum bilirubin reaches about 2 to 2.5 mg/dL. Choledochal cyst is a rare anomaly producing extrahepatic biliary obstruction with conjugated hyperbilirubinemia. Primary biliary cirrhosis results in conjugated hyperbilirubinemia, as does the rare Dubin-Johnson syndrome. Hepatitis A can often be mild but is not so transient, and it can be accompanied by a mild increase in conjugated and unconjugated bilirubin.
BP6 520–521   PBD6 850–851

39. **(C)** The symptoms are typical for acute calculous cholecystitis. Hepatitis is unlikely to produce acute pain and leukocytosis. Extrahepatic biliary atresia is seen in neonates and is characterized by obstructive jaundice. Sclerosing cholangitis is typically a chronic process that presents with jaundice and pruritus. Carcinomas of the gallbladder are not common and typically have a more insidious onset.
BP6 551–552   PBD6 893–895

40. **(B)** Cirrhosis is characterized by portal fibrosis with nodular regeneration and disruption of architecture of the entire liver. Chronic hepatitis and alcoholism are the most common causes for cirrhosis. Alcoholic hepatitis is characterized by liver cell necrosis with a neutrophil exudate around necrotic liver cells. There is some perivenular (central) and sinusoidal fibrosis, but there is no nodular regeneration. Acetaminophen in large quantities causes extensive hepatocyte necrosis. Chronic passive congestion can cause centrilobular necrosis and rarely can produce fibrosis, or so-called cardiac cirrhosis with fibrosis bridging central zonal regions. However, this is not a true cirrhosis, because nodular regeneration is usually absent.
BP6 523   PBD6 853-854

41. **(C)** This is Reye syndrome, an uncommon disease seen most often in young children. It can follow a viral illness and has been unconvincingly linked to the use of aspirin for the treatment of fever in this setting. Reye syndrome is caused by mitochondrial dysfunction that affects the liver, brain, and other organs. Death from hepatic failure is a dreaded complication. Accumulation of small droplets of fat in hepatocytes (microvesicular steatosis) is the typical histologic finding. This feature is not seen in any of the other conditions included in the list here. Extrahepatic biliary atresia is a rare neonatal disease. The PAS-positive globules are seen in α_1-antitrypsin deficiency, a condition that affects adults. Hereditary hemochromatosis manifests with complications in middle age after extensive iron deposition has occurred. The loss of intrahepatic bile ducts with primary biliary cirrhosis is also a rare disease of middle age.
BP6 542   PBD6 869

42. **(C)** Antibodies to HCV do not confer protection against reinfection. HCV RNA remains in the circulation, despite the presence of neutralizing antibodies. In infections with HAV, HBV, HDV, or HGV, development of IgG antibodies offers lifelong immunity. A hepatitis B vaccine exists for this purpose.
BP6 528   PBD6 860

43. **(B)** This is macrovesicular steatosis (fatty change) of the liver with early fibrosis. The most common cause of fatty liver and fibrosis is chronic alcoholism. Patients with chronic cholelithiasis can develop extrahepatic obstruction and secondary biliary cirrhosis. In these cases, there is no fat in the liver, but there is accumulation of bile. Skin pigmentation, diabetes, and ascites suggest hemochromatosis, in which there is pigment storage and cirrhosis. Pruritus and jaundice are features of biliary obstruction. Xanthomas result from cholesterol retention in primary biliary cirrhosis. Association with ulcerative colitis is a feature of primary sclerosing cholangitis.
BP6 517   PBD6 869-870

44. **(B)** The patient has serologic markers of hepatitis B (i.e., HBsAg positive), and the detection of hepatitis B core IgM antibody indicates acute infection. Most cases of HBV infection do not progress to chronic hepatitis, but a small number of cases are complicated by fulminant hepatitis or by progression to cirrhosis. In some patients, cirrhosis progresses to hepatocellular carcinoma, but given that most patients with hepatitis B recover, the risk for liver cancer in a given individual is very small. Donation of blood is *not* a risk to the donor, but testing for hepatitis B and C, among others, is done to lessen the risk to blood recipients. After recovery from hepatitis B, IgG antibodies against HBsAg may persist for life. They confer protection from reinfection.
BP6 527   PBD6 857-859

45. **(C)** He has alcoholic cirrhosis with portal hypertension. Venous collateral flow can be increased in esophageal submucosal veins, producing varices, and in abdominal wall, producing caput medusae. The coagulopathy from decreased liver function may lead to purpuric hemorrhages, but splinter hemorrhages of the nails are most characteristic for embolization from infective endocarditis. Liver failure with cirrhosis may lead to hepatic coma, but brain swelling with papilledema is not a major feature. Hyperreflexia but not diminution of deep tendon reflexes can occur when hepatic encephalopathy develops. Right-sided heart failure, in which liver can be enlarged because of passive congestion, is associated with distended jugular veins.
BP6 524   PBD6 853-854

46. **(B)** She has primary biliary cirrhosis, an uncommon autoimmune disorder with progressive intrahepatic bile duct destruction. Pruritus, conjugated hyperbilirubinemia, and increased alkaline phosphatase levels are indicative of obstructive jaundice resulting from bile duct destruction. Ninety percent or more of patients with this disease have antimitochondrial antibodies in the serum. Chronic hepatitis C is marked by hepatocyte necrosis, not bile duct destruction. An elevated sweat chloride is seen with cystic fibrosis, which can cause neonatal jaundice. An increased serum ferritin is seen in patients with hereditary hemochromatosis. Alpha$_1$-antitrypsin deficiency can affect the liver, causing chronic hepatitis and cirrhosis. These patients also develop panlobular emphysema.
BP6 543-544   PBD6 878-879

47. **(C)** The restrictive lung disease leads to cor pulmonale with right-sided congestive heart failure. This causes passive venous congestion in the liver that is most pronounced in the centrilobular areas. When the congestion is severe, the anoxia can cause centrilobular necrosis with transaminase elevation. The microscopic appearance is that of intense centrilobular congestion. Notice that the area around the portal tract is less congested.
BP6 546-547,   PBD6 882-883

48. **(G)** They have hereditary hemochromatosis, an autosomal recessive genetic disorder that results in increased dietary iron absorption. By middle age, there is excess iron storage in many organs, including liver, pancreas, heart, and joints. The resultant tissue injury causes cirrhosis, diabetes mellitus, and sometimes arthralgias.
BP6 538-539,   PBD6 873-874

49. **(J)** This is a classic case of acute alcoholic hepatitis. The picture shows globular eosinophilic cytoplasmic inclusions, called Mallory bodies. These inclusions are characteristic of, but not specific for, alcoholic hepatitis. There are also areas of hepatocyte necrosis surrounded by neutrophils. Some neutrophils can be seen in the picture.
BP6 535-538   PBD6 869-871

The Pancreas

PBD6 Chapter 20 - The Pancreas
BP6 Chapter 17 - The Pancreas

1. The test of choice to monitor diabetes control over the preceding 2 months is to measure the level of

- (A) Random plasma glucose
- (B) Fasting plasma glucose
- (C) Glycosylated hemoglobin
- (D) Glycosylated serum albumin
- (E) Serum fructosamine

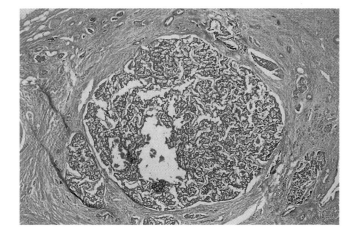

2. A 33-year-old female has had several "fainting spells" over the past 6 months. Each time, she has a prodrome of light-headedness followed by a brief loss of consciousness. Each time, she awakens with no loss of motor or sensory function. On the basis of the microscopic finding seen here, which of the following pancreatic lesions is most likely in this patient?

- (A) Adenocarcinoma
- (B) Acute pancreatitis
- (C) Islet cell adenoma
- (D) Pseudocyst
- (E) Fatty replacement

3. A 66-year-old female has had diabetes mellitus for more than 30 years. She now has decreasing visual acuity. There is no eye pain. Her intraocular pressure is measured as normal. Which of the following lesions is most likely to account for her visual problems?

- (A) Keratomalacia
- (B) Optic neuritis
- (C) Cytomegalovirus retinitis
- (D) Proliferative retinopathy
- (E) Glaucoma

For each of the clinical histories in questions 4 and 5, match the most closely associated finding that accompanies or complicates diabetes mellitus:

- (A) Acute myocardial infarction
- (B) Amyloidosis
- (C) Arteriolosclerosis
- (D) Gangrenous necrosis
- (E) Ketoacidosis
- (F) Hyperosmolar coma
- (G) Hypoglycemic coma
- (H) Insulitis
- (I) Mucormycosis
- (J) Necrotizing papillitis
- (K) Neurogenic bladder
- (L) Retinopathy

4. A 52-year-old male has had type 1 diabetes for the past 40 years. Increased oxidized low-density lipoprotein (LDL) cholesterol has led to abnormalities of his right popliteal artery. (   )

5. A 28-year-old male has been using insulin injections to control his diabetes mellitus for the past 10 years. He is unable to be wakened by his roommate one morning and is unconscious when brought to the emergency department. Laboratory findings include a high plasma level of insulin and a lack of detectable c-peptide. Urinalysis reveals no blood, protein, or glucose, but the ketone level is 4+. (   )

6. A 73-year-old female has had a 10-kg weight loss in the past 3 months. She is becoming increasingly icteric.

She also has some vague epigastric pain that is constant, along with nausea and episodes of bloating and diarrhea. Her total serum bilirubin concentration is 11.6 mg/dL, with a direct bilirubin level of 10.5 mg/dL. Which of the following conditions involving the pancreas is most likely to be present?

○ (A) Islet cell adenoma
○ (B) Chronic pancreatitis
○ (C) Cystic fibrosis
○ (D) Adenocarcinoma
○ (E) Pseudocyst

7.   A 58-year-old male has diabetes mellitus. This disease has been poorly controlled for many years. As a consequence, he has had nonenzymatic glycosylation of free amino groups of proteins in his body. This process is best illustrated by finding which of the following pathologic abnormalities?

○ (A) Peripheral neuropathy
○ (B) Amyloid replacement of islets
○ (C) Formation of retinal microaneurysms
○ (D) Accelerated atherogenesis
○ (E) Cataracts

8.   A 38-year-old female has had a low-volume watery diarrhea for the past 3 months. She now presents with midepigastric pain. Over-the-counter antacid medications do not relieve the pain. On upper endoscopy, she is found to have multiple 0.5- to 1.1-cm duodenal ulcerations. She is given drug treatment to inhibit acid secretion. Three months later, endoscopy reveals that the ulcerations are still present. Which of the following analytes in serum or plasma is most likely to be increased on laboratory testing?

○ (A) Insulin
○ (B) Somatostatin
○ (C) Glucagon
○ (D) Vasoactive intestinal polypeptide (VIP)
○ (E) Gastrin

9.   Which of the following features is common to type 1 and type 2 diabetes?

○ (A) Presence of islet cell antibodies
○ (B) Association with certain major histocompatibility complex (MHC) class II alleles
○ (C) Marked resistance to the action of insulin
○ (D) Nonenzymatic glycosylation of proteins
○ (E) Concordance rate of more than 90% in monozygotic twins

10.   A 40-year-old male has been taking daily insulin injections for the past 25 years. When he does not show up for work, a friend visits his house, finds him on the floor in an obtunded state, and calls an ambulance. On admission to the hospital, the patient has a hemoglobin A_{1C} concentration of 8.9%, a serum glucose level of 11 mg/dL, a serum osmolality of 295 mOsm/kg, and a urinalysis that reveals 4+ ketonuria with specific gravity of 1.010. Which

of the following statements best characterizes these findings?

○ (A) He is in poor control and has had an insulin overdose.
○ (B) He is in good control but has developed ketoacidosis.
○ (C) He is in poor control and is not taking his insulin.
○ (D) He is in good control but has not eaten food recently.
○ (E) He is in poor control and has developed hyperosmolar coma.

11.   A previously healthy, 36-year-old female has had several "fainting spells" in the past month. During these episodes, she becomes light-headed and then collapses, recovering in a few minutes, but experiencing diaphoresis and tachycardia. Which of the following laboratory results is most likely to be found during one of these episodes?

○ (A) Hypocalcemia
○ (B) Hypoglycemia
○ (C) Hypercarbia
○ (D) Ketonuria
○ (E) Hyperglycemia

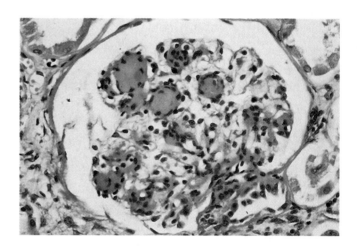

12.   A 35-year-old female is admitted to the hospital with severe anginal pain. An electrocardiogram reveals evidence of left ventricular infarction that is confirmed by elevated serum levels of creatine kinase (CK) and the CK-MB fraction. Additional investigation reveals a 2+ proteinuria and a modest elevation of the blood urea nitrogen level. A renal biopsy is performed and is illustrated here under high magnification. This patient is at a high risk for which of the following additional complications?

○ (A) Gallstones
○ (B) Gangrene of the foot
○ (C) Chronic pancreatitis
○ (D) Uric acid stones
○ (E) Renal cell carcinoma

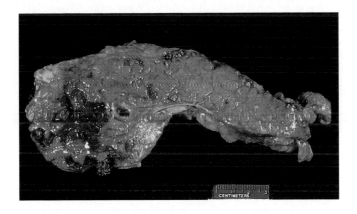

(F) Necrosis with neutrophilic infiltration and interstitial hemorrhage

(G) Normal islets of Langerhans within a fibrous stroma containing a few lymphocytes

(H) Poorly formed glandular structures with hyperchromatic and pleomorphic nuclei comprising a 5-cm mass in the head

(I) Small concretions within an irregularly dilated pancreatic duct

(J) Small round cells with a richly vascularized stroma comprising a 1-cm nodule in the body

13. A 52-year-old male has had severe abdominal pain for the past 2 days. Physical examination reveals boardlike rigidity of the abdominal musculature, making further examination difficult. There does not appear to be any abdominal distention. His pancreas looks similar to the one shown here. What is the most common predisposing factor in the development of this disorder?

(A) Coxsackievirus infection
(B) Hypertriglyceridemia
(C) Chronic alcoholism
(D) Vasculitis
(E) Thiazide diuretic therapy

14. The same patient described in question 13 is admitted to the hospital, and with supportive care, his acute condition subsides over the next week. Which of the following complications is most likely to occur in this patient?

(A) Pseudocyst formation
(B) Hemoperitoneum
(C) Small bowel infarction
(D) Gastric ulceration
(E) Hyperosmolar coma

15. Which of the following laboratory test findings best distinguishes type 1 diabetes mellitus from other forms of diabetes?

(A) Elevated hemoglobin A_{1C} level
(B) Ketoacidosis
(C) Glucosuria
(D) Decreased plasma insulin concentration
(E) Hyperglycemia

For each of the clinical histories in questions 16 and 17, match the most closely associated microscopic description of a pathologic process involving the pancreas:

(A) Amyloid deposition within the islets of Langerhans
(B) Extensive fibrosis and fatty replacement of the acinar parenchyma
(C) Hyperplasia of the islets of Langerhans with a normal surrounding acinar parenchyma
(D) Infiltration of T lymphocytes into the islets of Langerhans
(E) Necrosis with circumferential granulation tissue formation comprising a 4-cm mass in the tail

16. The prenatal course of a 25-year-old primigravida is uncomplicated. Soon after birth, her 4500-g male neonate with Apgar scores of 8 at 1 minute and 10 at 5 minutes develops irritability with seizure activity. Serum chemistry tests on the baby reveal a sodium level of 145 mmol/L, potassium level of 4.2 mmol/L, chloride level of 99 mmol/L, carbon dioxide concentration of 25 mmol/L, urea nitrogen level of 0.4 mg/dL, and glucose level of 18 mg/dL. (   )

17. A 12-year-old female is healthy with no complaints. There is no history of a significant illness. She has a serum glucose concentration of 81 mg/dL. However, she has HLA-DR3 and HLA-DR4 alleles. She has autoantibodies to glutamic acid decarboxylase. (   )

18. A 72-year-old female is admitted to the hospital in an obtunded condition. Her temperature is 37°C, pulse is 95 beats/min, respiration rate is 22/min, and blood pressure is 90/60 mm Hg. She appears to be dehydrated and has poor skin turgor. Her serum glucose level is 872 mg/dL. A urinalysis shows 4+ glucose but no ketones, protein, or blood. Which of the following factors is most important in the pathogenesis of this condition?

(A) HLA-DR3/HLA-DR4 genotype
(B) Insulin resistance
(C) Autoimmune insulitis
(D) Severe depletion of β cells in islets
(E) Virus-induced injury to β cells in islets

19. For the past 24 years, a man has had poorly controlled diabetes mellitus. He now has an increasing serum urea nitrogen and creatinine along with proteinuria. Which of the following pathologic findings on renal biopsy is most likely?

(A) Membranous glomerulonephritis
(B) Amyloid deposition
(C) Diffuse glomerulosclerosis
(D) Necrotizing vasculitis
(E) Polycystic change

20. A 38-year-old female with a long history of gallbladder disease has the sudden onset of severe mid-abdominal pain. An abdominal radiograph shows no free air, but there is marked soft tissue edema. At laparotomy, the pancreas is found to be markedly edematous with foci of reddish black discoloration interspersed throughout the parenchyma. Which of the following serum laboratory test findings is most likely?

○ (A) Hyperammonemia
○ (B) Increased amylase level
○ (C) Hypoglycemia
○ (D) Increased alanine aminotransferase (ALT) level
○ (E) Hypokalemia

21. A 56-year-old female dies suddenly and unexpectedly. She had a long history of diabetes mellitus. She is obese—about 40 kg over ideal body weight. Her only previous serious medical problem was a poorly healing ulcer on the sole of her left foot. Which of the following lesions is most likely to be found at autopsy?

○ (A) Subarachnoid hemorrhage
○ (B) Pulmonary thromboembolism
○ (C) Perforated duodenal ulcer
○ (D) Pancreatic adenocarcinoma
○ (E) Coronary artery thrombosis

22. A 39-year-old male has had numerous bouts of pneumonia for the past 35 years, caused by *Pseudomonas aeruginosa* and *Burkholderia cepacia*. He has had a mild to moderate volume diarrhea that has a high stool fat content. Laboratory testing reveals an elevated sweat chloride level. Which of the following pathologic findings would you expect to be present in the pancreas in this patient?

○ (A) Acute inflammation
○ (B) Pseudocyst
○ (C) Amyloidosis
○ (D) Acinar atrophy
○ (E) Adenocarcinoma

23. A 13-year-old female collapses while playing basketball. When brought to the emergency room, she is obtunded. She has hypotension, tachycardia, and deep, rapid, labored respirations. She has a serum sodium level of 151 mmol/L, potassium level of 4.6 mmol/L, chloride level of 98 mmol/L, bicarbonate level of 7 mmol/L, and glucose level of 521 mg/dL. A urinalysis reveals no protein, blood, or nitrite, but there are 4+ glucose and 4+ ketone levels. The most probable pathologic finding in the pancreas at the time of her collapse is

○ (A) Amyloid replacement of islets
○ (B) Chronic pancreatitis
○ (C) Eosinophil infiltration of islets
○ (D) Pancreatic duct obstruction
○ (E) Loss of islets of Langerhans

24. A 50-year-old male has a 35-year history of diabetes mellitus. During this time, his disease has been poorly controlled. He now has problems with sexual function, including difficulty attaining an erection. He is also plagued by a mild but recurrent, low-volume diarrhea and by difficulty with urination. These problems stem from which of the following mechanisms of cellular injury?

○ (A) Coagulative necrosis
○ (B) Sorbitol accumulation
○ (C) Nonenzymatic glycosylation
○ (D) Leukocytic infiltration
○ (E) Hyaline deposition

25. The most significant factor that leads to the metabolic derangements seen in type 2 diabetes mellitus is

○ (A) Lack of β cells in islets of Langerhans
○ (B) Chronic renal failure
○ (C) Peripheral insulin resistance
○ (D) Overproduction of amylin protein
○ (E) Development of autoantibodies to insulin

26. The pancreas of a 63-year-old male at autopsy is found to be grossly small and densely fibrotic. Microscopically, there is extensive atrophy of the acini with abundant collagenous interstitial fibrosis, but the islets of Langerhans appear normal. Inspissated proteinaceous secretions are present in branches of the pancreatic duct. Which of the following conditions best accounts for these findings?

○ (A) α_1-antitrypsin deficiency
○ (B) Hypercholesterolemia
○ (C) Chronic alcoholism
○ (D) Blunt trauma to the abdomen
○ (E) Cholelithiasis

ANSWERS

1. (C) Nonenzymatic glycosylation refers to the chemical process whereby glucose attaches to proteins without the aid of enzymes. The degree of glycosylation is proportionate to the level of blood glucose. Many proteins, including hemoglobin, undergo nonenzymatic glycosylation. Because red cells have a life span of about 120 days, the amount of glycosylated hemoglobin is a function of blood glucose level over the previous 120-day period. The level of glycosylated hemoglobin is not appreciably affected by short-term changes in plasma glucose levels.
BP6 567   PBD6 919

2. (C) This is a circumscribed cellular lesion in the pancreas, most suggestive of an islet cell adenoma. Secretion of insulin by these lesions causes hypoglycemia and the described symptoms. Many of these tumors are less than 1 cm in diameter, making them difficult to detect. Most patients who have an islet cell adenoma have only mild insulin hypersecretion. The laboratory finding of an increased insulin to glucose ratio is helpful. Surgical excision is necessary in cases with marked symptoms. Acute pancreatitis is unlikely to increase islet cell release of insulin. Adenocarcinomas of the pancreas are derived from ductal epithelium and have no endocrine function. Pseudocysts are complications of pancreatitis that are focal and do not produce insulin hypersecretion. Fatty replacement of the pancreas can occur with cystic fibrosis, but the islets also gradually diminish in number with time.
BP6 559   PBD6 926-927

3. (D) A variety of retinal lesions occur with diabetes mellitus. Retinopathy, cataracts, and glaucoma result in acquired blindness in some diabetics. Keratomalacia may be seen with vitamin A deficiency. Optic neuritis can be seen with systemic autoimmune diseases, with ischemia from

temporal arteritis, and from toxicity as a consequence of methanol poisoning. Cytomegalovirus retinitis is seen in immunocompromised patients, particularly those with acquired immunodeficiency syndrome (AIDS). Glaucoma is marked by an increased intraocular pressure.
BP6 571   PBD6 924, 1369–1370

4.   **(D)** Severe peripheral atherosclerotic disease is a common complication of long-standing diabetes mellitus. Atherosclerotic narrowing of the popliteal artery can cause ischemia and gangrene. The foot is often involved with gangrene, which may necessitate amputation.
BP6 567–569   PBD6 919–921

5.   **(G)** This patient has experienced hypoglycemic coma. The fact that he does not have detectable C-peptide indicates that there is no endogenous insulin production, as expected in type 1 diabetics. The high insulin level has resulted from the exogenous insulin that he takes for treating diabetes. However, he has not eaten enough to keep his glucose at an adequate level and has developed hypoglycemia. The lack of food intake has led to the ketosis.
BP6 572–574   PBD6 924–926

6.   **(D)** The weight loss and pain suggest a malignancy. The jaundice (a conjugated hyperbilirubinemia) comes from biliary tract obstruction by a mass in the head of the pancreas. Such a carcinoma may present with "painless jaundice" as well, but the carcinoma tends to invade the nerves around the pancreas, causing pain. An islet cell adenoma is not as common as pancreatic carcinoma, although a well-placed adenoma right near the ampulla could have a similar effect. However, weight loss with an adenoma is unlikely. Chronic pancreatitis does not usually obstruct the biliary tract. With cystic fibrosis, there is progressive pancreatic acinar atrophy without a mass effect. Most pseudocysts from pancreatitis are in the region of the body or tail of the pancreas.
BP6 561–562   PBD6 561–562

7.   **(D)** Nonenzymatic glycosylation of collagen accelerates atherosclerosis because it leads eventually to the formation of irreversible advanced glycosylation end products (AGEs), which accumulate over some period. Such changes in collagen in arterial walls aid in trapping low density lipoproteins (LDLs) and thus accelerate lipid deposition. The neuropathy, retinal microaneurysms, and cataracts common to diabetes result from sorbitol accumulation and subsequent osmotic cell injury. The amyloid replacement of islets is a feature of some cases of type 2 diabetes mellitus.
BP6 567   PBD6 919–920

8.   **(E)** This patient has the Zollinger-Ellison syndrome, with one or more islet cell adenomas of the pancreas secreting gastrin. This secretion leads to intractable peptic ulcer disease, with multiple duodenal or gastric ulcerations. Islet cell tumors may secrete a variety of hormonally active compounds. Glucagonomas and somatostatinomas may produce a syndrome with a mild diabetes mellitus. VIPomas may be associated with marked watery diarrhea, hypokalemia, and achlorhydria.
BP6 574–575   PBD6 927

9.   **(D)** Nonenzymatic glycosylation of proteins is a function of the level of blood glucose, rather than the cause of hyperglycemia. Type 1 and type 2 diabetes are characterized by hyperglycemia, but the underlying pathogenetic mechanisms are different. Type 1 diabetes is an autoimmune disease that is associated with certain alleles of the MHC class II molecules. It is characterized by a very high concordance rate and the presence of autoantibodies. Insulin resistance is a feature of type 2 diabetes.
BP6 567   PBD6 919–920

10.   **(A)** The increased hemoglobin A_{1C} level suggests that he has poorly controlled hyperglycemia. The profound hypoglycemia is consistent with overdose of insulin, and the ketonuria suggests that he has not been eating any food. If he had not been taking his insulin, the glucose should be higher, and if this were coupled with ketonuria, a diagnosis of ketoacidosis could be made. Because the serum osmolarity and the glucose are not increased, he does not have hyperosmolar coma.
BP6 572–573   PBD6 924–925

11.   **(B)** She has features of hypoglycemia. An islet cell tumor may be suspected as the cause of episodic hypoglycemia. Reactive hypoglycemia after meals may also be considered. Hypocalcemia gives rise to tetany, characterized by muscle spasms. Hypercarbia may result from decreased respiration. Ketonuria is a feature of type 1 diabetes mellitus and accompanies hyperglycemia.
BP6 574   PBD6 926–927

12.   **(B)** This is nodular glomerulosclerosis, a characteristic feature of renal involvement with advanced diabetes mellitus. Myocardial infarction in this premenopausal female strongly suggests an underlying predisposing condition such as diabetes mellitus. Proteinuria and evidence of renal failure support the likelihood of diabetes. Diabetics also are prone to early and accelerated atherosclerosis of peripheral vessels. Thrombotic occlusion of arteries in the leg places diabetics at a very high risk for developing gangrene. None of the other diseases have any association with diabetes.
BP6 569–572,   PBD6 920–928

13.   **(C)** This is acute hemorrhagic pancreatitis, with foci of chalky white fat necrosis. Although each of the listed predisposing factors can cause acute pancreatitis, chronic alcoholism is the most common. Gallstones also are present in many cases of pancreatitis. Eighty percent of cases are associated with biliary tract disease and alcoholism. Viral infection of the pancreas is a possible cause for pancreatitis, but it is uncommon. Hypertriglyceridemia is a rare cause for pancreatitis, because the triglyceride level must be in the range of 1000 mg/dL. A variety of drugs may produce a pancreatitis, including thiazides, but the number of cases of pancreatitis due to drugs is small compared with alcoholism and gallstones.
BP6 558–559   PBD6 904–907

14.   **(A)** During acute pancreatitis, the extent of necrosis may be so severe that a liquefied area becomes surrounded by granulation tissue, forming a cystic mass. However,

because there is no epithelial lining to the cyst, it is best called a pseudocyst. Although acute pancreatitis may be hemorrhagic, the hemorrhage is confined to the body of the pancreas and surrounding fibroadipose tissue. The inflammation is not likely to compromise the blood supply to abdominal organs and produce an infarction. Although the pancreas is inferior and posterior to the stomach, spread of inflammation to the stomach does not typically occur. The islets of Langerhans usually continue to function despite marked inflammation of the parenchyma. Therefore, lack of insulin is not a typical feature of pancreatitis.
BP6 558   PBD6 909

15.   **(B)** The markedly diminished insulin levels associated with type 1 diabetes, coupled with absolute or relative increases in glucagon, result in catabolism of adipose tissue. The released fatty acids can then become oxidized to form ketone bodies and produce ketoacidosis. Type 2 diabetes mellitus can have mild to moderately decreased insulin levels, but there is still sufficient insulin to prevent this complication. Elevated glucose levels occur in type 1 and type 2 diabetes mellitus, with resultant increases in the hemoglobin A_{1C} level and spillage of glucose into the urine.
BP6 572   PBD6 924-926

16.   **(C)** Maternal diabetes can result in hyperplasia of the fetal islets because of the maternal hyperglycemic environment. After birth, the hyperplastic islets continue to overfunction, resulting in neonatal hypoglycemia. Infants of diabetic mothers also tend to exhibit macrosomia because of the growth-promoting effects of increased insulin.
BP6 574   PBD6 927

17.   **(D)** The presence of HLA-DR3, HLA-DR4, or both is found in 95% of Caucasians with type 1 diabetes mellitus. Autoantibodies to islet cell antigens such as glutamic acid decarboxylase are present years before overt clinical diabetes develops. Similarly, an insulitis caused by T-cell infiltration occurs prior to the onset of symptoms or very early in the course of type 1 diabetes. The insulitis in type 1 diabetes is associated with increased expression of class I MHC molecules and aberrant expression of class II MHC molecules on the β cells of the islets. These changes are mediated by cytokines such as interferon-γ elaborated by CD4 cells (along with CD8 cells).
BP6 565   PBD6 916

18.   **(B)** This patient has type 2 diabetes with hyperosmolar, nonketotic coma. In type 2 diabetes, there is a decrease in plasma insulin or a relative lack of insulin, but there is still enough to prevent ketosis. The fundamental defect is insulin resistance. The resulting hyperglycemia tends to produce polyuria, leading to dehydration that further increases the serum glucose. If enough fluids are not ingested, dehydration drives the serum glucose to very high levels. Severe loss of β cells is a feature of autoimmune, or type 1, diabetes. The HLA-DR3/HLA-DR4, genotype predisposes to type 1 diabetes.
BP6 572   PBD6 926

19.   **(C)** Diffuse glomerulosclerosis and nodular glomerulosclerosis are changes characteristic for diabetic nephropa-

thy. This nephropathy takes years to develop, and renal function gradually diminishes. Membranous glomerulonephritis is most often idiopathic. Amyloidosis is uncommonly associated with diabetes mellitus. Although there are progressive vascular changes in the kidney with diabetes—notably large artery atherosclerosis and hyaline arteriolosclerosis—vasculitis is not a feature of diabetes. Polycystic changes are most likely to manifest in diabetics who have received long-term hemodialysis.
BP6 570   PBD6 923

20.   **(B)** The clinical feautes, along with preexisting gallbladder disease, are highly suggestive of acute pancreatitis. This is confirmed by the appearance of the pancreas. Serum amylase is rapidly elevated after an attack of acute pancreatitis. Serum and urine lipase levels are also elevated. These enzymes are released from necrotic pancreatic acini. Liver function test abnormalities may be seen in cases of gallstone pancreatitis. Hyperammonemia is a feature of liver failure. In acute pancreatitis, the islets of Langerhans still function but do not become hyperactive. An increased ALT level is more characteristic of liver cell injury. The serum potassium concentration does not drop with pancreatitis.
BP6 558-559   PBD6 904-907

21.   **(E)** The most common cause of death of diabetics is ischemic heart disease. Diabetics have accelerated, advanced atherosclerosis. Heart, kidneys, and brain are most often affected by ischemia from vascular narrowing, thrombosis, or thromboembolic disease. There can also be severe peripheral vascular disease, with poor tissue perfusion and poor wound healing, explaining her poorly healing foot ulcer. A diabetic could have a hemorrhagic cerebral infarction from a thromboembolus or a hypertensive hemorrhage, but these lesions are not known to involve the subarachnoid space. The advanced atherosclerosis of diabetes has minimal impact on the venous system. The risk for duodenal ulcers and for cancer is not appreciably greater in diabetics.
BP6 568   PBD6 922

22.   **(D)** This patient has cystic fibrosis, an autosomal recessive condition that results from an abnormal CFTR gene. The abnormal viscid secretions that occur with cystic fibrosis affect the pancreas, resulting in ductal obstruction that leads to acinar atrophy. Eventually, the exocrine function is gone. Acute and chronic pancreatitis do not typically occur in this setting, nor does the complication of inflammation known as a pseudocyst. Amyloid deposition may be seen in the islets of Langerhans in a type 2 diabetic, but generalized amyloid deposition of the pancreas is a rare event. Cystic fibrosis is not a risk factor for adenoma or carcinoma of the pancreas.
BP6 208-209   PBD6 479-480

23.   **(E)** Type 1 diabetes mellitus does not become overt until the β cells are markedly depleted and insulin levels are greatly reduced. In this case, the female is in ketoacidosis. Amyloid replacement of islets is a feature of type 2 diabetes mellitus, and ketoacidosis is not a feature of type 2 diabetes mellitus. Chronic pancreatitis diminishes exo-

crine pancreatic function but rarely destroys enough islets to result in overt diabetes mellitus. Inflammatory cells, mostly T cells, can be seen in the islets of patients with type 1 diabetes mellitus *before* the diabetes is clinically overt. However, eosinophils are rare, found usually in the islets of diabetic infants who fail to survive the immediate postnatal period. Pancreatic duct obstruction can produce an acute pancreatitis that is unlikely to affect the function of enough islets to cause diabetes mellitus.
BP6 564–565   PBD6 915–917

24.   **(B)** This patient has autonomic neuropathy caused by long-standing diabetes. It is thought that nerve cells do not require insulin for glucose uptake. In the presence of hyperglycemia, too much glucose diffuses into cell cytoplasm and accumulates. The excess glucose is metabolized by intracellular aldose reductase enzyme to sorbitol and then to fructose. This increased carbohydrate increases cellular osmolarity and increases free water influx, injuring the cell. Schwann cells are injured in this manner, leading to peripheral neuropathy. Coagulative necrosis in diabetics is most likely to result as a complication of atherosclerosis. Glycosylation tends to affect vascular walls and promote atherosclerosis. Infections with inflammation are more common in diabetics but do not lead to the characteristic neuropathy. Hyalinization affects small blood vessels, not nerves.
BP6 567   PBD6 920

25.   **(C)** Insulin resistance is the most important factor in the pathogenesis of type 2 diabetes mellitus. The number of insulin receptors are decreased and postreceptor insulin signaling is impaired, with reduced synthesis and translocation of glucose transport units (GLUTs), in fat and muscle. Insulin resistance leads to hyperglycemia. Obesity, affecting more than 80% of type 2 diabetics, appears to play a significant role in this process. In contrast, severe loss of β cells from autoimmune injury is responsible for greatly reduced insulin production in type 1 diabetes.
BP6 566–567   PBD6 917–918

26.   **(C)** This patient has chronic pancreatitis. Alcohol promotes intracellular proenzyme activation that leads to acinar cell injury. Chronic alcoholism also causes secretion of protein-rich pancreatic fluid, which is inspissated and deposited in small pancreatic ducts. Ductal obstruction predisposes to acinar injury. Ongoing or repeated injury leads to chronic pancreatitis. α_1-antitrypsin deficiency can produce liver disease with chronic hepatitis, cirrhosis, or both. Hypercholesterolemia can cause acute pancreatitis, as can cholelithiasis. Blunt abdominal trauma may produce hemorrhage, sometimes with a component of acute pancreatitis.
BP6 561   PBD6 907–909

The Kidney and the Lower Urinary Tract

BP6 Chapter 14 - The Kidney and Its
                Collecting System
PBD6 Chapter 21 - The Kidney
PBD6 Chapter 22 - The Lower Urinary Tract

1. A 24-year-old male is diagnosed with urolithiasis after passing a small radiopaque stone. He has no underlying illnesses and has been healthy all his life. Urinalysis shows no protein, glucose, ketones, or nitrite, with a pH of 7 and specific gravity of 1.020. He is advised to drink more water. He likes iced tea, and he consumes large quantities over the course of a hot summer. However, he continues to have urinary tract calculi. Which of the following types of calculi is he most likely to have on stone analysis?

○ (A) Uric acid
○ (B) Magnesium ammonium phosphate
○ (C) Calcium oxalate
○ (D) Cystine
○ (E) Mucoprotein

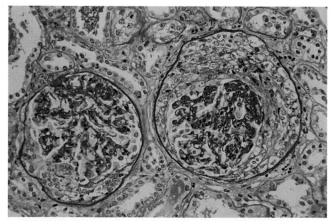

Courtesy of Dr. M. A. Venkatachalam, Department of Pathology, University of Texas Health Sciences Center, San Antonio, TX.

2. A 47-year-old male has had a decreased urine output over the past week. A urinalysis shows 1+ proteinuria, 4+ blood, no glucose, no ketones, and urobilinogen. The urine microscopic examination shows a few white blood cells (WBCs) and some red blood cells (RBCs) with RBC casts. A renal biopsy is performed, and the light microscopic appearance with periodic acid–Schiff (PAS) staining is shown here. Which of the following is the most likely clinical course in this patient?

○ (A) Acute renal failure that is reversible with supportive therapy
○ (B) Slowly developing renal failure that is unresponsive to corticosteroid treatment
○ (C) Rapidly progressive renal failure accompanied by hemoptysis
○ (D) Stable clinical course with intermittent hematuria
○ (E) Fever, leukocytosis, and endotoxic shock

3. A 3-year-old boy has been increasingly lethargic for the past 3 weeks. Physical examination finds the child has periorbital edema. A urine specimen shows 4+ proteinuria without blood, ketones, or glucose. What advice would you give to this child's parents?

○ (A) A relative should be found to provide a renal transplant.
○ (B) A course of antibiotic therapy is indicated.
○ (C) Rapid onset of renal failure is likely.
○ (D) Corticosteroid therapy should alleviate this problem.
○ (E) Other family members are at risk for this disease.

4. At autopsy, small (75-g) kidneys are found in a 58-year-old female. The cortical surfaces of both kidneys have a coarsely granular appearance. Microscopically, there are sclerotic glomeruli, a fibrotic interstitium, tubular atrophy, arterial thickening, and scattered lymphocytic infiltrates. Laboratory findings before death include elevated blood urea nitrogen (110 mg/dL) and creatinine (9.8 mg/dL) levels. Which of the following clinical findings was most likely in this patient?

○ (A) Rash
○ (B) Hypertension

○ (C) Hemoptysis
○ (D) Lens dislocation
○ (E) Pharyngitis

5.   A 72-year-old female has noticed a 2.5-cm, warty, ulcerated mass protruding from the external urethral meatus. This mass has been enlarging for the past 6 months. It causes local pain and irritation and is now bleeding. A biopsy of this lesion is most likely to show findings most consistent with a (an)

○ (A) Embryonal rhabdomyosarcoma
○ (B) Leiomyoma
○ (C) Papilloma
○ (D) Squamous cell carcinoma
○ (E) Syphilitic chancre

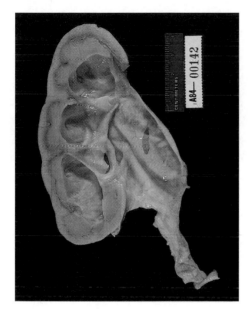

6.   The gross appearance of the right kidney shown here (the left was normal) at autopsy of a 62-year-old male is most suggestive of renal injury from

○ (A) Ureteral obstruction
○ (B) Benign nephrosclerosis
○ (C) Analgesic abuse
○ (D) Chronic pyelonephritis
○ (E) Diabetes mellitus

7.   A 25-year-old male has a history of celiac disease. Several days after an upper respiratory infection, he notices dark red-brown urine that persists for the next 3 days. His urine then becomes clear and yellow, only to become red-brown again in a month. His 24-hour urine protein level is now 200 mg. Which of the following alterations is most likely to be seen in the glomeruli on renal biopsy?

○ (A) Subepithelial deposits by electron microscopy
○ (B) Granular staining of the basement membrane by anti-IgG
○ (C) Mesangial IgA staining by immunofluorescence

○ (D) Diffuse proliferation and basement membrane thickening by light microscopy
○ (E) Thrombosis in the glomerular capillaries

8.   A 7-year-old child is recovering from impetigo caused by group A streptococcus and treated with a course of antibiotics. He develops malaise with nausea and a slight fever, and he passes dark brown urine. The serum anti streptolysin O (ASO) titer is 1:1024. Which of the following outcomes is most likely in this situation?

○ (A) Development of rheumatic heart disease
○ (B) Chronic renal failure
○ (C) Lower urinary tract infection
○ (D) Complete recovery without treatment
○ (E) Progression to crescentic glomerulonephritis

9.   A stone passed in the urine of a 28-year-old male is sent for analysis. The chemical composition is found to be calcium oxalate. The patient has had no previous major illnesses. Urinalysis shows a pH of 7, specific gravity of 1.015, 1+ blood, no protein, no glucose, and no ketones. Which of the following underlying conditions is he most likely to have?

○ (A) Gout
○ (B) Acute cystitis
○ (C) Diabetes mellitus
○ (D) Primary hyperparathyroidism
○ (E) Idiopathic hypercalciuria

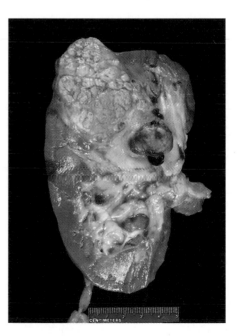

10.   A 56-year-old male presents with a month-long history of flank pain and hematuria. The gross appearance of the renal lesion in this patient is shown here. Which of the following laboratory test findings would you most expect?

○ (A) Elevated serum cortisol level
○ (B) Hematocrit of 63%
○ (C) Ketonuria

○ (D) Decreased creatinine clearance
○ (E) Increased plasma renin activity

11. A 15-year-old male presents with hematuria. He has previous diagnoses of deafness and corneal dystrophy. Urinalysis shows 1+ protein, no ketones, no glucose, 1+ blood, and no leukocytes. A renal biopsy reveals tubular epithelial foam cells by light microscopy. By electron microscopy, the glomerular basement membrane shows areas of attenuation, with splitting and lamination of lamina densa in other thickened areas. The most probable diagnosis is

○ (A) Acute tubular necrosis
○ (B) Berger disease
○ (C) Membranous glomerulonephritis
○ (D) Diabetic nephropathy
○ (E) Alport syndrome

12. Fever and skin rash develop in a 32-year-old man. Several days later, he has rising serum levels of urea nitrogen and creatinine along with oliguria. Urinalysis reveals 2+ proteinuria, 1+ hematuria, no glucose, no ketones, and no nitrite. The leukocyte esterase result is positive. Urine microscopic examination shows RBCs and WBCs, some of which are eosinophils. What is the most probable cause for this condition?

○ (A) Urinary tract infection
○ (B) Congestive heart failure
○ (C) Drug ingestion
○ (D) Streptococcal pharyngitis
○ (E) Poorly cooked ground beef

13. After a meal of cheeseburger, french fries, and ice cream, a 6-year-old girl develops some nausea, mild abdominal cramping, and minimal fever. A few days later, she experiences the sudden onset of hematuria and melena, and she quickly becomes oliguric. Renal biopsy shows small thrombi in glomerular capillary loops. Which of the following diseases has she most probably acquired?

○ (A) Postinfectious glomerulonephritis
○ (B) Wegener granulomatosis
○ (C) Hereditary nephritis
○ (D) Hemolytic-uremic syndrome
○ (E) IgA nephropathy

14. A 4-year-old girl presents with nephrotic syndrome. A renal biopsy is performed. There are no abnormal findings on light microscopic or immunofluorescence examination. Which of the following findings with electron microscopy is most likely in this biopsy?

○ (A) Subepithelial electron-dense humps
○ (B) Reduplication of glomerular basement membrane
○ (C) Areas of thickened and thinned basement membrane
○ (D) Increased mesangial matrix
○ (E) Effacement of podocyte foot processes

15. A 25-year-old female experiences the sudden onset of fever, malaise, and nausea. A routine urinalysis shows 1+ protein, no ketones, no glucose, and 4+ blood, with RBC casts seen on microscopic examination. There is marked

glomerular hypercellularity by light microscopy, with neutrophils in glomerular capillary loops. Immunofluorescence microscopy reveals granular deposition of IgG and C3 in glomerular capillary basement membranes. By electron microscopy, there are electron-dense subepithelial "humps." The most likely diagnosis is

○ (A) Goodpasture syndrome
○ (B) Systemic amyloidosis
○ (C) Membranous glomerulonephritis
○ (D) Diabetes mellitus
○ (E) Postinfectious glomerulonephritis

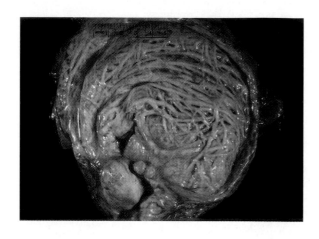

16. The gross appearance of the bladder at the autopsy of a 75-year-old male is seen here. Which of the following laboratory findings was most likely in this patient?

○ (A) Positive antinuclear antibody test
○ (B) Urine culture with *Mycobacterium tuberculosis*
○ (C) Hemoglobin concentration of 22.5 g/dL
○ (D) *Schistosoma hematobium* eggs in urine
○ (E) Elevated serum level of prostate-specific antigen (PSA)

17. A 50-year-old female has an episode of flank pain, and urinalysis reveals hematuria. An abdominal ultrasound reveals bilaterally enlarged kidneys that are completely replaced by 0.5- to 3-cm cysts. Which of the following complications is she most likely to suffer?

○ (A) Hypertension
○ (B) Renal cell carcinoma
○ (C) Nephrotic syndrome
○ (D) Microangiopathic hemolytic anemia
○ (E) Renal infarction

18. After acute blood loss incurred during a motor vehicle accident, a 26-year-old male remains hypotensive for several hours. Within the next week, his serum urea nitrogen concentration has risen to 48 mg/dL and creatinine level to 5 mg/dL, while his urine output is falling. He receives hemodialysis for the next 2 weeks, after which time he has marked polyuria, with 2 to 3 L of urine output per day. His course is then complicated by bronchopneumonia. His renal function gradually returns to normal. The

transient renal disease in this case is best characterized by which of the following histologic features?

○ (A) Glomerular crescents
○ (B) Interstitial lymphocytic infiltrates
○ (C) Arteriolar fibrinoid necrosis
○ (D) Nodular glomerulosclerosis
○ (E) Rupture of the basement membrane

19. A 60-year-old male has noticed blood in his urine on several occasions in the past month. He has no urinary frequency, dysuria, or nocturia. He now presents with fever and weakness. He has had no previous major illnesses. A dipstick urinalysis reveals 4+ blood, no protein, no glucose, and no ketones. Which of the following procedures would you recommend to be performed next?

○ (A) Straining urine for calculi
○ (B) Urine microbiologic culture
○ (C) Abdominal computed tomography (CT) for a renal mass
○ (D) Collection of 24-hour urine for protein
○ (E) Percutaneous renal biopsy

20. A 40-year-old man presents with edema and is found to have a 24-hour urine protein excretion of 7 g with a serum creatinine level of 1.2 mg/dL and no hematuria on urinalysis. Serologic test results for antinuclear antibody (ANA), antistreptolysin O (ASO), human immunodeficiency virus (HIV), and antineutrophil cytoplasmic antibody (ANCA) are all negative. Serum complement levels are normal. A renal biopsy is performed, and by light microscopy the glomeruli appear normal except for diffuse, uniform thickening of the glomerular capillary basement membranes. By immunofluorescence, there is granular peripheral staining of the basement membrane for IgG and C3. Given these clinical and histopathologic findings, the *most likely* finding by electron microscopy would be

○ (A) Subepithelial electron-dense deposits
○ (B) Subendothelial electron-dense deposits, with duplication of the basement membrane
○ (C) Mesangial electron-dense deposits only
○ (D) No deposits but marked podocyte foot process fusion
○ (E) No abnormality

21. A 50-year-old woman has had a fever and flank pain for the past 2 days. Urinalysis reveals no protein, no glucose, no ketones, and positive leukocyte esterase. Microscopic examination of the urine reveals numerous polymorphonuclear leukocytes along with occasional WBC casts. A urine culture is most likely to yield

○ (A) *M. tuberculosis*
○ (B) *Mycoplasma hominis*
○ (C) *Escherichia coli*
○ (D) Group A streptococcus
○ (E) *Cryptococcus neoformans*

For each of the clinical histories in questions 22 and 23, match the most closely associated laboratory finding:

(A) Anti-glomerular basement membrane antibody positive

(B) ANA positive
(C) ANCA positive
(D) ASO antibody positive
(E) C3 nephritic factor positive
(F) Hemoglobin A_{1C} level elevated
(G) Hepatitis B surface antigen positive
(H) HIV positive
(I) Hypercalcemia
(J) Hypergammaglobulinemia
(K) Hyperuricemia

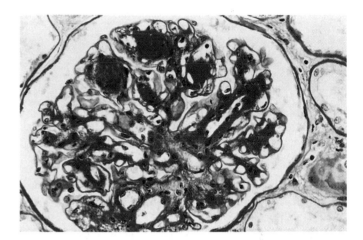

22. A 58-year-old male has mild hypertension. His serum urea nitrogen level that has progressively increased over the past 2 years and now is 45 mg/dL. Several years ago, he was found to have microalbuminuria, with excretion of 250 mg/day of albumin, but his 24-hour urine protein is now 2.8 g. The light microscopic appearance of his kidney is shown here with PAS staining. (   )

23. A 47-year-old female had a right mastectomy 3 years ago to remove an infiltrating ductal carcinoma. She now has bone pain, and a nuclear medicine scan reveals multiple areas of increased uptake in vertebrae, ribs, pelvis, and right femur. Urinalysis reveals a specific gravity of 1.010, and this remains unchanged after water deprivation for 12 hours. She undergoes several courses of chemotherapy over the next year. During that time, her serum urea nitrogen level progressively rises. (   )

24. A 65-year-old female experienced increasing malaise with nocturia and polyuria. Her blood pressure was 170/95 mm Hg. Urinalysis showed a pH of 7.5, specific gravity of 1.010, 1+ protein, and no glucose, blood, or ketones. She was found to have elevated levels of blood urea nitrogen and serum creatinine. Her clinical course was characterized by worsening renal failure, and she succumbed to a terminal bout of bronchopneumonia. At autopsy, her kidneys are shrunken but unequal in size, and they have deep, irregular scars on the surface. On sectioning, the calyces underlying the cortical scars are blunted and deformed. The most likely cause of renal failure in this case is

○ (A) Chronic glomerulonephritis
○ (B) Benign nephrosclerosis
○ (C) Chronic pyelonephritis
○ (D) Autosomal dominant polycystic kidney disease
○ (E) Systemic lupus erythematosus

25. A 29-year-old female presents with fever and sore throat and is diagnosed to have streptococcal pharyngitis. She is treated with ampicillin and recovers fully in 7 days. Two weeks later, she again develops fever and also a rash. She also notices slightly decreased urinary output. Urinalysis shows a pH of 6, specific gravity of 1.022, 1+ protein, 1+ blood, no glucose, and no ketones. Urine microscopic examination shows RBCs, WBCs (including eosinophils), but no casts or crystals. Which of the following renal complications is most likely to have occurred in this patient?

○ (A) Post-streptococcal glomerulonephritis
○ (B) Acute pyelonephritis
○ (C) Acute tubular necrosis
○ (D) Drug-induced interstitial nephritis
○ (E) Membranous glomerulopathy

26. Cystoscopy reveals a superficial, 1-cm papillary mass lesion in the dome of the bladder of a 57-year-old male. The mass is excised and reveals a urothelium with minimal cytologic and architectural atypia overlying a fibrovascular stalk. There is no involvement of the muscularis. Which of the following genetic alterations has most likely given rise to this lesion?

○ (A) 13q deletion
○ (B) *p53* mutation
○ (C) 9p deletion
○ (D) c-*abl* translocation
○ (E) K-*ras* activation

27. After a mild flulike illness, a 9-year-old male had an episode of hematuria. This subsided in a couple of days, but a month later, he notices red urine again and visits his physician. Urinalysis shows a pH of 7, specific gravity of 1.015, 1+ protein, 1+ blood, no ketones, no glucose, and no urobilinogen. His serum urea nitrogen level is 36 mg/dL, and the creatinine concentration is 3.2 mg/dL. A renal biopsy shows diffuse mesangial proliferation and electron-dense deposits in the mesangium. This disorder is most likely caused by

○ (A) Deposition of IgA-containing immune complexes
○ (B) Formation of antibodies against type IV collagen
○ (C) Virus-mediated injury to glomeruli
○ (D) Cytokine-mediated injury to the glomerular capillaries
○ (E) Congenital defects in the structure of glomerular basement membranes

28. A 35-year-old male is awakened at night by severe lower abdominal pain radiating to the groin. This pain is very intense and comes in waves. He is concerned about the appearance of blood in his urine the next morning. Which urinary tract disease does he most likely have?

○ (A) Acute cystitis
○ (B) Renal cell carcinoma
○ (C) Ureteral lithiasis
○ (D) Hydronephrosis
○ (E) Dominant polycystic kidney disease

29. A 4-year-old male presented with facial puffiness. He was found to have 3.8 g of protein in his 24-hour urine collection. There was no blood, glucose, or ketones in the urine, and microscopic examination showed no casts or crystals. Serum creatinine was normal. He received a course of corticosteroid therapy, and he improved. However, he had two more episodes of proteinuria over the next few years, each responsive to steroid therapy. Examination of a renal biopsy under the light microscope is most likely to reveal

○ (A) Diffusely hypercellular glomeruli with normal basement membranes
○ (B) Marked basement membrane thickening but no glomerular proliferation
○ (C) Normal cellularity and normal basement membranes
○ (D) Crescent formation in the Bowman space
○ (E) Diffuse hypercellularity with "tram track" appearance of basement membrane

30. A 49-year-old male presented with generalized edema. He had a 24-hour urine protein of 4.1 g with the presence of albumin and globulins. Extensive testing failed to reveal any systemic disease such as diabetes mellitus or systemic lupus erythematosus. He did not respond to a course of corticosteroid therapy. A renal biopsy revealed diffuse thickening of basement membranes. Immunofluorescence staining with antibody to the C3 component of complement was positive in a granular pattern in glomerular capillary loops. Several years later, he developed chronic renal failure. Which of the following immunologic mechanisms was most likely responsible for the glomerular changes?

○ (A) Antibodies that react with basement membrane collagen
○ (B) Antibodies against streptococci that cross-react with the basement membrane
○ (C) Release of cytokines by inflammatory cells
○ (D) Cytotoxic T cells directed against renal antigens
○ (E) Deposition of immune complexes on the basement membranes

31. Which of the following microscopic findings on urinalysis is most indicative of glomerulonephritis?

○ (A) Neutrophils
○ (B) Red cell casts
○ (C) Transitional cells
○ (D) Oxalate crystals
○ (E) Hyaline casts

32. A 42-year-old, HIV-positive male presents with mucocutaneous lesions consistent with *Candida* infection. Further workup reveals a blood pressure of 150/95 mm Hg, serum creatinine level of 2.5 mg/dl, 24-hour urine protein of 9 g, and urinalysis showing moderate numbers of red cells in the urine. A renal biopsy would most likely show

○ (A) Diffuse proliferative glomerulonephritis
○ (B) Focal segmental glomerulosclerosis
○ (C) Minimal change disease
○ (D) Membranoproliferative glomerulonephritis type I
○ (E) Crescentic glomerulonephritis

33. A 51-year-old woman has had recurrent urinary tract infections for years. On many of these occasions, *Proteus vulgaris* was cultured from her urine. Her most recent urinalysis shows a pH of 7.5, specific gravity of 1.020, 1+ blood, no protein, no glucose, and no ketones. Microscopic urinalysis shows many RBCs, many WBCs, and many triple phosphate crystals. Which of the following renal lesions is she most likely to have?

○ (A) Renal cell carcinoma
○ (B) Acute tubular necrosis
○ (C) Malignant nephrosclerosis
○ (D) Staghorn calculus
○ (E) Papillary necrosis

34. A 51-year-old diabetic female presents with fever and pain in the costovertebral angle. She also complains of dysuria and frequency. Urine examination reveals glucose but no ketones or proteins. Microscopic examination of urine shows numerous pus cells. Urine culture is positive for *E. coli*. Which of the following complications is most likely to develop in this setting?

○ (A) Acute tubular necrosis
○ (B) Necrotizing papillitis
○ (C) Crescentic glomerulonephritis
○ (D) Hydronephrosis
○ (E) Renal calculi

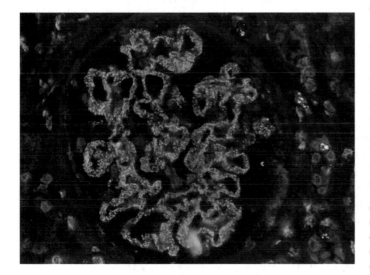

35. A 42-year-old male has experienced increasing malaise for the past month. He is bothered by edema in both hands and legs. Urinalysis shows a pH of 6.5, specific gravity of 1.017, 4+ protein, no blood, no glucose, no ketones, no casts, no RBCs, and 2 WBCs per high-power-field. The 24-hour urine protein is 4.2 g. A renal biopsy shows the pattern seen here with antibody to C3 on immunofluorescence. Which of the following underlying disease processes is he most likely to have?

○ (A) Chronic hepatitis B
○ (B) Acquired immunodeficiency syndrome
○ (C) Multiple myeloma
○ (D) Recurrent urinary tract infection
○ (E) Nephrolithiasis

36. After an acute myocardial infarction, a 58-year-old male is in stable condition. However, 2 days later, his urine output drops, and his serum urea nitrogen increases to 3.3 mg/dL. This oliguria persists for a few days and is followed by polyuria for 2 more days. He is then discharged from the hospital. What lesion best explains his renal abnormalities?

○ (A) Acute tubular necrosis
○ (B) Benign nephrosclerosis
○ (C) Acute renal infarction
○ (D) Hemolytic-uremic syndrome
○ (E) Rapidly progressive glomerulonephritis

37. Several members of a family have developed chronic renal failure by age 50. Most of them are males. These persons also have developed visual problems. Some younger family members have proteinuria and hematuria on urinalysis. A renal biopsy from one 20-year-old male shows prominent tubular foam cells and glomerular basement membrane thickening and thinning. Which of the following additional manifestations of this disease do you expect to find?

○ (A) Watery diarrhea
○ (B) Nerve deafness
○ (C) Presenile dementia
○ (D) Dilated cardiomyopathy
○ (E) Infertility

38. A 65-year-old male is now retiring from his job in which he had exposure to aniline dyes, including use of β-naphthylamine. He has an episode of hematuria not accompanied by any abdominal pain. Physical examination reveals no abnormal findings. A urinalysis reveals 4+ blood but no ketones, glucose, or protein. The urine microscopic examination reveals RBCs too numerous to count, 5 to 10 WBCs per high-power field, no crystals, and no casts. The urine culture result is negative. Which of the following conditions does he most likely have?

○ (A) Renal cell carcinoma
○ (B) Hemorrhagic cystitis
○ (C) Tubercular cystitis
○ (D) Transitional cell carcinoma of the bladder
○ (E) Squamous cell carcinoma of the urethra

For each of the clinical histories in questions 39 and 40, match the most closely associated disease involving the glomerulus:

(A) IgA nephropathy
(B) Membranoproliferative glomerulonephritis, type II
(C) Minimal change disease
(D) Focal segmental glomerulosclerosis
(E) Goodpasture syndrome
(F) Lupus nephritis
(G) Wegener granulomatosis
(H) Membranous glomerulonephritis
(I) Postinfectious glomerulonephritis
(J) Nodular glomerulosclerosis
(K) Hereditary nephritis

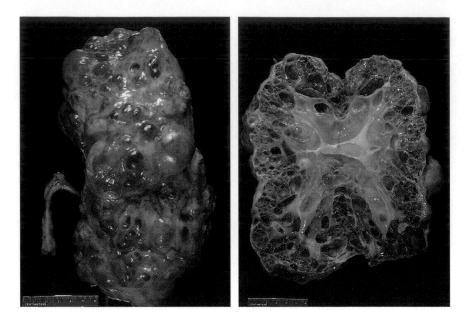

39. A 55-year-old female has had poorly controlled hyperglycemia for years. A urinalysis shows 1+ protein, no blood, 2+ glucose, no ketones, and no urobilinogen. A urine culture has more than 100,000 colony-forming units/mL of *Klebsiella pneumoniae*. (   )

40. A 44-year-old male developed oliguria over the past 3 days. His serum urea nitrogen level rises to 43 mg/dL. A renal biopsy reveals glomerular crescents and granulomatous vasculitis. The result of immunofluorescence with anti-IgG and anti-C3 antibodies is negative. The assay for serum C-ANCA is positive. (   )

41. A 28-year-old female presents with a 2-day history of dysuria with frequency and urgency. A urine culture grows more than 100,000 colonies/mL of *E. coli*. She is treated with antibiotic therapy. However, if she continues to suffer recurrences of this problem, she is at greatest risk for development of

○ (A) Diffuse glomerulosclerosis
○ (B) Chronic glomerulonephritis
○ (C) Amyloidosis
○ (D) Membranous glomerulonephritis
○ (E) Chronic pyelonephritis

42. A sexually active 26-year-old male complains of some pain with urination. Physical examination reveals no lesions of the penis. A urinalysis reveals no blood, ketones, protein, or glucose. The urine microscopic examination shows a few WBCs with no casts or crystals. Which of the following infectious agents is most likely to blame for these findings?

○ (A) *Chlamydia trachomatis*
○ (B) *M. tuberculosis*
○ (C) Herpes simplex virus
○ (D) *Candida albicans*
○ (E) *Treponema pallidum*

43. The kidney shown in the figure was present at autopsy of a 61-year-old female. Both of her kidneys had this appearance. Which of the following conditions was the most probable cause of death?

○ (A) Metastatic Wilms tumor
○ (B) Ruptured berry aneurysm
○ (C) Acute tubular necrosis
○ (D) Disseminated intravascular coagulation
○ (E) Pneumothorax

44. A 69-year-old male has ingested more than 3 g per day of analgesics, including phenacetin, aspirin, and acetaminophen, for the past 20 years to treat his chronic arthritis. He now has a blood pressure of 156/92 mm Hg. His serum urea nitrogen level is 68 mg/dL, and the creatinine level is 7.1 mg/dL. His hematocrit is 36%. Which of the following complications is he most likely to develop?

○ (A) Hydronephrosis
○ (B) Chronic glomerulonephritis
○ (C) Renal papillary necrosis
○ (D) Renal cell carcinoma
○ (E) Acute tubular necrosis

45. A blood pressure check on a 58-year-old female shows a reading of 168/109 mm Hg. Her urinalysis shows a pH of 7.0, specific gravity of 1.020, 1+ protein, no blood, no glucose, and no ketones. An abdominal ultrasound reveals that her kidneys are quite small and have no masses. Her ANA test result is negative. Her serum urea nitrogen level is 51 mg/dL, and the creatinine level is 4.7 mg/dL. Her hemoglobin A_{IC} concentration is within the reference range. Which of the following conditions is she most likely to have?

○ (A) Lupus nephritis
○ (B) Dominant polycystic kidney disease
○ (C) Chronic glomerulonephritis
○ (D) Diabetic glomerulosclerosis
○ (E) Amyloidosis

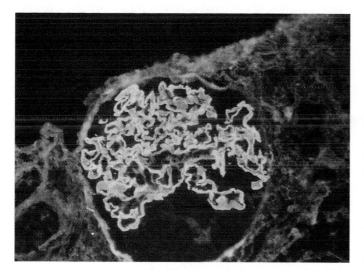

46. A renal biopsy is performed on a previously healthy, 21-year-old male who presented with acute onset of hematuria. His serum urea nitrogen level is 39 mg/dL, and the creatinine level is 4.1 mg/dL. The immunofluorescence pattern with antibody against human IgG is shown here. Which of the following serum laboratory test findings is most likely to be positive?

O (A) Antistreptolysin O antibody
O (B) HIV antibody
O (C) Antiglomerular basement membrane antibody
O (D) Hepatitis B surface antibody
O (E) C3 nephritic factor

47. Which of the following renal diseases is the most likely to be reversible in a 40-year-old male patient with elevated serum urea nitrogen and creatinine levels?

O (A) Analgesic nephropathy
O (B) Benign nephrosclerosis
O (C) Focal segmental glomerulosclerosis
O (D) Acute tubular necrosis
O (E) Diabetic nephropathy

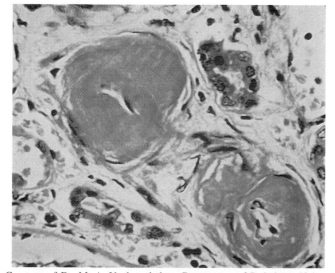

Courtesy of Dr. M. A. Venkatachalam, Department of Pathology, University of Texas Health Sciences Center, San Antonio, TX.

48. High-magnification appearance of the kidney at the autopsy of a 66-year-old female is shown in the figure. Grossly, both kidneys were decreased in size (about 120 g each) with a finely granular cortical surface. Which of the clinical abnormalities listed below most likely accompanied this lesion?

O (A) Oliguria
O (B) Benign hypertension
O (C) Malignant hypertension
O (D) Hematuria
O (E) Flank pain

49. A 39-year-old Vietnamese man who is otherwise healthy consults his physician for passage of blood in urine. Questioning reveals that the hematuria has occurred on and off for the past 4 years. Physical examination findings are unremarkable. His serum creatinine level is 1.6 mg/dl. Urinalysis reveals 4+ blood with no protein or glucose. Serologic test results for ANA and ANCA are negative. Which of the following alterations is most likely to be seen in the glomeruli?

O (A) Subepithelial electron-dense deposits by EM
O (B) Granular membranous IgG staining by immunofluorescence
O (C) Mesangial IgA staining by immunofluorescence
O (D) Diffuse proliferation and basement membrane thickening by light microscopy
O (E) Thrombosis in the glomerular capillaries

50. A 30-year-old female presents with recurrent urinary tract infections. A renal sonogram shows extensive scarring with pelvic and calyceal enlargement and cortical thinning. A renal biopsy reveals inflammatory infiltrates extending from medulla to cortex, with tubular destruction and fibrosis. Lymphocytes, plasma cells, and occasional neutrophils are present. These findings most likely resulted from

O (A) Benign nephrosclerosis
O (B) Vesicoureteral reflux
O (C) Lupus nephritis
O (D) Systemic amyloidosis
O (E) Congestive heart failure

For each of the clinical histories in questions 51 and 52, match the most closely associated gross pathologic appearance of the kidneys:

(A) Bilaterally enlarged kidneys replaced by 1- to 4-cm, fluid-filled cysts
(B) Bilaterally shrunken kidneys with uniformly finely granular cortical surfaces
(C) Decreased overall size of right kidney with normal-sized left kidney
(D) Irregular cortical scars in asymmetrically shrunken kidneys with marked calyceal dilatation
(E) Large "staghorn" calculus filling dilated calyces in the right kidney
(F) Marked bilateral renal pelvic and calyceal dilation with thinning of the cortices
(G) Normal-sized kidneys with smooth cortical surfaces
(H) Scattered petechial hemorrhages in slightly swollen kidneys

(I) Symmetrically enlarged kidneys composed of small, radially arranged cysts

(J) Wedge-shaped regions of yellow-white cortical necrosis involving both kidneys

51. A 32-year-old male with a history of intravenous drug use presents with a high fever, palpable spleen tip, bilateral costovertebral angle tenderness, and diastolic cardiac murmur. A blood culture is positive for *Staphylococcus aureus*. His serum urea nitrogen concentration is 15 mg/dL. A urinalysis reveals 2+ blood with no glucose, protein, or ketones. (   )

52. At autopsy, a 33-week gestational age stillborn has deformations resulting from marked oligohydramnios. Microscopically, the liver demonstrates multiple epithelium-lined cysts and a proliferation of bile ducts. (   )

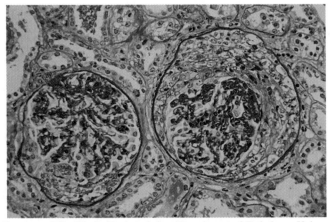

Courtesy of Dr. M. A. Venkatachalam, Department of Pathology, University of Texas Health Sciences Center, San Antonio, TX.

53. A 45-year-old male experienced the rapid onset of renal failure. The light microscopic appearance of the PAS-stained renal biopsy is shown here. Which of the following additional tests is extremely useful for further classification and treatment of the diseases that have similar changes?

○ (A) Antinuclear antibody titer
○ (B) Immunofluorescence with anti-IgG
○ (C) Human immunodeficiency virus titer
○ (D) Radiograph of the chest
○ (E) Rheumatoid factor

For each of the clinical histories in questions 54 and 55, match the most closely associated finding on urinalysis:

(A) Bence Jones proteinuria
(B) Eosinophils
(C) Glucosuria
(D) Hyaline casts
(E) Ketonuria
(F) Myoglobinuria
(G) Oval fat bodies
(H) Oxalate crystals
(I) RBC casts
(J) Triple phosphate crystals
(K) Uric acid crystals
(L) Waxy casts

54. A 28-year-old male has been diagnosed with acute myelogenous leukemia. After induction with a multiagent chemotherapy protocol, he has an episode of lower abdominal pain accompanied by passage of red-colored urine. He has no fever, dysuria, or urinary frequency. An abdominal radiograph reveals nothing remarkable. A urinalysis shows a pH of 5.5, specific gravity of 1.021, 2+ blood, no protein, no ketones, and no glucose. (   )

55. A 17-year-old female has had arthralgias and myalgias for the past several months. She recently noticed a decrease in urine output, and the urine is reddish brown. Her blood pressure has increased to 160/100 mm Hg. She is found to have a positive ANA test result along with a positive anti–double-stranded DNA test result. Her serum urea nitrogen concentration is 52 mg/dL. (   )

56. A 65-year-old female has a blood pressure of 150/95 mm Hg. She has experienced several transient ischemic attacks recently. Urinalysis reveals 1+ proteinuria, no glucose, no blood, and no ketones. On ultrasound, her kidneys are slightly decreased in size. Which of the following renal lesions is most likely?

○ (A) Crescentic glomerulonephritis
○ (B) Hyaline arteriolosclerosis
○ (C) Mesangial cell proliferation
○ (D) Arteriolar fibrinoid necrosis
○ (E) Acute tubular necrosis

57. A 44-year-old male experiences the onset of headache, nausea, and vomiting over 72 hours. Physical examination reveals bilateral papilledema. His blood pressure is 276/158 mm Hg. A urinalysis shows 2+ proteinuria, 1+ blood, no glucose, and no ketones. Which of the following renal lesions is most likely?

○ (A) Papillary necrosis
○ (B) Acute infarction
○ (C) Necrotizing arteriolitis
○ (D) Acute tubular necrosis
○ (E) Acute pyelonephritis

58. A 40-year-old previously healthy male is found at home, dead from a cocaine overdose. At autopsy, the medical examiner notices bilaterally enlarged kidneys that contain multiple, irregularly arranged cysts of different shapes and sizes. She asks you to review the case, and you also find intracerebral berry aneurysms and occasional liver cysts. You tell her the following:

○ (A) The individual probably had lesions related to chronic use of cocaine.
○ (B) The individual probably had infantile (autosomal recessive) polycystic kidney disease and was one of the rare ones to survive to adulthood.
○ (C) The individual probably had adult (autosomal dominant) polycystic kidney disease; no further action is necessary.
○ (D) The individual probably had adult polycystic kidney disease, and his family (i.e., children, siblings, and parents) should be evaluated for the same condition.
○ (E) The individual probably had an unfortunate combination of incidental findings unrelated to overdose.

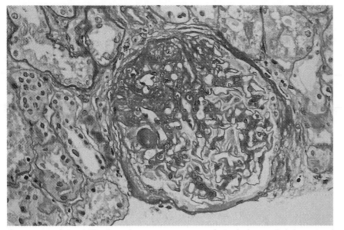

Courtesy of Dr. H. Rennke, Department of Pathology, Brigham and Women's Hospital, Boston, MA.

59. Approximately 50% of the glomeruli in a renal biopsy are affected by the lesion illustrated in the figure. This histologic picture is most consistent with which of the following clinical scenarios?

○ (A) A 9-year-old child with corticosteroid-resistant nephrotic syndrome

○ (B) A 4-year-old child with corticosteroid-responsive nephrotic syndrome

○ (C) A 16-year-old youth with a sore throat followed 3 weeks later by nephritic syndrome

○ (D) A 45-year-old male with 25-year history of diabetes mellitus

○ (E) A 60-year-old male with a 30-year history of hypertension and slow-onset renal failure

60. A 19-year-old female presents with fever and chills accompanied by right flank pain for the past 3 days. She is not diabetic, and her blood pressure is 150/90. Urinalysis shows a pH of 6.5 specific gravity of 1.018, no protein, no blood, no glucose, and no ketones. Urine microscopic examination shows many WBCs and WBC casts. Which of the following factors is most important in the pathogenesis of the renal disease affecting this patient?

○ (A) Age
○ (B) Sex
○ (C) Vesicoureteral reflux
○ (D) Blood pressure
○ (E) A focus of infection in the lungs

61. Several days after a home barbecue with hamburgers, hot dogs, chili, and ice cream, a 5-year-old girl develops cramping abdominal pain with diarrhea. A day later, she has melena, and she develops oliguria. Her peripheral blood smear shows schistocytes, and her serum D-dimer level is elevated. Which of the following infectious agents probably led to these events?

○ (A) *Candida albicans*
○ (B) *Proteus mirabilis*
○ (C) *Clostridium difficile*

○ (D) *Escherichia coli*
○ (E) *Staphylococcus aureus*

62. A 17-year-old male is involved in a motor vehicle accident in which he incurs severe blunt trauma to his extremities and abdomen. Over the next 3 days, he develops oliguria with dark brown urine. The urine is positive for myoglobin. His serum urea nitrogen level rises to 38 mg/dL. He is given hemodialysis over the next 3 weeks. His condition improves, although his urine output is in excess of 3 L per day a week before his urea nitrogen returns to normal. Which of the following renal lesions did he probably have?

○ (A) Malignant nephrosclerosis
○ (B) Renal vein thrombosis
○ (C) Membranous glomerulonephritis
○ (D) Acute pyelonephritis
○ (E) Acute tubular necrosis

63. A 45-year-old man has headaches, nausea, and vomiting that worsens over several days, and he starts "seeing spots" before his eyes. His blood pressure is 268/150 mm Hg. Urinalysis reveals 1+ protein, 2+ blood, no glucose, no ketones, and no leukocytes. His serum urea nitrogen and creatinine levels are elevated. Which of the following histologic findings for his kidneys is most likely?

○ (A) Nodular glomerulosclerosis
○ (B) Segmental tubular necrosis
○ (C) Hyperplastic arteriolosclerosis
○ (D) Mesangial IgA deposition
○ (E) Glomerular crescents

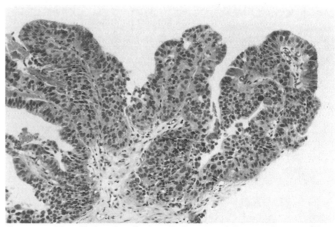

Courtesy of Dr. Christopher Corless, University of Oregon, Eugene, OR.

64. A 62-year-old male has had several episodes of hematuria in the past week. He does not report any increased urinary frequency or dysuria. A urinalysis shows 4+ blood. The urine culture is negative. A cystoscopy is performed, and a 2-cm, sessile, friable mass is seen on the right bladder dome. A biopsy is taken, and the microscopic appearance is shown here. Which of the following risk factors is most important in the pathogenesis of this bladder lesion?

○ (A) Smoking
○ (B) Schistosomiasis
○ (C) Diabetes mellitus
○ (D) Chronic bacterial cystitis
○ (E) Nodular prostatic hyperplasia

65. A 38-year-old female has been tired and lethargic for months. As part of a workup by her physician, she is found to be anemic and to have a serum creatinine level of 5.8 mg/dL. Urinalysis shows 2+ proteinuria. C3 nephritic factor is present in serum, and the ANA test result is negative. A renal biopsy is performed. The glomeruli are hypercellular, and there are prominent electron-dense deposits along the lamina densa of the glomerular basement membrane. Which of the following forms of glomerulonephritis is most likely?

○ (A) Postinfectious glomerulonephritis
○ (B) Rapidly progressive glomerulonephritis
○ (C) Membranoproliferative glomerulonephritis
○ (D) Chronic glomerulonephritis
○ (E) Membranous glomerulonephritis

ANSWERS

1. **(C)** Seventy-five percent of all renal stones are made up of calcium oxalate crystals. Patients with these stones tend to have hypercalciuria without hypercalcemia. Triple phosphate stones tend to occur in association with urinary tract infections, particularly with urease-positive bacteria such as *Proteus*. Uric acid stones and cystine stones are radiolucent and tend to form in acidic urine. Cystine stones are rare.
BP6 465   PBD6 989-990

2. **(C)** The glomeruli show epithelial crescents that are the morphologic correlates of rapidly progressive glomerulonephritis. These patients develop renal failure rapidly. One cause of rapidly progressive renal failure is Goodpasture syndrome, in which anti-glomerular basement membrane (anti-GBM) antibodies damage the glomeruli and lung alveoli, the latter giving rise to hemoptysis.
BP6 452-453   PBD6 951-952

3. **(D)** The most likely cause for nephrotic syndrome in a child is minimal change disease. For this reason, a course of corticosteroids is indicated, and 90% of cases respond. If there is no response, further workup, including renal biopsy, can be done. Few cases go on to chronic renal failure requiring dialysis or transplantation. The cause for minimal change disease is unknown. Children with minimal change disease do not develop rapid renal failure. There is no genetic tendency to minimal change disease.
BP6 447   PBD6 954-956

4. **(B)** These are findings of end-stage renal disease, with an appearance that is similar regardless of the cause (e.g., vascular disease or glomerular disease). With advanced renal destruction, hypertension almost always supervenes, even if it was absent at the onset of renal disease. Many such cases are called "chronic glomerulonephritis" for want of a better term. A rash might have preceded the postinfectious glomerulonephritis. Hemoptysis is seen with Goodpasture syndrome. Lens dislocation is a feature of Alport syndrome.
BP6 454-455   PBD6 963-964

5. **(D)** Carcinoma of the urethra is uncommon. It tends to occur in older women and is locally aggressive. An embryonal rhabdomyosarcoma (i.e., sarcoma botryoides) is a rare pediatric tumor. Benign tumors such as a leiomyoma or papilloma are typically well circumscribed and do not ulcerate. Syphilis produces indurated, painless lesions rather than ulcerated, warty masses.
PBD6 1009

6. **(A)** The ureteral, pelvic, and calyceal dilation results from long-standing obstruction leading to hydroureter and hydronephrosis. With benign nephrosclerosis, the kidneys become small with granular surfaces, but there is no dilation. The scarring that accompanies analgesic nephropathy or chronic pyelonephritis can be marked, with significant loss of renal parenchyma but without pelvic dilation. There are many renal complications of diabetes mellitus, mostly from vascular, glomerular, or interstitial injury, but there is no obstruction. Diabetes may be complicated by a neurogenic bladder, and this can lead to functional obstruction. However, in such cases, both kidneys and ureters should be affected.
BP6 465-466   PBD6 988-989

7. **(C)** IgA nephropathy, also known as Berger disease, can explain the presence of recurrent hematuria in a young adult. There is no nephrotic syndrome, and mesangial IgA deposition is characteristic. The initial episode of hematuria usually follows an upper respiratory infection. IgA nephropathy occurs with increased frequency in patients with celiac disease. Granular staining of basement membrane with IgG antibodies denotes immune complex deposition, as may occur in post infectious glomerulonephritis; these are seen as subepithelial deposits by electron microscopy. Patients with these changes present with nephritic syndrome. Diffuse proliferation and basement membrane thickening denotes membranoproliferative glomerulonephritis. IgG and C3 are deposited in the glomeruli in this condition.
BP6 453   PBD6 961-962

8. **(D)** The findings are characteristic for poststreptococcal glomerulonephritis. The strains of group A streptococcus that cause poststreptococcal glomerulonephritis are different from those that give rise to rheumatic fever. Most children with poststreptococcal glomerulonephritis recover, although perhaps 1% go on to a rapidly progressive glomerulonephritis. Progression to chronic renal failure may occur in 10% to 15% of affected adults. A urinary tract infection is not likely to accompany poststreptococcal glomerulonephritis, because the organisms that caused this immunologic reaction are gone when the disease appears.
BP6 451-452   PBD6 949-951

9. **(E)** The most common urinary tract stones are made up of calcium oxalate. Approximately 50% of patients with calcium oxalate stones have increased excretion of calcium without hypercalcemia. The basis of hypercalciuria is not clear. Most uric acid stones are formed in acidic urine and are not related to gout. It is thought that these patients have an unexplained tendency to excrete acidic urine. At low pII, uric acid is insoluble, and stones form. Infections can predispose to the formation of magnesium ammonium phosphate stones. Diabetes mellitus is not known as a cause for urinary tract lithiasis, although infections are more common. Hyperparathyroidism predisposes to formation of stones with calcium, but few patients with stones have this condition.
BP6 464-465   PBD6 989-990

10. **(B)** This is a renal cell carcinoma. About 5% to 10% of these tumors secrete erythropoietin, giving rise to polycythemia. Other substances can be secreted, including corticotropin (ACTH) to produce Cushing syndrome, but these are less frequently encountered than polycythemia. Ketonuria is a feature of type I diabetes mellitus, which is not associated with the development of renal neoplasms. Renal cell carcinomas are usually unilateral, and typically they do not destroy all of a kidney. There is no significant loss of renal function, and the serum urea nitrogen and creatinine levels are not elevated. Hypertension can be seen with some renal cell carcinomas, although not frequently.
BP6 466-467   PBD6 991-993

11. **(E)** Alport syndrome is one form of hereditary nephritis. Hematuria is the most common presenting feature. Patients progress to chronic renal failure in adulthood. Most patients have an X-linked dominant pattern of inheritance, but autosomal dominant and autosomal recessive pedigrees also exist. The foamy change in the tubular epithelial cells and ultrastructural alterations of the basement membrane are quite characteristic. The genetic defect involves type IV collagen synthesis. Acute tubular necrosis follows ischemic or toxic injuries to the kidney and does not involve glomeruli. Berger disease, or IgA nephropathy, is a form of glomerulonephritis without tubular epithelial changes. Membranous glomerulonephritis generally produces a nephrotic syndrome, and there is immune complex deposition in glomerular basement membrane. Nodular and diffuse glomerulosclerosis are typical changes of diabetic nephropathy.
BP6 454   PBD6 962-963

12. **(C)** These are typical findings for a drug-induced interstitial nephritis. A variety of drugs can give rise to this. The disease appears on average about two weeks after drug use is started. There are elements of type I (increased IgE) and type IV (skin test positivity to drug haptens) hypersensitivity. WBCs can be seen with a urinary tract infection but not eosinophils. Congestive heart failure can lead to acute tubular necrosis, but it is not associated with a rash or proteinuria. Poststreptococcal glomerulonephritis can account for proteinuria and hematuria but not the rash, because the strains of group A β-hemolytic streptococci that cause a skin infection are not nephritogenic and do not lead to glomerulonephritis. Hemolytic-uremic syndrome

can follow ingestion of strains of *E. coli* that may be found in ground beef.
BP6 458   PBD6 977-978

13. **(D)** Hemolytic-uremic syndrome is one of the most common causes for acute renal failure in children. It most commonly follows ingestion of meat infected with verocytotoxin-producing *E. coli*. The toxin damages endothelium, reducing nitric oxide, promoting vasoconstriction and necrosis, and promoting thrombosis. With supportive therapy, most patients recover in a few weeks, although perhaps one fourth go on to chronic renal failure. Postinfectious glomerulonephritis occurs several weeks after an infection, usually with group A β-hemolytic streptococci. Wegener granulomatosis is a vasculitis seen most often in adults. Hereditary nephritis may present in childhood but is progressive and not related to vascular disease. An IgA nephropathy is most often seen in young adults; it is not accompanied by vascular changes.
BP6 463   PBD6 985-986

14. **(E)** A child with nephrotic syndrome and no other clinical findings is most likely to have lipoid nephrosis, also called minimal change disease. The term minimal change disease applies to the paucity of pathologic findings. There is fusion of foot processes, which can be seen only by electron microscopy. Subepithelial electron-dense humps represent immune complexes and are seen in post infectious glomerulonephritis. Variability of the basement membrane thickening may be seen with Alport syndrome. The mesangial matrix is expanded in some forms of glomerulonephritis (e.g., IgA nephropathy) and other diseases, such as diabetes mellitus, but not in minimal change disease.
BP6 447   PBD6 954-956

15. **(E)** Postinfectious glomerulonephritis is one of many causes for a nephritic syndrome with hematuria and RBC casts. Most children recover completely, whereas one of six adults may progress to chronic renal failure. Some cases may follow a streptococcal pharyngitis (i.e., poststreptococcal glomerulonephritis). Goodpasture syndrome may also produce a nephritic syndrome, but there is linear deposition of antibody to glomerular basement membrane. Amyloidosis of the kidney mainly produces proteinuria without hematuria, as does membranous glomerulonephritis. Nodular and diffuse glomerulosclerosis are characteristic of diabetic nephropathy.
BP6 451   PBD6 949-951

16. **(E)** This is bladder hypertrophy from outlet obstruction. In an older male, this is most commonly caused by prostatic obstruction from hyperplasia or carcinoma. Mild elevations in the PSA can appear with prostatic hyperplasia, and greater increases in PSA suggest carcinoma. Autoimmune conditions can be associated with interstitial cystitis, but this does not cause bladder neck obstruction. Bladder outlet obstruction can increase the risk for infection, typically with bacterial organisms such as *E. coli,* not *M. tuberculosis*. Polycythemia can be the result of a paraneoplastic syndrome, but urothelial malignancies are unlikely to produce this. Renal cell carcinoma is a more

likely cause. Schistosomiasis leads to chronic inflammation and scarring.
PBD6 1008

17. **(A)** This woman has an autosomal dominant form of polycystic kidney disease. Hypertension and infection are the most frequent complications of this disorder. There is an increased risk for renal cell carcinoma in persons with dialysis-acquired cysts but not with polycystic kidney disease. Though there can be some proteinuria with many forms of chronic renal disease, nephrotic syndrome is not common with polycystic kidney disease. A microangiopathic hemolytic anemia may be seen with hemolytic-uremic syndrome. Vascular changes with resultant infarction are not seen in polycystic kidney disease.
BP6 463-464   PBD6 937-940

18. **(E)** This is the typical history for ischemic acute tubular necrosis, which is often accompanied by rupture of the basement membrane (i.e., tubulorrhexis). There is an initiating phase of a day or so, followed by a maintenance phase during which there is progressive oliguria and rising blood urea nitrogen levels, with salt and water overload. This is followed by a recovery phase during which there is a steady increase in urinary output and hypokalemia. Eventually, tubular function is restored. By treating this acute renal failure, nearly all patients recover. Crescents suggest a rapidly progressively glomerulonephritis that is unlikely to resolve. Interstitial infiltrates suggest a chronic tubulointerstitial process. Fibrinoid necrosis in arterioles is a feature of malignant nephrosclerosis, a serious condition that produces significant renal damage. Nodular glomerulosclerosis is a feature of diabetic nephropathy and is a progressive condition that leads to chronic renal failure.
BP6 460-461   PBD6 969-971

19. **(C)** Painless hematuria in an older adult suggests a renal neoplasm. The additional presence of constitutional symptoms, such as fever and weakness, should raise the suspicion of a renal cell carcinoma. Urinary tract calculi usually cause severe, colicky pain when they pass. Urinary tract infections do not present with recurrent hematuria without any fever or other signs of acute inflammation. Nephrotic syndrome with proteinuria is typically not associated with hematuria. A renal biopsy has a low yield without the acute onset of a renal disease and is a poor way to diagnose tumors.
BP6 468-469   PBD6 994

20. **(A)** This patient with nephrotic syndrome has clinical and histologic features of membranous glomerulonephritis. In most cases, this is an idiopathic disease caused by immune complex deposition on the glomerular basement membranes. Granular immunofluorescence with IgG and C3 supports this diagnosis. Under the electron microscope, electron-dense immune complexes are seen on the epithelial side of the basement membrane. Subendothelial electron-dense deposits with duplication of the basement membrane is a feature of type I membranoproliferative glomerulonephritis. Electron-dense deposits limited to the mesangium are seen in IgA nephropathy. Podocyte foot process fusion without any other abnormality occurs in lipoid nephrosis.
BP6 447-449   PBD6 953-955

21. **(C)** The clinical features are typical of urinary tract infection, and *E. coli* is the most common cause. The WBCs are characteristic of an acute inflammatory process. The presence of WBC casts indicates that the infection must have occurred in the kidney, because casts are formed in renal tubules. Most infections of the urinary tract start in the lower urinary tract and then ascend to the kidneys. Hematogenous spread is less common. *M. tuberculosis* is the cause for the rare "sterile pyuria." However, renal tuberculosis typically does not present as an acute febrile illness. *Mycoplasma* and *Cryptococcus* are rare urinary tract pathogens. Group A streptococcus is best known as an antecedent infection to post-streptococcal glomerulonephritis, an immunologically mediated disease in which the organisms are not present at the site of glomerular injury.
BP6 455-456   PBD6 974-975

22. **(F)** This is nodular and diffuse glomerulosclerosis, a classic lesion for diabetes mellitus. In diabetes mellitus, the level of glycosylated hemoglobin (Hb A1c) is elevated. Type I diabetics may initially have microalbuminuria, which predicts development of future overt diabetic nephropathy. There is progressive loss of renal function. These patients are often hypertensive and have hyaline arteriolosclerosis. The presence of overt proteinuria suggests progression to end-stage renal disease in 5 years.
BP6 570   PBD6 966-968

23. **(I)** She has findings characteristic for nephrocalcinosis from hypercalcemia. One of the most common causes for hypercalcemia in adults is metastatic disease. The hypercalcemia produces a chronic tubulointerstitial disease of the kidneys that is initially manifested by loss of concentrating ability. With continued hypercalcemia, there is progressive loss of renal function. Urinary tract stones formed of calcium oxalate may also be present.
PBD6 980

24. **(C)** The gross appearance of the kidney is characteristic of chronic pyelonephritis. The features are coarse and irregular scarring, resulting from ascending infection, blunting and deformity of calyces, and asymmetric involvement of the kidneys. The loss of tubules from scarring gives rise to reduced renal concentrating ability, and hence the patient had polyuria with a low specific gravity of the urine. Chronic glomerulonephritis, systemic lupus erythematosus, and benign nephrosclerosis give rise to bilateral symmetric involvement, and the affected kidneys are shrunken and finely granular. Dominant polycystic kidney disease shows large cysts that replace the renal parenchyma and greatly increase the size of the kidneys bilaterally.
BP6 457-458   PBD6 975-977

25. **(D)** These findings point to an acute drug-induced interstitial nephritis caused by ampicillin. This is an immunologic reaction, probably caused by a drug acting as a hapten. A poststreptococcal glomerulonephritis is not likely to be accompanied by a rash or eosinophils in the urine.

Acute pyelonephritis is an ascending infection; only un-commonly is it caused by hematogenous spread of bacteria from other sites. Acute tubular necrosis can give rise to acute renal failure. It is caused by hypoxia resulting from shock or from toxic injury caused by chemicals such as mercury. Membranous glomerulopathy is characterized by heavy proteinuria and nephrotic syndrome.
BP6 458   PBD6 977-978

26. **(C)** Chromosome 9 deletions (9p or 9q) are the only genetic changes present in superficial papillary tumors of the bladder. Additional alterations, including mutations in the retinoblastoma gene (13q) and *p53*, are present in inva-sive bladder tumors. The c-abl translocation is seen in leukemias and the K-*ras* oncogene is activated in a variety of adenocarcinomas.
PBD6 1007

27. **(A)** Development of recurrent hematuria following a viral illness in a child or young adult is typically associated with IgA nephropathy. In these patients, some defect in immune regulation causes excessive mucosal IgA synthesis in response to viral or other environmental antigens. IgA-containing complexes deposit in the mesangium and initiate glomerular injury. Antibodies against type IV collagen are formed in Goodpasture syndrome. Although viruses induce IgA synthesis, they do not cause direct glomerular damage. Defects in the structure of glomerular basement membrane are a feature of hereditary nephritis.
BP6 453-454   PBD6 961-962

28. **(C)** He has ureteral colic from the passage of a stone down the ureter. Dysuria may accompany acute cystitis, but not colicky pain. Flank pain may accompany a renal cell carcinoma, but the pain is usually dull. He is young for a renal carcinoma. Hydronephrosis is typically a "si-lent" disease that develops slowly and painlessly over years. A rupture of one of the many cysts in adult polycys-tic kidney disease can cause acute pain, but it is usually not colicky, and hematuria may not be present.
BP6 464-465   PBD6 989-990

29. **(C)** Steroid-responsive proteinuria in a child in the absence of renal failure is characteristic of minimal change disease. The renal biopsy in these cases shows no abnor-mality under the light microscope. Fusion of foot processes is seen under the electron microscope. Diffuse glomerular hypercellularity with normal basement membranes is usu-ally seen in acute poststreptococcal glomerulonephritis. This presents as a nephritic syndrome. Diffusely thickened basement membrane without proliferative changes in glo-meruli is seen in membranous glomerulonephritis. This typ-ically causes nephrotic syndrome in adults. Crescent forma-tion in glomeruli—crescentic glomerulonephritis—is associated with rapidly progressive renal failure. Glomeru-lar hypercellularity with thickening and splitting of the basement membrane is a feature of membranoproliferative glomerulonephritis. This disease presents with mixed ne-phrotic and nephritic syndrome and usually fails to respond to steroids.
BP6 447   PBD6 954-956

30. **(E)** He has idiopathic membranous glomerulopathy, giving rise to nephrotic syndrome. Diffuse basement mem-brane thickening, in the absence of proliferative changes, and granular deposits of IgG and C3 are typical of this condition. It is caused by the deposition of immune com-plexes on the basement membrane, which activates comple-ment. Antibodies that react with basement membrane give rise to a linear immunofluorescence pattern, as in Goodpas-ture syndrome. Membranous glomerulopathy has no associ-ation with streptococcal infections. There is also no evi-dence of cytokine- or T-cell–mediated damage in this disease. In 85% of patients with membranous glomerulopa-thy, the cause of immune complex deposition is unknown. In the remaining 15%, an associated systemic disease, such as systemic lupus erythematosus or some known cause for immune complex formation (e.g., drug reaction), exists.
BP6 447-449   PBD6 953-954

31. **(B)** Casts form in the tubules when there is protein-uria, resulting most commonly from glomerular injury. The presence of RBCs in the casts indicates bleeding into the tubules, where the red cells become attached to the casts. RBC casts almost always result from glomerular injury. Neutrophils can come from inflammation anywhere in the urinary tract, but most are from lower urinary tract infec-tions. The transitional epithelium extends only to the caly-ces. Oxalate crystals and hyaline casts in small numbers can be seen even in persons without renal disease.
BP6 440   PBD6 935-936

32. **(B)** HIV infection can cause a variety of renal mani-festations, but the most common is focal segmental glome-rulosclerosis. Diffuse proliferative glomerulonephritis can occur, although much less commonly. The other forms listed are not seen in conjunction with HIV infection.
BP6 449   PBD6 958

33. **(D)** Recurrent urinary tract infections with urea-split-ting organisms such as *Proteus* can lead to formation of magnesium ammonium phosphate stones. These stones are large, and they fill the dilated calyceal system. Because of their large size and projections into the calyces, such stones are sometimes called *staghorn calculi*. Infections are not a key feature of renal cell carcinoma. Cases of acute tubular necrosis typically occur from toxic or ischemic renal inju-ries. Malignant nephrosclerosis is primarily a vascular proc-ess that is not associated with infection. Papillary necrosis can complicate diabetes mellitus.
BP6 465   PBD6 989-990

34. **(B)** This diabetic patient has clinical features of acute pyelonephritis caused by *E. coli* infection. Papillary necro-sis is a complication of acute pyelonephritis, and diabetics are particularly prone to develop this. In the absence of diabetes, papillary necrosis develops when acute pyelone-phritis occurs along with urinary tract obstruction. This complication can also occur with chronic use of analgesics. Acute tubular necrosis typically occurs in acute renal fail-ure caused by hypoxia (e.g., shock) or toxic injury (e.g., mercury). Crescentic glomerulonephritis gives rise to rap-idly progressive renal failure. Hydronephrosis occurs when urinary outflow is obstructed in the renal pelvis or in the

ureter. Renal calculi can complicate conditions such as gout but not diabetes mellitus.
BP6 457   PBD6 979

35. **(A)** The most common cause for nephrotic syndrome in adults is membranous glomerulonephritis. About 85% of cases are idiopathic, but some cases follow infections (e.g., hepatitis, malaria) or are associated with malignancies or autoimmune diseases, among other causes. In some cases of AIDS, a nephropathy resembling focal segmental glomerulosclerosis can be seen. Multiple myeloma can be complicated by systemic amyloidosis, which can involve the kidney. Nephrolithiasis may lead to interstitial nephritis, not glomerular injury.
BP6 447–449   PBD6 953–955

36. **(A)** The most common cause for acute tubular necrosis is ischemic injury. The hypotension that develops after myocardial infarction causes decreased renal blood flow. Benign nephrosclerosis takes years to develop and is associated with benign essential hypertension. Emboli from mural thrombosis after myocardial infarction could reach the kidney to cause infarction, but most are small and focal. Hemolytic-uremic syndrome is a thrombotic microangiopathy that most often follows childhood enterotoxigenic *E. coli* infection. A rapidly progressive glomerulonephritis (RPGN) does not follow ischemic injury and does not resolve so quickly.
BP6 459–460   PBD6 969–971

37. **(B)** These findings are characteristic for Alport syndrome, a form of hereditary nephritis. Most cases are inherited as X-linked dominant, but autosomal dominant and autosomal recessive patterns of inheritance are also seen. Most commonly, males are severely affected. Vision, hearing, and renal function are affected, but other organ systems are not.
BP6 454   PBD6 962–963

38. **(D)** Exposure to arylamines results in a markedly increased risk for bladder cancer, which can occur decades after the first exposure. After absorption, aromatic amines are hydroxylated into an active form, detoxified by conjugation with glucuronic acid, and then excreted. Urinary glucuronidase then splits the nontoxic conjugated form into the active carcinogenic form. Renal cell carcinomas can also present as painless hematuria, but exposure to aniline dyes is not a risk factor. Hemorrhagic cystitis follows radiation injury or treatment with cytotoxic drugs such as cyclophosphamide. Tubercular cystitis is typically a complication of renal tuberculosis. Squamous cell carcinoma is the most common malignancy of the urethra, but it is rare and has no relation to carcinogens.
BP6 468–469   PBD6 1007

39. **(J)** This patient has diabetes mellitus. Nodular and diffuse glomerulosclerosis are often seen with long-standing diabetes mellitus. Infections with bacterial organisms also occur more frequently in patients with diabetes mellitus.
BP6 570   PBD6 966–967

40. **(G)** Wegener granulomatosis causes rapidly progressive glomerulonephritis characterized by epithelial crescents in Bowman's space. Several features differentiate Wegener granulomatosis from other forms of crescentic glomerulonephritis (e.g., Goodpasture syndrome). These are the presence of granulomatous vasculitis, the absence of immune complexes or anti-GBM antibodies, and the presence of C-ANCA.
BP6 452–453   PBD6 951–952

41. **(E)** Most cases of pyelonephritis result from ascending bacterial infections, which are more common in women. Recurrent urinary tract infections complicated by vesicoureteral reflux cause progressive interstitial damage and scarring. This can lead to chronic pyelonephritis with renal failure. Diffuse glomerulosclerosis is a feature of diabetes mellitus. Glomerular injury is not the major consequence of renal infections. Some cases of membranous glomerulonephritis are preceded by chronic infections such as hepatitis B or malaria, but recurrent urinary tract infections alone are not likely antecedents. Some chronic infections (e.g. lung abscess, pulmonary tuberculosis) can lead to reactive systemic amyloidosis that may involve the kidney. However, recurrent urinary tract infections do not cause amyloidosis.
BP6 455–457   PBD6 972–975

42. **(A)** This patient has urethritis. The most common cause for nongonococcal urethritis in males is *C. trachomatis*. This condition is more of a nuisance, but the behavior that led to this infection can put the patient at risk for other sexually transmitted diseases. Tuberculosis of the urinary tract is uncommon. Herpes simplex can produce painful vesicles on the skin. *Candida* infections are more typically seen with immunocompromised states or with long-term antibiotic therapy. A syphilitic chancre on the penis is a good indicator for *T. pallidum* infection.
PBD6 1009

43. **(B)** This is autosomal dominant polycystic kidney disease (DPKD), and several large cysts have completely replaced the kidney. In autosomal recessive polycystic kidney disease (which typically presents in fetal and neonatal life), the kidneys have a smooth external appearance, and on cut section, many small cysts give the kidney a sponge-like appearance. About 10% to 30% of affected patients with DPKD have an intracranial berry aneurysm, and some of these can rupture without warning. Wilms tumor does not arise in a polycystic kidney. Acute tubular necrosis is the result of ischemic or toxic renal injuries. Disseminated intravascular coagulation may complicate hemolytic-uremic syndrome. Pulmonary disease does not accompany adult polycystic kidney disease.
BP6 463–464   PBD6 937–940

44. **(C)** He has analgesic nephropathy, which damages the renal interstitium and can give rise to papillary necrosis. Hydronephrosis is not likely because there is no urinary tract obstruction in analgesic nephropathy. However, there is an increased risk for transitional cell carcinoma of

the renal pelvis. The toxic injury with analgesics is slowly progressive and not acute, as seen in acute tubular necrosis.
BP6 458-459   PBD6 978-979

45. **(C)** Chronic glomerulonephritis may follow specific forms of acute glomerulonephritis or in many cases develop insidiously with no known cause. With progressive glomerular injury and sclerosis, both kidneys become small, and their surfaces become granular. Hypertension often develops because of renal ischemia. Regardless of the initiating cause, these "end-stage" kidneys look morphologically identical. They have sclerotic glomeruli, thickened arteries, and chronic inflammation of interstitium. Because her ANA test result is negative, lupus is unlikely. Because her hemoglobin A_{1C} level is normal, she does not have diabetes mellitus. Polycystic kidney disease and amyloidosis should increase renal size.
BP6 454-455   PBD6 963-964

46. **(C)** This linear pattern of staining indicates anti-GBM antibody. Such antibodies are typically seen in Goodpasture syndrome. The ASO titer is increased with poststreptococcal glomerulonephritis, which typically has a granular pattern of immune complex deposition. HIV infection can lead to a nephropathy that resembles focal segmental glomerulosclerosis, in which IgM and C3 are deposited in the mesangial areas of affected glomeruli. Some cases of membranous glomerulonephritis are associated with hepatitis B virus infection, but the immune complex deposition is granular. The C3 nephritic factor can be a marker for type II membranoproliferative glomerulonephritis.
BP6 444   PBD6 943-944

47. **(D)** Acute tubular necrosis causes reversible acute renal failure. The tubular epithelium can regenerate after injury, although the patient may require interim hemodialysis. The chronic renal damage with analgesic abuse is not reversible but is progressive. Benign nephrosclerosis is also slowly progressive. Unlike minimal change disease, focal segmental glomerulosclerosis is unlikely to respond to corticosteroid therapy, and most patients progress to chronic renal failure. The renal changes with diabetes mellitus are chronic and progressive.
BP6 459-461   PBD6 969-971

48. **(B)** This is hyaline arteriolosclerosis; it is characteristically seen in patients with benign hypertension. Similar changes can also be seen with aging in the absence of hypertension. Oliguria is a sign of acute renal failure that does not complicate benign essential hypertension, a slowly progressive disease that is often clinically silent. Blood pressure screening is important for identifying patients with hypertension before significant organ damage has occurred. Malignant hypertension causes distinctive renal vascular lesions that include fibrinoid necrosis and hyperplastic arteriosclerosis. Hematuria may be seen in malignant hypertension from vascular injury but it is not a feature of benign hypertension. Flank pain is a symptom of acute pyelonephritis and some renal neoplasms.
BP6 461   PBD6 981-982

49. **(C)** IgA nephropathy is a frequent cause of recurrent gross or microscopic hematuria. In this condition, IgA is deposited in the mesangium. Subepithelial deposits of immune complexes occur in membranous glomerulopathy, giving rise to a granular pattern of immunofluorescence with anti-IgG. The clinical manifestations of membranous glomerulopathy are quite distinct. These patients present with the nephrotic syndrome. Diffuse proliferation and basement membrane thickening is seen in membranoproliferative glomerulonephritis, which also presents with nephrotic syndrome. Thrombosis in glomerular capillaries can occur with any severe damage to the glomerulus.
BP6 453-454   PBD6 961-962

50. **(B)** These are changes of chronic pyelonephritis. Urinary tract obstruction favors recurrent urinary tract infection. Vesicoureteral reflux propels infected urine from the urinary bladder to the ureters and renal pelvis and predisposes to infection. Benign nephrosclerosis is a vascular disease without a risk for infection. Lupus nephritis is associated with extensive inflammatory changes of glomeruli that are noninfectious. Amyloidosis can lead to progressive renal failure caused by amyloid deposition in the glomeruli. Amyloid does not evoke an inflammatory response. Congestive heart failure may predispose to acute tubular necrosis.
BP6 457-458   PBD6 975-976
BP6 452-453   PBD6 951-952

51. **(J)** He is septic, and the heart murmur strongly suggests an infective endocarditis. Cardiac lesions are the source for emboli (from valvular vegetations or mural thrombi) that can lodge in renal artery branches and produce areas of coagulative necrosis. These areas of acute infarction are typically wedge-shaped on cut section because of the vascular flow pattern.
PBD6 987-988

52. **(I)** This fetus has features of recessive polycystic kidney disease (RPKD) involving the liver. RPKD is a pediatric disease; by contrast, autosomal dominant polycystic kidney disease leads to presentation with renal failure in adults. Some less common forms of RPKD are accompanied by survival beyond infancy, and these patients develop congenital hepatic fibrosis.
PBD6 940

53. **(B)** The renal biopsy shows glomerular crescents, indicative of rapidly progressive glomerulonephritis. Crescentic glomerulonephritis is divided into three groups on the basis of immunofluorescence: type I (anti-GBM disease), type II (immune-complex disease), and type III (characterized by absence of anti-GBM antibodies or immune complexes). Each type has a different cause and treatment. The presence of anti-GBM antibodies suggests Goodpasture syndrome, and these patients need plasmapheresis. Type II crescentic glomerulonephritis can occur in systemic lupus erythematosus, in Henoch-Schönlein purpura, and after infections. Causes of type III crescentic glomerulonephritis include Wegener granulomatosis and microscopic polyangiitis. Immunofluorescence studies are critical for the classification and treatment of crescentic glomerulonephritis.

54. **(K)** The rapid cell turnover with acute leukemias and cell death from treatment result in hyperuricemia that can predispose to the formation of uric acid stones. Renal stones can produce colicky pain when they pass down the ureter and through the urethra, and the local trauma to the urothelium can produce hematuria. Uric acid stones form in acid urine. Unlike stones containing calcium, uric acid stones are radiolucent and do not show up on a plain radiograph.
BP6 465   PBD6 990

55. **(I)** She has findings of systemic lupus erythematosus, an autoimmune disease that often manifests with renal involvement. There are several forms of lupus nephritis, and they tend to produce a nephritic pattern of involvement. Because these patients have leakage of RBC from damaged glomeruli, as well as proteinuria, RBC casts are found in urine.
BP6 106-108   PBD6 220-222, 965

56. **(B)** Hyaline arteriosclerosis, characterized by thickening and hyalinization of small arteries and arterioles, is typically seen in patients with long-standing benign hypertension. Such a change also occurs with aging. Vascular narrowing causes ischemic changes that are slow and progressive. There is diffuse scarring and shrinkage of the kidneys. RBCs and RBC casts are a feature of crescentic glomerulonephritis, which is typically a rapidly progressive form of renal failure. Mesangial proliferation is also a feature of some forms of glomerulonephritis. Fibrinoid necrosis in arterioles is seen in malignant hypertension. Acute tubular necrosis is seen with anoxic or toxic injury to the renal tubular.
BP6 461   PBD6 981-982

57. **(C)** This patient has malignant hypertension. Necrotizing arteriolitis and hyperplastic arteriolosclerosis are the distinctive vascular lesions of malignant hypertension. Papillary necrosis is more likely to complicate diabetic nephropathy or analgesic nephropathy. Infarction of the kidney may result from emboli originating in the systemic circulation. However, malignant hypertension does not damage the large systemic vessels. Acute tubular necrosis is seen in hypoxic or toxic injury to the renal tubules. Acute pyelonephritis is a febrile illness, without severe blood pressure elevation.
BP6 461-462   PBD6 982-984

58. **(D)** The combination of cysts in the kidney and berry aneurysms in the brain is characteristic of adult autosomal dominant polycystic kidney disease. The cysts may also appear in liver and pancreas. Because of the autosomal dominant inheritance with high penetrance of the gene, first-degree relatives are at risk of having the same disorder and should be evaluated by ultrasound or other imaging techniques. This is particularly important because many patients remain asymptomatic until the onset of renal failure as adults.
BP6 463-464   PBD6 937-940

59. **(A)** This biopsy shows sclerosis of only a segment of the glomerulus (i.e., segmental lesion), and because only

50% of the glomeruli are affected, this is focal disease. Focal segmental glomerulosclerosis presents clinically with nephrotic syndrome that does not respond to corticosteroid therapy. In contrast, corticosteroid-responsive nephrotic syndrome in children is typically caused by minimal change disease; this is not associated with any glomerular change under the light microscope. Sore throat (i.e., pharyngitis) followed by nephritic syndrome is the typical clinical history for acute proliferative post-streptococcal glomerulonephritis. A diabetic with nephrotic syndrome is likely to show nodular glomerulosclerosis or diffuse thickening of basement membrane. Long-standing hypertension is most likely to cause hyalinization of most glomeruli.
BP6 449   PBD6 956-958

60. **(C)** This patient has acute pyelonephritis. Vesicoureteral reflux, acquired or congenital, is extremely important in the pathogenesis of ascending urinary tract infections. This allows bacteria to ascend from the urinary bladder into the ureter and the pelvis. In general, urinary tract infections are more common in females because of their shorter urethra, but in the absence of vesicoureteral reflux, the infections tend to remain localized in the urinary bladder. Hypertension can cause renal vascular narrowing and ultimately impair renal function, but it does not predispose to infections. Foci of infection in lungs can seed the kidney hematogenously, but this route is far less common than ascending infection.
BP6 455-456   PBD6 974-975

61. **(D)** This patient has the hemolytic-uremic syndrome. Some strains of *E. coli*, which can contaminate ground beef products, may elaborate a toxin that damages endothelium, leading to the hemolytic-uremic syndrome. This syndrome most often occurs in children and is one of the most common causes for acute renal failure in children. *Candida* urinary tract infections typically affect the urinary bladder. *Proteus* is a common cause for bacterial urinary tract infections. *C. difficile* is best known for causing a pseudomembranous enterocolitis, not renal lesions. *S. aureus* can cause urinary tract infections.
BP6 462-463   PBD6 985-986

62. **(E)** He suffered muscle injury with myoglobinemia and myoglobinuria. The large amount of excreted myoglobin produces a toxic acute tubular necrosis. With supportive care, the tubular epithelium can regenerate, and renal function can be restored. During the recovery phase of acute tubular necrosis, patients excrete large volumes of urine because the glomerular filtrate cannot be adequately reabsorbed by the damaged tubular epithelium. Trauma is not a cause for malignant hypertension. A bilateral renal vein thrombosis is not common. Glomerulonephritis does not occur from trauma. An infection is not likely to follow such a short course with such marked loss of renal function.
BP6 459-460   PBD6 969-971

63. **(C)** This is malignant hypertension, which may follow long-standing benign hypertension. Two types of vascular lesions are found in malignant hypertension. There

may be fibrinoid necrosis of arterioles; in addition, in inter-lobular arteries and arterioles, there is intimal thickening caused by proliferation of smooth muscle cells and colla-gen deposition. The proliferating smooth muscle cells are concentrically arranged, and these lesions, called hyperplas-tic arteriolosclerosis, cause severe narrowing of the lumen. The resultant ischemia elevates renin, which further pro-motes vasoconstriction to potentiate the injury. Nodular glomerulosclerosis is a feature of diabetes mellitus that slowly progresses over many years. Segmental tubular ne-crosis is seen in ischemic forms of acute tubular necrosis. An IgA nephropathy involves glomeruli but not typically the interstitium or vasculature. Glomerular crescents are a feature of a rapidly progressive glomerulonephritis. The blood pressure in this condition is not so markedly ele-vated.

BP6 461–462   PBD6 982–984

64.   **(A)** This is a high-grade transitional cell carcinoma of the bladder. Cigarette smoking, the most important influ-ence, is a risk factor in more than one half of men with such cancers. Schistosomiasis is also a risk factor for blad-der cancer, although typically squamous cell carcinoma. The increased risk for infection that occurs with diabetes mellitus and prostatic hyperplasia with the resultant acute and chronic cystitis does not predispose to transitional cell carcinoma.

BP6 468–469   PBD6 1004–1007

65.   **(C)** She has type II membranoproliferative glomeru-lonephritis, or dense-deposit disease, which usually leads to chronic renal failure. A postinfectious glomerulonephritis often has a hypercellular glomerulus with infiltration of polymorphonuclear leukocytes but no basement membrane thickening. A rapidly progressive glomerulonephritis is marked by crescents. Chronic glomerulonephritis is a term often used when there is sclerosis of many glomeruli but no clear cause. In membranous glomerulonephritis, there is just basement membrane thickening and small electron-dense deposits.

BP6 450–451   PBD6 958–960

The Male Genital Tract

BP6 Chapter 18 - The Male Genital System
PBD6 Chapter 23 - The Male Genital Tract

1. A 30-year-old male presents with a testicular mass that is suspected to be a malignant tumor. Abdominal computed tomography reveals enlargement of para-aortic lymph nodes, and multiple lung nodules are seen on a chest radiograph. Serum levels of chorionic gonadotropin (hCG) and α-fetoprotein (AFP) are markedly increased. Which of the following features is *not consistent* with the diagnosis of a classic seminoma?

O (A) Age
O (B) Presence of lung metastases
O (C) Enlargement of para-aortic nodes
O (D) Elevations in serum hCG and AFP levels
O (E) No history of cryptorchidism

2. For the past year, a 65-year-old male has had multiple, recurrent urinary tract infections, including acute cystitis and acute pyelonephritis. Before that time, he had no urinary tract problems. These findings should most strongly suggest which of the following underlying conditions?

O (A) Gonorrhea
O (B) Prostatic nodular hyperplasia
O (C) Phimosis
O (D) Epispadias
O (E) Adenocarcinoma of the prostate

For each of the clinical histories in questions 3 and 4, match the most closely associated microscopic description of a pathologic condition in the male genital tract:

(A) Back-to-back glands lined by cells with nuclei containing prominent nucleoli
(B) Congestion and edema with inflammatory infiltrates composed of neutrophils, macrophages, and lymphocytes
(C) Diffuse suppurative inflammation with gram-negative rods identified by gram staining
(D) Extensive interstitial hemorrhage and congestion with hemorrhagic infarction

(E) Full-thickness epithelial dysplasia with an intact underlying basement membrane
(F) Islands of cartilage, squamous epithelial pearls, and glands lined by tall columnar epithelium in a fibrous stroma
(G) Nests of large polyhedral cells with watery cytoplasm and large central nucleus containing one or two prominent nucleoli, surrounded by a lymphoid stroma
(H) Nodular arrangement of glands lined by two cell layers and surrounded by a fibrous stroma
(I) Rounded cells with abundant granular eosinophilic cytoplasm containing crystalloids of Reinke
(J) Syncytiotrophoblast and cytotrophoblast arranged in sheets with extensive hemorrhage and necrosis
(K) Thickened squamous epithelium with acanthosis, koilocytosis, and overlying hyperkeratosis

3. A 35-year-old male has noticed a slight enlargement of his right testis. He has also noticed bilateral breast enlargement over the past 6 months. An ultrasound scan reveals a discrete, rounded, 2-cm mass in the body of the testis. The testis is removed, and the mass is seen to have a uniform, brown cut surface. He is alive and well 10 years later. (   )

4. A 23-year-old sexually active male has been treated for *Neisseria gonorrhoeae* infection several times during the past 5 years. He now presents with multiple, sessile, 1- to 3-mm, nonulcerated papillary excrescences over the inner surface of the penile prepuce. The lesions have enlarged slowly during the past year. They are excised, but 2 years later, similar lesions are present. (   )

5. A 55-year-old male presents with a 6-month history of dysuria. The expressed prostatic secretions contain 30 leukocytes per high-power field. The most likely cause of these symptoms is

O (A) Benign prostatic hyperplasia
O (B) Acute bacterial prostatitis
O (C) Syphilitic prostatitis
O (D) Chronic abacterial prostatitis
O (E) Metastatic prostatic adenocarcinoma

6. An elevated serum AFP level in a 32-year-old male with an enlarged testis containing a 6-cm mass most strongly suggests the presence of which of the following cellular components in the mass?

○ (A) Yolk sac cells
○ (B) Leydig cells
○ (C) Seminoma cells
○ (D) Cytotrophoblasts
○ (E) Embryonal carcinoma cells

7. Retroperitoneal lymph node dissection is performed for metastatic testicular carcinoma in a 25-year-old male. The metastases were discovered before the primary site in the left testis, which was a hemorrhagic mass only 1.8 cm in diameter. Sections of the lymph nodes demonstrate a neoplasm with extensive necrosis and hemorrhage. Areas of viable tumor are composed of cuboidal cells intermingled with large, eosinophilic syncytial cells containing multiple, dark, pleomorphic nuclei. Immunohistochemical staining of the tumor is most likely to demonstrate which of the following antigenic components in the syncytial cells?

○ (A) Human chorionic gonadotrophin
○ (B) Alpha-fetoprotein (AFP)
○ (C) Vimentin
○ (D) CD20
○ (E) Embryonal carcinoma

8. During routine physical examination of a 70-year-old male, the prostate is found to be normal in size on palpation. He has a serum prostate-specific antigen (PSA) that is 17 ng/mL, four times the upper limit of normal and twice the value measured only 1 year ago. A routine urinalysis reveals no abnormalities. He is healthy, with no history of major illnesses. Which of the following histologic findings seen on a biopsy of the prostate is most likely to account for these findings?

○ (A) Hyperplastic nodules of the stroma and glands lined by two layers of epithelium
○ (B) Poorly differentiated glands lined by a single layer of epithelium and packed back to back
○ (C) Foci of chronic inflammatory cells in the stroma and in normal appearing glands
○ (D) Areas of liquefactive necrosis filled with neutrophils
○ (E) Multiple caseating granulomas

9. During a workup for infertility on a 35-year-old man and his 33-year-old wife, the man is found to have a sperm count in the low-normal range. On microscopic examination of the seminal fluid, the sperm are morphologically normal. A testicular biopsy is performed because this couple is desperate for an answer. The biopsy shows some patchy atrophy of seminiferous tubules, but remaining tubules show active spermatogenesis. The most probable cause for these findings is a previous history of

○ (A) Mumps
○ (B) Cryptorchidism
○ (C) Hydrocele
○ (D) Klinefelter syndrome
○ (E) Estrogen therapy

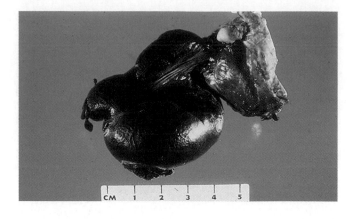

10. A 25-year-old male experiences sudden, severe pain in his scrotum one night. The pain continues unabated for hours. The excised testis is shown here. Which of the following conditions best explains these findings?

○ (A) Local invasion by a testicular tumor
○ (B) Parasitic infestation of the scrotum
○ (C) Obstruction to the flow of blood
○ (D) Obstruction to the flow of lymph
○ (E) Dissemination of tuberculosis from lungs to testis

11. A 2-year-old child is found to have a mass in the left testis that is 2.5 cm in diameter and well circumscribed. Histologically, this mass demonstrates sheets of cells and ill-defined glands composed of cuboidal cells, some of which contain eosinophilic hyaline globules. The analysis finds microcysts and primitive glomeruloid structures. AFP is demonstrated in the cytoplasm of the neoplastic cells by immunohistochemistry. The child most likely has

○ (A) Choriocarcinoma
○ (B) Seminoma
○ (C) Yolk sac tumor
○ (D) Teratoma
○ (E) Testosterone

12. The prepuce (i.e., foreskin) cannot be easily retracted over the glans penis of an uncircumcised 19-year-old male. He complains of local pain and irritation with difficult urination. Erections are painful. This condition is known as

○ (A) Epispadias
○ (B) Bowenoid papulosis
○ (C) Phimosis
○ (D) Genital candidiasis
○ (E) Paraphimosis

13. A routine physical examination performed on a 19-year-old male reveals that there is no left testis palpable in the scrotum. He is healthy, has had no major illnesses, and has normal sexual function. In counseling this patient, which of the following statements would be most appropriate for his condition?

○ (A) He will be unable to father children.
○ (B) He is at an increased risk for developing a testicular tumor.
○ (C) This is a finding common to more than one half of all males.
○ (D) This is an outcome of mumps infection as a child.
○ (E) This is an inherited disorder.

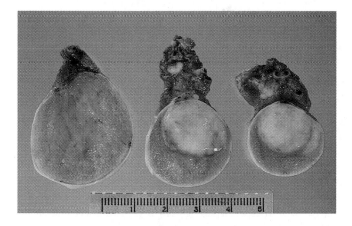

14. A 29-year-old male complains of a vague feeling of heaviness in the scrotum but no increase in pain. He is otherwise healthy. Physical examination reveals that the right testis is slightly larger than the left testis. An ultrasound scan indicates the presence of a circumscribed, 1.5-cm mass in the body of the right testis. The gross appearance of the mass is shown here. A biopsy reveals that the mass consists of uniform nests of cells with distinct cell borders, glycogen-rich cytoplasm, and round nuclei with prominent nucleoli. There are aggregates of lymphocytes between these nests of cells. Which of the following features is most characteristic for this lesion?

○ (A) Excellent response to radiation therapy
○ (B) Likelihood of extensive metastases early in the course
○ (C) Elevation of hCG levels in the serum
○ (D) Elevation of AFP levels in the serum
○ (E) Elevation of testosterone levels in the serum

15. A 5-year-old boy has a history of multiple bacterial urinary tract infections. Physical examination reveals an abnormal, constricted opening of the urethra on the ventral aspect of the penis, about 1.5 cm from the tip of the glans penis. There is also a cryptorchid testis on the right and an inguinal hernia on the left. His penile abnormality is best described as

○ (A) Hypospadias
○ (B) Phimosis
○ (C) Balanitis
○ (D) Epispadias
○ (E) Bowen disease

16. A 46-year-old male with a history of poorly controlled diabetes mellitus presents with painful, erosive, and markedly pruritic lesions on the glans penis, scrotum, and inguinal regions of the skin. These lesions are irregular, shallow, erythematous ulcerations that are 1 to 4 cm in diameter. Scrapings of the lesions examined under the microscope are most likely to demonstrate

○ (A) Burrows of *Sarcoptes scabiei*
○ (B) Budding cells with pseudohyphae
○ (C) Atypical cells with hyperchromatic nuclei
○ (D) Enlarged cells with intranuclear inclusions
○ (E) Spirochetes under darkfield examination

17. Pharmacologic agents that inhibit 5α-reductase and diminish dihydrotestosterone (DHT) synthesis in the prostate have the greatest effect on which of the following prostatic lesions?

○ (A) Acute prostatitis
○ (B) Adenocarcinoma
○ (C) Leiomyoma
○ (D) Chronic prostatitis
○ (E) Nodular hyperplasia

18. The right testis of a 33-year-old male is enlarged to twice normal size. The testis is removed, and the epididymis and the upper aspect of the right testis are involved with extensive granulomatous inflammation with epithelioid cells, Langhans giant cells, and caseous necrosis. The most common cause for these findings is

○ (A) Mumps
○ (B) Syphilis
○ (C) Tuberculosis
○ (D) Gonorrhea
○ (E) Sarcoidosis

19. A solitary, 0.8-cm, plaque-like erythematous area is identified on the distal shaft of the penis of a 48-year-old male. He has had no episodes of sexual intercourse for more than 1 month. A routine microbiologic culture with a Gram stain of the lesion reveals normal skin flora. A biopsy shows dysplasia involving the full thickness of the epithelium. The most likely diagnosis is

○ (A) Primary syphilis
○ (B) Balanitis
○ (C) Soft chancre
○ (D) Bowen disease
○ (E) Condyloma acuminatum

20. An 85-year-old male presented with a long history of urinary hesitancy and nocturia. Digital rectal examination revealed a hard, irregular prostate. Laboratory data revealed a serum alkaline phosphatase level of 300 U/L, serum prostatic acid phosphatase level of 8 ng/mL, and serum PSA level of 120 ng/mL. Blood urea nitrogen concentration is 44 mg/dL, and the serum creatinine level is 3.8 mg/dL. Which of the following clinical or laboratory features of this case most strongly suggests prostate cancer, rather than benign nodular hyperplasia?

○ (A) Age of the patient
○ (B) Symptoms of urethral obstruction
○ (C) The serum level of alkaline phosphatase
○ (D) The level of blood urea nitrogen
○ (E) PSA level

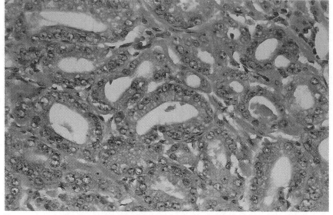

Courtesy of Dr. Kyle Molberg, Department of Pathology, University of Texas Southwestern Medical Center, Dallas, TX.

21. The microscopic appearance at high-power magnification from a transrectal needle biopsy of the prostate in a 63-year-old male is shown here. If this lesion is not treated, which of the following complications is most likely to occur?

- (A) Destructive lesions in the lumbar vertebrae
- (B) Recurrent urinary tract infections
- (C) Hydronephrosis
- (D) Gram-negative bacteremia
- (E) Sterility

22. A 59-year-old male notices a gradual enlargement of the scrotum over the course of a year. This is not painful but gives him a sensation of heaviness. There are no lesions of the overlying scrotal skin. He has no problems with sexual function. Physical examination reveals no obvious masses, but the scrotum bilaterally is enlarged, boggy, and soft, and the transillumination test result is positive. The most likely condition to explain these findings is

- (A) Varicocele
- (B) Elephantiasis
- (C) Orchitis
- (D) Seminoma
- (E) Hydrocele

23. An otherwise healthy 72-year-old male has increasing difficulty with urination. He has to get up several times each night because of a feeling of urgency, but each time, the urine volume is not great. He has difficulty starting and stopping urination. This problem has gotten worse over the last few years. His serum PSA level is slightly increased but stable over this time. A biopsy of the prostate is most likely to reveal which of the following?

- (A) Hyperplastic nodules of stroma and glands lined by two layers of epithelium
- (B) Poorly differentiated glands lined by a single layer of epithelium and packed back to back
- (C) Foci of chronic inflammatory cells in the stroma and in normal-appearing glands
- (D) Areas of liquefactive necrosis filled with neutrophils
- (E) Multiple areas of caseating granulomatous inflammation

24. Biopsy of an 8-cm mass in the left testis of a 30-

year-old male demonstrates areas of mature cartilage, keratinizing squamous epithelium, and colonic glandular epithelium. Serum hCG and AFP levels are elevated. Despite the benign appearance of the cells in the tumor, the surgeon tells the patient that he probably has a malignant testicular tumor. This conclusion is based on which of the following factors?

- (A) Size of the tumor
- (B) Age of the patient
- (C) Presence of colonic glandular epithelium
- (D) Elevation of hCG and AFP levels
- (E) Location in the left testis

ANSWERS

1. (D) Although a modest elevation of the hCG concentration can occur when a seminoma contains some syncytial giant cells, elevation of the AFP level never occurs with pure seminomas. Elevated levels of AFP and hCG effectively exclude the diagnosis of a pure seminoma and indicate the presence of a nonseminomatous tumor of the mixed type.
BP6 583–584   PBD6 1018–1023

2. (B) Of the diseases listed, prostatic hyperplasia is the most common in older adult males. By causing obstruction of the prostatic urethra, it can predispose to bacterial infections. Gonorrhea is more likely to be seen in younger, sexually active males, and obstruction is not a key feature. Phimosis can occur in uncircumcised males and can be congenital or acquired from inflammation, usually at a much younger age. Epispadias is a congenital condition. Prostatic adenocarcinomas are less likely than hyperplasia to cause obstructive symptoms.
BP6 585–586   PBD6 1028–1029

3. (I) This is a Leydig cell tumor of the testis. These tumors are most often benign, small masses that may go unnoticed, but some patients have gynecomastia from hormone production by the tumor. Most patients are young to middle-age men; sexual precocity may occur in the few children who have such tumors.
PBD6 1024

4. (K) This patient has condyloma acuminata, lesions typical of human papillomavirus (HPV) infection. Condyloma acuminatum is a benign but recurrent squamous epithelial proliferation because of infection with HPV, one of many sexually transmitted diseases that can occur in sexually active persons. Koilocytosis is particularly characteristic of HPV infection. Recurrent gonococcal infection indicates that he is sexually active. Gonococcal infection itself causes suppurative lesions in which there is liquefactive necrosis and a neutrophilic exudate.
PB6 596   PBD6 1012–1013

5. (D) The patient has more than 10 leukocytes per high-power field, indicating prostatitis. Chronic abacterial prosta-

titis is the most common form of prostatitis. Patients with this condition typically do not have a history of recurrent urinary tract infections. Nodular prostatic hyperplasia by itself is not an inflammatory process. Patients with acute bacterial prostatitis, most often caused by *Escherichia coli* infection, have systemic signs and symptoms of fever, chills, and dysuria; on rectal examination, the prostate is very tender. Syphilis is a disease of the external genitalia, although the epididymis of the testis may be involved. Prostate carcinomas generally do not have a significant amount of acute inflammation, and metastases are most often associated with pain; most prostatic conditions causing dysuria are benign.
BP6 584–585   PBD6 1026

6.   (A) AFP is a product of yolk sac cells that can be demonstrated by immunohistochemistry. Pure yolk sac tumors are rare in adults, but yolk sac components are common in mixed nonseminomatous tumors. Cytotrophoblasts do not produce a serum marker, but they may be present in a choriocarcinoma along with syncytiotrophoblasts that do produce hCG. Embryonal carcinoma cells by themselves do not produce any specific product. However, embryonal carcinoma cells are common in nonseminomatous tumors and are often mixed with other cell types.
BP6 584   PBD6 1020–1021

7.   (A) This is a choriocarcinoma, the most aggressive of the testicular carcinomas, which often metastasizes widely. The primitive syncytial cells mimic the syncytiotrophoblast of placental tissue and, therefore, stain for HCG. AFP is a marker that is more likely to be found in mixed tumors with a yolk sac component. Vimentin is more likely to be seen in sarcomas, which are rare in the testicular region. CD20 is a lymphoid marker. Testosterone is found in Leydig cells.
BP6 581–584   PBD6 2021

8.   (B) This is a significant elevation in the PSA level, and the increase over time is more indicative of carcinoma. Typically, prostatic carcinomas are adenocarcinomas that form small glands packed back to back; unlike hyperplastic glands, malignant glands are lined by a single layer of epithelium. Many adenocarcinomas of the prostate do not produce obstructive symptoms and may not be palpable on digital rectal examination. Hyperplasias can increase the PSA level, although not to high levels that increase significantly over time. Prostatitis, like hyperplasia, can slightly elevate the PSA level.
BP6 586–588   PBD6 1022–1023

9.   (A) Mumps is a common childhood infection that can produce parotitis, but in adults who have this infection orchitis is more frequent. The orchitis is usually not severe, and its involvement of the testis is patchy; therefore infertility is not a common outcome. Klinefelter syndrome and estrogen therapy can cause tubular atrophy, although it is generalized in both cases. Patchy loss of seminiferous tubules indicates a local inflammatory process. Cryptorchidism results from failure of the testis to descend into the scrotum normally, and the abnormally positioned testis becomes atrophic throughout. A hydrocele is a fluid collec-

tion outside the body of the testis and does not interfere with spermatogenesis.
BP6 580   PBD6 1017

10.   (C) The markedly hemorrhagic appearance results from testicular torsion with a greater obstruction to venous outflow than to arterial supply, producing a hemorrhagic infarction. An abnormally positioned or anchored testis in the scrotum is a risk factor for this condition. Testicular cancers do not obstruct blood flow. Parasitic infestation, typically filariasis, causes obstruction to the flow of lymphatics, leading to gradual enlargement of scrotum with thickening of the overlying skin. Tuberculosis can spread from the lung through the bloodstream, producing miliary tuberculosis, seen as multiple, pale, millet-sized lesions. Isolated spread to the epididymis or testis can also occur. It does not cause vascular obstruction.
PBD6 1017

11.   (C) Yolk sac tumors are typically seen in males younger than 3 years of age. The primitive glomeruloid structures are known as Schiller-Duval bodies. Choriocarcinomas contain large, hyperchromatic syncytiotrophoblastic cells. Seminomas have sheets and nests of cells resembling primitive germ cells, often with an intervening lymphoid stroma. Teratomas contain elements of mature cartilage, bone, or other endodermal, mesodermal, or ectodermal structures. Embryonal carcinomas that contain yolk sac cells contain AFP but are seen in adults and are composed of cords and sheets of primitive cells.
BP6 581–584   PBD6 1019–1021

12.   (C) Phimosis can be congenital, but it is more often a consequence of multiple episodes of balanitis (i.e., inflammation of the glans penis or foreskin). The balanitis leads to scarring that prevents retraction of the foreskin. Forcible retraction may result in vascular compromise with further inflammation and swelling, known as paraphimosis. Epispadias is a congenital condition in which the penile urethra opens onto the dorsal surface of the penis. Bowenoid papulosis is a premalignant lesion of the penile shaft resulting from viral infection. Candidiasis is most likely to produce shallow ulcerations that are intensely pruritic.
BP6 578   PBD6 1012

13.   (B) This condition is known as cryptorchidism, and it results from failure of the testis to descend from the abdominal cavity to the scrotum during fetal development. One or both testes may be involved. It is associated with increased risk of developing testicular cancer. An undescended testis eventually undergoes atrophy in childhood. Unilateral cryptorchidism does not usually lead to infertility, but it may be associated with atrophy of the contralateral descended testis. Mumps infection tends to produce patchy testicular atrophy, usually without infertility. Isolated cryptorchidism is a developmental defect that is usually sporadic and is not inherited in the germ line.
BP6 580   PBD6 1015–1016

14.   (A) This is the most common form of "pure" testicular germ cell tumor that may remain confined to the testis (stage I). The prognosis is good for most cases, even with

metastases, because seminomas are radiosensitive. The hCG levels may be slightly elevated in about 15% of patients with seminoma. An elevated hCG level suggests a component of syncytial cells, although very high levels suggest the existence of a choriocarcinoma. AFP levels are elevated in testicular tumors with a yolk sac component, and many tumors with an embryonal cell component also contain yolk sac cells. Testosterone is a product of Leydig cells, not germ cells.

BP6 581-583   PBD6 1018-1020

15.   **(A)** This is a congenital condition seen in about 1 of 300 male births. The inguinal hernia and the cryptorchidism are abnormalities that may accompany this condition. Phimosis is a constriction preventing retraction of the prepuce. It can be congenital but more likely is the result of inflammation of the foreskin of the penis, such as a balanitis, a form of local inflammation of the glans penis. Epispadias is a congenital abnormal opening of the urethra that is on the dorsal aspect of the penis. Bowen disease is seen in adults and is squamous cell carcinoma in situ of the penis.

BP6 578   PBD6 1012

16.   **(B)** Genital candidiasis can occur in persons without underlying illnesses, but it is far more common in those with diabetes mellitus. Warm, moist conditions at these sites favor fungal growth. Scabies mites are more likely to be found in linear burrows in epidermis scraped from extremities. Neoplasms may ulcerate, but such lesions are unlikely to be shallow or multiple without a mass lesion present. Intranuclear inclusions suggest a viral infection, but diabetes is not a risk for genital viral infections. These lesions are too large and numerous to be syphilitic chancres.

BP6 578   PBD6 1012

17.   **(E)** The presence of androgens is the major hormonal stimulus to glandular and stromal proliferation that results in nodular prostatic hyperplasia. Although testosterone production decreases with age, prostatic hyperplasia increases, probably because of an increased expression of hormonal receptors that enhance the effect of any DHT that is present.

BP6 585   PBD6 1027

18.   **(C)** Tuberculosis is an uncommon infection, but it can occur with disseminated disease. The infection typically starts in the epididymis and spreads to the body of the testis. Mumps produces a patchy orchitis with minimal inflammation that heals with patchy fibrosis. Syphilis is more likely to involve the testis, and there can be gummatous inflammation with neutrophils, necrosis, and some mononuclear cells. Gonococcal infections produce acute inflammation. Sarcoidosis produces noncaseating granulomas that are not likely to be found in the testis.

BP6 580   PBD6 1016-1017

19.   **(D)** Bowen disease is a form of squamous cell carcinoma in situ, and like carcinoma in situ elsewhere, it has a natural history of progression to invasive cancer if not treated. Poor hygiene and infection with HPV (particularly types 16 and 18) are factors that favor development of dysplasias and malignancies of genital epithelia. Syphilis is

a sexually transmitted disease that produces a hard chancre that heals in a matter of weeks. Balanitis is an inflammatory condition without dysplasia. A soft chancre may be seen with *Haemophilus ducreyi* infections. Condylomas are raised, whitish lesions.

BP6 578   PBD6 1013-1014

20.   **(E)** The presence of a hard, irregular nodule, along with the extremely high PSA level, points most clearly to prostate carcinoma. Modest elevations of the PSA concentration can occur in nodular hyperplasia of the prostate and prostatitis. Symptoms of urinary obstruction, although more prominent in nodular hyperplasia because of the location of the nodules in the periurethral region, are not sufficient to distinguish cancer from hyperplasia. Similarly, renal failure due to obstruction or infiltration, although most common with nodular hyperplasia, can occur in both conditions. Levels of alkaline phosphatase are elevated when prostate carcinoma gives rise to osteoblastic metastases. However, alkaline phosphatase, unlike PSA, is not a tissue-specific marker. It can be elevated in bone disease and in obstructive liver diseases.

BP6 586-588   PBD6 1032-1033

21.   **(A)** The back-to-back glands indicate prostatic adenocarcinoma. The neoplasm shown is well differentiated, and the nucleoli are prominent. Without treatment, prostatic carcinomas may metastasize, often to the vertebrae, where they can produce osteolytic or osteoblastic lesions. Recurrent urinary tract infections and hydronephrosis are complications of obstruction produced most commonly by nodular hyperplasia. Acute bacterial prostatitis can cause bacteremia. Sterility is rarely a complication of any prostatic lesion, benign or malignant. Impotence may follow radical surgery for prostate carcinoma.

BP6 587-588   PBD6 1030-1031

22.   **(E)** Hydrocele is one of the most common causes for scrotal enlargement. It consists of fluid collection within the tunica vaginalis. Most cases are idiopathic, although some may result from local inflammation. A varicocele is a collection of dilated veins (i.e., pampiniform plexus of veins) that may produce increased warmth that inhibits spermatogenesis. Elephantiasis is a complication of parasitic filarial infections involving the inguinal lymphatics. Orchitis involves the body of the testis without marked enlargement but with tenderness. A seminoma is typically a unilateral, firm mass.

BP6 579-580   PBD6 1025

23.   **(A)** The clinical features are typical of nodular hyperplasia of prostate. Mild elevation of the PSA level can occur with nodular hyperplasia. The area of the prostate that is most often involved with nodular hyperplasia to produce significant obstruction is in the inner (transitional and periurethral) zone. The hyperplastic nodules consist of proliferating glands, lined by two layers of cells, and the intervening fibromuscular stroma. Prostatitis may cause dysuria and increased frequency from inflammation, but it is less common in older males than hyperplasia, and it is less likely to produce obstructive symptoms. Adenocarcinomas of the prostate (choice B) are common in older men,

but they arise in the posterior zone of the prostate and are less likely to produce obstructive symptoms than is hyperplasia. Acute prostatitis (abscesses with neutrophils) produce much more dysuria and has symptoms of shorter duration. Tuberculosis can affect prostate, but it does not produce symptoms of obstruction.
BP6 584–585   PBD6 1028

24.   **(D)** The tumor has elements of all three germ layers and is a teratoma. It is uncommon for teratomas in adult males to be completely benign. The most common additional histologic component is embryonal carcinoma. The elevated levels of hCG and AFP indicate that this is a mixed tumor with additional elements of choriocarcinoma and yolk sac cells. The size of the tumor, age of the patient, location of the tumor (e.g., right, left, cryptorchid), and differentiation of the glandular epithelium are not markers of malignancy.
BP6 580–582   PBD6 1019–1022

The Female Genital Tract

PBD6 Chapter 24 - The Female Genital Tract
BP6 Chapter 19 - Female Genital System
and Breast

1.   A 24-year-old female experiences the sudden onset of severe lower abdominal pain. A physical examination reveals no masses, but there is severe right lower quadrant abdominal tenderness. A pelvic examination shows no lesions of the cervix or vagina. Bowel sounds are detected. An abdominal ultrasound reveals a focal 4-cm area of enlargement involving the proximal right fallopian tube. A dilation and curettage procedure reveals only decidua from the endometrial cavity. Which of the following laboratory test findings is most likely to be present?

O (A) Positive cervical culture for *Neisseria gonorrhoeae*
O (B) 69,XXY karyotype on decidual tissue
O (C) Positive serum pregnancy test result
O (D) Positive serologic test result for syphilis
O (E) Pap smear showing *Candida*

2.   A 30-year-old sexually active woman presents with a mucopurulent vaginal discharge. On pelvic examination, the cervix appears reddened around the os, but no erosions or mass lesions are present. A Pap smear shows numerous neutrophils but no dysplastic cells. A cervical biopsy demonstrates a marked follicular cervicitis. The most common infectious agent that produces these findings is

O (A) *Chlamydia trachomatis*
O (B) *Neisseria gonorrhoeae*
O (C) *Candida albicans*
O (D) *Trichomonas vaginalis*
O (E) Herpes simplex virus

3.   A 36-year-old female has a pelvic examination that reveals a symmetrically enlarged uterus, without apparent nodularity or a palpable mass. She has had menorrhagia

and pelvic pain for several months. She had a normal, uncomplicated pregnancy 10 years ago. A serum pregnancy test result is negative. The most probable cause for these findings is

O (A) Endometriosis
O (B) Leiomyoma
O (C) Endometrial hyperplasia
O (D) Adenomyosis
O (E) Chronic endometritis

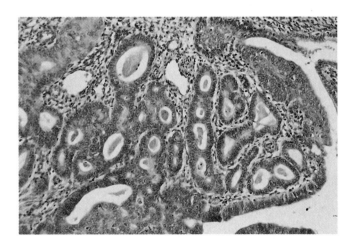

4.   A 45-year-old female has had menometrorrhagia for the past 3 months. An endometrial biopsy is performed, and the microscopic appearance of the endometrium is shown here. She then undergoes a dilation and curettage, and the bleeding stops, with no further problems. Which of the following conditions most likely helped to produce the findings in this case?

O (A) Ovarian mature cystic teratoma
O (B) Chronic endometritis
O (C) Failure of ovulation
O (D) Pregnancy
O (E) Use of oral contraceptives

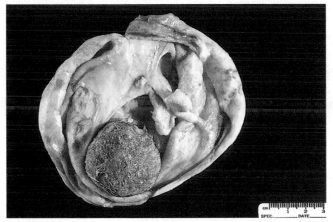

Courtesy of Dr. Christopher Crum, Brigham and Women's Hospital, Boston, MA.

5. A 31-year-old woman has had dull, constant abdominal pain for several months, and on physical examination, the only finding is a right adnexal mass. Pelvic computed tomography (CT) confirms the presence of a 7-cm circumscribed mass involving the ovary and reveals some irregular calcifications within this mass. The right tube and ovary with the mass are surgically excised. The gross appearance of the ovary, which has been opened, is shown here. The best diagnosis is

○ (A) Mucinous cystadenoma
○ (B) Choriocarcinoma
○ (C) Dysgerminoma
○ (D) Serous cystadenoma
○ (E) Mature cystic teratoma

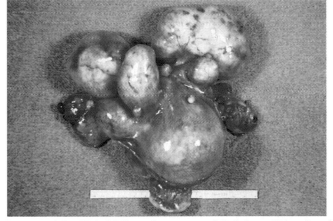

Courtesy of Dr. Kyle Molberg, Department of Pathology, University of Texas Southwestern Medical School, Dallas, TX.

6. A healthy 52-year-old female had a feeling of pelvic heaviness. There was no history of abnormal bleeding. Her physician palpated an enlarged, nodular uterus on bimanual pelvic examination. A Pap smear was normal. Pelvic ultrasound revealed multiple solid uterine masses with no evidence of necrosis or hemorrhage. A total abdominal hysterectomy was performed. Based on the gross appearance shown here, she is most likely to have

○ (A) Metastases
○ (B) Endometriosis
○ (C) An infiltrative leiomyosarcoma
○ (D) Multiple leiomyomas
○ (E) Adenomyosis

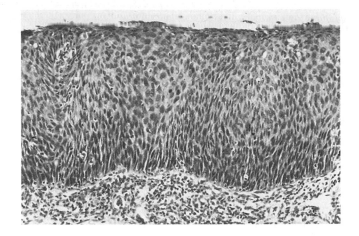

7. After an abnormal Pap smear result is obtained, an adult female has colposcopy and a biopsy. The microscopic appearance of the biopsy is seen here. Which of the following factors probably contributed the most to the development of the lesion depicted here?

○ (A) Diethylstilbestrol exposure
○ (B) Recurrent *Candida* infections
○ (C) Early age at first intercourse
○ (D) Multiple pregnancies
○ (E) Postmenopausal estrogen therapy

8. A 62-year-old, obese, nulliparous female has an episode of vaginal bleeding, producing only about 5 mL of blood. On pelvic examination, there appears to be no enlargement of the uterus. The cervix appears normal. A Pap smear yields cells that are consistent with adenocarcinoma. Which of the following conditions most likely contributed to this malignancy?

○ (A) Endometrial hyperplasia
○ (B) Chronic endometritis
○ (C) Use of oral contraceptives
○ (D) Human papillomavirus (HPV) infection
○ (E) Adenomyosis

9. A 36-year-old primigravida develops peripheral edema in the late second trimester. She is found to have a blood pressure of 155/95 mm Hg. A urinalysis demonstrates no blood, glucose, or ketones, but there is 2+ proteinuria. She delivers a normal, viable but low-birth-weight baby at 36 weeks. Her blood pressure returns to normal and she no longer has proteinuria. Examination of the placenta is most likely to demonstrate which of the following lesions?

○ (A) Chronic villitis
○ (B) Partial mole
○ (C) Hydrops
○ (D) Multiple infarcts
○ (E) Choriocarcinoma

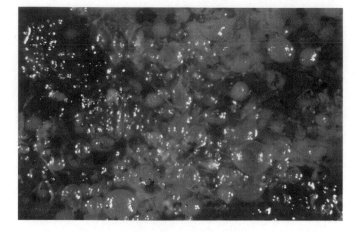

10. Shown here is the gross appearance of material obtained by dilation and curettage from a 22-year-old female who had some vaginal bleeding. She had marked nausea and vomiting for several weeks. On physical examination, the uterus measured large for dates. An ultrasound revealed a "snowstorm" appearance to the intrauterine contents, and no fetus was identified. Which of the following substances is most likely to be increased in her serum?

○ (A) Alpha-fetoprotein
○ (B) Thyroxine
○ (C) Estrogen
○ (D) Lactate dehydrogenase
○ (E) Beta-human chorionic gonadotropin

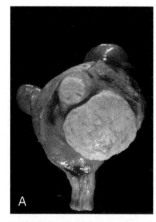

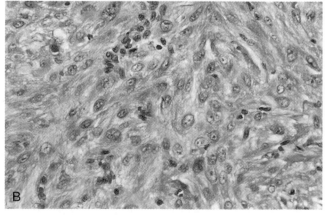

11. A total abdominal hysterectomy is performed in a 46-year-old postmenopausal female who presents with meno-

metrorrhagia. The gross (A) and microscopic (B) features of the uterus are illustrated here. These lesions are most likely to be

○ (A) Leiomyoma
○ (B) Leiomyosarcoma
○ (C) Endometrial polyp
○ (D) Adenomyosis
○ (E) Invasive mole

12. On two occasions in the past month, a 62-year-old childless woman noticed a blood-tinged vaginal discharge. Bimanual pelvic examination reveals a normal-sized uterus with no palpable adnexal masses. There are no cervical erosions or masses. Review of systems shows that she has hypertension and type I diabetes mellitus treated with insulin. An endometrial biopsy is most likely to show

○ (A) Adenomyosis
○ (B) Leiomyosarcoma
○ (C) Adenocarcinoma
○ (D) Squamous cell carcinoma
○ (E) Choriocarcinoma

13. At 15 weeks' gestation, a 23-year-old female has a spontaneous abortion. The male fetus is small for gestational age and is malformed, with syndactyly of the third and fourth digits of each hand. The placenta is also small and demonstrates scattered 0.5-cm, grapelike villi among morphologically normal villi. A chromosome analysis of placental tissue is most likely to show which of the following karyotypes?

○ (A) 69,XXY
○ (B) 46,XX
○ (C) 23,Y
○ (D) 45,X
○ (E) 47,XXY

14. A 54-year-old female has had weight loss accompanied by abdominal enlargement for the past 6 months. She is concerned because there is a family history of ovarian carcinoma. An abdominal ultrasound reveals a 10-cm cystic mass involving the left adnexal region, with scattered 1-cm peritoneal nodules. Peritoneal fluid cytology reveals the presence of malignant cells, consistent with a cystadenocarcinoma. Which of the following mutated genes is most likely a factor in the development of this neoplasm?

○ (A) *ras*
○ (B) *c-erb-B2 (HER2)*
○ (C) BRCA1
○ (D) *myc*
○ (E) *Rb1*

15. A 4-year-old female child presents with polypoid, grapelike masses projecting from the vagina. Histologic examination of the biopsy shows small round tumor cells, some of which have eosinophilic straplike cytoplasm. Immunohistochemical staining reveals the presence of desmin. This lesion is best classified as a (an)

O (A) Neuroblastoma
O (B) Embryonal rhabdomyosarcoma
O (C) Condyloma acuminatum
O (D) Vulvar intraepithelial neoplasm
O (E) Infiltrating squamous cell carcinoma

16.   An endometrial biopsy is performed on a 42-year-old woman who has had menometrorrhagia for the past 2 months. She has no history of irregular menstrual bleeding, and she has not yet reached menopause. The biopsy shows hyperplastic endometrium but no cellular atypia. An abdominal ultrasound reveals the presence of a right adnexal mass. The mass is most likely to represent a (an)

O (A) Mature cystic teratoma
O (B) Endometriosis
O (C) Corpus luteum cyst
O (D) Metastasis
O (E) Granulosa-theca cell tumor

17.   A 19-year-old female has had pelvic pain for a week. A pelvic examination shows mild erythema of the ectocervix. A Pap smear demonstrates many neutrophils but no dysplastic cells. A cervical culture grows *N. gonorrhoeae*. If this infection is not adequately treated, the patient will be at increased risk for

O (A) Ectopic pregnancy
O (B) Dysfunctional uterine bleeding
O (C) Cervical carcinoma
O (D) Endometrial hyperplasia
O (E) Endometriosis

18.   You obtain a routine Pap smear while performing a physical examination on a 28-year-old female. Gross inspection of the vulva, vagina, and cervix reveals no apparent lesions. The results of the Pap smear are consistent with cervical intraepithelial neoplasia (CIN) II. What is the major significance of this finding?

O (A) A cervicitis needs to be treated.
O (B) She has an increased risk for cervical carcinoma.
O (C) Condyloma acuminata are probably present.
O (D) An endocervical polyp needs to be excised.
O (E) She needs to discontinue oral contraceptives.

19.   A 50-year-old woman undergoes a total abdominal hysterectomy for an endometrial adenocarcinoma diagnosed by endometrial biopsy. Grossly, the uterus is normal in size, but sectioning through the uterus reveals a single, 1.5-cm, firm, tan-white, circumscribed subserosal nodule. This nodule is most likely to be a

O (A) Metastasis
O (B) Leiomyoma
O (C) Choriocarcinoma
O (D) Chocolate cyst
O (E) Malignant mixed müllerian tumor

20.   Which of the following conditions is most likely to be complicated by the development of disseminated intravascular coagulation (DIC) in a 25-year-old female?

O (A) Acute salpingitis
O (B) Hydatidiform mole
O (C) Mature cystic teratoma
O (D) Endometriosis
O (E) Eclampsia

21.   A 58-year-old female has had dull pain in the lower abdomen for the past 6 months, along with some minimal vaginal bleeding on three occasions. An abdominal ultrasound reveals a solid, 8-cm right adnexal mass. A total abdominal hysterectomy is performed, and the mass is diagnosed as an ovarian granulosa-theca cell tumor. Which of the following additional lesions is most likely to be seen in the surgical specimen?

O (A) Condyloma acuminata of the cervix
O (B) Endometrial hyperplasia
O (C) Metastases to the uterine serosa
O (D) Bilateral chronic salpingitis
O (E) Partial mole of the uterus

For each of the clinical histories in questions 22 through 24, match the most closely associated lesion of the female genital tract:

(A) Adenomyosis
(B) Cervical squamous cell carcinoma
(C) Condyloma acuminatum
(D) Endometriosis
(E) Endometrial adenocarcinoma
(F) Krukenberg tumor
(G) Ovarian mature cystic teratoma
(H) Ovarian papillary serous cystadenocarcinoma
 (I) Uterine leiomyoma
(J) Vulvar squamous cell carcinoma

22.   A 43-year-old female who had menarche at age 11 and who has had 12 lifetime sexual partners presents with a 6-month history of postcoital bleeding. A Pap smear performed 3 years previously was interpreted as a high-grade cervical intraepithelial neoplasm. In situ hybridization revealed infection of epithelial cells with HPV type 16 (HPV-16). (   )

23.   A 57-year-old, markedly obese, single, diabetic female presents with a 2-month history of vaginal bleeding. She went through menopause 7 years earlier and had not experienced menstrual periods since then. A recent Pap smear revealed atypical glandular cells of uncertain significance. (   )

24.   A 32-year-old female presents with cyclic abdominal pain that coincides with her menses. Attempts at becoming pregnant have failed over the past 5 years. Laparoscopic examination reveals numerous hemorrhagic 0.2- to 0.5-cm cysts over the peritoneal surfaces of the uterus and ovaries. (   )

25.   A Pap smear from a 21-year-old female yields cells with cytologic changes consistent with koilocytotic atypia. There is no necrosis or acute inflammation. Koilocytotic changes are most likely caused by infection with

○ (A) *Neisseria gonorrhoeae*
○ (B) *Chlamydia trachomatis*
○ (C) Human papillomavirus
○ (D) *Trichomonas vaginalis*
○ (E) Herpes simplex virus type 2

26. A 31-year-old female has had a whitish, globular vaginal discharge for the past week. On pelvic examination, the cervix appears erythematous, but there are no erosions or masses. A Pap smear reveals budding cells and pseudohyphae. No dysplastic cells are present. The infectious agent that is most likely to be present is

○ (A) *Trichomonas vaginalis*
○ (B) *Ureaplasma urealyticum*
○ (C) *Candida albicans*
○ (D) *Chlamydia trachomatis*
○ (E) *Neisseria gonorrhoeae*

27. A routine physical examination on a 57-year-old female reveals the presence of a 0.7-cm area of flat, white discoloration on the labia majora on the right. A biopsy shows dysplastic cells occupying about half the thickness of the squamous epithelium, with minimal underlying chronic inflammation. In situ hybridization reveals the presence of HPV-16 DNA in the epithelial cells. The condition that best accounts for these findings is

○ (A) Lichen sclerosus
○ (B) Condyloma acuminatum
○ (C) Squamous hyperplasia
○ (D) Vulvar intraepithelial neoplasia
○ (E) Chronic vulvitis

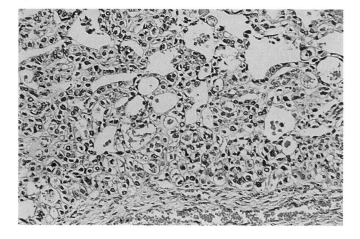

28. A 19-year-old female notes dyspareunia followed by some vaginal bleeding. On pelvic examination, a 2.5-cm, red, friable, nodular mass is seen on the anterior wall of the upper third of the vagina. A biopsy of this mass reveals the microscopic appearance shown here. Which of the following conditions contributed most to the origin of this neoplasm?

○ (A) Diethylstilbestrol exposure
○ (B) *Trichomonas vaginitis*
○ (C) Polycystic ovaries
○ (D) HPV infection
○ (E) Congenital adrenal hyperplasia

29. A 33-year-old female has been bothered by dyspareunia and dysuria for several years. Each time she visits a physician, a physical examination reveals no gross findings in the vulva, vagina, or cervix. A Pap smear reveals no abnormalities. She is referred to a psychiatrist, who finds no psychiatric problems or evidence for neurologic disease, but he does elicit a history of severe dysmenorrhea and pelvic pain on defecation and refers the patient to a gynecologist. Which of the following lesions is the gynecologist most likely to find with laparoscopy?

○ (A) Tubo-ovarian adhesions
○ (B) Red-blue to brown, 0.3-cm implants on the uterine serosa
○ (C) Multiple, 0.7- to 1.5-cm, firm, white peritoneal nodules
○ (D) Enlarged, edematous, and hemorrhagic right ovary
○ (E) Subserosal, 3-cm uterine leiomyoma

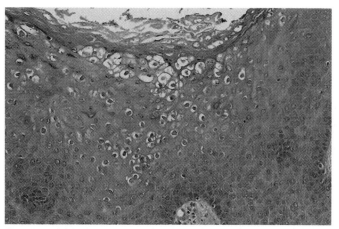

Courtesy of Dr. Jag Bhawan, Boston University School of Medicine, Boston, MA.

30. Several 0.5- to 2-cm, red-pink, flattened lesions with rough surfaces are present on the vulva and perineum of a 36-year-old woman. One of the larger lesions is excised and is shown microscopically. The appearance of these lesions is most likely indicative of infection with

○ (A) HPV
○ (B) *Chlamydia trachomatis*
○ (C) *Treponema pallidum*
○ (D) *Haemophilus ducreyi*
○ (E) *Candida albicans*

31. A routine Pap smear is obtained on a 45-year-old female who has not had a previous Pap smear. The results indicate that dysplastic cells are present, and the lesion is consistent with cervical intraepithelial neoplasia (CIN) III. The patient is referred to a gynecologist who performs colposcopy and takes several biopsies that all show CIN III. She undergoes conization of the cervix. Pathologic examination of the cone reveals a focus of microinvasion at the squamocolumnar junction. What would you advise this patient regarding these findings?

○ (A) A course of radiation therapy is indicated.
○ (B) A hysterectomy should be performed.

○ (C) A bone scan for metastatic lesions should be done.

○ (D) A pelvic exenteration will be necessary.

○ (E) No further therapy is indicated at this time.

32. A 20-year-old female had fairly regular menstrual cycles for several years following menarche. For the past year, she has had oligomenorrhea and has developed hirsutism. She has gained about 10 kg in the past 4 months. Each ovary is about twice normal size as seen on pelvic ultrasound, while the uterus is normal in size. The cervix appears normal on inspection at the time of physical examination. Which of the following conditions is most likely to be present?

○ (A) Immature teratomas

○ (B) Polycystic ovaries

○ (C) Krukenberg tumors

○ (D) Tubo-ovarian abscesses

○ (E) Cystadenocarcinomas

33. A 28-year-old female presents with fever, pelvic pain, and a feeling of pelvic heaviness for the past week. Pelvic examination reveals a palpable left adnexal mass. Laparoscopy is then performed and the left fallopian tube is found to be indistinct and part of a circumscribed, 5-cm, red-tan mass involving the left adnexa. The microbiologic agent most likely responsible for these findings is

○ (A) Human papillomavirus

○ (B) *Mycobacterium tuberculosis*

○ (C) *Treponema pallidum*

○ (D) *Neisseria gonorrhoeae*

○ (E) *Candida albicans*

34. A cervical biopsy is performed after an abnormal Pap smear result is obtained on a 42-year-old female. Her previous Pap smear was 10 years ago. The biopsy shows that dysplastic cells occupy the full thickness of the epithelium above the basement membrane. A cervical conization is performed because

○ (A) She has a high risk for invasive carcinoma.

○ (B) HPV infection cannot be treated.

○ (C) She is perimenopausal.

○ (D) CIN I is present.

○ (E) She has invasive cancer.

35. A 20-year-old female has had a bloody, brownish vaginal discharge for the past day. She now presents with shortness of breath. A chest radiograph demonstrates numerous 2- to 5-cm nodules in both lungs. A red-brown 3 cm mass is seen on the lateral wall of the vagina, and a biopsy of this mass reveals malignant cells resembling syncytiotrophoblasts. Serum level of which the following proteins is likely to be elevated in this patient?

○ (A) Human chorionic gonadotropin

○ (B) Alpha-fetoprotein

○ (C) Estrogen

○ (D) Androgen

○ (E) Thyroxine

36. An adolescent female started menstruation a year ago. However, she has abnormal uterine bleeding, with menstrual periods that are 2 to 7 days long and 2 to 6 weeks apart. The amount of bleeding varies considerably, from just minimal spotting to a very heavy flow. The most probable cause for these findings is

○ (A) Endometrial polyp

○ (B) Anovulatory cycles

○ (C) Ectopic pregnancy

○ (D) Uterine leiomyomata

○ (E) Endometrial carcinoma

For each of the patient histories in questions 37 through 39, match the most closely related neoplasm:

(A) Adenocarcinoma

(B) Brenner tumor

(C) Carcinoma in situ

(D) Choriocarcinoma

(E) Clear cell carcinoma

(F) Cystadenocarcinoma, serous

(G) Dysgerminoma

(H) Granulosa cell tumor

(I) Immature teratoma

(J) Leiomyosarcoma

(K) Malignant mixed müllerian tumor

(L) Mature cystic teratoma

(M) Sarcoma botryoides

(N) Sertoli-Leydig cell tumor

(O) Squamous cell carcinoma

37. The mother of a 4-year-old girl notes that her daughter has blood-stained underwear. The girl is examined by a nurse practitioner who notes a soft, lobulated, reddish mass that almost protrudes from the introitus. She is referred to a gynecologist, who finds no other lesions by physical examination. A biopsy is taken of the mass. (   )

38. An 18-year-old girl has a feeling of pelvic discomfort for several months. On pelvic examination, there is a 10-cm right adnexal mass. This circumscribed mass is solid on an abdominal CT scan. On surgical removal, the mass is found to be solid and white, with small areas of necrosis. Microscopically it contains mostly primitive mesenchymal cells along with some cartilage, muscle, and foci of neuroepithelial differentiation. (   )

39. A 35-year-old woman is found to have bilateral ovarian masses that are mainly cystic on pelvic ultrasound. Surgery is performed. These masses are grossly unilocular cysts filled with clear fluid, and they have papillary projections extending into the central lumen. Microscopically, the papillae are covered by atypical cuboidal cells that invade underlying stroma. Psammoma bodies are present. (   )

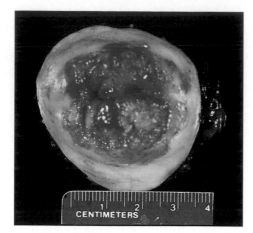

(C) Nests and sheets of epithelial cells with squamous differentiation in the subepithelial region

(D) Multiple irregular mucus-secreting glands in the subepithelial region

(E) Dense mononuclear infiltrate with a normally differentiating cervical epithelium

41. A 30-year-old female is healthy, with no significant findings on review of systems and on physical examination. A screening Pap smear shows cells consistent with CIN I. The causation of her CIN is most likely related to

(A) Intake of oral contraceptives

(B) Diethylstilbestrol exposure

(C) Vitamin B_{12} deficiency

(D) Treated squamous cell carcinoma

(E) Multiple sexual partners

40. On pelvic examination of a 45-year-old woman, there is a 3-cm lesion on the ectocervix, depicted in the figure. She had noticed a small amount of vaginal bleeding and a brownish, foul-smelling discharge for the past month. A histologic examination is most likely to show which of the following?

(A) Dysplastic changes affecting the lower one third of the cervical epithelium

(B) Dysplastic changes affecting the full thickness of the epithelium

42. The gross appearance (A) of the external genitalia of a 24-year-old female is shown below. The histologic appearance (B) of one of the lesions is also depicted. She has had this condition for several years, after she started taking vacations each year at a resort near Negril, Jamaica. Which of the following factors would you expect to contribute most to the development of her lesions?

(A) Lack of menstrual cycles

(B) Inheritance of a faulty tumor suppressor gene

(C) Poorly controlled diabetes mellitus

(D) Exposure to ultraviolet light

(E) Sexual intercourse

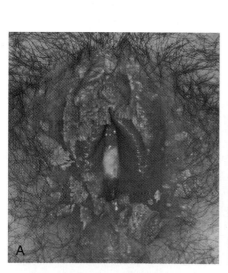

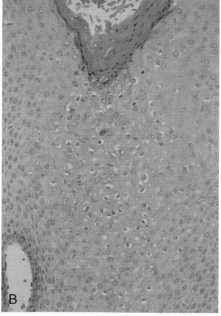

Courtesy of Dr. Alex Ferenczy, McGill University, Montreal, Quebec, Canada.

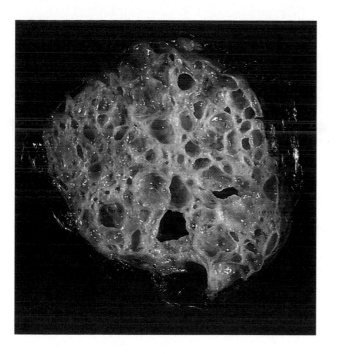

43. A 40-year-old female has noticed that her abdomen has progressively enlarged over the past 5 months, even although her diet has remained unchanged and she has been exercising more. Physical examination reveals no palpable masses, but a fluid wave is present. Paracentesis yields 500 mL of slightly cloudy fluid. Cytologic examination of this fluid reveals the presence of malignant cells. An abdominal ultrasound reveals a mass involving the right adnexal region. The uterus is normal in size. The gross appearance of the sectioned mass following surgical excision is shown here. Which of the following neoplasms is most likely?

O (A) Immature teratoma
O (B) Mucinous cystadenocarcinoma
O (C) Granulosa cell tumor
O (D) Choriocarcinoma
O (E) Dysgerminoma

ANSWERS

1. **(C)** She has an ectopic pregnancy. Identifiable conditions predisposing to ectopic pregnancy include chronic salpingitis (which may be caused by gonorrhea), intrauterine tumors, and endometriosis. In about one half of the cases there is no identifiable cause. Gestational trophoblastic disease, such as a complete or partial mole, developing outside of the uterus is rare. Syphilis is not likely to produce a tubal mass with acute symptoms (a gumma is a rare finding). *Candida* produces cervicitis and vaginitis and is rarely invasive or extensive in immunocompetent individuals.
BP6 620   PBD6 1079-1080

2. **(A)** The redness and presence of inflammatory cells in the cervical discharge, along with the biopsy findings, indicate that this woman has cervicitis. *C. trachomatis* is the most common cause for cervicitis in sexually active women. Gonorrhea, trichomoniasis, and candidiasis are also common. Herpetic infections are more likely to be seen in the perineal region.
BP6 603   PBD6 1038-1039

3. **(D)** When endometrial glands extend from the endometrium down into the myometrium, the condition is known as adenomyosis. The process may be just superficial, but on occasion, it can be extensive, in which case the uterus becomes enlarged from a reactive thickening of the myometrium up to two to four times in size. In endometriosis, endometrial glands and stroma are found outside the uterus in places such as peritoneum, ovaries, and ligaments. A leiomyoma is a myometrial tumor mass that, if large, produces a mass effect that is asymmetric. Endometrial hyperplasias do not increase the size of the uterus. Chronic endometritis does not extend to the myometrium and does not increase uterine size.
BP6 608   PBD6 1057

4. **(C)** This is endometrial hyperplasia, which results from excessive estrogenic stimulation. Such a lesion often occurs with failure of ovulation around the time of menopause. Estrogen-secreting ovarian tumors may also produce endometrial hyperplasia, but teratomas are not known for this phenomenon. Hyperplasias do not develop from endometritis. A secretory pattern of the endometrium is seen with pregnancy, not the proliferative pattern depicted here. The oral contraceptives in use have small doses of estrogenic compounds that do not lead to a hyperplasia.
BP6 610   PBD6 1059-1060

5. **(E)** This is a cystic tumor with a mass of hair in the lumen. This is the typical appearance of a mature cystic teratoma. Such a tumor is also known as a dermoid cyst because it is cystic and filled with hair and sebum derived from ectodermal structures. Dermoid cysts are benign tumors of germ cell origin, and they can contain various ectodermally, endodermally, and mesodermally derived tissues. A fibrothecoma is a solid, firm white stromal tumor. A choriocarcinoma is gestational in origin and is an aggressive neoplasm that usually has a hemorrhagic appearance. A dysgerminoma is the female equivalent of a male testicular seminoma and is a solid, lobulated, tan-white mass. A Brenner tumor is not common, and it is usually a solid, yellow mass.
BP6 617-619   PBD6 1073-1075

6. **(D)** These are well-circumscribed masses, suggesting the presence of multiple benign tumors. Leiomyomas are the most common benign tumors of the uterus. They are common; perhaps one third to one half of women have them. After menopause they generally do not continue to

enlarge. Metastases of this size and location are unlikely in a healthy-appearing person. The small implants of endometriosis rarely exceed 1 to 2 cm in diameter, and when a large mass is formed, it is cystic and filled with old blood (i.e., "chocolate cyst"). A leiomyosarcoma is a rare tumor and is usually a large, solitary mass. Endometrial glands and stroma that extend into the myometrium constitute adenomyosis, a process that tends to enlarge the uterus diffusely, without nodularity.
BP6 611　PBD6 1063-1064

7.　**(C)** This is cervical intraepithelial neoplasia (CIN) III because the full thickness of the cervical epithelium is involved with dysplasia. Such lesions arise more frequently in the setting of early intercourse, multiple sexual partners, and a male partner with multiple sexual partners. These factors are believed to increase the risk for HPV infection, particularly types 16 and 18. These HPVs are associated with dysplasias and carcinomas of the cervix. Diethylstilbestrol (DES) exposure in utero is strongly associated with clear cell adenocarcinomas of the vagina and cervix. Recurrent *Candida* infections are a nuisance, but they are not premalignant. Pregnancy does not play a role in development of cervical neoplasia. Most cervical dysplasias occur in premenopausal women. Estrogen therapy and use of oral contraceptives does not increase the risk for cervical dysplasia.
BP6 604-605　PBD6 1048-1051

8.　**(A)** She has an endometrial carcinoma. Estrogenic stimulation from anovulatory cycles, nulliparity, obesity, and exogenous estrogens (in higher amounts than found in birth control pills) gives rise to endometrial hyperplasia that can progress to endometrial carcinoma if the estrogenic stimulation continues. Atypical endometrial hyperplasias progress to endometrial cancer in about 25% of cases. Chronic endometritis does not give rise to cancer, nor does HPV infection (which is associated with squamous epithelial dysplasias and neoplasia). Adenomyosis is not a risk for endometrial carcinoma, and this condition increases the size of the uterus.
BP6 612　PBD6 1061-1062

9.　**(D)** She has toxemia of pregnancy. Her condition is best classified as pre-eclampsia because she has hypertension, proteinuria, and edema but no seizures. The placenta tends to be small because of reduced maternal blood flow with uteroplacental insufficiency. Infarctions and retroplacental hemorrhages can occur. Microscopically, the decidual arterioles may show acute atherosis and fibrinoid necrosis. A chronic villitis is characteristic of a congenital infection such as cytomegalovirus. A fetus is present with a partial mole but is malformed and rarely liveborn. Placental hydrops often accompanies fetal hydrops in conditions such as infections and fetal anemias. A fetus is not present with a choriocarcinoma.
BP6 622-623　PBD6 1082-1084

10.　**(E)** This is a hydatidiform mole, or complete mole, with enlarged grapelike villi that form the tumor mass in the endometrial cavity. These trophoblastic tumors secrete human chorionic gonadotropin. Molar pregnancies result from abnormal fertilization. In a complete mole, only paternal chromosomes are present. Alpha-fetoprotein is a marker for some germ cell tumors that contain yolk sac elements. Thyroxine could be produced by the rare struma ovarii, which is a teratoma composed predominantly of thyroid tissue. Estrogens can be elaborated by a variety of ovarian stromal tumors, including thecomas and granulosa cell tumors. Lactate dehydrogenase can be increased in many conditions such as liver and cardiac disease, but it is not known as a marker for genital tract lesions.
BP6 620-622　PBD6 1085-1086

11.　**(A)** The uterus shows two well-circumscribed, gray-white masses in the myometrium. Microscopically, the lesions show spindle-shaped cells in whorled bundles. The cells are uniform in size and shape, and mitotic figures are scarce. These features are characteristic of a benign neoplasm—a leiomyoma. Leiomyosarcomas are not so well demarcated, and their cut surface is not as homogeneous as that of leiomyomas. Microscopically, the spindle cells are much more pleomorphic, and there are numerous mitoses. Endometrial polyps are not uncommon in older women but generally are smaller than 3 cm and within the endometrial cavity. Adenomyosis is an extension of endometrial glands and stroma into the myometrium, generally resulting in symmetric uterine enlargement without mass effect. An invasive mole generally does not produce a large circumscribed mass, and molar pregnancy is not possible in postmenopausal women.
BP6 611　PBD6 1064-1065

12.　**(C)** Postmenopausal vaginal bleeding is a "red flag" for endometrial carcinoma. Such carcinomas often arise in the setting of endometrial hyperplasia. Increased estrogenic stimulation is thought to drive this process, and risk factors include obesity, diabetes mellitus, hypertension, and infertility. Adenomyosis is an extension of endometrial glands and stroma into the myometrium, generally resulting in symmetric uterine enlargement. Malignant mixed müllerian tumors are much less common than endometrial carcinomas but could produce the same findings. A leiomyosarcoma that is submucosal could produce vaginal bleeding, but the uterus should be enlarged, because leiomyosarcomas tend to be large masses. Squamous carcinomas of the endometrium are rare. Choriocarcinomas are gestational in origin.
BP6 612　PBD6 1061-1062

13.　**(A)** This is a partial hydatidiform mole, which results from triploidy. Unlike a complete mole, in which no fetus is present, a partial mole has a fetus because maternal chromosomes are present. Survival to term is rare. There may be some grapelike villi in a partial mole or none at all. The fetus is usually malformed. A 46,XX karyotype could be present in a complete mole or a normal male

fetus. The 23,Y karyotype is typical for a sperm. A fetus with Turner syndrome has a 45,X karyotype. Most fetuses with a complete loss of X chromosome undergo spontaneous abortion. Klinefelter syndrome has a 47,XXY karyotype, and the males are liveborn.
BP6 620–621   PBD6 1085–1086

14. **(C)** Some familial cases of ovarian carcinoma (usually serous cystadenocarcinoma) are associated with the homozygous loss of the *BRCA1* gene. This tumor suppressor gene also plays a role in the development of familial breast cancers. However, familial syndromes account for less than 5% of all ovarian cancers. Mutations of the *ras* and *myc* oncogenes occur in sporadic cancers. The *c-erb-B2* gene may be overexpressed in ovarian cancers. However, mutations of the gene do not give rise to familial tumors. The *Rb1* gene can be involved with familial forms of retinoblastoma and osteosarcoma.
BP6 614   PBD6 1067

15. **(B)** Embryonal rhabdomyosarcoma is an uncommon vaginal tumor found in children younger than 5 years of age. Because it forms polypoid, grapelike masses, it is sometimes called sarcoma botryoides. Histologically, it is a small, round, blue-cell tumor with skeletal muscle differentiation, attested to by the presence of muscle-specific proteins such as desmin. Neuroblastomas are also small blue-cell tumors, but they occur in the adrenals or extra-adrenal sympathetic chain. Condyloma acuminata are caused by HPV that is sexually transmitted and hence are rarely seen at this age. Vulvar intraepithelial neoplasm is a carcinoma in situ of the vulvar skin. It also occurs in older age groups. Invasive squamous cell carcinomas are rare at this age, and histologically, they show evidence of squamous epithelial differentiation.
BP6 602   PBD6 1046–1047

16. **(E)** The mass is probably producing estrogen that has led to an endometrial hyperplasia. Estrogen-producing tumors of the ovary are typically sex cord tumors such as a granulosa-theca cell tumor or a thecoma-fibroma, with the former more often being functional. Teratomas can have a variety of histologic elements but not estrogen-producing tissues. Endometriosis can give rise to an adnexal mass that enlarges over time. Endometrial glands are hormonally sensitive, but they do not produce hormones. A corpus luteum cyst is a relatively common finding, but such cysts are not likely to produce estrogens. Metastases to the ovary do occur but do not cause increased estrogen production.
BP6 610, 618   PBD6 1076–1077

17. **(A)** Gonorrheal infections can lead to salpingitis and pelvic inflammatory disease with scarring. This predisposes to ectopic pregnancy. Gonorrhea and other genital tract infections do not cause dysfunctional bleeding. Gonorrhea does not carry a risk for dysplasias or carcinomas the way that HPV infection does. Gonorrhea and other infections do not contribute to endometrial hyperplasia. The actual cause

for endometriosis is unknown, but infection does not appear to play a role in this process.
BP6 620   PBD6 1079–1080

18. **(B)** Dysplasias of the cervix should not be ignored, because there is a natural progression to more severe forms of dysplasias and to invasive carcinomas over time. Although not all cases progress, the physician should not take a chance that they will not. Dysplasias are strongly related to HPV infections. HPV DNA can be found in about 90% of cases. In about 10% to 15% of cases, there is no evidence for HPV, and other factors may play a role in the development of the dysplasia. A condyloma acuminatum is also an HPV-associated lesion, but it is usually caused by distinct, low-risk types of HPV. With such HPV infection, the Pap smear may show changes of CIN I. Endocervical polyps may produce some bleeding, but they typically show no dysplasia. Oral contraceptive use does not significantly affect the risk for dysplasia.
BP6 604–605   PBD6 1048–1051

19. **(B)** Leiomyomas (i.e., "fibroids") can be present in up to one third to one half of all women. They tend to enlarge during reproductive years and then stop growing or involute after menopause. Most of them are asymptomatic. They are a common incidental finding in a uterus removed for another reason. A solitary metastasis to the serosa would be unusual. A choriocarcinoma is unlikely in a postmenopausal woman. A chocolate cyst represents a focus of endometriosis in the ovary. It is typically a cystic lesion, with the center of the cyst being filled with chocolate-brown sludge. A malignant mixed müllerian tumor is typically a large, bulky mass.
BP6 611   PBD6 1063–1064

20. **(E)** Untreated pre-eclampsia and eclampsia carry a significant risk for development of DIC. Inadequate maternal blood flow to the placenta probably triggers an ischemic event that leads to release of thromboplastic substances. DIC is possible with infections, but the organisms that produce most cases of salpingitis (e.g., *C. trachomatis*, *N. gonorrhoeae*) are not the gram-negative bacteria best known for causing DIC. Complete moles are typically treated with curettage without complication. Ovarian tumors are not known for producing DIC. Endometriosis is a chronic condition not associated with DIC.
BP6 622–623   PBD6 1082–1084

21. **(B)** Most granulosa-theca cell tumors are hormonally active and secrete estrogens that can lead to endometrial hyperplasia or carcinoma. Most of these tumors are also benign. A condyloma acuminatum is related to HPV infection and is more likely to be seen in younger, sexually active persons. Chronic salpingitis is related in most cases to sexually transmitted infections, such as gonorrhea. A partial mole is an uncommon form of gestational trophoblastic disease seen only in women of reproductive age.
BP6 618   PBD6 1076–1077

22. **(B)** This woman has several risk factors for the development of cervical squamous cell carcinomas. These include multiple sexual partners, documented infection of the cervix with high-risk HPV-16, and prior diagnosis of a high-grade squamous intraepithelial neoplasm.
BP6 604-605   PBD6 1048-1049

23. **(E)** This woman has multiple risk factors for the development of endometrial cancer. These include obesity, diabetes, and nulliparity. All these are thought to contribute to the development of endometrial hyperplasias and carcinomas due to hyperestrinism.
BP6 612   PBD6 1061

24. **(D)** This woman has endometriosis. In this condition, functional endometrial glands are found outside the uterus. Common locations include ovaries, uterine ligaments, rectovaginal septum, and pelvic peritoneum. These glands respond to ovarian hormones, and hence there is cyclic abdominal pain coinciding with menstruation. Recurrent hemorrhages are followed by scarring and fibrous adhesions in the pelvis. This may cause distortion of the ovaries and fallopian tubes and lead to infertility.
BP6 608-609   PBD6 1057-1058

25. **(C)** HPV infection results in squamous epithelial changes marked by nuclear hyperchromatism and a clear perinuclear halo. These changes, called koilocytosis, can be seen in condylomas. Gonococci can cause acute cervicitis, characterized by an acute inflammatory infiltrate. *C. trachomatis* and *T. vaginalis* cause cervicitis, and there is a discharge containing inflammatory cells. Herpes simplex virus causes herpetic ulcers associated with the formation of inclusion-bearing, multinucleated syncytia.
BP6 604-605   PBD6 1049-1050

26. **(C)** The presence of pseudohyphae is indicative of a fungal infection. Candidal (monilial) vaginitis is common, because this organism is present in about 5% to 10% of adult women. The inflammation tends to be superficial, and there is typically no invasion of underlying tissues. *T. vaginalis* infections can produce a purulent vaginal discharge, but the organisms are protozoa, and they do not produce hyphae. *Ureaplasma* is a bacterial agent, as is *Chlamydia*, and both can produce cervicitis. *N. gonorrhoeae*, a gram-negative diplococcus, is the causative agent for gonorrhea.
BP6 602   PBD6 1038-1039

27. **(D)** The presence of dysplastic cells occupying one half of the thickness of the epithelium suggests the diagnosis of vulvar intraepithelial neoplasia (VIN). These lesions have been increasing in incidence, probably because of more HPV infections. Some of these lesions may go on to invasive cancers. Lichen sclerosus is a vulvar dystrophy characterized by thinning of the squamous epithelium and sclerosis of the dermis. A condyloma is usually a raised, nodular lesion. It is also caused by HPV, principally types 6 and 11. Squamous hyperplasia, another form of vulvar

dystrophy, can appear as an area of leukoplakia, just like VIN, but no dysplastic changes are present. Chronic inflammation does not produce dysplasia.
BP6 600   PBD6 1042-1044

28. **(A)** The microscopic appearance is that of a malignant tumor containing cells with a clear cytoplasm. Vaginal clear-cell carcinomas are associated with exposure of the mother to diethylstilbestrol during pregnancy. These tumors are generally first diagnosed in the late teenage years. Trichomonal infections do not give rise to neoplasia. Polycystic ovary disease can lead to hormonal imbalances from excess androgen production, but vaginal neoplasms do not arise in this setting. HPV infections are associated with squamous epithelial dysplasias and malignancies, not clear cell adenocarcinomas.
BP6 602   PBD6 1046

29. **(B)** These findings point to a diagnosis of endometriosis, which is the presence of endometrial glands and stroma outside of the uterus. The small implants of endometriosis undergo bleeding with menstrual cycles, resulting in local irritation and pain. The process is chronic and can be difficult to diagnose. Tubo-ovarian adhesions can be part of pelvic inflammatory disease in which the pain tends to be more constant. The finding of peritoneal nodules suggests metastases, which are usually not painful. An enlarged hemorrhagic ovary suggests ovarian torsion, which is an acute problem. A subserosal leiomyoma of this size is generally asymptomatic.
BP6 608-609   PBD6 1057-1058

30. **(A)** The epithelium shows typical features of infection with HPV. There is prominent perinuclear vacuolization (i.e., koilocytosis) and angulation of nuclei. These lesions, called condyloma acuminata, may occur anywhere on the anogenital surface, as single lesions or, more commonly, multiple lesions. They are not precancerous. Chlamydial infections may produce urethritis, cervicitis, and pelvic inflammatory disease. *T. pallidum* is the infectious agent of syphilis, characterized by the gross appearance of a "hard" chancre. *H. ducreyi* is the agent that produces the "soft" chancre of chancroid. Candidal infections produce a vaginitis or cervicitis with exudate and erythema.
BP6 599   PBD6 1042

31. **(E)** Microinvasive squamous cell carcinomas of the cervix are stage I lesions that have a survival rate approaching that for in situ lesions. Such minimal invasiveness does not warrant more aggressive therapies. The likelihood of metastasis or recurrence is minimal.
BP6 606-607   PBD6 1051-1053

32. **(B)** Polycystic ovarian disease is a disorder of unknown origin that is typically associated with oligomenorrhea, obesity, and hirsutism. It is believed to be caused by abnormal regulation of androgen synthesis. Teratomas are mass lesions that can be bilateral but are not usually sym-

metric. Krukenberg tumors represent metastatic disease involving the ovaries, usually from a gastrointestinal tract primary, and would be rare at age 20. Abscesses are usually unilateral and do not account for the hormonal changes. Cystadenocarcinoma can be bilateral. However, androgen production by ovarian tumors is very uncommon, except by the rare Sertoli-Leydig cell tumors.
BP6 614   PBD6 1066

33. **(D)** Gonorrhea is one of the most common causes for inflammation of the fallopian tube. When the incidence of gonorrhea decreases in a population, the proportion of cases of salpingitis caused by *Chlamydia* and *Mycoplasma* increases. The fallopian tube can become distended and adherent to the ovary and may even form a tubo-ovarian abscess. These are features of pelvic inflammatory disease. HPV infection is associated with genital tract squamous epithelial dysplasia and neoplasia. *M. tuberculosis* is an uncommon cause for salpingitis. *T. pallidum* infection causes syphilis, which does not produce florid inflammation with mass effect. *Candida* infections are typically limited to the vagina and cervix and are superficial, without invasion.
BP6 613   PBD6 1065

34. **(A)** She has cervical intraepithelial neoplasia (CIN) III, or carcinoma in situ, which may progress to invasive carcinoma in several years if not treated. HPV infection often drives this process, but the presence of HPV alone does not determine therapy. The HPV infection cannot be eradicated, but this is not the reason to treat dysplasias. A dysplasia requires treatment regardless of age. A CIN I lesion involves only part of the thickness of the cervical epithelium. Invasive cancers penetrate the basement membrane, and hence the cancer cells are seen below the basement membrane.
BP6 604-605   PBD6 1049-1051

35. **(A)** This patient has a choriocarcinoma, an aggressive malignant trophoblastic tumor. Metastases in the vaginal wall and lungs, along with a hemorrhagic appearance, are characteristic. The syncytiotrophoblastic cells produce human chorionic gonadotropin. The α-fetoprotein level is elevated in yolk sac tumors; estrogens are elevated in granulosa-theca cell tumors; androgens are elevated in Leydig cell tumors; and thyroxine can be elevated in specialized teratomas that contain thyroid tissue (e.g., struma ovarii).
BP6 622   PBD6 1087-1088

36. **(B)** Anovulatory cycles are a common cause for dysfunctional uterine bleeding in young women beginning menstruation or in women nearing menopause. There is prolonged estrogenic stimulation that is not followed by secretion of progesterone. Polyps are more common in older women. An ectopic pregnancy should present with acute findings and not have a prolonged course. Submucosal leiomyomas are a cause for bleeding that is not so variable, and such tumors are more likely to be seen in women who are older. An endometrial carcinoma is rare at this age.
BP6 609   PBD6 1056

37. **(M)** Sarcoma botryoides is a rare pediatric neoplasm seen in infancy to the age of 5. It is a form of embryonal rhabdomyosarcoma.
BP6 602   PBD6 1046-1047

38. **(I)** Immature teratomas are not cystic like mature teratomas. However, like all teratomas, tissues derived from multiple germ cell layers are present. The presence of neuroectodermal tissues is typical. The less differentiated the neuroepithelial elements and the more of them, the worse is the prognosis.
BP6 617   PBD6 1074-1075

39. **(F)** Serous cystadenocarcinomas are common ovarian tumors that are often bilateral. They account for more than one half of ovarian cancers. As the name indicates, they are cystic in appearance. Serous cystic tumors of the ovary may be benign, borderline, or malignant. Benign tumors have a smooth cyst wall with small or absent papillary projections. Borderline tumors have increasing amounts of papillary projections.
BP6 615-616   PBD6 1068-1070

40. **(C)** The illustrated lesion is large and ulcerative and is projecting into the vagina. It is most likely to be an invasive squamous cell carcinoma that has infiltrated into the subepithelial region. Dysplastic changes that are confined to the epithelium represent cervical intraepithelial neoplasms. Glandular invasive lesions indicate an adenocarcinoma. This cancer is much less common than squamous cell carcinoma of the cervix. Mononuclear infiltrates indicate chronic cervicitis.
BP6 606-607   PBD6 1051-1053

41. **(E)** CIN I represents minimal (mild) dysplasia and is potentially a reversible process. However, dysplasias are preneoplastic and may progress to carcinoma if not treated. The risk factors for cervical dysplasias and carcinoma include early age at first intercourse, multiple sexual partners, and a male partner with multiple previous sexual partners. These factors all increase the potential for infection with HPV. Use of oral contraceptives does not cause cervical dysplasia or carcinoma. Diethylstilbestrol exposure is a factor in the development of clear cell carcinomas of vagina and cervix. A B_{12} deficiency may manifest with some megaloblastic epithelial changes, not dysplasia. Treatment of carcinomas does not result in dysplasia.
BP6 604-605   PBD6 1049-1051

42. **(E)** These lesions represent condyloma acuminata, which are often multiple and can reach several centimeters in diameter. They are also known as genital warts or venereal warts and are the result of HPV infection acquired during sexual intercourse. The presence of HPV-infected cells is indicated by koilocytotic change. These cells have cytoplasmic vacuolation. Anovulatory cycles can lead to irregular menstrual periods but not vulvar skin changes. The best known association of a faulty tumor suppressor gene and a genital tract cancer is the BRCA-1 gene and ovarian carcinoma. Diabetics are more prone to infections,

typically bacterial or fungal, that do not produce nodular masses. There are portions of this data that are best left to the imagination of the reader to interpret.
BP6 599-600   PBD6 1042

43. **(B)** Mucinous tumors of the ovary are of epithelial origin and are less common than serous tumors. These tumors tend to be multiloculated. The appearance of ascites suggests metastases, which is most common with surface epithelial neoplasms of the ovary. Immature teratomas tend to be solid masses, as do granulosa cell tumors and dysgerminomas. Choriocarcinomas rarely reach this size because they metastasize early; they are typically hemorrhagic.
BP6 616-617   PBD6 1070-1071

The Breast

C H A P T E R
23

BP6 Chapter 19 - Female Genital System
and Breast
PBD6 Chapter 25 - The Breast

1. A 36-year-old female notices a bloody nipple discharge from her right breast. Which of the following breast lesions is most likely to account for this finding?

○ (A) Fibroadenoma
○ (B) Phyllodes tumor
○ (C) Acute mastitis
○ (D) Intraductal papilloma
○ (E) Sclerosing adenosis

2. In the third trimester of pregnancy, a 28-year-old woman discovers a lump in her right breast. Her physician palpates a 2-cm, discrete, freely movable mass beneath the nipple. After delivery of a term infant, the mass appears to decrease slightly in size. The infant breast-feeds without difficulty. This breast lesion is most likely to be a (an)

○ (A) Intraductal papilloma
○ (B) Phyllodes tumor
○ (C) Lobular carcinoma in situ
○ (D) Fibroadenoma
○ (E) Medullary carcinoma

3. A 30-year-old female suffered a traumatic blow to the right breast. Initially, there was a 3-cm contusion that resolved in a few weeks, but then she felt a firm lump below the place where the bruise was located. Which of the following lesions is the lump most likely to be?

○ (A) Fibroadenoma
○ (B) Sclerosing adenosis

○ (C) Fat necrosis
○ (D) Intraductal carcinoma
○ (E) Mammary duct ectasia

4. Over the past year, a 55-year-old male has developed bilateral breast enlargement. This enlargement is symmetric and is not painful. He is not obese. Which of the following underlying conditions best accounts for these findings?

○ (A) Micronodular cirrhosis
○ (B) Chronic glomerulonephritis
○ (C) Choriocarcinoma of testis
○ (D) ACTH-secreting pituitary adenoma
○ (E) Rheumatoid arthritis

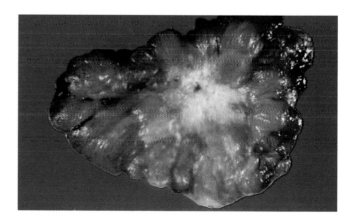

5. The gross appearance of the excisional biopsy from a 44-year-old female is shown here. Which of the following physical examination findings would you most expect to accompany the lesion?

○ (A) Axillary lymphadenopathy
○ (B) Bloody nipple discharge
○ (C) Painful breast enlargement
○ (D) Mass in the opposite breast
○ (E) Cushingoid face

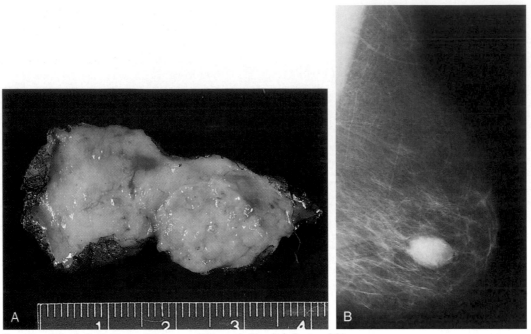

Courtesy of Dr. Jack G. Meyer, Brigham and Women's Hospital, Boston, MA.

6. A 25-year-old woman palpates a lump in her right breast. Her physician determines that there is a firm, circumscribed, 2-cm, lower outer quadrant mass. Based on the gross appearance (A) and the mammogram (B) shown here, the most likely diagnosis is

○ (A) Phyllodes tumor
○ (B) Fibrocystic changes
○ (C) Fibroadenoma
○ (D) Fat necrosis
○ (E) Infiltrating ductal carcinoma

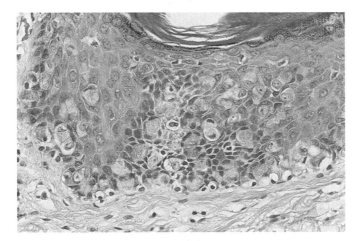

7. A skin biopsy of a 1-cm-diameter area of eczema over the left breast is performed on a 47-year-old female. The microscopic appearance of the biopsy shown here is most characteristic for which of the following breast lesions?

○ (A) Apocrine metaplasia
○ (B) Paget disease of breast
○ (C) Inflammatory carcinoma

○ (D) Lobular carcinoma in situ
○ (E) Fat necrosis

8. Several weeks after a normal term delivery, a 24-year-old female who is nursing her baby is bothered by some fissures in the skin around the left nipple. Over the next few days, the region around this nipple becomes erythematous and tender. A small abscess drains purulent exudate through a fissure. Which of the following organisms is most likely to be cultured from the exudate?

○ (A) *Listeria monocytogenes*
○ (B) *Streptococcus viridans*
○ (C) *Candida albicans*
○ (D) *Staphylococcus aureus*
○ (E) *Lactobacillus acidophilus*

9. Biopsy of a breast "lump" in a 27-year-old woman shows microscopic evidence of increased numbers of ducts. These are compressed because of proliferation of fibrous connective tissue. In some areas, there are dilated ducts with apocrine metaplasia. These findings are most typical for

○ (A) Traumatic fat necrosis
○ (B) Fibrocystic changes
○ (C) Mammary duct ectasia
○ (D) Fibroadenoma
○ (E) Infiltrating ductal carcinoma

10. A 44-year-old female notices some lumps in her right breast. Mammography reveals several 0.5- to 1-cm foci of irregular density in both breasts. A fine-needle aspirate of one lesion in the left breast shows malignant cells to be present, and a similar result is obtained for a right breast lesion. Which of the following breast carcinomas is most likely?

○ (A) Infiltrating ductal carcinoma
○ (B) Malignant phyllodes tumor

○ (C) Colloid carcinoma
○ (D) Medullary carcinoma
○ (E) Infiltrating lobular carcinoma

11.   A 56-year-old female has a mammogram that shows a small, irregular, 0.5-cm area of increased density along with scattered microcalcifications in the upper outer quadrant of the left breast. An excisional biopsy of the lesion demonstrates histologic findings of atypical lobular hyperplasia. Based on these findings, what is your best advice to the patient?

○ (A) She has the BRCA-1 genetic mutation.
○ (B) Her postmenopausal estrogen replacement therapy should be stopped.
○ (C) Her risk for breast carcinoma is increased.
○ (D) She should undergo bilateral simple mastectomies.
○ (E) She should stop smoking.

12.   For evaluation of the risk for breast cancer in women, which of the following factors is *least* important?

○ (A) Age at menarche
○ (B) Family history of breast cancer
○ (C) Age at menopause
○ (D) Age at first pregnancy
○ (E) Cigarette smoking

13.   A 35-year-old woman with normal menstrual cycles, whose last child was born 5 years ago, feels a poorly defined "lump" in her right breast. The lump is not painful, and it does not feel hard. If a right breast biopsy were to be performed, the most probable finding would be

○ (A) Fibrocystic changes
○ (B) Lobular carcinoma
○ (C) Acute mastitis
○ (D) Fibroadenoma
○ (E) No pathologic diagnosis

14.   A 51-year-old female develops a 7-cm area of tender, firm, erythematous skin with swelling of the right breast, accompanied by nipple retraction and right axillary lymphadenopathy. A biopsy of this right breast is most likely to show

○ (A) Atypical epithelial hyperplasia
○ (B) Phyllodes tumor
○ (C) Fat necrosis
○ (D) Sclerosing adenosis
○ (E) Infiltrating ductal carcinoma

15.   Which of the following risk factors plays the most important role in the development of male breast carcinoma?

○ (A) Obesity
○ (B) Age older than 70 years
○ (C) Long-term digoxin therapy
○ (D) Klinefelter syndrome
○ (E) Chronic alcoholism

16.   A mammogram performed on a 47-year-old female shows an irregular area of density about 1.5 cm in diameter in the upper outer quadrant of the right breast. Some scattered microcalcifications are present in this density. A biopsy from the area of the mammographic density shows ducts with atypical epithelial hyperplasia. What should you tell the patient?

○ (A) Your risk for breast cancer is significantly increased.
○ (B) A radical mastectomy should be performed.
○ (C) A biopsy of the opposite breast should be performed.
○ (D) Antibiotic therapy is indicated to treat this lesion.
○ (E) You have inherited the BRCA-1 oncogene.

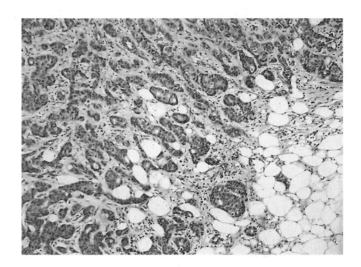

17.   A 25-year-old Jewish female presents with a lump in her right breast. The microscopic picture of a biopsy from this lesion is depicted in the figure. Family history reveals that her mother, maternal aunt, and maternal grandmother have had similar lesions. As the word of her illness spreads through the family, her younger sister, who is 18 years old, requests that her physician determine if she is genetically susceptible to developing a similar disease. Her physician is most likely to order an analysis of which of the following genes?

○ (A) c-*erb*-B2
○ (B) c-*myc*
○ (C) BRCA-1
○ (D) *Rb1*
○ (E) Estrogen receptor gene

18.   A biopsy of a breast carcinoma is analyzed to determine the presence and amount of estrogen receptor (ER) and progesterone receptor (PR) in the carcinoma cells. Establishing the ER-PR status is most useful for predicting

○ (A) Response to chemotherapy
○ (B) Immunogenicity of the tumor
○ (C) Risk for familial breast cancer
○ (D) Tumor stage
○ (E) Presence of metastases

19.   A mammography performed on a 50-year-old African-American female shows an irregular, 1-cm density in the right breast. A fine-needle aspirate of the lesion shows malignant cells. An excision of the mass is performed, along with axillary lymph node sampling. The microscopic

features of this neoplasm are consistent with intraductal carcinoma, and there are no lymph node metastases. Which of the following statements provides the most appropriate advice to the patient?

○ (A) You will probably not survive 5 years.
○ (B) Another cancer is probably present in the opposite breast.
○ (C) Distant metastases are unlikely to be found.
○ (D) Your family members should be screened for BRCA-1 and BRCA-2 mutations.
○ (E) Flow cytometric analysis of the neoplasm can determine whether chemotherapy is warranted.

20. Which of the following is the single most important prognostic factor in carcinoma of the female breast?

○ (A) Age
○ (B) Histologic subtype
○ (C) DNA content
○ (D) Axillary lymph node metastases
○ (E) Expression of stromal proteases in tumor cells

21. A 29-year-old woman and her 32-year-old sister have had bilateral mastectomies for infiltrating ductal carcinoma of the breast. Which of the following risk factors is most important in explaining the origin of these breast cancers?

○ (A) Oral contraceptive use
○ (B) Inheritance of a mutant p53 allele
○ (C) Obesity
○ (D) Multiparity
○ (E) Smoking

For each of the patient histories in questions 22 and 23, select the most closely associated breast neoplasm:

(A) Colloid carcinoma
(B) Fibroadenoma
(C) Infiltrating ductal carcinoma
(D) Infiltrating lobular carcinoma
(E) Intraductal carcinoma
(F) Intraductal papilloma
(G) Lobular carcinoma in situ
(H) Medullary carcinoma
(I) Paget disease of breast
(J) Papillary carcinoma
(K) Papilloma
(L) Phyllodes tumor

22. A firm area in the right breast of a 63-year-old female has a cordlike feel on physical examination. Mammography reveals a right breast density that contains microcalcifications. An excisional breast biopsy is performed. Pressure on the biopsy specimen causes soft, white material to be extruded from small ducts. Microscopically, the ducts contain large, atypical cells that form a cribriform pattern. (   )

23. A 4-cm mass is found in a 39-year-old female, and she undergoes simple mastectomy with axillary lymph node sampling. Grossly, sectioning the mass reveals a soft, tan, fleshy surface. Histologically, the mass is composed of large cells with vesicular nuclei and prominent nucleoli. There is a marked lymphocytic infiltrate within the tumor,

and the tumor has a discrete, noninfiltrative border. No axillary node metastases are seen. The tumor cells are ER and PR negative. (   )

ANSWERS

1. **(D)** Intraductal papillomas are usually solitary and less than 1 cm, but they are located within large lactiferous sinuses or ducts, and they have a tendency to bleed. Fibroadenomas contain ducts with stroma and are not highly vascular; these lesions are not located within ducts. Phyllodes tumors also arise from intralobular stroma and can be malignant. They do not invade ducts to cause bleeding. Abscesses complicating mastitis organize with a fibrous wall. Sclerosing adenosis, a lesion occurring with fibrocystic changes, has abundant collagen, not vascularity.
BP6 629   PBD6 1104–1105

2. **(D)** Fibroadenomas are common, and they may enlarge in pregnancy or late in each menstrual cycle. Most intraductal papillomas are smaller than 1 cm, and they are not influenced by hormonal changes. Phyllodes tumors are uncommon, and they tend to be larger than 4 cm. Lobular carcinoma in situ (LCIS) is typically an ill-defined lesion without a mass effect. Medullary carcinomas tend to be large, and they comprise only about 1% of all breast carcinomas.
BP6 628   PBD6 1102–1103

3. **(C)** Fat necrosis typically occurs with trauma to the breast. The damaged, necrotic fat is phagocytosed by macrophages, which become lipid laden. The lesion resolves in weeks to months into a collagenous scar. A fibroadenoma is a neoplasm, and tumors are not induced by trauma. Sclerosing adenosis is a feature of fibrocystic changes, a common cause for nontraumatic breast lumps. An intraductal carcinoma may not even be palpable. Mammary duct ectasia from inspissated secretions can induce chronic inflammation and fibrosis that can mimic a carcinoma.
BP6 628   PBD6 1097–1098

4. **(A)** Most often a consequence of chronic alcoholism, micronodular cirrhosis impairs hepatic estrogen metabolism, which can lead to gynecomastia. Chronic renal failure is not likely to have this consequence. Choriocarcinomas of testis produce hCG, not estrogens. ACTH-secreting pituitary adenomas cause truncal obesity because of Cushing syndrome. Rheumatoid nodules can appear in a variety of locations with rheumatoid arthritis, but they occur uncommonly in breast and are unlikely to be bilateral.
BP6 635   PBD6 1117

5. **(A)** This irregular, infiltrative mass is an infiltrating ductal carcinoma, the most common form of breast cancer. Breast carcinomas are most likely to metastasize to regional lymph nodes. A bloody nipple discharge most often results from an intraductal papilloma. Pain with breast enlargement suggests inflammation. Lobular carcinomas are

more often bilateral, but are less common overall than infiltrating ductal carcinoma. Lymph node metastases can be present in all forms of breast cancer. Breast cancers are uncommonly associated with ectopic corticotropin secretion or Cushing syndrome.
BP6 631–633   PBD6 1110

6. **(C)** Such a discrete mass at this age is most likely a fibroadenoma. Phyllodes tumors are typically much larger and are far less common. Fibrocystic changes are generally more irregular lesions, not discrete masses. Fat necrosis and infiltrating cancers are masses with irregular outlines.
BP6 628   PBD6 1102–1103

7. **(B)** The large cells with clear, mucinous cytoplasm that are infiltrating into the skin are "Paget cells." These cells are malignant and are extending to the skin from an underlying breast carcinoma. Apocrine metaplasia affects the cells lining the cystically dilated ducts in fibrocystic change. "Inflammatory carcinoma" does not refer to a specific histologic type of breast cancer, but, rather, to the involvement of dermal lymphatics by infiltrating carcinoma. In lobular carcinoma in situ (LCIS), terminal ducts or acini are filled with neoplastic cells. The overlying skin is unaffected. The macrophages in fat necrosis do not infiltrate the skin and do not have the atypical nuclei seen here.
BP6 632   PBD6 1108–1109

8. **(D)** Staphylococcal acute mastitis typically produces localized abscesses, while streptococcal infections tend to spread throughout the breast. Listeriosis can be spread by contaminated food (including milk) products, not from human milk. *Candida* may cause some local skin irritation but is not likely to become invasive in nonimmunosuppressed individuals. *L. acidophilus* is the organism used to produce fermented nonhuman milk.
BP6 627   PBD6 1096

9. **(B)** Fibrocystic changes account for the largest category of breast "lumps." They are characterized by ductal proliferation, ductal dilation (sometimes with apocrine metaplasia), and fibrosis. Fat necrosis may produce a localized, firm lesion that mimics carcinoma, but histologically macrophages and neutrophils are seen surrounding necrotic adipocytes, and healing leaves a fibrous scar. Inspissated duct secretions may produce duct ectasia with a surrounding lymphoplasmacytic infiltrate. A fibroadenoma is a discrete mass formed by a proliferation of fibrous stroma with compressed ductules. Carcinomas have proliferations of atypical neoplastic cells that fill ducts and can invade stroma.
BP6 626   PBD6 1098–1100

10. **(E)** Of all the primary malignancies of the breast, lobular carcinoma is most likely to be bilateral. Invasive lesions may have been preceded for several years by LCIS. Lobular carcinoma may be mixed with ductal carcinoma, and it may be difficult to distinguish them histologically.
BP6 633   PBD6 1110–1111

11. **(C)** Atypical lobular hyperplasia increases the risk for future breast cancer fivefold. The BRCA-1 mutation ac-

counts for perhaps 10% to 20% of familial breast carcinomas and only a few percent of all breast cancers. Mastectomies are probably not warranted at this time, but close follow-up is needed. Smoking and exogenous estrogen therapy are not well-established risk factors for breast cancer.
BP6 629–630   PBD6 1105–1106

12. **(E)** Cigarette smoking, diet, drug use, and obesity are not well-established factors that influence the risk for breast cancer. All others listed are known risk factors.
BP6 629   PBD6 1105–1106

13. **(A)** Statistically, the largest category of breast lumps (40% of all lumps) results from fibrocystic changes. These lesions are probably related to cyclic breast changes over time with menstrual cycles. About 30% of the time, no specific pathologic diagnosis can be made for the lump. Carcinomas often produce palpable masses, and these represent about 10% of lumps. Fibroadenomas constitute 7% of lumps but are usually discrete and firm masses. Acute mastitis does not usually manifest as a lump, and it is most often a complication during lactation.
BP6 624   PBD6 1096

14. **(E)** The gross appearance of the skin is consistent with invasion of dermal lymphatics by carcinoma—the so-called inflammatory carcinoma. Nipple retraction and axillary lymphadenopathy also favor an invasive ductal carcinoma. Atypical ductal hyperplasia may increase the risk for carcinoma but does not produce skin changes. A phyllodes tumor can be large and sometimes tender, but the overlying skin is typically not affected, and spread to lymph nodes is uncommon. The feel of fat necrosis can mimic carcinoma, but the skin is not involved. Sclerosing adenosis is a feature of benign fibrocystic changes and has no skin involvement.
BP6 633   PBD6 1114

15. **(B)** Male breast cancers are rare, and they occur primarily among the elderly. Unlike female breast cancers, a family history does not have major significance. Causes of gynecomastia, including drug therapy with digitalis compounds, Klinefelter syndrome, obesity, and hyperestrinism from chronic alcoholism, are not major risks for male breast carcinoma.
BP6 635   PBD6 1118

16. **(A)** Fibrocystic changes without any epithelial hyperplasia do not suggest an increased risk for breast cancer. Moderate to florid hyperplasia increases the risk up to twofold, and atypical changes push the risk to fivefold. This risk is not great enough to suggest radical or simple mastectomy at this time. The left breast should be biopsied only if it has a lesion. These changes are not the result of infection. The BRCA-1 gene accounts for a small percentage of breast cancers, particularly those in families in which cancer onset occurs at a young age.
BP6 626–627   PBD6 1099–1100

17. **(C)** The biopsy shows an invasive breast cancer. Given the young age of the patient and the strong family

history of breast cancer, it is reasonable to assume that she has inherited an altered gene that predisposes to breast cancer. There are two known breast cancer susceptibility genes: BRCA-1 and BRCA-2. Both are cancer suppressor genes. Specific mutations of BRCA-1 are common in some ethnic groups, such as Ashkenazi Jews. c-*erb-B2* is a growth factor receptor gene that is amplified in certain breast cancers and is a marker of poor prognosis, not susceptibility. Inheritance of *Rb1* mutations predisposes to retinoblastoma and osteosarcomas, not breast carcinomas. ERs are expressed in 50% to 75% of breast cancers. Their presence bodes well for therapy with receptor antagonists. There is no known relation between estrogen receptor gene structure and susceptibility to breast cancer.
BP6 630-631   PBD6 1106-1107, 1110

18. **(A)** The ER-PR status helps to determine whether chemotherapy with antiestrogen compounds such as tamoxifen will be effective. However, the correlation is not perfect. The ER and PR do not affect immunogenicity and are not targets for immunotherapy. In contrast, immunotherapy targeted to the overexpressed c-*erb-B2* gene is being used. The prognosis may be predicted from a number of factors, including histologic type, histologic grade, degree of aneuploidy, and tumor stage.
BP6 634   PBD6 1115

19. **(C)** This in situ carcinoma is highly unlikely to metastasize, and the 5-year survival rate is very high. Of various histologic types of breast cancer, lobular carcinomas are the most likely to be present in the opposite breast. Patients with BRCA-1 or BRCA-2 mutations can have familial breast carcinomas. In these patients, there is usually a strong family history, and the age of onset may be early. The occurrence of a sporadic breast cancer in a racial group that is not at high risk for familial cancer does not warrant mutational analysis of BRCA-1 and BRCA-2.

Flow cytometry is useful to suggest prognosis, not treatment.
BP6 633-635   PBD6 1113-1115

20. **(D)** Many factors affect the course of breast cancer. However, the involvement of axillary lymph nodes is the most important prognostic factor. With no spread to axillary nodes, the 10-year disease survival rate is close to 80%. It falls to between 35% and 40% with one to three positive nodes and to 15% with more than 10 positive nodes.
BP6 634   PBD6 1115

21. **(B)** Bilateral breast cancer in very young women in the same family suggests a germ-line mutation in a tumor suppressor gene. The affected genes may be BRCA-1, BRCA-2, or p53. The BRCA-1 and BRCA-2 genes account for most hereditary breast cancers. Establishment of other risk factors is not as secure. Multiparity actually reduces breast cancer risk.
BP6 630   PBD6 1105

22. **(E)** Intraductal carcinomas may not produce a palpable mass. The necrosis of the neoplastic cells in the ducts leads to calcification, and the necrotic cells can be extruded from the ducts, giving rise to the term comedocarcinoma. Such intraductal carcinomas represent about a fourth of all breast cancers. If not excised, such lesions become invasive.
BP6 631   PBD6 1107-1108

23. **(H)** Medullary carcinomas account for about 1% to 5% of all breast carcinomas. They tend to occur at a younger age than most other breast cancers. Despite poor prognostic indicators, such as absence of ERs or PRs, they have better prognosis than most other breast cancers. Perhaps the infiltrating lymphocytes are helpful.
BP6 633   PBD6 1111

The Endocrine System

BP6 Chapter 20 - The Endocrine System
PBD6 Chapter 26 - The Endocrine System

1. A 2-year-old child has had failure to thrive. The child is short, with coarse facial features, a protruding tongue, and an umbilical hernia. Profound mental retardation is apparent as the child matures. These findings are best explained by a lack of

○ (A) Cortisol
○ (B) Norepinephrine
○ (C) Somatostatin
○ (D) Thyroxine (T_4)
○ (E) Insulin

2. A 5-year-boy develops secondary sex characteristics, including pubic hair development and enlargement of the penis. Which of the following morphologic features is most likely to be seen in his adrenal glands?

○ (A) Bilateral adrenal cortical hyperplasia
○ (B) Bilateral adrenal cortical atrophy
○ (C) A nodule in the adrenal medulla
○ (D) Normal size and architecture
○ (E) A nodule in the adrenal cortex composed of zona glomerulosa cells

3. Which of the following tests should be done *first* when assessing the functional status of the thyroid gland?

○ (A) A total T_4 level
○ (B) Total triiodothyronine (T_3) level
○ (C) Thyroid-stimulating hormone (TSH) level
○ (D) Fine-needle aspiration
○ (E) Radioiodine scan

4. Which of the following laboratory tests should be performed on a serum specimen in the immediate postoperative period after a subtotal thyroidectomy for a follicular neoplasm?

○ (A) Calcitonin
○ (B) Thyroid stimulating hormone (TSH)

○ (C) Parathyroid hormone (PTH)
○ (D) Anti-thyroglobulin antibody
○ (E) Calcium

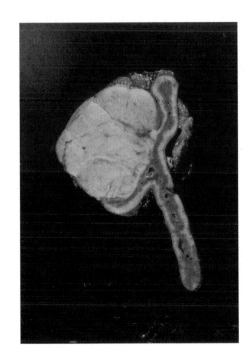

5. A 28-year-old healthy male presented with headaches of recent onset. Physical examination revealed blood pressure of 170/110 mm Hg on several separate occasions, but the remainder of the physical examination findings were normal. An abdominal computed tomography (CT) scan revealed an enlarged right adrenal gland that was surgically removed and is depicted here. Laboratory investigations before surgery would have most likely revealed which of the following?

○ (A) Hyponatremia
○ (B) Hyperglycemia
○ (C) Low serum renin level
○ (D) Hyperkalemia
○ (E) Low serum corticotropin level

For each of the patient descriptions in questions 6 and 7, select the most likely accompanying morphologic changes observed in the thyroid gland:

(A) Diffuse enlargement of the thyroid with destruction of follicles, lymphoid aggregates, and Hürthle cell metaplasia

(B) Diffuse enlargement of the thyroid with papillary projections in thyroid follicles and lymphoid aggregates in the stroma

(C) Irregular, nodular enlargement of the thyroid with areas of hemorrhage, cystic changes, and a nodule with hyperplastic follicles

(D) Single, circumscribed nodule in the thyroid that contains well-differentiated follicles and appears "hot" on a scintiscan

(E) Single, circumscribed nodule in the thyroid that reveals papillae, follicles, and psammoma bodies and epithelial cells that show hypochromatic "empty" nuclei, with nuclear folds and grooves

(F) Multiple nodules in both lobes of thyroid that show nests of cells separated by hyaline stroma that is birefringent under polarized light after staining with Congo red

(G) Isolated circumscribed nodule in the thyroid that reveals well-differentiated follicles, with invasion of the capsule and blood vessels, but no psammoma bodies and with nuclei that are hyperchromatic

6. A 60-year-old female felt a "lump" on the right side of her neck for several months, and thyroidectomy was performed. Six months later, she presents with a pathologic fracture of the right femur. A radioiodine scan reveals uptake localized to the region of the fracture. (   )

7. A 40-year-old male presents with loss of weight, increased appetite, and double vision. Physical examination reveals tachycardia, a fine tremor, and bilateral proptosis with corneal ulceration. His TSH level is only 0.1 μU/mL. A radioiodine scan demonstrates increased diffuse uptake throughout the thyroid. (   )

8. A 40-year-old male presents with headache, weakness, and weight gain. Physical examination reveals puffiness of the face and a blood pressure of 160/75 mm Hg while lying down. Initial laboratory tests reveal a fasting plasma glucose level of 200 mg/dL, serum sodium level of 150 mmol/L, and serum potassium level of 3.1 mmol/L. His plasma cortisol concentration is 38 μg/dL at 8:00 AM and 37 μg/dL at 6:00 PM. Administration of low and high doses of dexamethasone fail to suppress the plasma cortisol level and excretion of urinary 17-hydroxycorticosteroids. His plasma corticotropin level is 0.8 pg/mL. In this patient, which of the following lesions is most likely?

(A) An adenoma of the right adrenal cortex with atrophy of the contralateral adrenal cortex

(B) Small cell carcinoma of the lung with bilateral hyperplasia of the adrenal cortex

(C) A corticotroph adenoma of the anterior pituitary with bilateral hyperplasia of the adrenal cortex

(D) An adenoma of the right adrenal cortex without atrophy of contralateral adrenal cortex

(E) A corticotroph adenoma of the anterior pituitary, medullary carcinoma of thyroid, and bilateral nodular hyperplasia of the adrenal cortex

9. A 69-year-old male has become progressively obtunded over the past week. On admission to the hospital, he is found to have papilledema on physical examination. There is no peripheral edema. A head CT scan reveals no mass lesions, but the ventricles are narrowed. Laboratory findings include a serum sodium level of 115 mmol/L, potassium level of 4.2 mmol/L, chloride level of 85 mmol/L, and bicarbonate level of 23 mmol/L. His serum glucose concentration is 80 mg/dL, urea nitrogen level is 19 mg/dL, and creatinine level is 1.7 mg/dL. Which of the following neoplasms is he most likely to have?

(A) Pituitary adenoma
(B) Adrenal cortical carcinoma
(C) Renal cell carcinoma
(D) Pheochromocytoma
(E) Pulmonary small cell carcinoma

10. A 40-year-old male presents with weakness and easy fatigability. A screening blood chemistry panel reveals that the serum calcium concentration is 11.5 mg/dL. When rechecked, the serum calcium level is the same, the serum inorganic phosphorus level is 2.4 mg/dL, and the serum parathyroid hormone level is *near the top* of the reference range at 58 pg/mL. A radionuclide bone scan fails to reveal any areas of increased uptake, suggesting an absence of bony metastases. With additional investigation, his physicians feel confident that he does not have a malignant neoplasm. The most likely cause for this clinical picture is

(A) Chronic renal failure
(B) Parathyroid adenoma
(C) Parathyroid carcinoma
(D) Parathyroid hyperplasia
(E) Hypervitaminosis D

11. A 23-year-old female died suddenly and unexpectedly after complaining only of a mild sore throat the day before. At autopsy, her adrenal glands are enlarged and have extensive bilateral cortical hemorrhage. Infection with which of the following organisms best accounts for these findings?

(A) *Mycobacterium tuberculosis*
(B) *Streptococcus pneumoniae*
(C) *Neisseria meningitidis*
(D) *Histoplasma capsulatum*
(E) Cytomegalovirus

12. A 45-year-old female has a feeling of fullness in her neck but no other complaints. Physical examination confirms diffuse enlargement of the thyroid gland without any apparent masses. This enlargement has been gradual and painless for more than a year. Tests for thyroid function reveal a normal free thyroxine (free T_4) and a slightly increased level of TSH. The most likely cause for these findings is

○ (A) Toxic multinodular goiter
○ (B) Papillary carcinoma
○ (C) Subacute granulomatous thyroiditis
○ (D) Hashimoto thyroiditis
○ (E) Diffuse nontoxic goiter

13. A 37-year-old woman complains that she has had difficulty swallowing for about a week, accompanied by a feeling of fullness in the anterior neck. She has a slight fever. Palpation of the thyroid elicits pain. Her serum free T_4 level is increased. When seen by an endocrinologist 2 months later, after waiting for an appointment, she no longer has these complaints, and the free T_4 level is normal. The condition that best explains these findings is

○ (A) Medullary carcinoma
○ (B) Subacute thyroiditis
○ (C) Toxic multinodular goiter
○ (D) Toxic follicular adenoma
○ (E) Hashimoto thyroiditis

14. A 40-year-old female has a multicentric thyroid neoplasm that is composed of polygonal to spindle-shaped cells forming nests and trabeculae. There is a prominent, pink hyaline stroma that stains positively with Congo red. Electron microscopy reveals variable numbers of intracytoplasmic, membrane-bound, electron-dense granules. Which of the following immunohistochemical stains is most likely to be useful in corroborating the diagnosis of this neoplasm?

○ (A) Calcitonin
○ (B) Cathepsin D
○ (C) Parathormone
○ (D) Vimentin
○ (E) Cytokeratin

15. A 42-year-old male was found to have a blood pressure of 165/105 mm Hg on several occasions in the past 5 months. He has gained weight, predominantly in a truncal distribution. He exhibits proximal muscle weakness. Laboratory findings include a fasting serum glucose concentration of 155 mg/dL, an 8 AM serum cortisol level that is elevated at 54 μg/dL, and an elevated serum concentration of corticotropin. Which of the following tests is most likely to be helpful in establishing the diagnosis?

○ (A) Magnetic resonance imaging (MRI) of the brain
○ (B) Abdominal CT scan of the adrenals
○ (C) Serum assay for glycosylated hemoglobin
○ (D) Biopsy of the gastrocnemius
○ (E) Assay for urinary catecholamine metabolites

16. A 27-year-old female experienced an acute pancreatitis, and laboratory testing pointed to hypercalcemia as the cause. She also had an increased serum parathyroid hormone level. She was taken to surgery, and four enlarged parathyroid glands were found. They were excised, with reimplantation of one half of one gland. Her serum calcium concentration returned to normal. Three years later, she had an episode of upper gastrointestinal hemorrhage, and endoscopy with biopsy revealed multiple benign gastric ulcerations. Abdominal MRI reveal multiple, 1- to 2-cm mass lesions in the pancreas, and multiple gastrinomas were found at surgery. Two years after this operation, she presents with galactorrhea. Which of the following lesions is she most likely to have now?

○ (A) Medullary carcinoma of thyroid
○ (B) Adrenal pheochromocytoma
○ (C) Small cell anaplastic carcinoma of lung
○ (D) Endometrial carcinoma
○ (E) Pituitary adenoma

17. A neonate is found to have the following laboratory findings: a low serum cortisol level, high serum testosterone level, low serum sodium level, and high serum potassium level. The baby has a metabolic acidosis. Hypotension with cardiovascular collapse ensues within 48 hours of birth. An abdominal ultrasound reveals bilaterally enlarged adrenal glands. Which of the following enzyme deficiency states does the baby probably have?

○ (A) Aromatase
○ (B) 11-Hydroxylase
○ (C) 21-Hydroxylase
○ (D) 17α-hydroxylase
○ (E) Oxidase

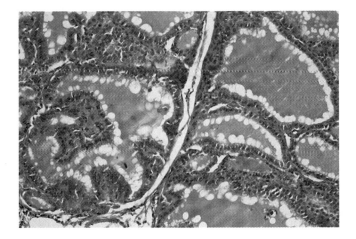

18. A 22-year-old female presents with a 7-kg weight loss without dieting over the last 4 months. She has experienced increasing anxiety and nervousness without apparent changes in her job or home life. Physical examination reveals a diffusely enlarged thyroid gland. Radioiodine uptake shows a diffuse increase in uptake. The microscopic appearance of the lesion leading to these findings is shown here at high power. This lesion is most likely caused by

○ (A) Antibodies against TSH receptor
○ (B) Dietary deficiency of iodine
○ (C) Mutation in the RET protooncogene
○ (D) Maternal deficiency in T_4
○ (E) Irradiation to the neck

19. A small (1-cm) nodule is palpable in the right lower pole of the thyroid gland of a 43-year-old male. Fine-needle aspiration is performed, and the nodule has the cytologic features of a follicular neoplasm. By radionucleotide scanning, this nodule does not pick up radioactive iodine, and no other nodules are present. Based on these findings, laboratory investigations are most likely to show

- (A) Anti–TSH receptor immunoglobulins
- (B) High free T_4 and low TSH
- (C) Normal free T_4 and TSH
- (D) Low free T_4 and elevated TSH
- (E) Anti-microsomal antibody

20. A middle-aged man has experienced diarrhea, nervousness, palpitations, and increased irritability for the past 5 months. Proptosis and lid lag are among physical examination findings. Which of the following laboratory findings is most likely?

- (A) Increased plasma insulin level
- (B) Increased serum T_4 level
- (C) Increased serum TSH level
- (D) Increased serum cortisol level
- (E) Increased serum corticotropin level

For each of the patient histories in questions 21 and 22, match the most closely related laboratory finding:

- (A) Decreased serum free T_4 level
- (B) Increased urinary homovanillic acid (HVA) level
- (C) Decreased serum calcium level
- (D) Decreased serum potassium level
- (E) Increased serum gastrin level
- (F) Decreased serum sodium level
- (G) Increased urinary free catecholamines level
- (H) Decreased serum TSH level
- (I) Increased serum corticotropin level
- (J) Increased serum parathormone level
- (K) Increased serum growth hormone level
- (L) High titer serum anti-microsomal antibody
- (M) Increased serum prolactin level
- (N) Urine *Neisseria meningitidis* antigen
- (O) Increased serum cortisol level

21. Exophthalmos with weak extraocular muscle movement occurs in a 20-year-old female and her identical twin sister. Their conditions develop within 3 years of each other. (   )

22. A neonate is found to have an enlarged abdomen, and an abdominal ultrasound scan reveals a right retroperitoneal mass involving the adrenal gland. (   )

23. A 55-year-old male experiences marked lethargy, and physical examination reveals hyperpigmentation of his skin. The serum cortisol concentration is low, and the serum corticotropin level is high. Which of the following diseases is *most likely* to accompany this disorder?

- (A) Systemic lupus erythematosus (SLE)
- (B) Hashimoto thyroiditis
- (C) Diabetes mellitus, type II

- (D) Ulcerative colitis
- (E) Polyarteritis nodosa

24. A 40-year-old female experienced a feeling of fullness in her neck, and physical examination revealed an enlarged, asymmetric thyroid with one distinct palpable nodule in the left lobe. At surgery, a frozen section revealed carcinoma, and a thyroidectomy was performed. Subsequent pathologic examination of the thyroid gland revealed a multicentric carcinoma with a stroma of amyloid. Several years later, she is diagnosed with multicentric extra-adrenal pheochromocytomas. The endocrinologist says that her family members may be at risk for development of similar tumors and advises that they be screened for mutations in which of the following genes?

- (A) RET
- (B) *Rb1*
- (C) *p53*
- (D) BRCA-1
- (E) NF-1

25. A 20-year-old obese female presents with chronic headache and visual deterioration. A head CT scan reveals an expansion of the sella turcica without significant bony destruction. The endocrine laboratory evaluation is normal except for a serum prolactin level of 70 ng/mL. Craniotomy is performed, and the sellar mass is removed. On histologic examination, the mass reveals a monomorphous population of cells that fail to stain for growth hormone, TSH, follicle-stimulating hormone (FSH), corticotropin, or prolactin. Serum calcium and blood glucose concentrations are normal. Which of the following lesions is most consistent with these clinical and laboratory findings?

- (A) Nonsecretory adenoma with "stalk effect"
- (B) Multiple endocrine neoplasia type I (MEN I)
- (C) Chronic renal failure
- (D) Craniopharyngioma
- (E) MEN II

26. A 45-year-old male feels a small lump on the left side of his neck. He feels fine and has no other complaints. His physician palpates a firm, painless, 1.5-cm cervical lymph node. The thyroid gland is not enlarged. A chest radiograph is unremarkable. Laboratory test findings, including thyroid function tests, are normal. A fine-needle aspirate of the thyroid gland is most likely to show findings consistent with

- (A) Papillary carcinoma
- (B) Metastatic adenocarcinoma
- (C) Medullary carcinoma
- (D) Follicular carcinoma
- (E) Anaplastic carcinoma

27. A 23-year-old male presents for evaluation of headaches, polyuria, and "problems seeing." Your evaluation includes CT and MRI of the head, which reveal a large, partially calcified, cystic mass involving the sellar and suprasellar areas. Laboratory evaluation reveals a serum prolactin concentration of 60 ng/mL and a serum sodium level of 152 mEq/L. Serum calcium, phosphate, and glucose levels are normal. The mass is excised. Histologic exami-

nation of the mass reveals a mixture of squamous epithelial elements and lipid-rich debris containing cholesterol crystals. Which of the following lesions is most consistent with the clinical laboratory findings in this patient?

○ (A) A craniopharyngioma that has destroyed the posterior pituitary
○ (B) A prolactin-secreting macroadenoma
○ (C) MEN I
○ (D) Metastases from a lung neoplasm involving the sella and brain
○ (E) MEN II

28.   A 0.7-cm microadenoma of the adenohypophysis is seen by head MRI in a 25-year-old female. Which of the following complications is she most likely to have?

○ (A) Amenorrhea with galactorrhea
○ (B) Hyperthyroidism
○ (C) Acromegaly
○ (D) Cushing disease
○ (E) Syndrome of inappropriate antidiuretic hormone (SIADH)

29.   A 60-year-old woman experienced back pain with a compressed fracture of T11, easy bruisability, and cutaneous striae over the lower abdomen. She also experienced mental depression, for which she took antidepressants. She died from a disseminated cytomegalovirus infection. At autopsy, both adrenal glands demonstrate cortical atrophy. Her pituitary gland is normal in appearance grossly and microscopically. Which of the following conditions is most likely to explain these findings?

○ (A) Addison disease
○ (B) Corticosteroid therapy
○ (C) 21-Hydroxylase deficiency
○ (D) Cushing disease
○ (E) Waterhouse-Friderichsen syndrome

30.   A 45-year-old female complained of headaches for about a month. She then suffered a generalized seizure and became obtunded. Her serum calcium concentration was found to be markedly elevated at 15.4 mg/dL, with a serum phosphorus level of only 1.9 mg/dL. The serum albumin level was 4.2 g/dL. A chest radiograph showed multiple lung masses, and there appeared to be lytic lesions of the vertebral column. Which of the following conditions best accounts for these findings?

○ (A) Parathyroid carcinoma
○ (B) Renal failure
○ (C) Metastatic breast cancer
○ (D) Vitamin D toxicity
○ (E) Tuberculosis

31.   The figure shows the microscopic appearance of the thyroid gland of a 46-year-old female who experienced painless, diffuse enlargement of her thyroid gland that was accompanied by clinical hypothyroidism. Which of the following antibodies is most likely to be present in her serum?

○ (A) Anti-microsomal antibody
○ (B) Anti-mitochondrial antibody
○ (C) Anti-ribonucleoprotein antibody

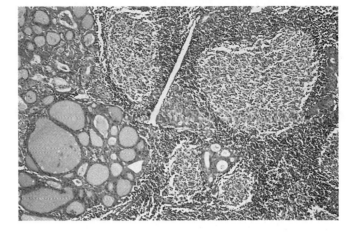

○ (D) Anti–double-stranded DNA antibody
○ (E) Anti–gastric parietal cell antibody

For each of the patient descriptions in questions 32 and 33, select the most likely accompanying morphologic changes observed in the adrenal gland:

(A) Bilateral cortical nodular hyperplasia
(B) Solitary, 2-cm, well-circumscribed cortical mass associated with atrophy of the contralateral adrenal cortex
(C) Solitary, 1-cm, well-circumscribed right cortical mass without atrophy of the contralateral adrenal cortex
(D) Bilateral adrenal cortical atrophy involving predominantly the zona fasciculata and zona reticularis
(E) Bilateral lymphocytic infiltration with atrophy of all cortical zones
(F) Bilateral hemorrhagic necrosis
(G) Bilateral caseating granulomas
(H) Bilateral masses that have nearly obliterated the cortices and medullae
(I) A large, 12-cm, yellow-tan mass with extensive necrosis arising in the left adrenal cortex
(J) Bilateral, 2- to 4-cm masses arising in the adrenal medullae

32.   A 32-year-old woman with systemic lupus erythematosus has been treated with corticosteroid therapy for several years because of lupus nephritis. While on vacation, she undergoes an emergency appendectomy for acute appendicitis. Postoperatively, she remains somnolent and develops severe nausea and vomiting, followed by hypotension. (   )

33.   A 27-year-old male presents for evaluation of headaches. He is also found to have a right thyroid mass. The serum calcitonin level is found to be elevated, and subsequent thyroidectomy reveals multiple tumor nodules in both lobes of the thyroid, composed of nests of neoplastic cells separated by amyloid-rich stroma. Further evaluation reveals the presence of an adrenal lesion. (   )

34.   A radiograph of the foot demonstrates increased amount of soft tissue beneath the calcaneus in a 40-year-old woman, who also notices that her gloves from the

previous winter no longer fit her hands. She is found to have glucose intolerance and an increased hemoglobin A_{1C} level, hypertension, and congestive heart failure. Which of the following laboratory test results is most likely to indicate the cause for these findings?

○ (A) Elevated serum prolactin level
○ (B) Failure of growth hormone suppression by glucose administration
○ (C) Increased serum cortisol level
○ (D) Abnormal glucose tolerance test result
○ (E) Increased serum TSH level

35. A 44-year-old Caucasian female attorney complains of listlessness and weakness that has increased over the past few months, and she has had chronic diarrhea along with a weight loss of 5 kg. She also notices that her skin seems darker, even though she has been mostly indoors because she is too tired to go outside and do anything. Laboratory findings include a serum sodium level of 120 mmol/L, potassium level of 5.1 mmol/L, glucose level of 58 mg/dL, urea nitrogen level of 18 mg/dL, and creatinine level of 0.8 mg/dL. Her serum corticotropin level is markedly elevated. Her blood pressure is 85/50 mm Hg. Which of the following morphologic changes in her adrenal glands is most likely to account for these findings?

○ (A) Bilateral adrenal cortical hyperplasia
○ (B) Bilateral adrenal hemorrhagic necrosis
○ (C) Bilateral lymphocytic adrenalitis with cortical atrophy
○ (D) Bilateral granulomatous adrenalitis
○ (E) Bilateral metastases from an occult colon carcinoma

For the patient history in question 36, match the most closely related endocrinologic syndrome:

(A) Addison disease
(B) Waterhouse-Friderichsen syndrome
(C) SIADH
(D) Wermer syndrome
(E) Sipple syndrome
(F) Graves disease
(G) Plummer syndrome
(H) DiGeorge syndrome
(I) Cushing syndrome
(J) Cushing disease
(K) Adrenogenital syndrome
(L) Conn syndrome

36. An infant exhibits neuromuscular irritability and seizure activity, and the serum calcium concentration is very low. The baby has had multiple fungal and viral infections since birth. Fluorescent in situ hybridization (FISH) analysis reveals del 22q11. (   )

37. Serum electrolyte measurements for a 67-year-old female show a sodium level of 118 mmol/L, potassium level of 6.0 mmol/L, chloride level of 95 mmol/L, carbon dioxide level of 21 mmol/L, and glucose level of 49 mg/dL. Her 8 AM serum cortisol concentration is 9 ng/mL. She has experienced malaise and has had a 10-kg weight loss over the past 4 months. An abdominal CT scan reveals bilaterally enlarged adrenal glands. A chest radiograph reveals a 6-cm perihilar mass on the right with prominent hilar lymphadenopathy. Which of the following conditions best accounts for these findings?

○ (A) Meningococcemia
○ (B) Pituitary adenoma
○ (C) Amyloidosis
○ (D) Metastatic carcinoma
○ (E) Ectopic corticotropin syndrome

38. A 42-year-old male presents with a history of polyuria and polydipsia. His history reveals that he fell off a ladder and hit his head. Laboratory investigations reveal hypernatremia and increased serum osmolality. The specific gravity of the urine is 1.002. These manifestations are most likely caused by a deficiency of

○ (A) Oxytocin
○ (B) ADH
○ (C) Corticotropin
○ (D) Prolactin
○ (E) Melatonin

39. A 37-year-old female states that, although most of the time she feels fine, she has experienced episodes of palpitations, tachycardia, tremor, diaphoresis, and headache for 3 months. When her symptoms are worse, her blood pressure is in the range of 155/90 mm Hg. She collapses suddenly one day and is brought to the hospital, where her ventricular fibrillation is successfully converted to sinus rhythm. Which of the following laboratory test findings is most likely to be seen in this patient?

○ (A) Increased urinary homovanillic acid (HVA) level
○ (B) Decreased serum potassium level
○ (C) Increased serum free T_4 level
○ (D) Increased urinary free catecholamines
○ (E) Decreased serum glucose level

40. A 60-year-old woman has been feeling tired and sluggish for more than a year. Her thyroid gland is not palpable on physical examination. She has a decreased serum level of T_4, but her serum TSH concentration is greatly increased. Which of the following factors is important in the pathogenesis of this condition?

○ (A) Irradiation to the neck during childhood
○ (B) Anti-microsomal and anti-thyroglobulin antibodies
○ (C) Prolonged iodine deficiency
○ (D) Mutations in the RET protooncogene
○ (E) Recent viral upper respiratory tract infection

41. A 68-year-old male has end-stage renal disease as a consequence of dominant polycystic kidney disease (DPKD). He has undergone hemodialysis three times per week for the past 6 years. Which of the following endocrine lesions is the most likely complication of his chronic renal failure?

○ (A) Multinodular goiter
○ (B) Islet cell hyperplasia
○ (C) Adrenal atrophy
○ (D) Parathyroid hyperplasia
○ (E) Pituitary microadenoma

42. A 44-year-old male without previous illnesses presents with a 3-week history of progressive hoarseness, shortness of breath, and stridor. He is found to have a firm, large, tender thyroid mass that by CT scan extends posterior to the trachea and into the upper mediastinum. A fine-needle aspirate shows pleomorphic spindle cells. He is taken to surgery, and the mass is resected. The mass infiltrates into adjacent skeletal muscle. Four of seven cervical lymph nodes have metastases. Pulmonary metastases are also identified by a chest radiograph. Which of the following neoplasms is most likely?

○ (A) Non-Hodgkin lymphoma
○ (B) Follicular carcinoma
○ (C) Medullary carcinoma
○ (D) Papillary carcinoma
○ (E) Anaplastic carcinoma

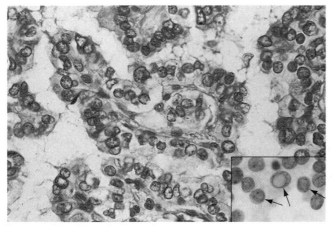

Courtesy of Dr. Edmund Cibas, Brigham and Women's Hospital, Boston.

43. The high-power microscopic appearance of a thyroid nodule shown here is from a 44-year-old male. His serum free T_4 and TSH levels are normal. No thyroid autoantibodies are detectable in the serum. This is most consistent with a past history of

○ (A) Dietary iodine deficiency
○ (B) Irradiation to the neck
○ (C) Consumption of goitrogens
○ (D) Removal of a tumor from the adrenal medulla
○ (E) Viral infection

ANSWERS

1. **(D)** The child has cretinism. This condition is uncommon when there is routine testing and treatment at birth for hypothyroidism. Hypothyroidism that develops in older children and adults is known as myxedema. A lack of cortisol from primary adrenal failure leads to Addison disease, or a 21-hydroxylase deficiency could produce congenital adrenal hyperplasia. There is no deficiency state for norepinephrine or somatostatin. An absolute deficiency of insulin leads to type I diabetes mellitus.
BP6 645   PBD6 1133

2. **(A)** This patient has precocious puberty, caused most likely by the adrenogenital syndrome. It is caused most commonly by a deficiency of 21-hydroxylase. The lack of this enzyme reduces cortisol production, driving corticotropin production that leads to adrenal hyperplasia and production of sex steroid hormones. This condition is rare. Bilateral adrenal cortical atrophy is typically seen in cases of Addison disease or after exogenous glucocorticoid therapy. A nodule in the adrenal medulla, if functional, produces catecholamines, and the patients, who are older, present with hypertension. A nodule in the adrenal cortex that has zona glomerulosa cells produces primary hyperaldosteronism.
BP6 659   PBD6 1157-1159

3. **(C)** The TSH level gives an indication of whether there is a primary disease involving the thyroid. If the patient appears hypothyroid and a primary thyroid disease (e.g., Hashimoto thyroiditis) is suspected, the TSH level is elevated. If the patient appears hyperthyroid and a primary thyroid disease (e.g., Graves disease) is suspected, the TSH level is decreased. A total T_4 level is low with hypothyroidism and high with most forms of hyperthyroidism, but it does not necessarily implicate the thyroid gland as the cause. Hyperthyroidism due to an elevated T_3 level is much less common than an elevated T_4 level. Fine-needle aspiration and isotopic scans are employed to study mass lesions of the thyroid, which typically do not alter thyroid function. Hyperfunction or hypofunction of the thyroid because of diseases of the pituitary gland is uncommon.
BP6 643-645   PBD6 1130-1133

4. **(E)** Inadvertent removal of or damage to the parathyroid glands during thyroid surgery can cause hypocalcemia due to hypoparathyroidism. This is the most common cause of hypoparathyroidism. Persons with hypocalcemia exhibit neuromuscular irritability, carpopedal spasm, and possibly, seizures. Calcitonin quantitation is not a useful measure for determining the status of calcium metabolism. The TSH concentration may increase if the patient becomes hypothyroid after surgery and is not receiving thyroid hormone replacement, but this is not an immediate problem. PTH levels become decreased if the parathyroid glands are inadvertently removed during thyroid surgery, but the calcium level gives the best immediate indicator of hypoparathyroidism, and this test is more readily available in the laboratory. Anti-thyroglobulin antibody levels are of no use in diagnosing surgical diseases of the thyroid.
BP6 655   PBD6 1151

5. **(C)** The gross specimen shows a tumor in the adrenal cortex. In young, otherwise healthy individuals who present with hypertension, a surgically curable cause of hypertension must be sought. This patient had an adrenal cortical adenoma that secreted aldosterone (i.e., Conn syndrome). Hyperaldosteronism reduces the synthesis of renin by the juxtaglomerular apparatus in the kidney. Adrenal adenomas may be nonfunctional or secrete glucocorticoids or mineralocorticoids. Had this been a glucocorticoid-secreting ade-

noma, the patient could have hypertension, but there also would be clinical features of Cushing syndrome. Aldosterone does not exhibit feedback suppression of the anterior pituitary, and corticotropin levels therefore are not affected. Patients with hyperaldosteronism have low serum potassium levels and sodium retention. There is no effect on blood glucose.
BP6 658–659   PBD6 1155–1157

6. **(G)** She has a follicular carcinoma, which may be difficult to differentiate from follicular adenoma, but in this case, the invasion indicates malignancy. Follicular carcinomas are often indolent, but they may metastasize. They are much less likely than papillary carcinomas to involve lymph nodes, but they are more likely to metastasize to distant sites such as bone, lung, and liver. If the metastatic lesions are functional, they will pick up radioactive iodine.
BP6 651–652   PBD6 1144–1145

7. **(B)** The clinical findings point to hyperthyroidism, and the increased, diffuse uptake corroborates Graves disease as a likely cause, because the TSH level is quite low. The thyroid stimulating immunoglobulins that appear with this autoimmune condition result in diffuse thyroid enlargement and hyperfunction.
BP6 645–646   PBD6 1136–1137

8. **(A)** The clinical and laboratory features of this case point to Cushing syndrome. The dexamethasone suppression test is used to localize the source of excess cortisol. When low- and high-dose dexamethasone trials fail to suppress cortisol secretion, a pituitary corticotropin-secreting adenoma as the source of excess glucocorticoids is unlikely. The choice then is an ectopic source of corticotropin, such as a lung cancer, or a tumor of the adrenal cortex that is secreting glucocorticoids. The plasma corticotropin level distinguishes between these two possibilities. Corticotropin levels are high if there is an ectopic source, whereas glucocorticoid secretion from an adrenal neoplasm suppresses corticotropin production by the pituitary, which leads to atrophy of the contralateral adrenal cortex. An adrenal cortical adenoma that secretes aldosterone does not cause atrophy of the contralateral adrenal cortex.
BP6 656–657   PBD6 1152–1154

9. **(E)** He has syndrome of inappropriate antidiuretic hormone (SIADH) secretion, which results in increased free water resorption by the kidney and hyponatremia. SIADH is most often a paraneoplastic effect, and oat cell carcinoma of the lung is the most likely candidate among candidate malignant neoplasms. Anterior pituitary adenomas do not produce ADH. Adrenal cortical carcinomas may secrete cortisol or sex steroids, not ADH. Renal cell carcinomas are known for a variety of paraneoplastic effects, but SIADH is not high on the list. Pheochromocytomas secrete catecholamines.
BP6 643   PBD6 1129

10. **(B)** When a patient presents with hypercalcemia, a disorder of the parathyroid glands, malignancy at a visceral location must be considered. Hypercalcemia of malignancy can be caused by osteolytic metastases or a paraneoplastic syndrome from secretion of parathyroid hormone (PTH)–related protein by the tumor. If a malignant neoplasm can be excluded, an intrinsic abnormality of the parathyroid glands must be sought. The most common cause of primary hyperparathyroidism is parathyroid adenoma. Secondary hyperparathyroidism, most commonly resulting from renal failure, is excluded when the serum inorganic phosphate is low, because phosphate is retained with renal failure. Hypervitaminosis D can cause hypercalcemia because of increased calcium absorption, but in these cases, the PTH levels are expected to be near the low end of the reference range because of feedback suppression. Serum PTH levels near the high end of the reference range indicate autonomous PTH secretion not regulated by hypercalcemia.
BP6 653–655   PBD6 1148–1150

11. **(C)** This is the typical adrenal finding with Waterhouse-Friderichsen syndrome, and meningococcemia is the most likely cause for such a rapid course. Chronic adrenocortical insufficiency can result from disseminated tuberculosis and from fungal infections, such as histoplasmosis, that involve the adrenal glands. *S. pneumoniae* can produce a septicemia but is unlikely to specifically involve the adrenal glands. Cytomegalovirus infections of the adrenal can be seen in immunocompromised states and may be severe enough to produce diminished adrenal function, although not acute failure.
BP6 661–662   PBD6 1160

12. **(E)** Diffuse nontoxic goiter is most often caused by dietary iodine deficiency. Such a condition is said to be endemic in regions of the world where there is a deficiency of iodine (e.g., inland mountainous areas). Otherwise, it may occur sporadically. As in this case, the patients are typically euthyroid. Plummer syndrome, or toxic multinodular goiter, occurs when there is a hyperfunctioning nodule in a goiter. Papillary carcinomas most often produce a mass effect or metastases and do not affect thyroid function. Subacute granulomatous thyroiditis may lead to diffuse enlargement, and there may be transient hyperthyroidism, but the disease typically runs a course of no more than 6 to 8 weeks. A lymphocytic thyroiditis, such as Hashimoto thyroiditis, may initially produce thyroid enlargement, but atrophy occurs over time.
BP6 646–647   PBD6 1138–1139

13. **(B)** Subacute thyroiditis is a self-limited condition that may be of viral origin, because many cases are preceded by an upper respiratory infection. The transient hyperthyroidism results from inflammatory destruction of the thyroid follicles and release of thyroid hormone. The released colloid acts as a foreign body to produce florid granulomatous inflammation in the thyroid. Thyroid neoplasms are not typically associated with signs and symptoms of inflammation. A toxic goiter likewise produces no signs of inflammation. Hashimoto thyroiditis may transiently enlarge the thyroid, but there is usually no pain or hyperthyroidism.
BP6 649   PBD6 1135–1136

14. **(A)** This is a medullary carcinoma, which is derived from the C-cells, or parafollicular cells, of the thyroid that synthesize calcitonin. An amyloid stroma is a common feature of this tumor. These tumors occur sporadically in about 80% of cases, but they can be part of MEN II and III. Cathepsin D is a marker useful for some breast carcinomas. Staining for PTH is useful to determine if a parathyroid carcinoma is present. Vimentin is a marker for sarcomatous neoplasms, and cytokeratin is a useful marker to determine if a neoplasm is epithelial.
BP6 652   PBD6 1146–1147

15. **(A)** This patient has Cushing syndrome. If the cortisol concentration is increased along with the corticotropin level, the pituitary is producing it, or there is an ectopic source such as a lung carcinoma. MRI to determine the size of the pituitary is the logical investigation because over 50% of Cushing patients have a pituitary adenoma. If the source of cortisol is primary adrenal hyperplasia or an adrenal neoplasm, the corticotropin level should be suppressed. A CT scan to determine adrenal size is therefore of no value. Because the patient has hyperglycemia, the glycosylated hemoglobin level is increased. This finding can confirm diabetes but cannot indicate the cause of hyperglycemia. The changes in muscle are not specific for different causes of Cushing syndrome. Urinary catecholamines are useful for the diagnosis of pheochromocytoma. Although patients with pheochromocytoma can have hypertension, they do not have other changes of Cushing syndrome.
BP6 656–658   PBD6 1153–1154

16. **(E)** She has MEN I. This is also known as Wermer syndrome. Remember the "three Ps" with neoplasia or hyperplasia of pancreas, pituitary, and parathyroids. Endometrial carcinomas can arise in patients who have unopposed estrogen secretion, as may occur in estrogen-producing ovarian tumors. These are not part of MEN I. Medullary carcinomas are part of MEN II or III. Small cell carcinomas of the lung are known for a variety of paraneoplastic syndromes, but not usually hypercalcemia. It is also very doubtful that she would have lived 5 years with such a neoplasm. If her hypercalcemia had been a paraneoplastic syndrome, the parathyroid glands would not have been enlarged, nor would the serum calcium level have returned to normal after surgery.
BP6 664–665   PBD6 1166–1167

17. **(C)** The 21-hydroxylase deficiency leads to a salt-wasting form of adrenogenital syndrome, because the enzyme deficiency blocks formation of aldosterone and cortisol. The 11-hydroxylase deficiency blocks cortisol and aldosterone production as well, although intermediate metabolites with some glucocorticoid activity are synthesized. Aromatase is involved with conversion of androstenedione to estrone, a side pathway that does not affect cortisol production. The 17α-hydroxylase deficiency would lead to reduction of cortisol and sex steroid synthesis. Oxidase is the final enzyme in the pathway to aldosterone production.
BP6 659–660   PBD6 1157–1159

18. **(A)** Most solitary cold thyroid nodules in younger persons are likely to be neoplastic, and most of these are benign follicular adenomas that do not affect thyroid function. If the nodule were hyperfunctioning to produce hyperthyroidism, it should appear "hot" on the scan. Anti-TSH receptor immunoglobulins may be seen with Graves disease, as may high T_4 and low TSH levels, but this is a diffuse disease of the thyroid. Anti-microsomal and anti-thyroglobulin antibodies are seen in Hashimoto thyroiditis, but thyroiditis is a diffuse process and unlikely to produce a solitary nodule. Decreasing function of the thyroid as Hashimoto thyroiditis progresses can lead to a decreasing T_4 and increasing TSH levels, typical of primary thyroid failure.
BP6 649–650   PBD6 1140–1142

19. **(C)** The tall columnar epithelium with papillary infoldings and scalloping of the colloid is characteristic of Graves disease, which leads to hyperthyroidism. This disease is caused by autoantibodies that bind to the TSH receptor and mimic the action of TSH. Dietary iodine deficiency can cause diffuse compensatory enlargement of thyroid, but it does not cause hyperthyroidism. Mutations in the RET protooncogene occur in papillary carcinoma of thyroid and in medullary carcinomas of thyroid. These neoplasms do not cause diffuse enlargement of the gland, hyperthyroidism, or diffuse increase in radioiodine uptake. Tumors usually produce "cold nodules" with radioiodine scans. Irradiation of the neck is a predisposing factor for papillary carcinoma of thyroid.
BP6 644   PBD6 1236–1238

20. **(B)** These findings indicate hyperthyroidism, most probably Graves disease; therefore, serum T_4 will be increased. The serum TSH level is decreased in Graves disease because of feedback inhibition. Hypoglycemia from an increased insulin concentration can lead to fainting with hypotension and palpitations. A pituitary adenoma secreting TSH may also produce hyperthyroidism, but this condition is far less common than Graves disease. Cushing syndrome, with increased cortisol, may result in hypertension and mood changes but not ocular changes. An increased corticotropin level also may lead to hypercortisolism.
BP6 645–646   PBD6 1131–1132

21. **(H)** Exophthalmos is a feature seen in about 40% of persons with Graves disease. The hyperfunctioning thyroid gland leads to an increased T_4 level, with positive feedback on the pituitary to decrease secretion of TSH. There is about 50% concordance of Graves disease among identical twins. The autoimmune character of this disorder is evidenced by an association with HLA-DR3.
BP6 645–646   PBD6 1136–1138

22. **(B)** Neuroblastomas are pediatric neoplasms, and they arise most commonly in the retroperitoneum in the adrenals or in extra-adrenal paraganglia. They are primitive "small blue cell" tumors that can produce high levels of catecholamines, and their metabolites, such as HVA, can be detected.
BP6 211   PBD6 485–487, 1166

23. **(B)** Addison disease (i.e., primary chronic adrenocortical insufficiency) most often results from an idiopathic autoimmune condition (in places where the incidence of active tuberculosis is low). Autoimmune adrenalitis is associated with the appearance of other autoimmune diseases in about one half of cases. Such autoimmune phenomena are likely to be seen in other endocrine organs like the thyroid gland. Other presumed autoimmune diseases such as SLE, ulcerative colitis, and vasculitides are not generally forerunners to adrenal failure, although treatment of these conditions with corticosteroids can lead to iatrogenic adrenal atrophy.
BP6 661   PBD6 1160–1162

24. **(A)** She has MEN II. These patients have medullary carcinomas of thyroid, pheochromocytomas, and parathyroid adenomas. This syndrome is associated with germ-line mutations in the RET protooncogene. Family members who inherit the same mutation are at increased risk for similar cancers. Genetic screening followed by increased surveillance of affected individuals is advised. The remaining four genes are tumor suppressor genes, and germ-line mutations for each are associated with increased risk of distinct tumors such as retinoblastoma and osteosarcomas (with Rb1), breast and ovarian cancers (with BRCA-1), and neurofibromatosis (with NF-1). Inherited mutations of p53 (e.g., Li-Fraumeni syndrome) predispose to a large variety of tumors, not just thyroid and adrenal neoplasms.
BP6 665   PBD6 1166–1167

25. **(A)** The hyperprolactinemia is a "stalk section" effect, with loss of a hypothalamic inhibiting factor for prolactin secretion. This can occur from an enlarging sellar mass that also produces headache and the visual disturbances from pressure on the optic chiasm. There is generally enough residual adenohypophysis to prevent panhypopituitarism. Those with MEN I have pituitary adenomas, as well as lesions in the pancreas and parathyroid. Chronic renal failure can cause hyperprolactinemia but not a sellar mass. A craniopharyngioma is a destructive sellar mass. MEN II does not involve the pituitary.
BP6 643   PBD6 1126

26. **(A)** Some papillary carcinomas may initially present with metastases, and local lymph nodes are the most common sites for metastases. The primary site may not be detectable as a palpable nodule. Papillary carcinoma is the most common thyroid malignancy. Metastases to thyroid are uncommon. Both medullary and follicular carcinomas tend to spread hematogenously. Anaplastic carcinomas are uncommon but are very aggressive, locally invasive lesions.
BP6 650–651   PBD6 1143–1144

27. **(A)** Craniopharyngiomas are uncommon neoplasms, usually suprasellar in location and found in young persons. They are thought to arise from embryologic remnants of the Rathke pouch in the region of the pituitary. These are aggressive neoplasms that infiltrate and destroy surrounding tissues, making complete excision difficult. Despite their aggressive behavior, they are composed of benign-appearing squamoid or primitive tooth structures. The rise in prolactin occurs as a "stalk section" effect, and the hyper-

natremia results from diabetes insipidus caused by destruction of the hypothalamus, posterior pituitary, or both. Prolactinomas, like pituitary adenomas in general, may enlarge the sella but are not typically suprasellar or destructive of surrounding structures. MEN I does include pituitary adenomas but not craniopharyngiomas. A metastasis to this location in a young person is highly unlikely. MEN II does not involve the pituitary.
PBD6 1129

28. **(A)** Prolactinomas are more common than the other hormone-secreting pituitary adenomas. Microadenomas may not be detected because pressure effects on surrounding structures are absent, but they may come to attention because of their hormonal effects.
BP6 639–641   PBD6 1125–1126

29. **(B)** She has evidence of Cushing syndrome, and the accompanying adrenal atrophy suggests an exogenous source for cortisol. Corticosteroid therapy has many side effects, including immunosuppression, osteoporosis, depression, and reduced collagen synthesis. 21-Hydroxylase deficiency, the rare congenital pediatric condition, is associated with adrenal hyperplasia. Cushing disease results from a pituitary adenoma that is secreting corticotropin, and the adrenals should be large in such a case. Acute adrenal failure with Waterhouse-Friderichsen syndrome is accompanied by massive adrenal hemorrhage and most often results from severe infection, typically with meningococcemia. Addison disease is associated with bilateral adrenal cortical atrophy, most often because of autoimmunity. These patients show symptoms and signs of adrenal failure not present in this case.
BP6 656–662   PBD6 1153–1155

30. **(C)** The most common cause for clinically significant hypercalcemia in adults is a malignancy. Metastatic disease from common primaries such as breast, lung, and kidney tumors is much more frequent than parathyroid carcinoma, which tends to be local but aggressive. Parathyroid carcinomas are an uncommon cause for hyperparathyroidism, and bone metastases are rare from parathyroid carcinomas. Chronic renal failure causes phosphate retention that tends to depresses the serum calcium level and leads to secondary hyperparathyroidism; therefore serum calcium level is maintained at near normal levels. Vitamin D toxicity can theoretically lead to hypercalcemia, but this condition is uncommon. Tuberculosis is another granulomatous disease that may be associated with hypercalcemia, but lytic bone lesions are uncommon.
BP6 654–655   PBD6 1148–1149

31. **(A)** Notice the lymphoid follicles and the large, pink Hürthle cells in this photomicrograph. This patient has Hashimoto thyroiditis. The anti-microsomal and anti-thyroglobulin antibody titers are typically increased in cases of Hashimoto thyroiditis *when thyroid enlargement is still present*. In the later, "burnt-out" phase of Hashimoto thyroiditis, the antibodies may not be detectable—only the hypothyroidism. Increased anti-mitochondrial antibody is indicative of primary biliary cirrhosis. Anti-riboneucleoprotein antibodies are seen with some of the collagen vascular diseases. Anti–double-stranded DNA antibody is specific

for SLE. Anti–parietal cell antibody occurs in atrophic gastritis that gives rise to pernicious anemia. Although pernicious anemia may coexist with Hashimoto thyroiditis and other endocrinopathies, this is uncommon.
BP6 648   PBD6 1134–1135

32. **(D)** She has findings of acute adrenocortical insufficiency. Chronic corticosteroid therapy shuts off corticotropin stimulation to the adrenals, leading to adrenal atrophy. When this history is not elicited and the patient is not continued on the corticosteroid therapy, a crisis ensues, made worse by the stress of surgery.
BP6 661–662   PBD6 1159

33. **(J)** The findings suggest type II or possibly type III MEN. His headaches may be caused by hypertension from pheochromocytoma. More than 70% of pheochromocytomas are bilateral when familial. His thyroid mass is a medullary carcinoma, which also tends to be multifocal in this syndrome.
BP6 665   PBD6 1167

34. **(B)** Failure to suppress growth hormone (GH) levels by glucose infusion suggests autonomic GH production. The patient's symptoms suggest acromegaly, and a GH-secreting adenoma is most likely. Acromegaly causes an overall increase in soft tissue in adults because of the anabolic effects of the increase in growth hormone. Because the epiphyses of the long bones are closed in adults, there is no increase in height, or gigantism, that would be seen in children with a pituitary adenoma secreting excessive growth hormone. A prolactinoma would cause amenorrhea and galactorrhea. Cushing syndrome from an adrenal tumor could be accompanied by glucose intolerance, hypertension, and truncal obesity, but there is no overall increase in soft tissues. She probably has an abnormal glucose tolerance test result, but this does not give an indication of the underlying cause for diabetes mellitus. A TSH-secreting adenoma of the pituitary can give rise to hyperthyroidism. The increased metabolic rate found with hyperthyroidism is most likely to lead to weight loss, and glucose intolerance is not a feature of hyperthyroidism. Functional pituitary tumors may be detected clinically before they become large enough to cause pressure symptoms such as visual disturbances.
BP6 641   PBD6 1126

35. **(C)** She has chronic adrenal insufficiency (i.e., Addison disease) with decreased cortisol production and decreased mineralocorticoid activity. The skin hyperpigmentation results from increased corticotropin precursor hormone production, which stimulates melanocytes. The most common cause of Addison disease in areas where tuberculosis is not endemic is autoimmune adrenalitis. This process causes gradual destruction of the adrenal cortex, mediated most likely by infiltrating lymphocytes. Bilateral hemorrhages and resultant destruction of the adrenal glands are typically caused by meningococcemia, and this presents as acute adrenocortical insufficiency. Metastases, typically from a lung carcinoma, can cause adrenal cortical destruction, but this is less common than autoimmune adrenalitis.
BP6 662   PBD6 1160–1162

36. **(H)** DiGeorge syndrome is a developmental defect that results from failure of development of the third and fourth pharyngeal pouches. The latter give rise to the thymus, the parathyroids, and some clear cells of the thyroid. Congenital anomalies in the nearby esophagus and heart may also occur. These patients have a T-cell immunodeficiency and hypoparathyroidism. Hypocalcemia is responsible for the neuromuscular irritability and seizures, and 90% of the patients have deletion of chromosome 22q11.
BP6 655   PBD6 1151

37. **(D)** The lung mass suggests a primary carcinoma, and the bilaterally enlarged adrenals can be explained by adrenal metastases. Destruction of the adrenal cortex is responsible for malaise and the low serum cortisol concentration, as well as the electrolyte disturbances. The Waterhouse-Friderichsen syndrome from *N. meningitidis* infection may increase the adrenal size from marked hemorrhage (two to three times the normal size), but this does not explain the lung mass, and this syndrome has an abrupt onset. A pituitary adenoma secreting corticotropin could increase adrenal size bilaterally, but there should be hypercortisolism. Amyloidosis may increase adrenal size but does not produce a lung mass. With the ectopic corticotropin syndrome, a lung cancer is a likely finding, and the adrenal glands are typically enlarged, but there should be hypercortisolism.
BP6 658   PBD6 1161

38. **(B)** He has developed diabetes insipidus with a lack of ADH. There is failure of resorption of free water in the renal collecting tubules—hence the dilute urine. Oxytocin is involved with lactation. Corticotropin stimulates the adrenal glands, mainly with the effect of increasing cortisol secretion. Prolactin and melatonin deficiencies have no identifiable specific clinical effect in a male.
BP6 643   PBD6 1129

39. **(D)** These findings suggest a pheochromocytoma of the adrenal medulla. This is a rare neoplasm, but in cases of episodic hypertension, this diagnosis should be considered. Screening for urinary free catecholamines, metanephrines, and vanillylmandelic acid (VMA) can help to make the diagnosis. The level of HVA is increased with neuroblastoma, a pediatric tumor. Serum potassium may be decreased with aldosterone-secreting adrenal adenomas. An increased T_4 level occurs in patients with Graves disease, and this disease can cause tachycardia, tremors, and cardiac arrhythmia. However, episodic hypertension is not a feature of thyrotoxicosis. Hypoglycemia may be seen with Addison disease and islet cell tumors.
BP6 663–664   PBD6 1164–1165

40. **(B)** This patient has hypothyroidism, most likely Hashimoto thyroiditis. Autoantibodies are present in the serum. Many of these cases are not diagnosed as such, but patients simply present with hypothyroidism, which is the late, "burnt-out" phase of this autoimmune inflammatory condition. It is one of the most common causes for hypothyroidism in adults. An iodine deficiency can lead to hypothyroidism, but a goiter should be present. Irradiation of the thyroid gland can give rise to hypothyroidism, but it is unlikely that irradiation given in childhood would give rise

to hypothyroidism at the age of 60 years. Irradiation can also predispose to the development of papillary carcinoma, but these tumors do not affect thyroid hormone secretion. Mutations in the RET protooncogene are associated with papillary carcinoma and medullary carcinoma of the thyroid. A history of a viral infection may precede subacute thyroiditis, which is typically a self-limited disease lasting for weeks to a couple of months.
BP6 648   PBD6 1134–1135

41.   **(D)** Secondary hyperparathyroidism results from decreased phosphate excretion by the kidneys. The resultant hyperphosphatemia depresses serum calcium level and stimulates parathyroid gland activity. Because of reduced renal parenchymal function, there is also less active vitamin D, which leads to decreased dietary calcium absorption. Renal failure does not lead to any other endocrine lesions.
BP6 655   PBD6 1150–1151

42.   **(E)** The large size, histologic features, and aggressive nature of this neoplasm are in keeping with anaplastic carcinoma. The prognosis is poor. Malignant lymphomas do not have spindle cells and do not tend to be infiltrative. Other thyroid malignancies tend to form solitary or multifocal (in papillary and medullary carcinomas) masses without spindle cells, and they are less likely to be extensively invasive, although metastases may occur, particularly to local lymph nodes in the case of papillary carcinoma.
BP6 652   PBD6 1147

43.   **(B)** The nodule shows a papillary architecture, with cells having clear nuclei. This pattern is typical of a papillary carcinoma. There is no such thing as a papillary adenoma. The enlarged clear nuclei are typical for papillary carcinoma. These nuclear changes, even if the pattern is follicular, confirm the diagnosis of papillary carcinoma. Irradiation of the thyroid is a risk factor for papillary carcinoma. Iodine deficiency gives rise to uniform thyroid enlargement because the secretion of TSH increases when there is reduced synthesis of T_4. Goitrogens interfere with thyroid hormone synthesis and have an effect similar to iodine deficiency. An adrenal pheochromocytoma can occur along with medullary carcinoma of thyroid in MEN II or III. Viral infections can cause a subacute thyroiditis, not carcinoma.
BP6 651   PBD6 1143–1144

The Skin

BD6 Chapter 27 - The Skin
PBD6 Chapter 22 - The Skin

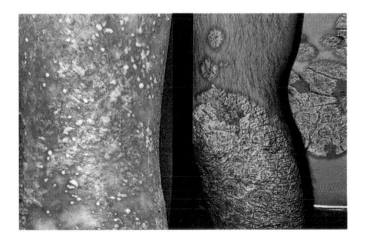

1. A 29-year-old male has had waxing and waning of the lesions depicted in the figure over the past decade. His scalp, lumbosacral region, and glans penis are also affected. In addition, he has a chronic arthritis involving his hips and knees. Which of the following physical examination findings would you most expect for this patient?

- (A) Guaiac-positive stool
- (B) Friction rub
- (C) Hyperreflexia
- (D) Damage to the nails
- (E) Renal failure

2. In which part of the world has the incidence of malignant melanoma of the skin increased the most in the past 25 years?

- (A) Edinburgh, Scotland
- (B) Cairo, Egypt
- (C) Brisbane, Australia
- (D) Tahiti, French Polynesia
- (E) Hong Kong, China

3. A 64-year-old male noticed the development over the past 3 months of thickened, darkly pigmented skin in axillae and flexural areas of the neck and groin. These areas are neither painful nor pruritic. A punch biopsy of axillary skin reveals undulating epidermal acanthosis with hyperkeratosis and basal layer hyperpigmentation. Which of the following underlying diseases is he most likely to have?

- (A) Systemic lupus erythematosus (SLE)
- (B) Mastocytosis
- (C) Acquired immunodeficiency syndrome (AIDS)
- (D) Colonic adenocarcinoma
- (E) Langerhans cell histiocytosis

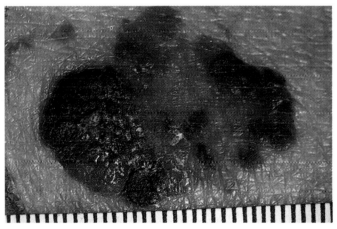

4. A 51-year-old male noticed the skin lesion shown here on his upper, outer right arm. The lesion had recently increased in size. Which of the following occupations is this man most likely to have had earlier in life?

- (A) Chemist
- (B) Lifeguard
- (C) Miner
- (D) Auto mechanic
- (E) Radiation oncologist

For the clinical histories in questions 5 and 6, match the most closely associated inflammatory condition of the skin:

(A) Acne vulgaris
(B) Bullous pemphigoid

(C) Contact dermatitis
(D) Dermatitis herpetiformis
(E) Discoid lupus erythematosus
(F) Erythema multiforme
(G) Erythema nodosum
(H) Impetigo
(I) Lichen planus
(J) Pemphigus
(K) Psoriasis
(L) Urticaria

5. A 35-year-old man has an outbreak of very pruritic, 0.4- to 0.7-cm vesicles over extensor surfaces of elbows and knees. He has a history of malabsorption with celiac disease but has had no skin problems before. A 3-mm punch biopsy of one of the skin lesions over the elbow is taken. It shows accumulation of neutrophils at the tips of dermal papillae and formation of small blisters because of separation at the dermoepidermal junction. Immunofluorescence studies performed on this biopsy shows granular deposits of IgA localized to tips of dermal papillae. (   )

6. Over the course of a week, a 6-year-old boy develops 1- to 2-cm erythematous macules and 0.5- to 1.0-cm pustules on his face. During the next 2 days, some of the pustules break, forming shallow erosions covered by a honey-colored crust. New lesions then form around the crust. The boy's 40-year-old uncle develops similar lesions after visiting for a week during this illness. (   )

7. Biopsy of an 0.8-cm, red, rough-surfaced lesion on the forehead of a 50-year-old female yields a diagnosis of actinic keratosis. What advice would you give this patient?

○ (A) Reduce dietary fat intake.
○ (B) Wear a hat outdoors.
○ (C) Stop taking aspirin for headaches.
○ (D) Apply a hydrocortisone cream to your face.
○ (E) This condition is related to aging.

8. A 10-year-old child has developed multiple excoriations of the skin of her hands. The child reports that she scratches her hands because they itch. Physical examination reveals several 0.2- to 0.6-cm linear streaks in the interdigital regions. Treatment with a topical lindane lotion resolves this condition. Which of the following organisms is most likely responsible for these findings?

○ (A) *Ixodes dammini*
○ (B) *Tinea corporis*
○ (C) *Staphylococcus aureus*
○ (D) Molluscum contagiosum
○ (E) *Sarcoptes scabiei*

9. A solitary, 0.4-cm, flesh-colored nodule has been present on the upper trunk of a 35-year-old male for the past 6 weeks. The dome-shaped lesion is umbilicated, and a curdlike material can be expressed from the center. This material is smeared on a slide, and Giemsa stain reveals many pink, homogenous, cytoplasmic inclusions. The lesion regresses over the next 2 months. Which of the following infectious agents is most likely the cause for this lesion?

○ (A) Human papillomavirus
○ (B) *Staphylococcus aureus*
○ (C) Molluscum contagiosum
○ (D) *Histoplasma capsulatum*
○ (E) Herpes zoster virus

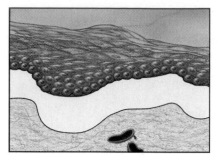

10. Many skin disorders give rise to vesicles or bullae (i.e., blisters) in the skin. The location of the bulla often helps the diagnosis of the condition. Which of the following disorders is most likely to produce the type of blister that is schematically illustrated here?

○ (A) Impetigo
○ (B) Pemphigus vulgaris
○ (C) Bullous pemphigoid
○ (D) Acute eczematous dermatitis
○ (E) Urticaria

11. A 2.1-cm, pigmented lesion is excised from the back of a 39-year-old female, who noticed that this lesion has become more nodular in appearance within the past 2 months. Microscopic examination of this lesion reveals a malignant melanoma, composed of epithelioid cells, that extends 2 mm down to the reticular dermis. There is a band of lymphocytes beneath the melanoma. Which of the following statements is most appropriate to make to this patient?

○ (A) Your body's immune system will prevent metastases.
○ (B) The prognosis is poor.
○ (C) Other family members are at risk for this condition.
○ (D) The primary site for this lesion is probably the eye.
○ (E) Nevi elsewhere on your body may become malignant.

12. On oral examination, a dentist notices that his 39-year-old female patient has scattered, white, 0.2- to 1.5-cm, reticulated areas on the buccal mucosa. She says that these lesions have been present for a year. She also has some 0.3-cm, pruritic, purple papules on each elbow. A biopsy of a skin lesion shows a bandlike infiltrate of lymphocytes at the dermal-epidermal junction along with degeneration of basal keratinocytes. What would you advise the patient regarding these lesions?

○ (A) A squamous cell carcinoma is likely to develop.
○ (B) You have systemic lupus erythematosus.
○ (C) A skin test for tuberculosis needs to be performed.

○ (D) You should stop taking all medications.
○ (E) These lesions will probably resolve over time.

For each of the clinical histories in questions 13 and 14, match the most closely associated infectious agent that can directly or indirectly result in the appearance of skin lesions:

(A) *Borrelia burgdorferi*
(B) Dermatophytic fungus
(C) Group A β-hemolytic *Streptococcus*
(D) Herpes simplex virus
(E) Herpes zoster virus
(F) Human papillomavirus
(G) *Malassezia furfur*
(H) Molluscum contagiosum
(I) *Mycobacterium leprae*
(J) *Propionibacterium acnes*
(K) *Sarcoptes scabiei*
(L) *Staphylococcus aureus*

13. "Athlete's foot," consisting of diffuse, erythematous, scaling skin lesions between the toes, has afflicted a 22-year-old male for the past 2 months. (   )

14. Variably sized 0.3- to 1.2-cm macules are seen over the upper trunk of a 32-year-old female. The macules are lighter than the surrounding skin and have a fine peripheral scale. These lesions have waxed and waned for several months. There is no pain or erythema. (   )

15. A 30-year-old male is known for his large appetite. At a luncheon meeting, he sees that all of the cookies contain nuts, which the other diners know he will not eat because he will develop blotchy erythematous, slightly edematous plaques on the skin that are pruritic. These plaques will fade over a couple of hours' time. Which of the following sensitized cells releases a mediator responsible for these skin lesions?

○ (A) Mast cell
○ (B) Neutrophil
○ (C) Natural killer cell
○ (D) CD4 lymphocyte
○ (E) Plasma cells

16. Macular to slightly raised, plaquelike, 0.4- to 1.7-cm, dark brown pigmented lesions are present on sun-exposed and non–sun-exposed areas of skin of a 17-year-old female. These lesions have irregular contours and show some variability in pigmentation. Detailed physical examination reveals that she has hundreds of such lesions on her body. She says that her 15-year-old brother also has similar spots. Which of the following statements would most accurately explain the significance of these lesions to the patient?

○ (A) These are benign lesions that will remain like this for years.
○ (B) These indicate an underlying visceral melanoma that is spreading to the skin.
○ (C) They represent areas of skin damaged by too much exposure to sun.

○ (D) These are inherited lesions that have a high risk of developing into melanomas.
○ (E) She and her brother have a reaction to some environmental antigen in their home.

17. A flesh-colored, dome-shaped, 1.2-cm nodule has appeared on the right ear lobe of a 60-year-old man in the past month. A central keratin-filled crater is surrounded by proliferating squamous epithelium. This lesion regresses over the next month and then disappears. Which of the following diagnoses is most appropriate for this lesion?

○ (A) Squamous cell carcinoma
○ (B) Basal cell carcinoma
○ (C) Seborrheic keratosis
○ (D) Actinic keratosis
○ (E) Keratoacanthoma

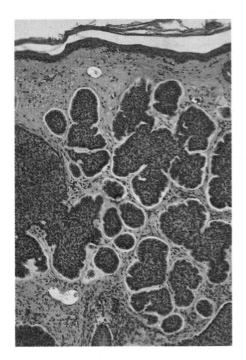

18. Near the lateral limbus of the right eye of a 68-year-old male is a pearly, 0.3-cm nodule on the upper eyelid. Multiple frozen sections are performed to minimize the extent of the resection of this lesion. The microscopic appearance of this lesion is shown here at low magnification. What is the diagnosis?

○ (A) Malignant melanoma
○ (B) Dermatofibroma
○ (C) Actinic keratosis
○ (D) Nevocellular nevus
○ (E) Basal cell carcinoma

19. A 5-year-old girl has scattered, 1- to 3-mm, light brown macules on her face, trunk, and extremities. These macules become more numerous in the summer months but fade over the winter. Each of these macules is best described as

○ (A) Vitiligo
○ (B) Lentigo

○ (C) Freckle
○ (D) Nevus
○ (E) Melasma

20. A 19-year-old male has facial lesions consisting of 0.3- to 0.9-cm comedones, erythematous papules, nodules, and pustules. These lesions have waxed and waned for several years. Other family members have been affected by this condition at a similar age. The lesions became worse on a cruise to the Caribbean. Which of the following organisms is most likely to play a key role in the pathogenesis of these lesions?

○ (A) *Staphylococcus aureus*
○ (B) Herpes simplex virus type 1
○ (C) Group A β-hemolytic *Streptococcus*
○ (D) *Mycobacterium leprae*
○ (E) *Propionibacterium acnes*

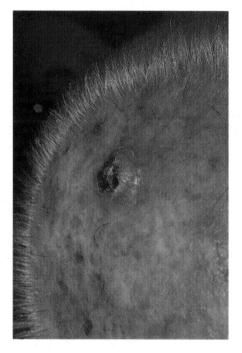

21. Five years after an orthotopic heart transplant, a 53-year-old male has developed multiple skin lesions on his face and upper trunk that are similar to the one depicted here. Some of the larger lesions have ulcerated. A biopsy of one of these skin lesions is most likely to show

○ (A) Psoriasis
○ (B) Lichen planus
○ (C) Dermatofibroma
○ (D) Squamous cell carcinoma
○ (E) Erythema multiforme

22. A 39-year-old female has developed 0.2- to 1-cm vesicles and bullae on her skin over the past week. These lesions are located over her scalp, both axillae, groin, and knees. Many ruptured lesions have left a shallow erosion with a dried crust of serum. A biopsy of an axillary lesion shows epidermal acantholysis, with the formation of an intraepidermal blister. The basal cell layer is intact. Which of the following additional tests is most likely to explain the pathogenesis of her disease?

○ (A) Immunofluorescent staining of skin with anti-IgG
○ (B) Viral culture of fluid from a skin vesicle
○ (C) Determination of serum IgE level
○ (D) Positive cytokeratin immunostaining of skin
○ (E) Darkfield microscopy of vesicular fluid

23. A 25-year-old male with acute respiratory failure has a bronchoalveolar lavage that yields *Pneumocystis carinii* by direct fluorescent antigen testing. After initiation of therapy, he develops "target lesions" composed of red macules with a pale, vesicular center. The lesions are 2 to 5 cm in diameter, and they are symmetrically distributed over his upper arms and chest. Which of the following drugs is most likely to be implicated in the development of his skin lesions?

○ (A) Hydrocortisone
○ (B) Diphenhydramine
○ (C) Trimethoprim-sulfamethoxazole
○ (D) Acetaminophen
○ (E) Dapsone

For each of the clinical histories in questions 24 and 25, match the most closely associated lesion involving the skin:

(A) Basal cell carcinoma
(B) Condyloma acuminatum
(C) Dermatofibroma
(D) Intradermal nevus
(E) Keratoacanthoma
(F) Melanoma
(G) Molluscum contagiosum
(H) Neurofibroma
(I) Seborrheic keratosis
(J) Squamous cell carcinoma
(K) Verruca vulgaris
(L) Xanthoma

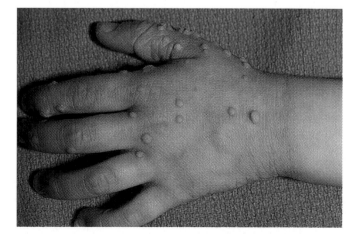

24. The lesions seen here on the hand of a 28-year-old male have been slowly enlarging for the past 3 years. They have not changed in color. There is no pain associated with these lesions. (   )

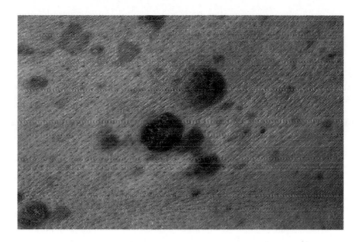

25. Biopsy of one of the lesions pictured here from the trunk of a 75-year-old male shows sheets of lightly pigmented basaloid cells that surround keratin-filled cysts. This lesion is sharply demarcated from the surrounding epidermis.

26. After a week in the hospital for treatment of an upper respiratory infection complicated by pneumonia, a 43-year-old female develops skin lesions that are 2 to 4 mm in diameter. These lesions are red, papulovesicular, oozing, and crusted and are located on her trunk and extremities. The lesions begin to disappear after she is discharged from the hospital a week later. What is the most likely pathogenesis for her skin lesions?

- ○ (A) Type I hypersensitivity
- ○ (B) Drug reaction
- ○ (C) Bacterial septicemia
- ○ (D) Photosensitivity
- ○ (E) Human papillomavirus infection

27. An enlarging, conical "cutaneous horn" that has been present for more than a year projects 0.5 cm from a 0.7-cm base on the left lateral cheek of the face of a 58-year-old farmer. This lesion is excised, and microscopic examination shows basal cell hyperplasia. Some of the basal cells show nuclear atypicalities. This is associated with marked hyperkeratosis and parakeratosis. Which of the following lesions best accounts for these findings?

- ○ (A) Verruca vulgaris
- ○ (B) Keratoacanthoma
- ○ (C) Dysplastic nevus
- ○ (D) Actinic keratosis
- ○ (E) Seborrheic keratosis

ANSWERS

1. **(D)** This is psoriasis, a chronic skin condition with marked epithelial hyperplasia and parakeratotic scaling. Nail changes such as yellow-brown discoloration, pitting, dimpling, and separation of the nail plate from the nail bed (i.e., onycholysis) affect about one third of patients. Other manifestations of psoriasis include arthritis (resembling rheumatoid arthritis), myopathy, enteropathy, and spondylitic heart disease. Gastrointestinal mucosal involvement with hemorrhage is not a feature of psoriasis. A friction rub from a fibrinous pericarditis does not occur with psoriasis, because mesothelial surfaces are not involved, and renal failure is not typically the result of psoriasis either. **BP6 701   PBD6 1198–1199**

2. **(C)** The driving force behind a worldwide increase in melanoma has been increased sun exposure. The Australian population is mainly derived from light-skinned Europeans who migrated to Australia. Indigenous, dark-skinned, populations do not have the same risk. **BP6 711   PBD6 1177**

3. **(D)** He has findings typical of acanthosis nigricans, a cutaneous marker for benign and malignant neoplasms. The skin lesions often precede signs and symptoms of associated cancers. They are believed to arise from the action of epidermal growth-promoting factors made by neoplasms. The rashes that develop with SLE are the result of antigen-antibody complex deposition and often exhibit photosensitivity. Skin lesions of mastocytosis in adults often exhibit urticaria. There are a variety of skin lesions with AIDS, including disseminated infections and a variety of papulosquamous dermatoses, although not pigmented lesions. Involvement of the skin with Langerhans cell histiocytoses typically occurs in children and produces reddish papules or nodules or erythematous scaling plaques because of the histiocytic infiltrates in the dermis. **PBD6 1180**

4. **(B)** This is a malignant melanoma with irregular borders and variability of pigmentation. Any change in a pigmented lesion suggests the possibility of melanoma. A few melanomas are familial, arising from such conditions as dysplastic nevus syndrome. However, most melanomas occur sporadically and are related to sun exposure, as may occur in a lifeguard. **BP6 711–712   PBD6 1177–1179**

5. **(D)** The clinical and histologic findings are typical of dermatitis herpetiformis. The IgA or IgG antibodies formed against the gliadin protein in gluten that is ingested cross-react with reticulin. This is a component of the anchoring fibrils that attach the epidermal basement membrane to the superficial dermis. This explains the localization of the IgA to the tips of dermal papillae and the site of inflammation. A gluten-free diet may relieve the symptoms. **BP6 704   PBD6 1204–1205**

6. **(H)** Impetigo is a superficial infection of skin that produces shallow erosions. These erosions are covered with exuded serum that dries to give the characteristic honey-colored crust. Cultures of the lesions of impetigo usually grow coagulase-positive *S. aureus* or group A β-hemolytic *Streptococcus*. The lesions are highly infectious. **PBD6 1210**

7. **(B)** Actinic keratoses are premalignant lesions related to sun exposure. Decreasing dietary fat is always a good idea, but this will not do much for your face. Drugs can cause acute eczematous dermatitis and erythema multiforme in many cases. Hydrocortisone can alleviate the symptoms of many dermatologic conditions, but it cannot reverse actinic damage. Older persons are more likely to have actinic keratoses because of more cumulative sun exposure, not because of aging alone.

BP6 707   PBD6 1184

8. **(E)** The small scabies mites burrow through the stratum corneum to produce the linear lesions, and the mites along with their eggs and feces produce intense pruritus. Scabies is easily transmitted by contact and typically occurs in local outbreaks. *I. dammini* is the tick that is the vector for *B. burgdorferi* organisms that cause Lyme disease with erythema chronicum migrans. *T. corporis* is a superficial fungal infection that can produce erythema and crusting. The erythematous macules and pustules of impetigo in children are often caused by staphylococcal and group A streptococcal infection. Molluscum contagiosum is a poxvirus that produces a localized, firm nodule.

PBD6 1211-1212

9. **(C)** The pink cytoplasmic inclusions called "molluscum bodies" are characteristic for this lesion. Immunocompromised persons may have multiple lesions and larger lesions. The infectious agent is a poxvirus. Human papillomavirus (not a toad) is implicated in the appearance of verruca vulgaris, or the common wart. *S. aureus* is implicated in the formation of the lesions of impetigo. Disseminated fungal infections are uncommon except in immunocompromised patients. Herpes zoster virus is the agent that results in "shingles," characterized by a dermatomal distribution of clear, painful vesicles.

PBD6 1209

10. **(C)** This is a subepidermal bulla. Bullous pemphigoid results from antibody-mediated damage to the basal cell–basement membrane attachment plaques (i.e., hemidesmosomes). The bulla formed is subepidermal. In contrast, the antibodies in pemphigus vulgaris attack the desmosomes that attach the epidermal keratinocytes together. Loosening of these junctions leads to acantholysis, and an intraepidermal blister is formed just above the basal layer (suprabasal). In impetigo, there is infection of the superficial layer of the skin, and the blister is just under the stratum corneum (subcorneal). In urticaria, the allergic reaction causes increased vascular permeability in dermal capillaries. This produces superficial dermal edema, not a bulla.

BP6 702-704   PBD6 1201-1204

11. **(B)** Extension deep into the reticular dermis is indicative of vertical (nodular) growth. When a melanoma exhibits a nodular growth pattern, rather than a radial pattern, there is a high likelihood that a clone of neoplastic cells has arisen that is more aggressive and is more likely to metastasize. Although there is a lymphocytic response to this tumor, it is not sufficient to destroy or contain it completely. Most melanomas are sporadic, nonfamilial, and related to sun exposure. Melanomas of the eye are much less common than melanomas of the skin. Benign skin nevi do not have a tendency to become malignant.

BP6 711-712   PBD6 1177-1179

12. **(E)** This patient has the classic "pruritic, purple, polygonal papules" of lichen planus, with the distinctive bandlike infiltrate of lymphocytes at the dermal-epidermal junction. The lesions of lichen planus are typically self-limited, although the course can run several years. Oral lesions may persist longer. There is no risk for malignancy. Although a lymphocytic infiltrate is present, an infectious or autoimmune cause is not implicated. A drug eruption should not last this long. Lesions of erythema multiforme are more likely to follow infections, drugs, autoimmune diseases, and malignancies.

BP6 702   PBD6 1199-1200

13. **(B)** Superficial dermatophyte infections are common and are caused by a variety of fungal species, including *Trichophyton*, *Epidermophyton*, and *Microsporum*. Those that involve the foot produce the condition known as *Tinea pedis*.

PBD6 1210

14. **(G)** Tinea versicolor is a relatively common condition caused by a superficial fungal infection with *M. furfur*. The lesions can be lighter or darker than the surrounding skin.

PBD6 1210

15. **(A)** He has "hives," or urticaria, from an allergy to an antigen in nuts. This causes a type I hypersensitivity reaction whereby IgE antibodies are bound to the IgE receptor on mast cells. IgE-sensitized mast cells degranulate when the antigen is encountered. Neutrophils may become attracted to this site, but they are not the sensitized cells. Natural killer cells mediate antibody-dependent cell-mediated cytotoxicity (ADCC) and lyse major histocompatability complex (MHC) class I–deficient target cells. Plasma cells secrete the IgE antibodies but do not release the mediators for allergic reactions.

BP6 698-699   PBD6 1194

16. **(D)** The clinical appearance, distribution, and occurrence in two siblings suggests that these lesions represent the dysplastic nevus syndrome. Dysplastic nevi are precursors of malignant melanoma.

BP6 710   PBD6 1176-1177

17. **(E)** The gross and microscopic appearance is typical of keratoacanthoma. These are self-limited lesions that often regress on their own. Those that do not regress should be suspected of being squamous cell carcinomas. The typical squamous cell carcinoma does not regress. Basal cell carcinomas may also be raised lesions, but they also do not regress. A seborrheic keratosis tends to be a flatter (although raised), rough-surfaced, pigmented lesion that slowly enlarges over time. An actinic keratosis tends to be a flat, pigmented lesion that is tan to brown to red.

BP6 705-706   PBD6 1181

18. **(E)** Basal cell carcinomas arise as pearly papules on the sun-exposed parts of the skin, particularly the face. They slowly infiltrate surrounding tissues, gradually enlarging. Although it rarely metastasizes, a basal cell carcinoma can have serious local effects, particularly in the region of the eye. Melanomas are usually pigmented, although some

are not, and they are composed of polygonal or spindle cells that tend to grow in sheets and infiltrate to produce a grossly irregular border to the lesion. A dermatofibroma is a benign lesion of the dermis composed of cells resembling fibroblasts. An actinic keratosis is a premalignant lesion of the epidermis, without invasion. A nevus is a small, localized, benign lesion.
BP6 709   PBD6 1186-1187

19.   **(C)** Freckles are relatively common. Persons with a light complexion or red hair are more likely to have them. These lesions may be cosmetically unpleasant, but they have no significance. The areas of skin known as vitiligo are depigmented. Lentigo describes brown macules whose pigmentation is not related to sun exposure. Melasma is most often a masklike area of facial hyperpigmentation associated with pregnancy. Nevi do not wax and wane with sun exposure.
PBD6 1174

20.   **(E)** He has acne vulgaris. Teenagers and young adults are more often affected than other age groups, and males are more often affected than females. *P. acnes* breaks down sebaceous gland oils to produce irritative fatty acids, and this may promote the process. *S. aureus* and group A streptococci are implicated in the inflammatory skin condition known as impetigo. Herpes simplex virus produces vesicular skin eruptions. *M. leprae* is the causative agent for leprosy, which is a chronic condition that can produce depigmentation and areas of skin anesthesia.
PBD6 1206-1207

21.   **(D)** Risk factors for squamous cell carcinoma include ultraviolet light exposure, scarring from burn injury, irradiation, and immunosuppression. This patient was immunosuppressed to prevent graft rejection. Squamous cell carcinomas also arise in rare disorders of DNA repair, such as xeroderma pigmentosa. Psoriasis is an inflammatory dermatosis that can be associated with underlying arthritis, myopathy, enteropathy, or spondylitic heart disease. Lichen planus is a self-limited inflammatory disorder that manifests as "purple, pruritic, polygonal papules," not as elevated ulcerated lesions. A dermatofibroma is typically solitary, firm, and dermal in location. Erythema multiforme is a hypersensitivity response to infections or drugs. These lesions take multiple forms, including papules, macules, vesicles, and bullae.
BP6 708   PBD6 1184-1186

22.   **(A)** These lesions are probably pemphigus vulgaris, a rare form of type II hypersensitivity reaction. In this disorder, IgG autoantibodies to the intercellular cement substance are formed. They disrupt intercellular bridges, causing the epidermal cells to detach from each other (i.e., acantholysis). This action then causes the formation of an intraepidermal blister. Staining with anti-IgG illuminates intercellular junctions at sites of incipient acantholysis. Herpes simplex viral infections can produce crops of vesicles, but such a wide distribution would be unusual. Type I

hypersensitivity with urticaria does not produce an acantholytic vesicle. Keratinocytes, being epithelial, always are positive for cytokeratin. Darkfield microscopy is used almost exclusively to find spirochetes in cases of syphilis.
BP6 702-703   PBD6 1201-1202

23.   **(C)** He has erythema multiforme, a hypersensitivity response to certain infections and drugs. It can follow ingestion of drugs such as sulfonamides and penicillin. Other inciting factors include herpes simplex virus, mycoplasmal, and fungal infections; malignant diseases; and collagen vascular diseases such as SLE. Hydrocortisone and diphenhydramine are often used to treat skin eruptions. Acetaminophen and dapsone are less likely to produce erythema multiforme, but many drugs can cause skin rashes and eruptions.
BP6 700   PBD6 1197-1198

24.   **(K)** Such "warts" are common. They are the result of infection with one of many types of human papillomavirus. They do not become malignant.
BP6 705-707   PBD6 1208-1209

25.   **(I)** These flat, round, pigmented, and sharply demarcated lesions are benign tumors called seborrheic keratosis. They are made up of pigmented basaloid cells. Seborrheic keratosis is common in older persons. These lesions gradually enlarge, are not painful, and do not ulcerate. They mainly produce a cosmetic problem.
BP6 705-706   PBD6 1179-1180

26.   **(B)** The time course fits best with a drug reaction producing an acute erythematous dermatitis. Urticaria from type I hypersensitivity is not as severe or as long lasting. Sepsis rarely involves the skin with an erythematous dermatitis. Photosensitivity may be enhanced by drugs, but ultraviolet light is the key component in light that produces photodermatitis. This is not likely to be encountered in indoor lighting in the hospital room. Human papillomavirus infection is associated with formation of verruca vulgaris (i.e., common wart).
BP6 699   PBD6 1194-1196

27.   **(D)** Actinic keratosis occurs on sun-exposed areas and is considered a precursor of squamous cell carcinoma. When the atypical basal cells occupy the entire thickness of the epidermis, the lesion transforms into a carcinoma in situ. The presence of a hyperkeratotic layer is characteristic. Occasionally, so much keratin is produced that a "cutaneous horn" is formed. A verruca vulgaris may also be a raised lesion, but it is usually more pebbly, and there is no squamous atypia. Superficial epidermal cells show vacuolation or koilocytosis. A keratoacanthoma is a dome-shaped nodule with a central keratin-filled crater that is surrounded by epithelial cells. Microscopically, it may mimic a squamous cell carcinoma. A dysplastic nevus is typically a flat, pigmented lesion. A seborrheic keratosis can be raised, but it usually appears as a coinlike plaque.
BP6 707   PBD6 1184-1185

CHAPTER 26

Bones, Joints, and Soft Tissue Tumors

BP6 Chapter 21 - The Musculoskeletal
System
PBD6 Chapter 28 - Bones, Joints, and Soft
Tissue Tumors

1. A 60-year-old female presents with lower back pain of 1 month's duration. A routine urinalysis, complete blood count, and serum electrolyte panel are all unremarkable. Twenty years earlier, she was treated for Hodgkin disease with abdominal irradiation and chemotherapy, and there has been no evidence of a recurrence during regular follow-up visits. Magnetic resonance imaging (MRI) reveals a 10 × 15 cm, ovoid mass of the left retroperitoneum. The condition most likely is

- (A) Desmoid tumor
- (B) Recurrent Hodgkin disease
- (C) Rhabdomyosarcoma
- (D) Leiomyosarcoma
- (E) Malignant fibrous histiocytoma

2. A 60-year-old male with a diagnosis of chronic myeloid leukemia is treated with intensive chemotherapy. He goes into remission but develops inflammation of the wrist joint. Aspiration of the swollen wrist joint reveals needle-shaped crystals. Which of the following processes played an important role in the pathogenesis of joint inflammation?

- (A) Damage to the articular cartilage by chemotherapeutic agents
- (B) Infiltration of the synovium by leukemic cells
- (C) Synovial proliferation from cytokine secretion by leukemic cells
- (D) Excessive production of uric acid from dying leukemic cells
- (E) Hemorrhages into the joint because of deranged platelet function

3. If you were an osteoclast in a callus near the cortex of the right tibial diaphysis of a skier sitting in the lodge because of a tibial fracture, what would you want to do?

- (A) Form collagen
- (B) Resorb bone
- (C) Synthesize osteoid
- (D) Elaborate cytokines
- (E) Divide

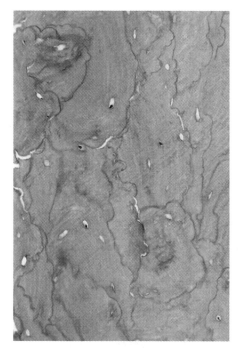

4. A 70-year-old male complains of right hip and thigh pain of several months' duration. Radiographs of the pelvis and right leg reveal sclerotic, thickened cortical bone with a narrowed joint space near the acetabulum. The serum alkaline phosphatase level is elevated, but serum calcium and phosphorus concentrations are normal. The microscopic appearance of a bone biopsy is illustrated. The most likely condition accounting for these findings is

- (A) Osteochondroma
- (B) Osteomalacia
- (C) Osteoarthritis
- (D) Osteitis fibrosa cystica
- (E) Osteitis deformans (i.e., Paget disease)

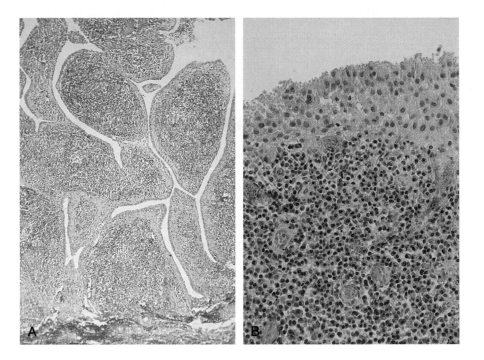

5. A 35-year-old female has experienced malaise, fatigue, and joint pain for several months. The joint involvement is symmetric, and most of the affected joints are in the hands and feet. The involved joints are swollen and warm to the touch. She has progressive loss of joint motion, along with a "swan neck" joint deformity and ulnar deviation of the hands. Examination of the excised joint capsule tissue is seen microscopically in the above figure. Which of the following laboratory test findings is most likely to be found?

○ (A) Positive *Borrelia burgdorferi* serology
○ (B) Positive acid-fast stain of joint tissue
○ (C) Positive rheumatoid factor in serum
○ (D) Hyperuricemia
○ (E) Calcium pyrophosphate crystals in a joint aspirate

6. A 79-year-old male was diagnosed with Paget disease of bone many years ago. Sites of involvement include vertebral bodies, ischium, and skull. Which of the following complications is he most likely to suffer as a result of this condition?

○ (A) Ankylosing spondylitis
○ (B) Osteoid osteoma
○ (C) Fibrous dysplasia
○ (D) Osteosarcoma
○ (E) Enchondroma

7. A 6-year-old boy complains of some discomfort in his right upper neck and a firm, 5-cm mass is palpable that is not painful or warm. The histologic appearance of this mass after a biopsy is shown in the following figure. Which of the following immunohistochemical stains is most likely to be positive in this lesion?

○ (A) Vimentin
○ (B) Neuron-specific enolase

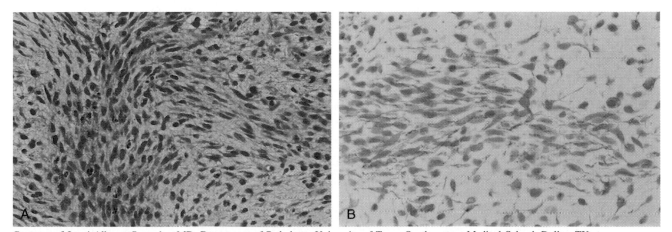

Courtesy of Jorgé Albores-Saavedra, MD. Department of Pathology, University of Texas Southwestern Medical School, Dallas, TX.

○ (C) Cytokeratin
○ (D) Factor VIII
○ (E) CD3

8. Three weeks after a contusion to the upper left arm, a 26-year-old male develops a painful, 2-cm, well-circumscribed, subcutaneous mass. Which of the following lesions do you most expect to be present?

○ (A) Malignant fibrous histiocytoma
○ (B) Organizing abscess
○ (C) Nodular fasciitis
○ (D) Superficial fibromatosis
○ (E) Lipoma

9. Several days after an episode of urethritis, a 28-year-old male develops acute pain and swelling of his left knee. A joint aspirate from the knee reveals numerous neutrophils, and the Gram stain of the fluid demonstrates gram-negative intracellular diplococci. No crystals are seen. Which of the following infectious agents is most likely responsible for this condition?

○ (A) *Borrelia burgdorferi*
○ (B) *Treponema pallidum*
○ (C) *Neisseria gonorrhoeae*
○ (D) *Staphylococcus aureus*
○ (E) *Haemophilus influenzae*

10. In a 75-year-old male, which of the following processes contributes most to the occurrence of osteoporosis?

○ (A) Decreased production of osteoid by osteoblasts
○ (B) Increased resorption of bone by osteoclasts
○ (C) Increased sensitivity of bone to the effects of parathyroid hormone
○ (D) Increased secretion of interleukin (IL)-1, IL-6, and tumor necrosis factor-α (TNF-α) by monocytes in the bone marrow
○ (E) Synthesis of chemically abnormal osteoid

11. A 47-year-old male presents with a 4-month history of dull pain in the mid-section of his right thigh. The pain is constant and is made slightly worse with movement. A radiograph reveals no fracture, but there appears to be an ill-defined soft tissue mass. MRI shows a $10 \times 8 \times 7$ cm mass below the quadriceps. The lesion most likely is

○ (A) Nodular fasciitis
○ (B) Liposarcoma
○ (C) Osteosarcoma
○ (D) Rhabdomyosarcoma
○ (E) Hemangioma

12. A 66-year-old male has experienced pain about the left knee for the past 6 weeks. No lesion is palpable, and there is no loss of range of motion. He can recall no trauma to his leg. MRI reveals a fairly well circumscribed, 4-cm mass superior and inferior to the patella in soft tissue, without bony erosion. A biopsy reveals a biphasic pattern of spindle cells and epithelial cells forming glands. Karyotypic analysis of tumor cells shows a t(X;18) translation. The most likely diagnosis is

○ (A) Leiomyosarcoma
○ (B) Synovial sarcoma
○ (C) Desmoid tumor
○ (D) Mesothelioma
○ (E) Osteoblastoma

13. After a minor fall, a 63-year-old woman sustains a complete right femoral neck fracture. Of the following conditions, the most significant contributing factor for this fracture is

○ (A) Chronic osteomyelitis
○ (B) Vitamin D deficiency
○ (C) Postmenopausal bone loss
○ (D) Parathyroid adenoma
○ (E) Multiple myeloma

14. A 51-year-old man has pain in the right knee, lower back, right distal fifth finger, and neck. He notices that the joints feel stiff in the morning. Some joint crepitus is audible on moving the knee. Serum calcium, phosphorus, alkaline phosphatase, and uric acid levels are normal. The most likely diagnosis for this constellation of findings is

○ (A) Paget disease of bone
○ (B) Osteoarthritis
○ (C) Gout
○ (D) Multiple myeloma
○ (E) Rheumatoid arthritis

15. A 30-year-old male presented with abdominal cramps and bloody diarrhea. Stool cultures were positive for *Shigella flexneri*. The episode resolved spontaneously within a week after its onset. Six weeks later, he contacted his physician again because of increasingly severe low back pain. Examination revealed stiffness of the lumbar joints and tenderness affecting the sacroiliac joints. He was treated with nonsteroidal anti-inflammatory drugs. Several months later the back pain recurred, and he complained of redness of the right eye and blurred vision. Which of the following laboratory investigations would most likely be positive in this patient?

○ (A) Rheumatoid factor
○ (B) Isolation of *Chlamydia trachomatis* from the conjunctiva
○ (C) Antibodies against Epstein-Barr virus (EBV)
○ (D) HLA-B27 genotype
○ (E) Antibodies against *Borrelia burgdorferi*

16. A 7-year-old boy incurred an open compound fracture of the right tibia and fibula in a fall from the barn loft to the floor below. The fracture was set by external manipulation, and the skin wound was sutured, but nothing more was done. One year later, he continues to have pain in his right leg, and a draining sinus tract has developed. A radiograph of the lower leg is most likely to show

○ (A) Osteolysis with osteosclerosis
○ (B) A mass with bony destruction
○ (C) A cortical nidus with surrounding sclerosis
○ (D) Involucrum and sequestrum
○ (E) Soft tissue swelling

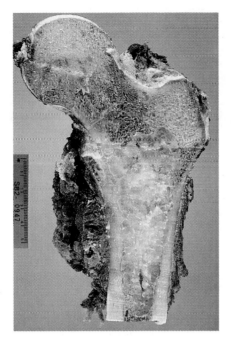

17. A 45-year-old male has experienced pain about the hip and upper thigh for several months. A radiograph reveals an upper femoral mass lesion. The proximal femur is excised and on sectioning has the gross appearance shown here. The cells that proliferate in this lesion are most likely to be

O (A) Osteoblasts
O (B) Chondroblasts
O (C) Osteoclasts
O (D) Primitive neuroectodermal cells
O (E) Plasma cells

18. An 18-year-old male presents with pain about the right knee. There are no physical examination findings other than local pain over the region of the distal femur. A radiograph demonstrates an ill-defined mass involving the metaphyseal region of the distal right femur, and there is elevation of the adjacent periosteum. A bone biopsy shows large, hyperchromatic, pleomorphic spindle cells forming an osteoid matrix. These findings are most typical for

O (A) Ewing sarcoma
O (B) Chondrosarcoma
O (C) Giant cell tumor of bone
O (D) Fibrous dysplasia
O (E) Osteosarcoma

19. A 38-year-old man who is otherwise healthy has experienced chronic leg pain for several months. A radiograph of the right lower leg shows a 4-cm cystic area in the right tibial diaphysis, without erosion of the cortex or soft tissue mass. Biopsy reveals increased numbers of osteoclasts in this lesion, along with fibroblast proliferation. The underlying condition that best accounts for these findings is

O (A) Secondary hyperparathyroidism
O (B) Paget disease of bone
O (C) Chronic osteomyelitis
O (D) Parathyroid adenoma
O (E) Giant cell tumor of bone

20. A 9-year-old boy has pain in the right hip region. A radiograph reveals changes of osteomyelitis involving the femoral metaphysis, with extension to the subperiosteal region and abscess formation. Which of the following organisms is most often responsible for this clinical picture?

O (A) *Staphylococcus aureus*
O (B) *Haemophilus influenzae*
O (C) *Salmonella*, nontyphi
O (D) Group B *Streptococcus*
O (E) *Neisseria gonorrhoeae*

21. A 37-year-old female has a contracture involving the third digit of her left hand that prevents her from fully extending this finger. The lesion has gradually developed over the past 6 months. A firm, hard, cordlike, 1 × 3 cm area is palpable beneath the skin of the left palm. Histologically, this mass is most likely to be composed of

O (A) Atypical spindle cells
O (B) Granulation tissue
O (C) Lipoblasts
O (D) Collagen
O (E) Dystrophic calcification

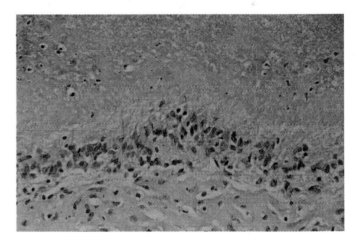

22. A 57-year-old female is found on physical examination to have bilateral ulnar deviation, along with "swan-neck" deformities of several fingers of her hands. She states that these deformities have been increasing in severity for the past 10 years. She presents with a subcutaneous nodule on the ulnar aspect of the right forearm. A biopsy of the nodule shows the microscopic appearance that is depicted. Which of the following mechanisms plays a primary role in the causation of joint injury in this disease?

O (A) Activation of neutrophils by phagocytosis of urate crystals
O (B) Inflammation of synovium caused by infection with *Borrelia burgdorferi*

○ (C) Autoimmune attack by CD4⁺ T cells
○ (D) Synthesis of antibodies against HLA-B27 antigen
○ (E) Granulomatous response to long-standing *T. pallidum* infection

For each of the patient histories in questions 23 through 25, match the most closely associated bone tumor or tumor-like condition:

(A) Brown tumor of bone
(B) Chondrosarcoma
(C) Enchondroma
(D) Ewing sarcoma
(E) Fibrous dysplasia
(F) Giant cell tumor
(G) Metastatic carcinoma
(H) Osteoblastoma
(I) Osteochondroma
(J) Osteoid osteoma
(K) Osteosarcoma
(L) Plasmacytoma

23. When a 12-year-old girl complains of episodic knee pain, her mother gives her aspirin. However, persistence of these symptoms results in a radiograph being taken, which shows a well-defined, 1-cm lucent area located in the proximal tibia that is surrounded by a thin rim of bony sclerosis. (   )

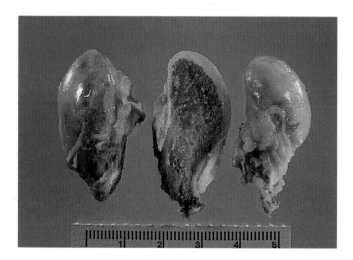

24. Some local pain about the right knee of a 23-year-old man results in a radiograph being taken, which shows a 3-cm, broad-based excrescence projecting from the upper tibial metaphysis. The lesion is excised. The gross sectioned lesion is shown here. (   )

25. A 13-year-old boy presents with pain in the right leg, and a radiograph of the right femur reveals an expansile 6-cm mass in the diaphysis. Biopsy of this mass reveals sheets of primitive cells with small, fairly uniform nuclei and only scant cytoplasm. Karyotypic analysis of tumor cells reveals a t(11;22) translocation. (   )

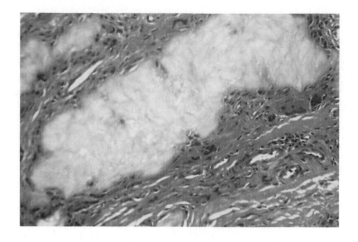

26. A 51-year-old man has noticed episodes of intense local pain lasting for several hours in his left foot. Each episode follows a meal in which he consumes a bottle of wine. Physical examination identifies the metatarsophalangeal joint as the focus of this pain, but there is minimal loss of joint mobility. A 1-cm subcutaneous nodule present on the extensor surface of the left elbow is excised and has the microscopic appearance seen here. An aspirate from the left metatarsophalangeal joint is most likely to yield

○ (A) Monosodium urate crystals
○ (B) Calcium pyrophosphate crystals
○ (C) Hydroxyapatite crystals
○ (D) Cholesterol crystals
○ (E) Charcot-Leyden crystals

27. Which of the following strategies can provide the best overall long-term reduction in risk of fracture from osteoporosis in women?

○ (A) Supplement the diet with calcium and vitamin D after menopause.
○ (B) Begin estrogen replacement therapy after a fracture.
○ (C) Avoid corticosteroid therapy for any inflammatory conditions.
○ (D) Increase bone mass with exercise in childhood and young adulthood.
○ (E) Limit alcohol use, and avoid use of tobacco.

28. A 15-year-old male experiences severe pain in his right leg after a gymnastic floor exercise. Radiographs reveal a pathologic fracture across a discrete, 3-cm lower femoral diaphyseal lesion that has central lucency with a thin sclerotic rim. A bone biopsy of the affected region shows trabeculae of woven bone scattered in a background of fibroblastic proliferation. The lesion is completely intramedullary and well circumscribed. The most likely bone lesion to account for these findings is

○ (A) Osteoid osteoma
○ (B) Enchondroma
○ (C) Osteogenic sarcoma
○ (D) Ewing sarcoma
○ (E) Monostotic fibrous dysplasia

29. A neonate is septic, with a temperature of 38.9°C. Examination reveals irritability on moving the left leg. The baby was born at term with normal birth weight. No congenital anomalies are identified. A radiograph of the left leg shows changes suggesting acute osteomyelitis in the upper end of the left femur. The most likely cause of this clinical picture is infection with

○ (A) *Staphylococcus aureus*
○ (B) *Neisseria gonorrhoeae*
○ (C) Group B streptococcus
○ (D) *Salmonella* species
○ (E) *Streptococcus pneumoniae*

30. A 43-year-old female had chronic arthritis involving the left shoulder and right hip. Several months later, she developed pain in her right knee and ankle, but this resolved. A radiograph demonstrates extensive erosion of the humeral head. Biopsy of synovium reveals a marked lymphoplasmacytic infiltrate and arteritis with endothelial proliferation. The infectious agent most likely responsible for these findings is

○ (A) Group B streptococcus
○ (B) *Neisseria gonorrhoeae*
○ (C) *Treponema pallidum*
○ (D) *Borrelia burgdorferi*
○ (E) *Mycobacterium tuberculosis*

31. At the lateral right wrist of a 55-year-old male is a painless nodule with overlying ulcerated skin. Beneath the eroded skin is a chalky white deposit of soft material surrounded by erythematous soft tissue. He has a history of episodes of acute arthritis affecting the ankle, heels, and knee joints. This clinical picture and gross appearance is most consistent with which of the following lesions?

○ (A) Tophus
○ (B) Pannus
○ (C) Osteophyte
○ (D) Purulent exudate
○ (E) Erythema chronicum migrans

32. A soft, 2-cm nodule is palpable in the subcutis of the right flank of a 32-year-old male. The excised mass is circumscribed and has a uniformly yellow cut surface. Your best advice to this patient is

○ (A) This mass is benign and will not recur.
○ (B) More of these lesions will develop over time.
○ (C) Metastases are likely to regional lymph nodes.
○ (D) Other members of your family should be examined for similar lesions.
○ (E) Antibiotic therapy will be needed.

33. A 30-year-old man has experienced pain in the region of his left knee for more than 1 month. A radiograph shows a 7-cm mass involving the distal femoral epiphyseal region, and a biopsy shows multinucleated cells in a stroma predominantly composed of spindle-shaped mononuclear cells. The most likely diagnosis is

○ (A) Ewing sarcoma
○ (B) Osteoblastoma
○ (C) Enchondroma
○ (D) Osteitis fibrosa cystica
○ (E) Giant cell tumor

34. A 55-year-old, previously healthy man has had episodes of pain and swelling of the right first metatarsal-phalangeal joint for the past year. These flare-ups usually occur after consumption of alcohol, typically port wine. A joint aspirate during one of these episodes yields needle-shaped crystals and many neutrophils in a small amount of fluid. Which of the following laboratory test findings is most likely?

○ (A) Increased serum parathyroid hormone level
○ (B) Elevated serum urea nitrogen level
○ (C) Hyperuricemia
○ (D) Markedly elevated levels of serum transaminases
○ (E) Elevated rheumatoid factor titer

35. A 39-year-old male has experienced back pain for several months, and a radiograph of the spine shows a compressed fracture at the L2 level. Computed tomography (CT) of the abdomen reveals an abscess involving the right psoas muscle. The most probable infectious cause for these findings is

○ (A) *Treponema pallidum*
○ (B) *Mycobacterium tuberculosis*
○ (C) *Streptococcus pyogenes*
○ (D) *Borrelia burgdorferi*
○ (E) *Cryptococcus neoformans*

For each of the clinical histories in questions 36 and 37, match the most closely associated laboratory finding:

(A) Antinuclear antibody titer in serum of 1:1024
(B) *B. burgdorferi* serologic positivity
(C) Calcium level of 14.5 mg/dL in serum
(D) *C. trachomatis*–positive urine culture
(E) Ferritin level of 7245 ng/mL in serum
(F) Hemoglobin S concentration of 96% on electrophoresis
(G) Parathyroid hormone level of 72 pg/mL in serum
(H) Rheumatoid factor titer in serum of 1:512
(I) Positive serologic test result for syphilis
(J) Urea nitrogen level of 110 mg/dL in serum
(K) Uric acid level of 15.8 mg/dL in serum

36. A 10-year-old girl has developed worsening pain in her knees and ankles for the past 3 months, and she now has difficulty walking. These joints are warm and swollen on examination. She recently developed a high fever and rash. Microbiologic culture of a joint aspirate from the right knee is negative. The joint fluid has increased numbers of lymphocytes but few neutrophils. This condition subsides over the next year, and she has no residual joint deformity. (   )

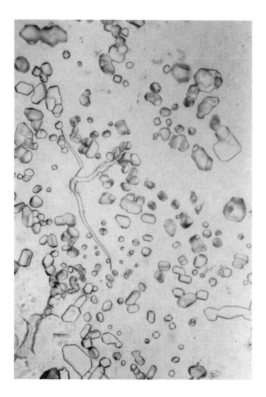

37. A 48-year-old male has had increasing left knee pain for several years. This joint is now slightly swollen and warm to touch. A joint aspirate is performed, and a cell count reveals increased neutrophils. A smear preparation of this fluid is depicted here. He experiences reduced knee joint mobility over the next several years. He also develops congestive heart failure, diabetes mellitus, and hepatic cirrhosis. (   )

38. A 75-year-old female presents with pain and limitation of movement affecting the right hip joint. These symptoms have been present for the past 15 years but have become disabling within the last 1 year. Physical examination reveals some tenderness and swelling of the distal interphalangeal joints of the right hand. A nodular bony outgrowth can be felt in the distal interphalangeal joint of the right index finger. All other joints are normal. There is no evidence of any systemic disease, and examination findings of cardiovascular and respiratory systems are unremarkable. A radiograph of the affected hip shows narrowing of joint space and subchondral sclerosis. Laboratory studies fail to reveal rheumatoid factor or antinuclear antibodies. Her serum uric acid level is 5 mg/dL. Which of the following factors is considered to be important in the pathogenesis of this disease?

○ (A) Infiltration of the synovial membrane by activated CD4$^+$ T cells
○ (B) A partial deficiency of the enzyme hypoxanthine guanine phosphoribosyl transferase (HGPRT)
○ (C) Inheritance of HLA-B27 antigens
○ (D) Defects in the function of chondrocytes of the articular cartilage
○ (E) Inherited defects in the synthesis of type I collagen

39. A 15-year-old male previously diagnosed with sickle cell anemia has been hospitalized in the past as a result of painful crises. He has had pain in his right hip region for the past week. A bone radiograph demonstrates changes of acute osteomyelitis in the metaphysis of the right proximal femur. Which of the following infectious agents is most likely responsible for these findings?

○ (A) *S. aureus*
○ (B) *N. gonorrhoeae*
○ (C) Group B *Streptococcus*
○ (D) *Salmonella* species
○ (E) *Klebsiella pneumoniae*

ANSWERS

1. (E) Although sarcomas in general are uncommon, malignant fibrous histiocytoma is one of the more common varieties of soft tissue sarcoma in adults, and it is the most common type of postirradiation sarcoma. A desmoid tumor is a deep fibromatosis of abdomen or extremities that can be locally aggressive or recur after excision. However, it is not a true neoplasm and does not metastasize. Rhabdomyosarcomas generally occur in the pediatric age group. A leiomyosarcoma is more likely to arise in the uterus or gastrointestinal tract.
BP6 693   PBD6 1264–1265

2. (D) This patient has secondary gout. When patients with leukemia, especially those with a high leukocyte count (as occurs in chronic myeloid leukemia), are treated with chemotherapeutic agents, there is massive lysis of nuclei, and large amounts of urate are produced. The hyperuricemia leads to deposition of crystals in the joint space that triggers a local inflammatory response. Articular cartilage damage can be seen in any form of chronic arthritis, but is a prominent feature of osteoarthritis. Synovial proliferation is also a nonspecific change that is prominent in rheumatoid arthritis. Joint hemorrhages can be seen in patients with thrombocytopenia, but they typically occur in patients with hemophilia.
BP6 683   PBD6 1254

3. (B) Bone remodeling is accomplished when osteoblasts produce new bone and osteoclasts resorb it. This is an ongoing process in all bones, but the process is speeded up in fracture callus. Collagen is produced by fibroblasts. Osteoid is produced by osteoblasts. Cytokines can be elaborated by macrophages and other inflammatory cells within the callus. Osteoprogenitor cells give rise to osteoblasts. Osteoclasts are derived from the same hematopoietic progenitor cells that give rise to macrophages and monocytes.
PBD6 1216–1218

4. (E) The biopsy shows a mosaic pattern of lamellar bone characteristic of Paget disease. This disease has three phases. Early in the course, there is a lytic phase, followed by the more classic mixed phase with osteosclerosis and

osteolysis, leading to the appearance of a "mosaic" of ir-regular bone. A sclerotic "burnt-out" phase then ensues. An osteochondroma is a tumor-like projection of bone capped by cartilage that protrudes from the metaphyseal region of a long bone. Osteomalacia results in osteopenia from vita-min D deficiency in an adult. Osteoarthritis produces chronic pain from joint erosion. Osteitis fibrosa cystica is seen with hyperparathyroidism.
BP6 673-674   PBD6 1225-1227

5.   (C) She has rheumatoid arthritis, a form of autoim-mune disease. The immunologically mediated damage leads to chronic inflammation with pannus formation that gradu-ally erodes and destroys the joints, resulting in joint defor-mity. Typically, the joint involvement is bilateral and sym-metric, and small joints are often involved. Lyme disease, caused by *B. burgdorferi* infection, can produce a chronic arthritis that can destroy cartilage, but larger joints are usually involved. Tuberculous arthritis is rare. Hyperurice-mia gives rise to gout. With gout, joint destruction and deformity is caused by tophaceous deposits of sodium urate crystals with a granulomatous inflammatory reaction. Cal-cium pyrophosphate crystal deposition disease, also known as pseudogout, may on occasion result in large, chalky, crystalline deposits; mostly, there is a neutrophilic re-sponse.
BP6 109-111   PBD6 1248-1251

6.   (D) In 5% to 10% of patients with severe polyostotic Paget disease, osteosarcomas can arise years later in bone involved by the disease. Ankylosing spondylitis involves the spine and carries no risk for malignancy. An osteoid osteoma is a small cortical bone lesion that can produce severe pain in children and young adults. Fibrous dysplasia is a focal developmental defect of bone seen at a younger age. An enchondroma does not arise in the setting of Paget disease.
BP6 675   PBD6 1225-1227

7.   (A) This is a rhabdomyosarcoma, the most common sarcoma in the pediatric age range. Sarcomas mark with antibody to vimentin, an intermediate cytoplasmic filament, by immunoperoxidase staining. Neuron-specific enolase is a marker of neoplasms with neural differentiation. Cytokera-tin is a marker for tumors of epithelial origin (e.g., carcino-mas). Factor VIII marks endothelial cells and related neo-plasms. CD3 is a T lymphocyte marker.
BP6 694   PBD6 1265-1266

8.   (C) This is a reactive fibroblastic proliferation that is seen in upper extremities and trunk of young adults, some-times occurring after trauma. Malignant fibrous histiocy-toma is a sarcoma of retroperitoneum and deep soft tissues of extremities in older adults. A contusion is not likely to lead to abscess formation because there is no disruption of the skin to allow entry of infectious agents. Superficial fibromatosis is a deforming lesion of fascial planes that develops over a long period. A lipoma is a common be-nign soft tissue tumor that is not painful and does not follow trauma.
BP6 692   PBD6 1261-1262

9.   (C) Gonorrhea should be considered the most likely cause of an acute suppurative arthritis in sexually active persons. *B. burgdorferi* causes Lyme disease, characterized by chronic arthritis that may mimic rheumatoid arthritis. Syphilitic gummas in the tertiary phase of syphilis may produce joint deformity. However, there is no preceding urethritis. Tertiary syphilis may be preceded years earlier by a syphilitic chancre. *S. aureus* is the most common cause for osteomyelitis, but the Gram stain should show gram-positive cocci. *H. influenzae* is a short, gram-negative rod that can cause osteomyelitis in children.
BP6 686   PBD6 1232-1233

10.   (A) With advancing age, the ability of osteoblasts to divide and to lay down osteoid is reduced, giving rise to senile osteoporosis. In contrast, postmenopausal osteoporo-sis is characterized by hormone-dependent acceleration of bone loss. Estrogen deficiency results in increased secretion of IL-1, IL-6, and TNF-α by monocytes-macrophages. These cytokines recruit and activate osteoclasts and hence resorption of bone is favored. In older females, therefore, bone loss is contributed to by both reduced synthesis and increased reabsorption. Nonhormonal drugs such as alen-dronate are designed to reduce osteoclast resorption of bone. There are no age-associated changes in the sensitivity to parathyroid hormone action or composition of osteoid.
BP6 669-670   PBD6 1223-1224

11.   (B) A large soft tissue mass suggests a malignancy, most likely a sarcoma. Liposarcomas are located in deep soft tissues, can be indolent, and reach a large size. They are the most common sarcomas of adulthood. Osteosarco-mas generally occur in young adults younger than 20 years of age and typically arise in the metaphysis. Nodular fasci-itis is a reactive fibroblastic lesion of young adults, most common on upper extremities and trunk, that can develop several weeks after local trauma. A rhabdomyosarcoma is most often a pediatric tumor of head and neck, genitouri-nary tract, or retroperitoneum. Hemangiomas, when present in extremities of adults, tend to be small, circumscribed lesions on the skin.
BP6 692   PBD6 1261

12.   (B) Synovial sarcomas account for 10% of all adult sarcomas and can be found around a joint or in deep soft tissues, because they arise from mesenchymal cells, not synovium. Most synovial sarcomas show the t(X;18) trans-location. Leiomyosarcomas do not have a biphasic pattern microscopically and are rarely seen in soft tissues. A des-moid tumor is a fibromatosis composed of fibroblasts and collagen. A mesothelioma can be biphasic, but it more typically arises in the pleura. An osteoblastoma is a bone neoplasm that arises in the epiphyseal region.
BP6 695   PBD6 1266-1267

13.   (C) Osteoporosis is the most common cause of frac-tures in postmenopausal women. The most significant bone loss occurs in the first decade after the onset of meno-pause, but bone loss continues relentlessly with age. A chronic osteomyelitis is not a common cause of fractures. Vitamin D deficiency may lead to osteomalacia in adults, but this condition is much less common than osteoporosis.

Metabolic bone disease from hyperparathyroidism is uncommon. The lytic lesions of myeloma can occur anywhere but most often in the vertebrae, where they may cause compression fractures.
BP6 669-670   PBD6 1222-1224

14.   **(B)** Osteoarthritis is a common problem of aging, and a variety of joints, from large, weight-bearing joints to small joints, can be involved. Joint stiffness in the morning is also a common feature. Paget disease does not cause arthritis and is marked by an increase in the alkaline phosphatase concentration. Gouty arthritis occurs in patients with elevated serum levels of uric acid. Multiple myeloma can produce lytic lesions in bone but does not typically involve joints. Rheumatoid arthritis can involve large or small joints. It is typically associated with symmetric involvement of small joints of hands and feet.
BP6 681-682   PBD6 1246-1248

15.   **(D)** This patient developed arthritis affecting the lumbar and sacroiliac joints several weeks after *Shigella* dysentery. He subsequently developed conjunctivitis and, most likely, uveitis. This symptom complex is classic of a cluster of related disorders called seronegative spondyloarthropathies. These include ankylosing spondylitis, Reiter syndrome, psoriatic arthritis, and enteropathic arthritis (this case). A feature common to all these is a very strong association with the HLA-B27 genotype. Despite some similarities with rheumatoid arthritis, these patients are invariably negative for rheumatoid factor. Urethritis caused by *C. trachomatis* can trigger Reiter syndrome, another form of seronegative spondyloarthropathy. However, such infection precedes the onset of arthritis. There is no relation between infection with *B. burgdorferi*, the causative agent of Lyme disease, and reactive arthritis in HLA-B27– positive individuals. Similarly, EBV infection is not a trigger for these disorders.
BP6 111   PBD6 1252

16.   **(D)** This patient has chronic osteomyelitis. The most likely sequence of events is the occurrence of a compound fracture that became infected by direct extension of bacteria into the bone. The subsequent care for this patient was inadequate, and chronic osteomyelitis developed. Infection of the bone and the associated vascular compromise caused bone necrosis, giving rise to a dead piece of bone, called sequestrum. With chronicity, a shell of reactive new bone, called involucrum, is formed around the dead bone. Osteolysis and osteosclerosis are features of bone remodeling with Paget disease of bone. A mass suggests a malignancy, and the most common neoplasm to develop in a sinus tract draining from osteomyelitis is squamous cell carcinoma, but this is uncommon. A nidus with surrounding sclerosis suggests an osteoid osteoma. Soft tissue swelling should resolve soon after the fracture is stabilized.
BP6 672   PBD6 1232-1233

17.   **(B)** The glistening, gray-blue appearance is typical for cartilage, and this lesion most likely represents a neoplastic proliferation of chondroblasts. The tumor has infiltrated the medullary cavity and invaded the overlying cor-

tex and hence is malignant. This is a chondrosarcoma. Most chondrosarcomas are low grade. There is a broad age range, unlike many other bone tumors that tend to occur in children or in young adults. Most chondrosarcomas arise toward central portions of the skeleton. Osteosarcomas are derived from osteoblasts. They are usually seen in younger persons and do not have a bluish-white appearance because they are marked by osteoid production. Giant cell tumors arise during third to fifth decades; they involve epiphyses and metaphyses. Grossly, they are large, red-brown, cystic tumors. Giant cells resembling osteoclasts are present in giant cell tumors of the bone. These tumors are believed to arise from cells of monocyte-macrophage lineage. Plasma cells give rise to multiple myeloma. Myelomas are dark red, rounded, lytic lesions that are often multiple.
BP6 678   PBD6 1240-1241

18.   **(E)** The osteoid production by a sarcoma is diagnostic of osteosarcoma. The metaphyseal location in a long bone, particularly in the region of the knee, is consistent with osteosarcoma, as is presentation in a young person. Ewing sarcoma is composed of small, round, blue cells without osteoid production, and these neoplasms are typically diaphyseal in location. A chondrosarcoma does not make osteoid. Most chondrosarcomas occur at an older age. Giant cell tumors of bone are most common between the ages of 20 and 40 years; they are composed of giant cells and a mononuclear cell stroma without osteoid production. Fibrous dysplasia is a localized "developmental arrest" of bone formation with irregular woven bone spicules in a fibroblastic stroma.
BP6 676-677   PBD6 1236-1237

19.   **(D)** Parathyroid adenomas secrete parathyroid hormone (PTH) and cause primary hyperparathyroidism. Excessive secretion of PTH activates osteoclastic reabsorption of bone. Microfractures within the areas of bone reabsorption give rise to hemorrhages. This causes an influx of macrophages and, ultimately, reactive fibrosis. These lesions are cystic, and they are sometimes called "brown tumor of bone." Because they contain osteoclasts and fibroblasts, these lesions can be confused with primary bone neoplasms such as giant cell tumor of bone. Secondary hyperparathyroidism is seen in persons with chronic renal failure. This patient is too young for Paget disease of bone, which may be osteolytic in its early phase. Chronic osteomyelitis rarely produces such a discrete lesion. A giant cell tumor of bone should be in the epiphyseal region.
BP6 672   PBD6 1228

20.   **(A)** Pyogenic osteomyelitis may arise from hematogenous dissemination of an infection. In a pediatric population with no history of previous illnesses, *S. aureus* is the most common causative organism. *Salmonella* infection involving bone is more common in persons with sickle cell anemia. *H. influenzae* and group B streptococcal infections are most common in the neonatal period. Gonorrhea may occasionally disseminate and involve the bones (i.e., osteomyelitis) or joints (i.e., septic arthritis) of sexually active persons.
BP6 672   PBD6 1232-1233

21. **(D)** She has superficial fibromatosis that has produced a lesion best known as a Dupuytren contracture. These lesions contain mature fibroblasts surrounded by dense collagen. A hard, firm lesion of this size is unlikely to be a malignancy. An injury with granulation tissue should give rise to a stable scar, without such severe retraction. Dystrophic calcification refers to calcification that occurs in necrotic tissues; it is not commonly a localized mass.
BP6 692–693   PBD6 1262–1263

22. **(C)** This patient has classic features of chronic rheumatoid arthritis. These include bilateral symmetric involvement of joints, destruction of joints with characteristic deformities, and presence of rheumatoid nodules. Subcutaneous rheumatoid nodules such as this one are typically found over extensor surfaces. Although the pathogenesis of rheumatoid arthritis is complex, it is believed that the tissue injury is mediated by an autoimmune reaction in which $CD4^+$ T cells play a pivotal role. These cells secrete cytokines that have a cascade of effects on B cells, macrophages, and endothelial cells. B cells are driven to form rheumatoid factors that form immune complexes in the joint; macrophages secrete cytokines that activate cartilage cells, fibroblasts, and synovial cells; and endothelial cell activation promotes accumulation of inflammatory cells in the synovium. Together, these processes form a pannus and eventually cause joint destruction. Activation of neutrophils by urate crystals is involved in the pathogenesis of gouty arthritis. Infection by *B. burgdorferi* causes Lyme disease. Although this can mimic rheumatoid arthritis, symmetric involvement of small joints and rheumatoid nodules are not seen. HLA-B27 has no association with rheumatoid arthritis. In contrast, chondrocyte activation and subsequent injury play an important role in osteoarthritis. Infectious granulomatous inflammation involving bone and joint is uncommon and not likely to be symmetric. Tertiary syphilis may produce gummatous necrosis.
BP6 109–110   PBD6 1248–1250

23. **(J)** This patient has an osteoid osteoma, a benign tumor of the bone that occurs in young adults. Pain disproportionate to the size of the tumor is characteristic. If such a lesion is larger than 2 cm, it is classified as an osteoblastoma. It can be treated by curettement.
BP6 676   PBD6 1235

24. **(I)** This is an osteochondroma. Notice the glistening cartilaginous cap. This tumor-like condition, also called exostosis, is benign. It results from a proliferation of mature bone capped by cartilage. When skeletal growth ceases, osteochondromas tend to cease proliferation as well. They may produce local irritation and pain.
BP6 677 PBD6 1237–1238

25. **(D)** The diaphysial location, histologic appearance, and t(11;22) translocations are characteristic of a Ewing tumor. This tumor occurs most commonly between the ages of 10 and 15 years. The t(11;22) translocation is present in about 85% of Ewing sarcomas and the related primitive neuroectodermal (PNET) tumors.
BP6 679–680   PBD6 1244

26. **(A)** The histologic picture shows a central amorphous aggregate of urate crystals surrounded by reactive fibroblasts and mononuclear inflammatory cells. This is a gouty tophus. He has gouty arthritis, and the big toe is a common location. The acute, severe pain tends to occur sporadically and may be precipitated by alcohol consumption. Calcium pyrophosphate crystals are characteristic for pseudogout, which can mimic a variety of joint diseases but most often involves the knees. Hydroxyapatite crystals appear with degenerative osteoarthritis, which tends to involve larger joints. Cholesterol crystals appear after resolution of hemorrhage into a joint space. Charcot-Leyden crystals are formed from breakdown of eosinophils and may be found in the sputum of patients with bronchial asthma.
BP6 682–686   PBD6 1253–1257

27. **(D)** The total bone mass is an important determinant of the subsequent risk for osteoporosis and its complications. A proactive regimen of exercise that puts stress on bones to increase mass before the inevitable loss after age 30 is most likely to reduce the subsequent risk of osteoporosis. Dietary supplements after menopause are not harmful but at best can only partially slow down the loss of bone with aging. Likewise, postmenopausal estrogen or raloxifene therapy can help to preserve bone mass. By the time a fracture has occurred, there has already been significant bone loss. Corticosteroid therapy is just one of many risk factors for osteoporosis, but short courses of corticosteroids have minimal effects on bone formation. Alcohol and tobacco use are not major risks for osteoporosis.
BP6 669–670   PBD6 1222–1224

28. **(E)** This patient has a single focus of fibrous dysplasia. This benign tumor-like condition is uncommon. The histologic appearance of woven bone in the middle of benign-looking fibroblasts is characteristic. Seventy percent of cases are monostotic, and the ribs, femur, tibia, mandible, and calvarium are the most frequent sites of involvement. Local deformity and, occasionally, fracture can occur. Polyostotic fibrous dysplasia may involve craniofacial, pelvic, and shoulder girdle regions, leading to severe deformity and fracture. An osteoid osteoma has a small central nidus with surrounding sclerosis. An enchondroma typically appears in more distal bones and is composed of cartilage. An osteosarcoma is typically a large destructive lesion without central lucency. A Ewing sarcoma usually occurs in the diaphyseal region of the long bones, and is histologically identified by sheets of small, round cells.
BP6 680   PBD6 1242–1243

29. **(C)** Infections with group B streptococcus and *E. coli* are common in the neonatal period. Both can cause congenital infections. *S. aureus* is the most common cause for osteomyelitis, but these patients are usually adults. Gonorrhea as a cause for acute osteomyelitis should be considered in sexually active young adults. *Salmonella* osteomyelitis is most characteristic for persons with sickle cell anemia. Pneumococcal osteomyelitis is uncommon.
BP6 672   PBD6 1232–1233

30. **(D)** This form of chronic arthritis is the late, or stage 3, manifestation of Lyme disease. The presence of a lym-

phoplasmacytic infiltrate with endothelial proliferation is characteristic (but not diagnostic) of Lyme arthritis. The infectious agent, *B. burgdorferi*, is a spirochete that is spread through the deer tick. This stage is reached about 2 to 3 years after the initial tick bite, and joint involvement can appear in about 80% of patients. Group B streptococcus may produce an acute osteomyelitis or arthritis in neonates. *N. gonorrhoeae* can cause an acute suppurative arthritis. In both of these conditions, the inflammatory infiltrate contains a preponderance of neutrophils. *T. pallidum* may produce gummatous necrosis that can involve large joints. Tuberculous arthritis may involve large, weight-bearing joints, and it can be progressive, giving rise to ankylosis. The histologic features of tuberculous arthritis include caseating granulomas.
BP6 686-687   PBD6 1253

31.   **(A)** Tophi are large collections of monosodium urate crystals that can appear in joints or soft tissues of persons with gout. Large superficial tophi can erode the overlying skin. There is an inflammatory reaction to the crystals, but the tophi are generally painless. A pannus is seen within the joint in rheumatoid arthritis and is composed of inflamed synovium and soft tissue. An osteophyte is a bony spur that develops at the joint margin with osteoarthritis. A purulent exudate with many polymorphonuclear lymphocytes would be expected with an acute arthritis. Erythema chronicum migrans is a skin lesion seen with Lyme disease that does not tend to ulcerate.
BP6 684-686   PBD6 1256-1257

32.   **(A)** This is a lipoma, the most common benign soft tissue neoplasm. Such masses are extremely well differentiated and discrete. Multiple lipomas may be seen in some familial cases, but these are rare. These benign tumors do not metastasize; moreover, mesenchymal neoplasms do not often metastasize through lymphatics. Recurrences of some atypical lipomas or liposarcomas can occur, but benign lipomas do not recur. Secondary infection of this uncomplicated excision procedure is unlikely.
BP6 691-692   PBD6 1260-1261

33.   **(E)** Most cases of giant cell tumor arise in the epiphyses of long bones of young adults between the ages of 20 and 40 years, with a slight female predominance. They may recur after curettage. Although most are histologically and biologically benign, in rare cases, a sarcoma can arise in a giant cell tumor of bone. A Ewing sarcoma is seen in the diaphyseal region and it usually presents within the first two decades of life. An osteoblastoma usually involves the spine. Enchondromas are most often peripheral skeletal lesions involving the metaphyseal region of small tubular bones of hands and feet. Osteitis fibrosa cystica is a complication of hyperparathyroidism.
BP6 679   PBD6 1244-1245

34.   **(C)** Acute inflammation of the first metatarsophalangeal joint, caused by precipitation of uric acid crystals in the joint space, is quite typical of gout. Hyperuricemia is a sine qua non for the development of gout. However, all patients with hyperuricemia do not develop gout. Other, ill-defined-factors also play a role in pathogenesis. Involve-

ment of the big toe is classic, but other joints may be involved. An increased parathyroid hormone level indicates primary hyperparathyroidism, which is not likely to produce joint disease. An elevated serum urea nitrogen is present with renal failure, which may produce secondary hyperparathyroidism. Although attacks of gout are often precipitated by a heavy bout of alcohol consumption, liver damage (elevated transaminases) is not a feature of gouty arthritis. Gout is not associated with rheumatoid arthritis.
BP6 682-686   PBD6 1253-1257

35.   **(B)** The presence of a destructive lesion in the vertebrae with extension of the disease along the psoas muscle is quite characteristic of tubercular osteomyelitis. Tuberculosis of bones usually results from hematogenous spread from an infection in the lung. Long bones and vertebrae are the favored sites for tuberculosis involving the skeletal system. *T. pallidum* may produce gummatous necrosis in the tertiary stage, but this involves soft tissues more than bone. Streptococcal osteomyelitis is uncommon. *B. burgdorferi* is the causative agent for Lyme disease, which produces an arthritis. Dissemination of *C. neoformans* infections from the lungs occurs most commonly in immunocompromised patients but infrequently produces osteomyelitis.
BP6 673   PBD6 1233

36.   **(A)** She has findings typical for juvenile rheumatoid arthritis, which, unlike the adult type of rheumatoid arthritis, is more likely to be self-limited and nondeforming. Juvenile rheumatoid arthritis typically is rheumatoid factor negative but antinuclear antibody positive. Compared with rheumatoid arthritis, the juvenile form is more likely to have systemic manifestations in other organs.
BP6 111   PBD6 1251-1252

37.   **(E)** These are calcium pyrophosphate crystals that are deposited in the articular matrix. With progression of the disease, the crystals can seed the joint space. However, there are rare inherited forms. Secondary forms of the disease can be associated with systemic diseases such as hemochromatosis. This patient has evidence of hemochromatosis—skin pigmentation, heart failure, diabetes, and cirrhosis. With progression of disease, the crystals can seed the joint space.
PBD6 873, 1257

38.   **(D)** The progressive involvement of large, weight-bearing joints, along with osteophytes in the interphalangeal joints in an elderly female is characteristic of osteoarthritis. The absence of rheumatoid factor and the asymmetric joint involvement renders the diagnosis of rheumatoid arthritis unlikely. Osteoarthritis is a disease of unknown cause in which chondrocytes play a primary role. In early stages, chondrocytes proliferate. This is accompanied by changes in the cartilage matrix from secretion of IL-1 and TNF-α by chondrocytes. Eventually, the osteoarthritic cartilage is degraded. The loss of articular cartilage causes reactive subchondral sclerosis. Infiltration of the synovium with CD4$^+$ T cells is seen in rheumatoid arthritis. A partial deficiency of HGPRT gives rise to hyperuricemia and gout. HLA-B27 is associated with ankylosing spondylitis and other seronegative spondyloarthropathies.

Inherited defects in type I collagen give rise to a group of disorders called osteogenesis imperfecta. These rare disorders may be lethal in utero or in some cases give rise to premature osteoarthritis.

BP6 681–682   PBD6 1246–1248

39. **(D)** *S. aureus* infection is responsible for 80% to 90% of all cases of osteomyelitis in which an organism can be cultured. However, *Salmonella* osteomyelitis is especially common in patients with sickle cell anemia. Gonorrhea can cause acute osteomyelitis in sexually active young adults. Group B streptococcal infections causing osteomyelitis are most common in neonates. *K. pneumoniae* osteomyelitis may rarely be seen in adults with urinary tract infections caused by this organism.

BP6 672   PBD6 1232–1233

Peripheral Nerve and Skeletal Muscle

BP6 Chapter 21 - The Musculoskeletal
System
PBD6 Chapter 29 - Peripheral Nerve and
Skeletal Muscle

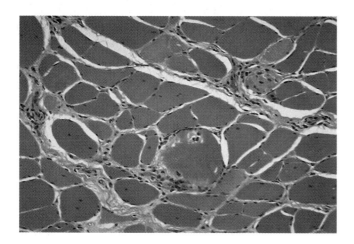

1. A 5-year-old boy displays muscular weakness. He is unable to play with the other children, quickly becoming tired and unable to keep up. The serum creatine kinase level is elevated. A muscle biopsy is performed, and it has the appearance shown here at low magnification. Which of the following laboratory test findings would be most appropriate to determine the diagnosis?

O (A) Serum acetylcholinesterase antibody titer
O (B) Immunohistochemical staining for dystrophin
O (C) Eosinophil count in blood
O (D) Presence of oligoclonal bands of immunoglobulin in cerebrospinal fluid
O (E) Polymerase chain reaction (PCR) to detect expansion of CGG repeats on Xq27.3

2. A 25-year-old female has been experiencing episodes of numbness and tingling in her right and left hands for several months. This problem typically occurs near the end of the day and makes it difficult to use her computer keyboard. The thumb and first two fingers are most affected. There is no pain or swelling, and she does not recall any trauma to her upper extremities. Which of the following conditions most likely caused her problem?

O (A) Repetitive stress injury
O (B) Diabetes mellitus
O (C) Amyotrophic lateral sclerosis
O (D) Acute intermittent porphyria
O (E) Varicella zoster infection

3. A 63-year-old man has been on hemodialysis for chronic renal failure and has developed symmetrically decreased sensation in his lower extremities over several years. He has no decrease in strength or abnormality of gait. The most likely cause for these findings is

O (A) Guillain-Barré syndrome
O (B) Cerebral astrocytoma
O (C) Cerebral infarction
O (D) Diabetes mellitus
O (E) Multiple sclerosis

4. A 17-year-old male has had generalized muscle pain with fever for the past week. Over the past 2 days, he has developed increasing muscular weakness and diarrhea. A complete blood count (CBC) shows a hemoglobin concentration of 14.6 g/dL, hematocrit of 44.3%, mean corpuscular volume (MCV) of 90 fL, platelet count of 275,000/μL, and white blood cell (WBC) count 16,700/μL, with differential count of 68 segmented neutrophils, 6 band cells, 10 lymphocytes, 4 monocytes, and 12 eosinophils per 100 WBCs. Which of the following conditions is he most likely to have?

O (A) Duchenne muscular dystrophy
O (B) Polymyositis
O (C) Poliomyelitis
O (D) Trichinosis
O (E) Diabetes mellitus

For each of the clinical histories in questions 5 and 6, select the most closely associated condition affecting skeletal muscle:

(A) Amyotrophic lateral sclerosis
(B) Becker muscular dystrophy
(C) Dermatomyositis
(D) Duchenne muscular dystrophy
(E) Lambert-Eaton syndrome
(F) McArdle disease
(G) Mitochondrial myopathy
(H) Myasthenia gravis
(I) Polymyositis
(J) Trichinosis
(K) Werdnig-Hoffmann disease

5. A 35-year-old man has experienced increasing weakness of pelvic and shoulder girdle muscles over several years' time. A Western blot analysis of the affected muscles showed reduced amounts of dystrophin with an abnormal molecular weight. (   )

6. A chest radiograph of a 40-year-old asymptomatic male reveals focal small calcifications in the diaphragmatic leaves. (   )

7. A 56-year-old male complains of double vision and eyelid drooping, particularly toward the end of the day. He also has difficulty chewing his food at dinner time. These problems have persisted for more than 1 month. He was diagnosed with Sjögren syndrome more than a decade ago. Which of the following laboratory test findings is most likely to be present?

○ (A) Elevated serum creatine kinase level
○ (B) Acetylcholine receptor antibody positivity
○ (C) Peripheral blood eosinophilia
○ (D) Increased serum cortisol level
○ (E) Anti-histidyl t-RNA synthetase (anti-Jo-1) titer of 1:512

8. A 72-year-old male has had weight loss along with proximal muscular weakness and difficulty with urination over several months, and administration of anticholinesterase agents has not produced clinical improvement. Laboratory testing reveals that he does not have serum antibodies to acetylcholine receptor. Which of the following underlying conditions is he most likely to have?

○ (A) Chronic hepatitis C
○ (B) Duchenne muscular dystrophy
○ (C) Small cell carcinoma of lung
○ (D) Lead poisoning
○ (E) Diabetes mellitus

9. A 56-year-old female has had increasing generalized muscle weakness for the past 2 months. On physical examination, she has 3/5 motor strength in both upper and lower extremities. She is afebrile but has a blood pressure of 155/90 mm Hg. A gastrocnemius muscle biopsy is performed, and histochemical staining of the biopsy shows type II

muscle fiber atrophy. Which of the following conditions is she most likely to have?

○ (A) Cushing syndrome
○ (B) McArdle disease
○ (C) Duchenne muscular dystrophy
○ (D) Myasthenia gravis
○ (E) Polymyositis

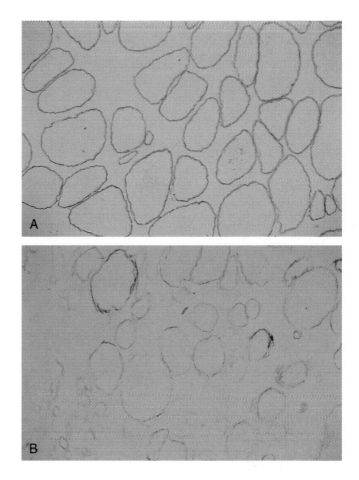

10. A 44-year-old male, who has worsening congestive heart failure for the past year, has muscular weakness involving upper arms and legs. A deltoid muscle biopsy is performed, and the immunohistochemical staining pattern with antibody to dystrophin is shown here (A, normal; B, patient). Which of the following conditions does he most likely have?

○ (A) Werdnig-Hoffmann disease
○ (B) Polymyositis
○ (C) Becker muscular dystrophy
○ (D) Amyotrophic lateral sclerosis
○ (E) Myasthenia gravis

11. A 40-year-old male had an influenza-like illness from which he recovered in a week. A few days later, he experienced a rapidly progressive ascending motor weakness that required intubation and mechanical ventilation. A lumbar puncture yielded clear, colorless cerebrospinal fluid under normal pressure that had a slightly elevated protein concen-

tration but normal glucose level and only a few mononuclear cells. He recovered in several weeks. If lymphocytic infiltrates were to be seen in peripheral nerves along with segmental demyelination at the time he initially presented, the most likely diagnosis would be

○ (A) Guillain-Barré syndrome
○ (B) Multiple sclerosis
○ (C) Amyotrophic lateral sclerosis
○ (D) Varicella zoster virus infection
○ (E) Vitamin B_{12} deficiency

12. A 35-year-old female has been experiencing muscular weakness for several weeks. When she drives her automobile for long distances, she notices difficulty keeping her eyes open because her eyelids droop, and she experiences double vision. While working at her job as a secretary, these problems get worse as the day progresses. Which of the following laboratory test findings is most likely to be present in this patient?

○ (A) Increased serum level of acetylcholine receptor antibody
○ (B) Loss of staining of muscle for dystrophin
○ (C) Increased serum creatine kinase level
○ (D) Elevated serum antinuclear antibody level
○ (E) Increased cerebrospinal fluid protein concentration

13. A 55-year-old male with a shallow, nonhealing ulceration of the left medial malleolus is found to have distal, symmetric decreased sensation in his lower extremities. He also has had multiple urinary tract infections resulting from difficulty in completely emptying his bladder. He is impotent as well. Which of the following pathologic findings is most likely to be present in his peripheral nerves?

○ (A) Wallerian degeneration
○ (B) Acute inflammation
○ (C) Onion bulb formation
○ (D) Endoneurial lymphocytic infiltration
○ (E) Axonal neuropathy

14. A 42-year-old male has had increasing, progressive muscular weakness involving both arms and legs for the past 2 years. A quadriceps muscle biopsy reveals a pattern of grouped atrophy of the myofibers. Which of the following conditions is he most likely to have?

○ (A) Werdnig-Hoffmann disease
○ (B) Amyotrophic lateral sclerosis
○ (C) Becker-type muscular dystrophy
○ (D) Myasthenia gravis
○ (E) Mitochondrial myopathy

ANSWERS

1. **(B)** The onset of muscle weakness in childhood suggests an inherited muscular dystrophy. Biopsy shows variation in muscle fiber size along with increased connective tissue between the fibers. This morphology, along with the sex of the child, strongly suggests X-linked muscular dys-

trophy. An immunohistochemical stain for dystrophin would demonstrate an absence of dystrophin, confirming the diagnosis of Duchcnnc muscular dystrophy. Antibodies to the acetylcholine receptor are found in myasthenia gravis, which is characterized by weakness in muscles after repetitive use. Eosinophilia may be seen in allergic or parasitic disorders, including trichinosis. Oligoclonal Ig bands in the cerebrospinal fluid are a feature of multiple sclerosis. Expansion of CGG repeats on Xq27.3 is diagnostic of familial mental retardation.
BP6 689-690   PBD6 1281-1282

2. **(A)** She has carpal tunnel syndrome, a form of compression neuropathy, which results from entrapment of the median nerve beneath the flexor retinaculum at the wrist. Women are more commonly affected than men. The problem is often bilateral because the causes affect both carpal tunnels. The most common cause is excessive usage of the wrist, which occurs with repetitive usage of any piece of equipment. Conditions such as hypothyroidism, amyloidosis, and edema with pregnancy also diminish the space in the carpal tunnel. Diabetes mellitus leads to a distal symmetric sensorimotor neuropathy. Amyotrophic lateral sclerosis results in progressive symmetric weakness from loss of motor neurons. Acute intermittent porphyria can lead to a hereditary form of motor and sensory neuropathy.
BP6 742-743   PBD6 1280

3. **(D)** The most common cause for a predominantly sensory peripheral neuropathy is diabetes mellitus. Long-standing diabetes also gives rise to renal failure. Guillain-Barré syndrome produces a rapidly ascending paralysis. Sensorimotor disturbances are typically not seen with intracranial mass lesions such as astrocytomas. A cerebral infarction could lead to decreased motor and sometimes to sensory loss, although not in a symmetric pattern. The demyelinating lesions of multiple sclerosis can produce many signs and symptoms, but symmetric lesions should suggest another disease process.
BP6 742-743   PBD6 1279

4. **(D)** Muscle pain with fever and eosinophilia suggests a parasitic infestation of skeletal muscles, most likely trichinosis. This occurs from ingesting poorly cooked infected meat. Duchenne muscular dystrophy is a noninflammatory myopathy that begins in early childhood. Polymyositis is an autoimmune condition with muscle inflammation but no eosinophilia. Poliomyelitis can lead to muscle weakness but is noninflammatory. Diabetes mellitus can lead to peripheral vascular disease and gangrene, but this would be rare at age 17.
BP6 689   PBD6 394-395

5. **(B)** This patient had Becker muscular dystrophy. This congenital condition is similar to Duchenne muscular dystrophy in that it has an X-linked pattern of inheritance and there is a mutation in the dystrophin gene. However, in Becker muscular dystrophy dystrophin is abnormal (not absent), resulting in less severe muscle disease than in Duchenne muscular dystrophy. Patients are typically middle-aged males at presentation.
BP6 689-690   PBD6 1281-1282

6. **(J)** Most cases of trichinosis, caused by ingestion of uncooked or poorly cooked meat containing *Trichinella spiralis* organisms, are asymptomatic, because few organisms are ingested. One clue to past infection is the appearance of the calcified encysted organisms in muscle. The most active muscles, such as the diaphragm, tend to be involved preferentially.
BP6 689   PBD6 394–395

7. **(B)** He has myasthenia gravis, with muscular weakness from loss of motor end-plate function. It is caused by an antibody-mediated loss of acetylcholine receptors at neuromuscular junctions. Myopathic diseases such as muscular dystrophies are accompanied by increases in serum creatine kinase. Parasitic infection with *T. spiralis* can lead to eosinophilia. Generalized muscle weakness with type II muscle fiber atrophy occurs with glucocorticoid excess. The anti-Jo-1 antibody is seen with polymyositis.
BP6 88–689   PBD6 1289

8. **(C)** He has a paraneoplastic syndrome called Lambert-Eaton myasthenic syndrome, which, like many of the paraneoplastic syndromes, is most often associated with small cell carcinoma of the lung. Persons with chronic viral hepatitis may have generalized malaise and weakness that is not related to specific muscle disease. Duchenne muscular dystrophy is an X-linked disease that manifests early in childhood. Lead poisoning leads to a neuropathy. Diabetes mellitus may also produce peripheral neuropathy.
PBD6 1289

9. **(A)** Type II atrophy can be seen with glucocorticoid excess and after prolonged immobilization. With routine light microscopy, it may be difficult to distinguish from denervation atrophy, and histochemical staining for ATPase must be performed. There is a deficiency of myophosphorylase enzyme with McArdle disease, leading to muscle pain and cramping with vigorous exercise. Duchenne muscular dystrophy is an X-linked condition, making it rare in females, with onset in early childhood. Antibodies to the acetylcholine receptor cause the muscular weakness in myasthenia gravis. Polymyositis is an inflammatory condition affecting all fiber types.
BP6 688   PBD6 1288–1289

10. **(C)** The biopsy shows reduced amounts of dystrophin, suggesting Becker muscular dystrophy. In Duchenne muscular dystrophy, dystrophin is absent because of gene deletion. In keeping with the diagnosis of Becker muscular dystrophy, the patient is older and not severely affected. Both are X-linked conditions. Werdnig-Hoffmann disease is one form of spinal muscular atrophy. It has onset at birth, and it results from genetically determined loss of anterior horn cells. Polymyositis is an autoimmune disease that results from T-cell–mediated attack on muscle fibers. It shows muscle fiber degeneration with inflammation. Amyotrophic lateral sclerosis is a denervation atrophy seen in adults with loss of anterior horn cells in spinal cord and cranial nerve nuclei. Myasthenia gravis occurs from acetyl-choline receptor antibody and there is minimal structural change to the muscle.
BP6 689–690   PBD6 1281–1282

11. **(A)** This history is typical of Guillain-Barré syndrome. This uncommon disorder most often follows a viral or mycoplasmal infection. It is believed to be an allergic reaction to the viral infection. The paralysis of respiratory muscles is life threatening, although many patients recover after weeks of ventilatory support. A variety of presentations are possible with multiple sclerosis, but the plaques of demyelination are generally not large or diffuse enough to cause paralysis of respiratory muscles. Amyotrophic lateral sclerosis slowly and progressively results in muscular weakness that may eventually require mechanical ventilation. Varicella zoster virus infection is most often responsible for skin involvement in a dermatomal distribution from a spinal nerve root. Vitamin B$_{12}$ deficiency results in progressive subacute combined degeneration of the cord with sensorimotor disturbances in extremities.
BP6 743   PBD6 1275–1276

12. **(A)** The clinical findings are highly suggestive of myasthenia gravis, a condition caused by antibodies to the acetylcholine receptor. Muscles with repetitive use are most affected. As the course of untreated disease progresses, larger muscle groups and respiratory muscles can be affected. Thymic abnormalities, including thymomas, are associated with myasthenia gravis. Lack of dystrophin on muscle fibers is typical for Duchenne muscular dystrophy. An increased creatine kinase can be seen in many types of muscle diseases, because myofibers are rich in creatine kinase. A positive ANA test result suggests an underlying autoimmune disease.
BP6 688–689   PBD6 1289

13. **(E)** These are features of a peripheral neuropathy with diabetes mellitus. Motor and sensory nerves are involved, and there may also be an autonomic neuropathy. Histologically, there is an axonal neuropathy with segmental demyelination. Difficulty in emptying the urinary bladder and impotence are results of autonomic neuropathy. Longer nerves are affected first, explaining the lower leg involvement and accounting for many cases of "diabetic foot" with trauma and subsequent ulceration. Wallerian degeneration typically occurs with traumatic transection of a nerve. Acute inflammation is not generally seen with neuropathies. Lymphocytic infiltrates may be seen with Guillain-Barré syndrome. Onion bulb formation is a feature of the hereditary neuropathy known as Refsum disease.
BP6 572   PBD6 1279

14. **(B)** Also known as Lou Gehrig disease, amyotrophic lateral sclerosis (ALS) was named for the famous New York Yankee first baseman afflicted with this disorder. Lower and upper motor neurons can be affected, resulting in a denervation-type pattern of muscular atrophy, because an individual neuron innervates a group of muscle fibers.
BP6 687–688   PBD6 1273, 1338

The Central Nervous System

PB6 Chapter 23 The Nervous System
PBD6 Chapter 30 The Central Nervous System

○ (A) Folate
○ (B) Niacin
○ (C) Cobalamin
○ (D) Pyridoxine
○ (E) Thiamine

1. A 46-year-old male injection drug user is admitted with a 1-day history of increasing headache and high fever. Head computed tomography (CT) does not reveal a mass lesion or midline shift. A lumbar puncture is performed; the cerebrospinal fluid (CSF) protein concentration is increased, but the glucose level is decreased. Which of the following infectious agents is most likely to account for these findings?

○ (A) J-C strain of papovavirus
○ (B) *Mycobacterium tuberculosis*
○ (C) *Staphylococcus aureus*
○ (D) Herpes simplex virus
○ (E) *Toxoplasma gondii*

2. A 63-year-old woman is observed by her family to be forgetful. This worsens over several weeks. She is unable to care for herself a month later, and she has difficulty ambulating. She develops myoclonus. A head CT scan shows only minimal cerebral atrophy, nearly consistent for age. An electroencephalogram (EEG) shows low-amplitude, slow background activity with periodic complexes and occasional repetitive, sharp waves with intervals of 0.5 to 1 second. Which of the following histologic abnormalities is most likely to be seen in cerebral cortex?

○ (A) Numerous neuritic plaques
○ (B) Plaques of demyelination
○ (C) Lewy bodies
○ (D) Microglial nodules
○ (E) Spongiform encephalopathy

3. A long history of chronic alcoholism is elicited by the nurse practitioner examining a 49-year-old male who presents with an acute psychosis. She notices that he has difficulty with a finger-to-nose test, and there is paralysis of the lateral rectus muscles. These findings are typically the result of a nutritional deficiency of

4. A 39-year-old male with a history of human immuno-deficiency virus (HIV) infection presents with a severe headache. A lumbar puncture reveals a few mononuclear cells, no neutrophils, no red blood cells (RBCs), a normal glucose level, and a normal protein concentration. An India ink preparation of the CSF is depicted. The organism most likely to produce these findings is

○ (A) *Staphylococcus aureus*
○ (B) *Mycobacterium tuberculosis*
○ (C) *Listeria monocytogenes*
○ (D) *Toxoplasma gondii*
○ (E) *Cryptococcus neoformans*

5. A 40-year-old, healthy male presented with sudden onset of a grand mal seizure. A head CT scan showed five sharply circumscribed, nonenhancing mass lesions, ranging from 1 to 2.5 cm in diameter and located in the cerebral hemispheres at the gray-white junction of the parietal and frontal lobes. Which underlying disease process is he most likely to have?

○ (A) Acquired immunodeficiency syndrome (AIDS)
○ (B) Metastatic malignant melanoma
○ (C) Infective endocarditis
○ (D) Neurofibromatosis type I
○ (E) Cysticercosis

6. A 25-year-old, previously healthy female has the acute onset of confusion and disorientation followed by a seizure. On admission to the hospital, her serum and urine drug screen results are negative. She is not febrile, and her blood pressure is 110/65 mm Hg. No papilledema is observed. However, a CT scan of the head reveals hemorrhage in the left temporal lobe. Lumbar puncture is performed, and examination of the CSF reveals only a few mononuclear cells, with normal glucose and protein levels. What is the cause of her condition?

○ (A) Cytomegalovirus (CMV)
○ (B) *Neisseria meningitidis*
○ (C) Herpes simplex virus
○ (D) Eastern equine encephalitis virus
○ (E) *Aspergillus niger*

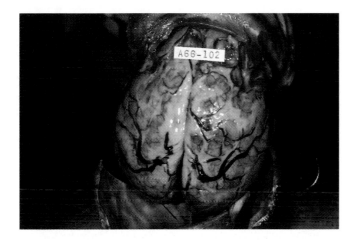

7. A healthy 20-year-old male has a mild pharyngitis followed a few days later by the sudden onset of a severe headache. Physical examination reveals nuchal rigidity. His vital signs reveal a temperature of 38.8°C, respiration of 26/min, pulse of 98/min, and blood pressure of 95/45 mm Hg. The gross appearance of the surface of the brain is shown here. The infectious agent most likely to have caused this clinical and histologic picture is

○ (A) *Cryptococcus neoformans*
○ (B) *Mycobacterium tuberculosis*
○ (C) *Toxoplasma gondii*
○ (D) Poliovirus
○ (E) *Neisseria meningitidis*

8. A 53-year-old male with a long history of chronic alcoholism has a flapping tremor of his outstretched hands. Which of the following laboratory test findings is most likely to account for this physical finding?

○ (A) Hyponatremia
○ (B) Hypoglycemia

○ (C) Elevated hemoglobin A_{1C} level
○ (D) Elevated carboxyhemoglobin level
○ (E) Hyperammonemia

9. A 68-year-old patient had a 7-year history of progressive dementia and died. At autopsy, there is cerebral atrophy in a predominantly frontal and parietal lobe distribution. Microscopic examination of the brain reveals numerous neuritic plaques in the hippocampus, amygdala, and the neocortex. Small peripheral cerebral arteries demonstrate amyloid in their media by Congo red staining. Which of the following is an important risk factor for the development of this disease?

○ (A) HLA-DR3/DR4
○ (B) Expansion of CAG repeats on chromosome 4p16
○ (C) Inheritance of the epsilon 4 allele at the ApoE 4 gene
○ (D) Inheritance of a mutant prion gene
○ (E) A deficiency of thiamine

10. A 72-year-old woman trips on a toy truck left at the top of a flight of stairs by one of the grandchildren. She falls down the stairs but does not lose consciousness. About 36 hours later, she develops a headache with confusion. When seen in the emergency room, she is still conscious, and there is a scalp contusion observed on the occiput. The most likely location for an intracranial hemorrhage in this situation is

○ (A) Pontine
○ (B) Subarachnoid
○ (C) Basal ganglia
○ (D) Epidural
○ (E) Subdural

11. A previously healthy 26-year-old medical student has headaches for several weeks. She has increasing malaise. A head CT scan shows no abnormalities. A lumbar puncture yields clear, colorless CSF with normal glucose and minimally elevated protein levels. A few lymphocytes are present, but no neutrophils. A CSF gram stain is negative, as is the India ink preparation. Her condition gradually improves over the next several months. Serum serologic tests are most likely to reveal an elevated titer of antibodies to

○ (A) *Toxoplasma gondii*
○ (B) *Listeria monocytogenes*
○ (C) *Cryptococcus neoformans*
○ (D) *Neisseria meningitidis*
○ (E) Echovirus

12. A 45-year-old man has been healthy all his life until the recent onset of headaches. A cerebral angiogram demonstrates a 7-mm saccular aneurysm at the trifurcation of the right middle cerebral artery. Which of the following events is most likely to result from this lesion?

○ (A) Epidural hematoma
○ (B) Subarachnoid hemorrhage
○ (C) Subdural hematoma
○ (D) Cerebellar tonsillar herniation
○ (E) Hydrocephalus

13. A 55-year-old man died following a 6-year-long illness. At autopsy, the brain and spinal cord are grossly normal. Microscopic sections reveal gliosis in the motor cortex, pallor of the lateral corticospinal tracts, and neuronal loss in the anterior horns of the spinal cord. The underlying cause of death in this case is most likely to be

○ (A) Becker muscular dystrophy
○ (B) Neurofibromatosis, type II
○ (C) Guillain-Barré syndrome
○ (D) Creutzfeldt-Jakob disease
○ (E) Amyotrophic lateral sclerosis

14. A 19-year-old snowboarder wearing protective equipment consisting of a baseball cap, baggy shorts, and a letterman's jacket flew off a jump and hit a tree. He was initially unconscious but then "came to" and wanted to try another run, but his friends thought it best to call for help. On the way to the emergency room, he became comatose. Skull radiographs revealed a linear fracture of the temporal-parietal region on the left. A serum drug screen was positive for cannabinoids. This clinical picture is most consistent with which of the following lesions?

○ (A) Contusion of frontal lobes
○ (B) Epidural hematoma
○ (C) Ruptured berry aneurysm
○ (D) Acute leptomeningitis
○ (E) Acute subdural hematoma

15. An 18-year-old female university student has 14 scattered, 2- to 5-cm, flat, hyperpigmented skin lesions with irregular borders on her extremities and torso. She had decreased left vision a year ago, and an optic nerve glioma was excised. She now presents with a mass involving the right wrist. The histologic examination of the mass is most likely to show

○ (A) Schwannoma
○ (B) Lipoma
○ (C) Fibrosarcoma
○ (D) Meningioma
○ (E) Hemangioma

16. A 62-year-old male has difficulty with voluntary movements because of muscular rigidity. He has an expressionless facies. When sitting, his hands have a "pill-rolling" tremor. Which of the following pathologic findings would best characterize his underlying disease condition?

○ (A) Hippocampal neurofibrillary tangles
○ (B) Neuronal loss with gliosis in caudate
○ (C) Hemosiderosis and gliosis of mammillary bodies
○ (D) Loss of pigmented neurons in substantia nigra
○ (E) Alzheimer type II gliosis in basal ganglia

17. An 18-year-old boy involved in a motor vehicle accident suffered severe head trauma. He died soon after arrival in the emergency room. At autopsy, a midbrain hemorrhage, arranged in a linear, ventral-to-dorsal direction, was found along with bilateral uncal and cerebral herniation. This type of hemorrhage results from which of the following mechanisms?

○ (A) Tearing of the bridging veins
○ (B) Rupture of the middle meningeal artery

○ (C) Kinking of the branches of basilar artery
○ (D) Rupture of saccular (berry) aneurysms
○ (E) Sudden decrease in blood pressure

18. A 5-cm mass beneath dura that compresses the underlying left lateral parietal lobe is found incidentally on head CT scan performed on a 38-year-old woman who fell and hit her head. She is taken to surgery, and after removal by the neurosurgeon, the mass is seen histologically to be composed of elongated cells with pale, oblong nuclei and pink cytoplasm with occasional psammoma bodies. The neoplasm of the central nervous system (CNS) that best explains these findings is

○ (A) Meningioma
○ (B) Tuberculoma
○ (C) Medulloblastoma
○ (D) Schwannoma
○ (E) Ependymoma

19. A 47-year-old woman is observed by her family to be more forgetful in the past few months. She is also emotionally labile and cries a lot. She has some choreiform movements of her extremities. She is disturbed by these developments, because her mother died a few years after experiencing the same symptoms. Which of the following underlying genetically determined conditions is most likely to be present?

○ (A) Decreased hexosaminidase A enzyme level
○ (B) Mutation in presenilin genes
○ (C) Trisomy 21
○ (D) An abnormal prion protein
○ (E) Increased trinucleotide CAG repeats

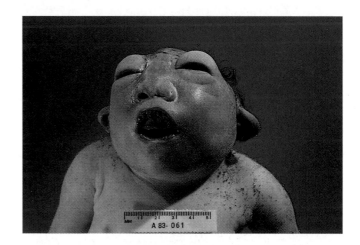

20. Which of the following laboratory test findings is most likely to be associated with the gross appearance of the 36-week-gestational-age fetus shown here?

○ (A) Hyperbilirubinemia
○ (B) High maternal CMV IgM titer
○ (C) Elevated maternal serum α-fetoprotein level
○ (D) Elevated maternal hemoglobin A_{1C} level
○ (E) 47,XX,+21 karyotype

21. On admission to the hospital, a 71-year-old woman with a history of head trauma has a serum sodium concen-

tration of 115 mmol/L. This is quickly corrected over the next couple of hours with intravenous fluids and electrolyte therapy along with diuretics. However, she then becomes obtunded. No papilledema is seen on funduscopic examination. Which of the following complications has probably occurred?

○ (A) Cerebellar tonsillar herniation
○ (B) Intraventricular hemorrhage
○ (C) Subacute combined degeneration of the cord
○ (D) Wernicke-Korsakoff syndrome
○ (E) Central pontine myelinolysis

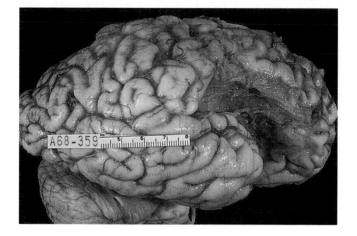

22. A 68-year-old woman lost consciousness and fell to the ground. When she became arousable, she could not move her left arm or leg and had difficulty speaking. The gross appearance of the brain is shown here at autopsy about 6 months later. The depicted lesion most likely represents

○ (A) Organizing subdural hematoma
○ (B) Arteriovenous malformation
○ (C) Recent cerebral infarction
○ (D) Contusion from blunt trauma
○ (E) Remote cerebral infarction

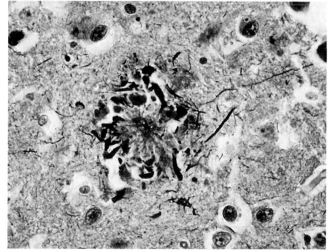

Courtesy of Eileen Bigio, MD, Department of Pathology, University of Texas Southwestern Medical School, Dallas, TX.

23. The high-power photomicrograph shown here of a specimen with Bielschowsky silver stain demonstrates a

prominent finding in the cerebral cortex of a 75-year-old male. He is most likely to have clinically exhibited

○ (A) Symmetric muscular weakness
○ (B) Gait disturbances
○ (C) Progressive dementia
○ (D) Grand mal seizures
○ (E) Choreiform movements

24. A baby is stillborn at 34 weeks' gestation to a 33-year-old gravida 3 para 2 woman, whose two previous pregnancies had resulted in normal term infants. The baby is observed to be hydropic. Autopsy of the fetus reveals marked organomegaly, and the brain has extensive necrosis in a periventricular pattern. Which of the following congenital infections is most likely to have accounted for these findings?

○ (A) *Listeria monocytogenes*
○ (B) Human immunodeficiency virus
○ (C) Herpes simplex virus
○ (D) Cytomegalovirus
○ (E) Group B streptococcus

25. A 25-year-old male complained of headaches and decreased mental function for several months. He then experienced the onset of generalized seizures, and this persisted for several weeks. A head CT scan reveals a 2-cm mass in the right cerebral hemisphere. A sterotactic biopsy of this lesion shows only gliosis, along with evidence for recent and remote hemorrhage. The mass is removed, and histologic examination shows it is composed of a conglomerate of tortuous vessels of various sizes, surrounded by gliosis. The best diagnosis is

○ (A) Arteriovenous malformation
○ (B) Organizing abscess
○ (C) Angiosarcoma
○ (D) Prior head trauma
○ (E) Ruptured saccular aneurysm

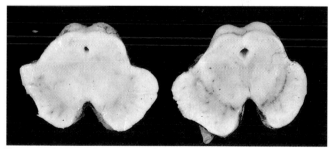

Courtesy of Eileen Bigio, MD, Department of Pathology, University of Texas Southwestern Medical School, Dallas, TX.

26. A 55-year-old male began having increasing difficulty with voluntary movements. The gross appearance of the midbrain of this patient is shown here on the left. On the right is a section through normal midbrain. Which of the following additional clinical features is most closely associated with the depicted lesion?

○ (A) Pill-rolling tremor at rest
○ (B) Symmetric weakness in the extremities
○ (C) Choreiform movements
○ (D) Difficulty with short-term memory
○ (E) Paraplegia

27.   A 43-year-old female has had a headache for a couple of weeks along with a fever. She has been healthy, except for a recent severe respiratory tract infection. A head CT scan shows a sharply demarcated, 3-cm, ring-enhancing lesion in the right occipital region. A lumbar puncture is performed, and the CSF obtained shows a cell count of 4 lymphocytes and 8 neutrophils, along with increased protein and normal glucose levels. The best diagnosis is

- O (A) Glioblastoma multiforme
- O (B) Multiple sclerosis
- O (C) Subacute infarction
- O (D) Cerebral abscess
- O (E) Metastatic carcinoma

28.   An elderly man has had several episodes in the past few months of neurologic dysfunction with dysarthria, a feeling of weakness in his hands, and dizziness. These episodes usually last less than an hour, and then he feels fine again. However, he suddenly loses consciousness while walking to the bathroom in his house and falls to the floor. On regaining consciousness several minutes later, he is unable to move his right arm and he is unable to speak clearly. Which of the following pathologic findings in his brain would best explain these problems?

- O (A) Frontal lobe astrocytoma
- O (B) Subdural hematoma
- O (C) Cerebral atherosclerosis
- O (D) Arteriovenous malformation
- O (E) Meningoencephalitis

29.   A 26-year-old male developed difficulty seeing from his left eye. Later that same year, he experienced some difficulty writing with his right hand. Over the next 5 years, he experienced paresthesias of his left arm and difficulty walking. Which of the following findings is most likely to be present in the CSF?

- O (A) Cryptococcal antigen
- O (B) Oligoclonal bands of immunoglobulins
- O (C) Malignant cells
- O (D) Xanthochromia
- O (E) Antitreponemal antibodies

30.   A 42-year-old male has had increasing difficulty with activities of daily living for the past year, mainly because of choreiform movements. His family has also observed that he has exhibited behavioral changes, although his memory remains intact. His older brother is similarly affected. The most likely finding in the CNS to explain these changes is

- O (A) Loss of pigmented neurons in the substantia nigra
- O (B) Congophilic angiopathy of the cerebral cortex
- O (C) Atrophy and gliosis of the caudate nuclei
- O (D) Loss of motor neurons in the cerebral cortex and brain stem
- O (E) Multiple lacunar infarcts within the basal ganglia

31.   A 12-year-old female presented with progressively diminishing neurologic function over several years. While in the hospital, she succumbed to pneumonia. At autopsy, the brain is atrophic, and the centrum semiovale and central white matter are shrunken, gray, and translucent on gross examination. Microscopically, there is widespread myelin loss with sparing of subcortical U fibers. Which of the following degenerative CNS diseases is most likely to explain her course?

- O (A) Metachromatic leukodystrophy
- O (B) Progressive multifocal leukoencephalopathy
- O (C) Acute disseminated encephalomyelitis
- O (D) Tay-Sachs disease
- O (E) Multiple sclerosis

32.   An 80-year-old nursing home resident is admitted to the hospital because of the recent onset of fluctuating levels of consciousness. Head MRI reveals an acute subdural hematoma on the right. The most likely cause for this finding is

- O (A) Tear of bridging veins
- O (B) Rupture of saccular aneurysm
- O (C) Bleeding from an arteriovenous malformation
- O (D) Laceration of the middle meningeal artery
- O (E) Thrombosis of the middle cerebral artery

33.   While working at her desk as an accountant, a 50-year-old female experiences a sudden, severe headache. In the emergency room, she is observed to have nuchal rigidity. A lumbar puncture shows numerous RBCs in the CSF, but there are no neutrophils, a few mononuclear cells, and a normal glucose level, with a negative result for the Gram stain. Which of the following events has probably occurred?

- O (A) Middle cerebral artery thromboembolism
- O (B) Tear of subdural bridging veins
- O (C) Ruptured intracranial berry aneurysm
- O (D) Bleeding from cerebral amyloid angiopathy
- O (E) Hypertensive basal ganglia hemorrhage

34.   Several 1- to 3-cm, ring-enhancing lesions are seen by MRI in the cerebral grey matter bilaterally in a 20-year-old male who has a history of HIV infection. A stereotaxic biopsy is most likely to reveal

- O (A) Large atypical lymphocytes
- O (B) Budding cells with pseudohyphae
- O (C) Spongiform encephalopathy
- O (D) *Toxoplasma* pseudocysts
- O (E) Squamous cell carcinoma

35.   A 5-year-old boy has experienced ataxia and complained of headaches for the past week. He then has the sudden onset of vomiting and becomes comatose. A head CT scan reveals the presence of a 4-cm mass in the region of the cerebellar vermis along with dilation of the cerebral ventricles. A lumbar puncture yields CSF that cytologically reveals small cells with dark blue nuclei and scant cytoplasm. Which of the following neoplasms is most likely to explain these findings?

- O (A) Schwannoma
- O (B) Ependymoma
- O (C) Glioblastoma multiforme
- O (D) Medulloblastoma
- O (E) Metastatic carcinoma

36. A 27-year-old woman is examined by a neurologist for decreased vision in her left eye. Clinical history reveals an episode of weakness several months earlier, which she attributed to job stress and fatigue. The neurologic examination reveals mild residual weakness in her right lower extremity. A spinal fluid tap reveals increased IgG levels with prominent oligoclonal bands in the CSF. A brain MRI scan reveals small, scattered, 0.5-cm areas consistent with demyelination, mostly located in periventricular white matter. What should the neurologist tell the patient?

O (A) No further neurologic problems will be experienced.
O (B) Relapses and remissions will occur over many years.
O (C) This disease can be passed on to children.
O (D) Further debilitation and death will occur within 5 years.
O (E) A test for HIV will be positive.

37. A hemorrhagic infarct is found at autopsy in the right parietal region of a 60-year-old male. Microscopically, a small thromboembolus is found in a peripheral cerebral artery branch at the gray-white junction near the infarct. Which underlying disease process is he most likely to have?

O (A) Hypertension with chronic renal failure
O (B) Rheumatic heart disease with left atrial mural thrombosis
O (C) Chronic alcoholism with micronodular cirrhosis
O (D) AIDS with a low CD4 count
O (E) Papillary thyroid carcinoma with metastases to bone

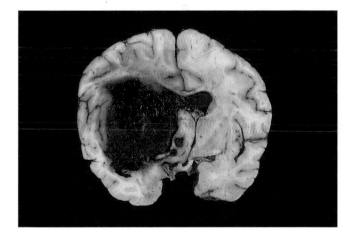

38. A 55-year-old man suddenly lost consciousness while driving his truck, but he was traveling at a slow speed and came to a stop without a collision. When paramedics arrived, he could not be aroused. The gross appearance of the brain from autopsy is shown here. Which of the following underlying conditions is most likely to have led to this lesion?

O (A) Thromboembolism
O (B) Metastatic carcinoma
O (C) Multiple sclerosis
O (D) Systemic hypertension
O (E) Chronic alcoholism

39. Papilledema is identified on funduscopic examination of an adult female who has complained of a severe headache for 2 days. A day later, she has right pupillary dilation and impaired ocular movement. She then becomes obtunded. Which of the following lesions best explains these findings?

O (A) Hydrocephalus ex vacuo
O (B) Transtentorial uncal herniation
O (C) Ruptured intracranial berry aneurysm
O (D) Chronic subdural hematoma
O (E) Occipital lobe infarction

For each of the clinical histories in questions 40 and 41, match the neoplasm:

(A) Hemangioblastoma
(B) Medulloblastoma
(C) Craniopharyngioma
(D) Pituitary adenoma
(E) Ependymoma
(F) Oligodendroglioma
(G) Schwannoma
(H) Meningioma
(I) Glioblastoma multiforme
(J) Non-Hodgkin lymphoma
(K) Metastatic carcinoma
(L) Melanoma

40. A 56-year-old male presents with a single episode of a grand mal seizure. MRI of the brain shows three mass lesions, 1 to 3 cm in diameter, located at the gray-white junction in the cerebral hemispheres. (   )

41. A 10-year-old boy has persistent headaches and ataxia. A head CT scan reveals a 4-cm mass involving the cerebellar vermis. Cerebral ventricles are enlarged. Abnormal cells are found in the CSF by lumbar puncture. (   )

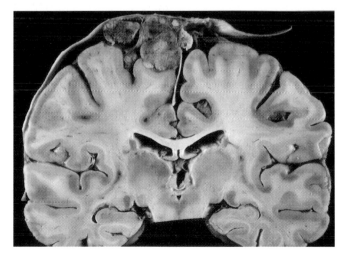

42. A 45-year-old female presents with unilateral headaches. The lesion found on head CT scan is represented on this gross photograph of the brain. Which of the following is most likely?

O (A) Meningioma
O (B) Astrocytoma
O (C) Ependymoma
O (D) Metastasis
O (E) Tuberculoma

43. A 72-year-old woman has experienced progressive memory problems for several years. For the past year, she has gotten lost while walking around her own neighborhood and has been unable to find her way home. Lately, she has been unable to find the bathroom in her own house, and she cannot recognize family members. Examination of her brain at autopsy would most likely reveal

○ (A) Many Lewy bodies in the substantia nigra
○ (B) Atrophy and gliosis of the caudate nuclei
○ (C) Neocortical neuronal Pick bodies
○ (D) Oligodendroglial cytoplasmic inclusions
○ (E) Numerous neocortical senile plaques

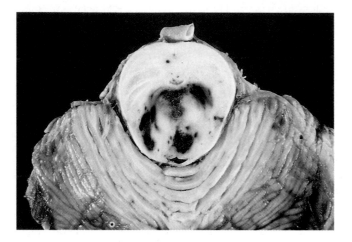

44. The gross appearance shown here was observed on sectioning the brain from a 45-year-old male who died from acute meningitis with *Streptococcus pneumoniae*. Based on this appearance, which of the following complications has likely resulted from his infection?

○ (A) Uncal herniation
○ (B) Hydrocephalus
○ (C) Abscess formation
○ (D) Subarachnoid hemorrhage
○ (E) Laminar cortical necrosis

45. A 41-year-old woman complains of diminished hearing on the left for several months. A head CT scan shows a sharply circumscribed, 4-cm mass located adjacent to the left pons that extends into left inferior cerebellar hemisphere. This lesion is most likely a (an)

○ (A) Meningioma
○ (B) Astrocytoma
○ (C) Schwannoma
○ (D) Medulloblastoma
○ (E) Ependymoma

46. A 48-year-old male has noticed speech difficulties for 2 months. A head CT scan reveals a large, irregular, 6-cm mass involving the centrum semiovale of the right cerebral hemisphere and extending across the corpus callosum. Biopsy of the mass shows areas of necrosis surrounded by nuclear pseudopalisading. The neoplastic cells within the mass are very hyperchromatic. He most likely has

○ (A) Medulloblastoma
○ (B) Glioblastoma multiforme
○ (C) Metastatic lung carcinoma
○ (D) Malignant melanoma
○ (E) Cystic astrocytoma

47. A 37-year-old male with a positive HIV-1 serologic test had increasing memory problems for the past year and became depressed. He also developed problems with motor function so that he was unable to stand and walk. He died from *Pneumocystis carinii* pneumonia. At autopsy, his brain appears atrophic, with no focal lesions identified. Which of the following microscopic findings would most likely be found in the brain?

○ (A) Plaques of demyelination in periventricular white matter
○ (B) Neocortical senile plaques and neurofibrillary tangles
○ (C) Multiple lacunar infarcts in basal ganglia
○ (D) Spongiform change involving cerebellum and neocortex
○ (E) White matter microglial nodules with multinucleate cells

48. Examination of a term newborn reveals a small lower lumbar skin dimple with a protruding tuft of hair. A radiograph shows that the underlying L4 vertebra has lack of closure of the posterior arches. This condition is best diagnosed as

○ (A) Dandy-Walker malformation
○ (B) Spina bifida occulta
○ (C) Tuberous sclerosis
○ (D) Arnold-Chiari malformation
○ (E) Meningomyelocele

49. A 5-year-old boy has been irritable for the past 2 days. He has a temperature of 39.1°C. A lumbar puncture is performed, and the CSF shows numerous neutrophils, a slightly increased protein level, and a decreased glucose concentration. A Gram stain of the CSF is most likely to show

○ (A) No organisms
○ (B) Gram-positive cocci
○ (C) Gram-negative diplococci
○ (D) Short gram-positive rods
○ (E) Gram-negative bacilli

50. A 55-year-old male who had been healthy all his life is now afflicted with progressive, symmetric muscular weakness. This first involved the head and neck region, such that he had difficulty in speaking, in making eye movements, and with swallowing. In the past year, the weakness in upper and lower extremities has increased, and he can no longer stand, walk, or feed himself. He most likely has

○ (A) Amyotrophic lateral sclerosis
○ (B) Huntington disease
○ (C) Multiple sclerosis
○ (D) Guillain-Barré syndrome
○ (E) Parkinson disease

51. A neonate was born prematurely after 28 weeks' gestation to a 22-year-old primigravida. The baby was initially stable but then became severely hypoxemic and developed seizure activity. Eight months later, the infant is diagnosed with an obstructive hydrocephalus. This clinical picture resulted from which of the following conditions?

○ (A) Germinal matrix hemorrhage
○ (B) Down syndrome
○ (C) Kernicterus
○ (D) Congenital CMV infection
○ (E) Medulloblastoma

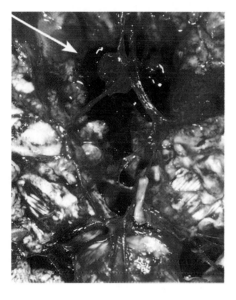

52. A 79-year-old woman was driving her car when she experienced the sudden onset of a severe headache. She pulled into a service station, stopped the car, and then slumped over the wheel. She was taken to the emergency room, where she remained comatose and died hours later. The most likely cause for the gross appearance of her brain seen here is

○ (A) Hemorrhage in a glioblastoma multiforme
○ (B) Thromboembolization with cerebral infarction
○ (C) Rupture of the bridging veins
○ (D) Rupture of a berry aneurysm
○ (E) Hyaline arteriolosclerosis with hemorrhage

ANSWERS

1. **(C)** Headache, fever, a high CSF protein level, and a low glucose concentration all point to bacterial meningitis. *S. aureus* is a common infection in injection drug users. He does not have a mass lesion of toxoplasmosis or focal lesions of progressive multifocal leukoencephalopathy (PML) that may be associated with AIDS. PML is associated with the J-C papovavirus. A tuberculous meningitis has a more insidious onset. Herpes simplex produces encephalitis, not a meningitis. Toxoplasmosis, seen in immunocompromised patients, produces parenchymal abscesses, not meningitis.
BP6 726–727   PBD6 1314–1315

2. **(E)** She has a rapidly progressive dementia that is most consistent with Creutzfeldt-Jakob disease (CJD). This is one of a group of diseases called spongiform encephalopathies because they produce a vacuolated appearance of the cortex. CJD occurs in sporadic or familial forms and is believed to be caused by prions. Her age and clinical findings are classic for the sporadic type of CJD. Cases of variant CJD (vCJD), possibly linked to exposure to bovine spongiform encephalopathy (BSE), are seen in much younger patients and do not have the characteristic EEG findings. Neuritic plaques are seen with Alzheimer disease, which has a course over many years. The demyelinating plaques of multiple sclerosis develop over years, as do the Lewy bodies of Parkinson disease and diffuse Lewy body disease. Microglial nodules can be seen in persons with AIDS.
BP6 730–731   PBD6 1323–1324

3. **(E)** This patient has Wernicke disease, resulting from a deficiency of vitamin B_1 (thiamine). It is uncommon in persons who have a varied diet, but persons with a history of chronic alcoholism may not have a well-balanced diet. The mammillary bodies and the periaqueductal gray matter are often involved with capillary proliferation, hemorrhage, necrosis, and hemosiderin deposition. This gives rise to paralysis of extraocular muscles. When memory problems with confabulation are observed, the term *Wernicke-Korsakoff syndrome* is used. Dementia may be seen with niacin deficiency. Folate deficiency does not produce CNS signs. A deficiency of pyridoxine may result in a peripheral neuropathy. Subacute combined degeneration of the cord may be seen with B_{12} (cobalamin) deficiency.
BP6 738   PBD6 1341

4. **(E)** His immunocompromised state results in infection with *C. neoformans*, which is distributed worldwide. Most infections with *Cryptococcus* probably start in the lung, but the CNS is the second most common area for involvement, and meningitis is the most typical manifestation. Cryptococci can be visualized by an India ink test because the thick, gelatinous capsule of the fungus does not stain black with the dye. Septicemia with *S. aureus* and disseminated *M. tuberculosis* infections are common with AIDS but do not commonly produce lesions in the CNS. *Listeria* is infrequently seen with AIDS and can cause meningitis, but the organisms are not seen with India ink. *T. gondii* is a frequent cause of CNS disease with AIDS, but the small organisms are found in parenchymal abscesses, not in the CSF.
BP6 727–728   PBD6 1322

5. **(B)** Metastases are typically multiple and are found at the gray-white junction, where peripheral arteries branch and narrow acutely. Malignant melanomas, when they me-

tastasize, are often widely disseminated, with multiple mass lesions in organ sites of involvement. Although AIDS is not associated with metastatic disease to the brain, primary infections such as toxoplasmosis could produce focal lesions, although not just at the gray-white junction, and they should be ring enhancing. Septic emboli from endocarditis could be found in a similar distribution, but the patient should be septic, and abscesses often show enhancement on CT or MRI. Cysticerci are irregularly distributed in the parenchyma and are typically 1 cm in diameter or smaller. The neurofibromas and schwannomas of neurofibromatosis type I are peripheral, not cortical.
BP6 735 PBD6 1351

6. **(C)** Hemorrhagic lesions of the temporal lobes are characteristic for herpes simplex virus infections, and the few cases that occur are usually sporadic, occurring in apparently healthy persons. CMV is seen in neonates and in immunocompromised adults but does not produce hemorrhagic lesions. Meningococcal infections produce a meningitis. Arboviral infections produce focal lesions that may sometimes have an associated vasculitis with hemorrhage; the CSF protein is usually elevated, and there is a neutrophilic pleocytosis. The lesions of aspergillosis can be hemorrhagic but are typically seen in persons who are immunocompromised.
BP6 729 PBD6 1318-1319

7. **(E)** The clinical signs and symptoms are typical of acute meningitis, and there is a purulent exudate on the cerebral convexities, indicative of bacterial infection. At his age, a common etiologic agent is *N. meningitidis*. Cryptococcosis should be considered in immunocompromised patients. Tuberculous meningitis does not manifest so acutely, and the exudate is typically on the base of the brain. Immunocompromised patients also get cerebral toxoplasmosis, but the lesions are parenchymal abscesses, not meningitis. Poliovirus could follow a pharyngitis, but it has an insidious onset of increasing paralysis from loss of motor neurons. It does not cause meningitis.
BP6 726-727 PBD6 1314-1315

8. **(E)** He has asterixis, a condition resulting from hepatic encephalopathy that can occur with severe liver disease from a variety of causes. Hyperammonemia is a feature of liver failure. Hyponatremia from diabetes insipidus may result in obtundation. Severe hypoglycemia can damage neurons in the hippocampus and neocortex. The elevated hemoglobin A_{1C} level suggests a diagnosis of diabetes mellitus, and diabetics are most prone to peripheral neuropathies and autonomic neuropathies. Carbon monoxide poisoning can produce obtundation and coma.
PBD6 1342

9. **(C)** The clinical history of dementia, along with the presence of numerous neuritic plaques and amyloid deposition in blood vessel wall, is characteristic of Alzheimer disease. The epsilon 4 allele of the ApoE 4 gene increases the risk of developing Alzheimer disease by unknown mechanisms. There is no association between HLA genes and this disease. Expansion of CAG repeats on 4p16 causes Huntington disease. Mutant prion genes give rise to spongiform encephalopathies, such as Creutzfeldt-Jacob

disease. Deficiency of thiamine in alcoholics causes Wernicke-Korsakoff syndrome.
BP6 739 PBD6 1329-1333

10. **(E)** She has a subdural hematoma resulting from tearing of the bridging veins beneath the dura. These veins are at risk for tearing with head trauma, particularly in the elderly, in whom some degree of cerebral atrophy may be present, thereby exposing these veins to potential traumatic tearing. Pontine hemorrhages are likely to be Duret hemorrhages. Subarachnoid hemorrhage could occur in a region of contusions with trauma. Basal ganglia hemorrhages are most often associated with hypertension. Epidural hemorrhages are most often preceded by a blow to the head that tears the middle meningeal artery, and there is commonly a "lucid" interval between initial loss of consciousness with the trauma and the later accumulation of blood.
BP6 722 PBD6 1305

11. **(E)** This is an acute lymphocytic meningitis, which is most typically caused by a virus. It may also be called aseptic meningitis because routine Gram stain and bacterial cultures are negative. Most cases are self-limited, occur in immunocompetent persons, and resolve without significant sequelae. Listerial and meningococcal infections are seen sporadically and should have a neutrophilic response. Cryptococcal and toxoplasmal infections can occur in immunocompromised patients, but the India ink test should be positive in the former, and the CT scan should show focal lesions in the latter.
BP6 727 PBD6 1315

12. **(B)** Intracranial aneurysms are typically saccular and slowly enlarge over time. Those that reach 4 to 7 mm in diameter are at greatest risk for rupture. Rupture occurs into the subarachnoid space at the base of the brain where the cerebral arterial distribution originates around the circle of Willis and where saccular aneurysms are most likely to arise. Epidural hematomas arise from a tear of the middle meningeal artery, typically from head trauma. Trauma may also cause a tear of bridging veins that produces a subdural hematoma. The bleeding that results from a berry aneurysm is not likely to cause a mass effect and herniation, and the aneurysm itself is too small to do this as well. In some cases of survival after rupture of a berry aneurysm, a noncommunicating hydrocephalus could result from organization of the subarachnoid hemorrhage.
BP6 720 PBD6 1311-1312

13. **(E)** There is loss of upper motor neurons with amyotrophic lateral sclerosis, leading to progressive muscular weakness from grouped atrophy of skeletal muscle fibers (i.e., denervation atrophy). Becker muscular dystrophy can produce progressive weakness from the decreased dystrophin in muscle in middle-aged males, but the CNS is not involved. In neurofibromatosis, mass lesions, including neurofibromas, schwannomas, meningiomas, and gliomas, may be seen. Guillain-Barré syndrome is a form of rapidly ascending paralysis that occurs over weeks. Creutzfeldt-Jakob disease is a rapidly progressive form of dementia that results in death in less than a year in most cases.
BP6 741 PBD6 1338

14. **(B)** The "lucid" interval is classic for an epidural hematoma. An acute subdural hematoma and a ruptured aneurysm do not typically have this lucid interval but instead have sudden and progressive worsening of symptoms. Contusions do not progressively worsen. A leptomeningitis is not associated with trauma. The cannabinoids no doubt enhanced his performance. Because cannabinoids are stored in adipose tissue and released irregularly for up to a month after the last use (or even after "second-hand" exposure in a smoke-filled room), low levels can be detected for weeks or may appear and disappear.
BP6 721–722   PBD6 1304–1305

15. **(A)** The multiple pigmented skin lesions and optic nerve glioma strongly suggest the diagnosis of neurofibromatosis type I. Patients with this condition, inherited as an autosomal dominant, have multiple large café-au-lait spots on the skin, and there is a propensity for development of multiple nerve sheath tumors—schwannomas or neurofibromas. CNS gliomas may also occur. The nerve sheath tumors may become malignant and metastasize, most commonly to the lungs.
BP6 725,743   PBD6 1354

16. **(D)** He has Parkinson disease. The most characteristic feature is loss of dopamine-secreting pigmented neurons in the substantia nigra of the midbrain. Some patients with Parkinson disease may also have dementia, and Lewy bodies may be found. Neurofibrillary tangles in neocortex are a feature of Alzheimer disease. Huntington disease involves the caudate. Wernicke-Korsakoff syndrome caused by vitamin B_1 deficiency involves the mammillary bodies. Hemorrhages in this area eventually give rise to the deposition of hemosiderin. Alzheimer type II gliosis is seen with chronic alcoholism.
BP6 740–741   PBD6 1333–1334

17. **(C)** During herniation of the brain stem, branches of the basilar artery are kinked. This gives rise to hemorrhagic infarcts in the midbrain and pons. Such infarcts, also called Duret hemorrhage, have a typical ventral-to-dorsal orientation, and they occur in the midline or paramedian regions. Tearing of bridging veins gives rise to subdural hematomas. Rupture of the middle meningeal artery gives rise to epidural hematomas. Hemorrhage from berry aneurysms is subarachnoid in location. Sudden global hypoxia resulting from hypotension gives rise to widespread brain infarction.
BP6 716–722   PBD6 1298, 1304–1312

18. **(A)** Meningiomas are typically circumscribed lesions that arise from meningothelial cells of the arachnoid and appear grossly attached to the overlying dura. They are most often seen in adult women. A parasagittal, sphenoid ridge, or subfrontal location is typical. Tuberculomas from disseminated tuberculosis are rare and usually occur at the base of the brain. Medulloblastomas are childhood tumors of the posterior fossa. The most typical location for a schwannoma is at the cerebellopontine angle involving the eighth nerve. Ependymomas arise in ventricles.
BP6 734–735   PBD6 1350–1351

19. **(E)** She has Huntington disease, a progressive degenerative disorder affecting the caudate nuclei. This disease is caused by an abnormal expansion of the trinucleotide CAG in the Huntington gene, found on chromosome 4. The more repeats, the earlier is the onset of the disease. Tay-Sachs disease of infancy and childhood is caused by a deficiency of hexosaminidase A. Mutations in presenilin genes causes familial Alzheimer disease. The risk for Alzheimer disease increases with increased levels of apoprotein E. Trisomy 21 results in mental retardation present from birth. About 10% of Creutzfeldt-Jakob disease cases be genetically determined with inheritance of an abnormal prion protein that leads to spongiform encephalopathy in later adult life.
BP6 741   PBD6 1335–1338

20. **(C)** This is anencephaly, a form of severe neural tube defect that results from failure of formation of the fetal cranial vault. This is one of the most common CNS malformations seen at birth. The defect allows fetal α-fetoprotein to enter amniotic fluid and from there reach the maternal circulation. Neural tube defects are not associated with neonatal jaundice. CMV can produce extensive parenchymal necrosis but not loss of the fetal cranial vault. Diabetes mellitus, suggested by an elevated hemoglobin A_{1C} level, can increase the risk for malformations (e.g., holoprosencephaly in the CNS) but not neural tube defects. Down syndrome (trisomy 21) can be associated with brachycephaly but rarely with anencephaly.
BP 723-724   PBD6 1299–1300

21. **(E)** The rapid correction of hyponatremia is one of the common antecedents to the demyelination in the basis pontis. Herniation is unlikely, because cerebral edema would cause papilledema. Intracranial hemorrhages should not result from electrolyte and fluid disturbances. A subacute combined degeneration of the cord happens slowly as a consequence of vitamin B_{12} deficiency. The Wernicke-Korsakoff syndrome is now a rare accompaniment to chronic alcoholism that affects mammillary bodies and periaqueductal gray matter.
BP6 737   PBD6 1329

22. **(E)** This is a remote cerebral infarction. There is a large cystic area that has resulted from resolution of an area of liquefactive necrosis after vascular injury in the distribution of the middle cerebral artery. A recent infarction may appear softened, but it takes weeks to months for macrophages to clear the debris of liquefactive necrosis to leave a cystic space. A vascular malformation has irregular vascular channels that give a mass effect with a dark red to bluish appearance. A contusion could produce some minimal focal loss of cortex with brown hemosiderin staining. An organizing subdural hematoma would leave a uniform area of compression with flattening of the hemisphere.
BP6 718   PBD6 1308–1309

23. **(C)** This lesion is a senile (or neuritic) plaque that shows a rim of dystrophic neuritis surrounding an amyloid core. Increased numbers of neuritic neocortical plaques for age are a diagnostic feature of Alzheimer disease, the most common form of dementia. Symmetric muscular weakness suggests amyotrophic lateral sclerosis. Gait disturbances oc-

cur with Parkinson disease. Seizures can be associated with many lesions, but often a pathologic finding is not discernible. Choreiform movements suggest Huntington disease.
BP6 739–740 PBD6 1329–1331

24. **(D)** CMV infection is one of the congenital TORCH infections, and it can become widely disseminated to affect the CNS. Periventricular necrosis is characteristic of CMV infection. Failure of the heart in utero causes hydrops fetalis. Listeriosis can produce focal microabscesses in a variety of organs, but there is generally minimal necrosis. HIV infections have no significant CNS findings in the perinatal period. Herpes simplex infection of neonates typically occurs during passage through the infected birth canal of the mother, not in utero. Group B streptococcal infections cause premature rupture of membranes and sepsis without significant CNS findings.
BP6 729 PBD6 376, 1319

25. **(A)** Arteriovenous malformations are most often seen in the cerebral hemisphere of a young adult. They can be removed by a neurosurgeon. There may be slow leakage of blood from the lesion over time, resulting in the clinical symptoms and the gliosis seen on biopsy. An abscess would have an organizing wall with collagen and gliosis but no prominent larger vessels. An angiosarcoma is not a primary lesion in the brain parenchyma. Head trauma generally produces contusions and hematomas on the surface but not hemorrhages in the brain parenchyma. A ruptured aneurysm can in some cases extend upward into parenchyma, but with this complication, the outcome is always fatal.
BP6 721 PBD6 1313

26. **(A)** There is loss of pigmented dopaminergic neurons in the substantia nigra of the midbrain, which is most characteristic for Parkinson disease. Pill-rolling tremors at rest are typical of this disorder. Symmetric weakness suggests a motor neuron disease. Paraplegia suggests a disruption in the motor pathways, such as an infarction. Choreiform movements suggest Huntington disease, which involves the caudate, not the substantia nigra. Short-term memory problems suggest hippocampal lesions.
BP6 740–741 PBD6 1333–1334

27. **(D)** An abscess is most often a complication of an infection, such as pneumonia that occurred days to weeks earlier. The bacteria spread hematogenously. As the abscess organizes, it is ringed by fibroblasts that lay down collagen, a feature characteristic of an abscess in the CNS. A neoplasm may be ring enhancing on occasion, but a glioblastoma multiforme is not well demarcated, and metastases are typically multifocal. A multiple sclerosis plaque is not this large and does not typically have ring enhancement. An infarct should produce sudden signs and symptoms that improve with time, and the CSF protein should not be increased.
BP6 728–729 PBD6 1315–1316

28. **(C)** The brief episodes of neurologic dysfunction represent transient ischemic attacks (TIAs) that are a prodrome to a stroke in many cases. Atherosclerotic cerebrovascular

disease is a common antecedent to cerebral infarction. A neoplasm is unlikely to produce such sudden symptoms and signs. A subdural hematoma, which most frequently results from a fall with head trauma, is unlikely to develop in a few minutes, and it does not explain the TIAs. A vascular malformation most often is symptomatic from bleeding in young adults. Meningoencephalitis may produce general features such as headache, confusion, and seizures but not sudden localizing signs.
BP6 718 PBD6 1308–1310

29. **(B)** This shifting spectrum of clinical findings over time in a young adult suggests the diagnosis of multiple sclerosis. The plaques of demyelination that give rise to the differing symptoms can be found in a variety of locations, but they most often occur in periventricular white matter. CSF immunoglobulins are increased, and most patients show oligoclonal bands of IgG. Cryptococcal meningitis should have a more acute presentation with meningeal signs. Primary or malignant brain tumors are not common at that age and should not have such a long course without serious sequelae. Xanthochromia from hemorrhage should suggest a more acute problem. Neurosyphilis is rare at his age and should not have localizing signs.
BP6 736 PBD6 1326–1327

30. **(C)** The findings point to Huntington disease, which has an autosomal dominant inheritance pattern and an onset in middle age. It results from increased trinucleotide repeat mutations in the Huntington gene on chromosome 4. There is atrophy with loss of neurons and gliosis in the caudate, putamen, and globus pallidus. The loss of pigmented neurons is typical for Parkinson disease. Congophilic angiopathy can be seen with Alzheimer disease. Loss of motor neurons is a feature of amyotrophic lateral sclerosis. Multiple lacunar infarcts may be seen with chronic hypertension.
BP6 741 PBD6 1335–1336

31. **(A)** In the pediatric age range, some inherited form of CNS disease accounting for a progressively worsening course should be suspected. The leukodystrophies affect white matter extensively with myelin loss and abnormal accumulations of myelin. A variety of lysosomal enzyme defects lead to these disorders, characterized by failure of generation or maintenance of myelin. However, there are no discrete plaques of demyelination as seen with multiple sclerosis. Sparing of subcortical myelin (U fiber) is often seen in leukodystrophies. Progressive multifocal leukoencephalopathy is an infectious lesion of immunocompromised adults. Tay-Sachs disease affects infants. Acute disseminated encephalomyelitis is a postinfectious process with an abrupt onset.
BP6 737 PBD6 1340

32. **(A)** Tearing of bridging veins gives rise to an acute subdural hematoma. This almost always results from head trauma in which there has been a fall to the ground. The risk for hemorrhage is greater in the elderly because of cerebral atrophy that leaves the bridging veins beneath the dura at the vertex more vulnerable to traumatic tearing. When saccular (berry) aneurysms rupture, the bleeding is typically subarachnoid and at the base of the brain. An

arteriovenous (vascular) malformation is often within the parenchyma of a hemisphere, and bleeding from them occurs more often in young adults. A tear of the middle meningeal artery can occur with head trauma (a blow to the head) but results in an acute epidural hematoma. Thrombosis of an intracranial artery may result in an infarction, and some of these may be hemorrhagic, but the hemorrhage typically does not extend into subarachnoid or subdural locations.
BP6 722   PBD6 1305

33.   **(C)** About 1 person in 100 has a saccular (berry) aneurysm. Although present from birth as a congenital defect in the arterial media at intracerebral artery branch points, it can manifest later in life with aneurysmal dilation and possible rupture. These aneurysms are the most common cause for spontaneous subarachnoid hemorrhage in adults. Thromboemboli can cause infarctions, most often in the distribution of the middle cerebral artery in cortex, and embolic infarcts may be hemorrhagic, but the blood does not typically reach the CSF. A subdural hematoma results from tear of bridging veins. The bleeding from amyloid angiopathy is in peripheral cortex. A hypertensive hemorrhage tends to remain in the brain parenchyma.
BP6 720   PBD6 1311-1312

34.   **(D)** Toxoplasmosis is one of the more common opportunistic infections seen in the CNS in patients with AIDS. Toxoplasmosis produces abscesses that organize on the periphery to produce a bright ring on CT and MRI scans. Lymphomas can also produce this picture, but they generally occur as fewer, larger masses or just a solitary mass. *Candida* infections of the CNS are rare, and disseminated candidiasis with AIDS is uncommon. A spongiform encephalopathy, such as Creutzfeldt-Jakob disease, typically has no grossly visible or radiographic findings. Metastatic carcinoma is uncommon at this age.
BP6 729   PBD6 1323

35.   **(D)** The clinical features, location, and cytologic findings all point to the diagnosis of medulloblastoma. Most intracranial neoplasms in children are located in the posterior fossa. The medulloblastoma, one of the "blue cell tumors" of childhood, arises in the midline, and the cells can seed into the CSF. Schwannomas are benign neoplasms that do not seed the CSF. Ependymomas can be seen in children, but they typically arise in the ventricles. A glioblastoma multiforme could also seed the CSF, but this neoplasm is seen in adults. Metastatic disease is uncommon in children.
BP6 734   PBD6 1346-1348

36.   **(B)** She has multiple sclerosis with plaques of demyelination. The course of multiple sclerosis is variable, with many relapses and remissions, and some patients are affected more than others. Some patients may have minimal problems, but most can be expected to have further neurologic problems. Severe neurologic impairment and death are unlikely, and most patients live for decades. There is no defined inheritance pattern. Multiple sclerosis is not related to HIV infection. The neurologic problems with HIV infection are related mainly to dementia.
BP6 736   BPD6 1326-1327

37.   **(B)** Thromboembolic disease leading to cerebral infarcts most often results from a cardiac disease (e.g., endocarditis, mural thrombosis, prosthetic valvular thrombosis). Hypertension is associated with basal ganglia, pontine, and cerebellar hemorrhages and with small lacunar infarcts in basal ganglia. Head trauma with hemorrhage is more common with chronic alcoholism. AIDS is not associated with significant cardiovascular or cerebrovascular diseases. Metastatic carcinomas may be found at the gray-white junction but do not typically produce infarction.
BP6 718-719   PBD6 1308-1310

38.   **(D)** Hypertensive hemorrhages are most likely to arise in the basal ganglia, the thalamus, cerebral white matter, pons, or the cerebellum. Multiple hemorrhages are uncommon. The small vessels weakened by hyaline arteriolosclerosis are prone to rupture. Metastases are typically multiple and peripheral at the gray-white junction. The plaques of multiple sclerosis occur in white matter and do not bleed. Chronic alcoholism predisposes to falls with subdural hematomas or contusions.
BP6 719   PBD6 1310

39.   **(B)** The papilledema and the herniation are a consequence of brain swelling. The herniation of the uncus results in a third cranial nerve palsy as the nerve is compressed. Rupture of a berry aneurysm produces subarachnoid hemorrhage at the base of the brain, which is less likely to result in a mass effect. There is no pressure effect with hydrocephalus ex vacuo, which is a consequence of atrophy. A chronic subdural hemorrhage accumulates slowly enough that herniation may not occur. An infarct is not likely to have significant associated brain swelling.
BP6 716   PBD6 1298

40.   **(K)** Multiple discrete neoplasms in the CNS are more likely to be metastases than a primary brain tumor. Tumor cells may reach the brain in the form of emboli through the cerebral arterial circulation. Most embolic events involve the gray-white junction, where there is narrowing and acute branching of the vessels, trapping emboli. The distribution of the middle cerebral artery, which receives the most blood, would be the most likely location.
BP6 735   PBD6 1351

41.   **(B)** Most malignant neoplasms of the brain in children are in the posterior fossa. The two most common neoplasms at this site are cystic cerebellar astrocytoma and medulloblastoma.
BP6 733-734   PBD6 1348-1349

42.   **(A)** This tan-yellow mass is a meningioma, a benign tumor that arises in meningothelial cells beneath the dura. Gliomas are most often found within a cerebral hemisphere in an adult. Ependymomas are seen within ventricles or on the distal spinal cord. The parasagittal location is unusual for a metastatic lesion, although some malignancies such as breast carcinomas may involve the dura in a diffuse fashion. Tuberculomas are rare complications of disseminated tuberculosis and often appear at the base of the brain.
BP6 734-735   PBD6 1350-1351

43. **(E)** She has Alzheimer disease, a progressive dementia marked by plaques and neurofibrillary tangles. This is the most common form of dementia. Other forms of dementia include diffuse Lewy body disease, Huntington disease, Pick disease, and various forms of multisystem atrophy. The number of senile plaques normally increases with age, but persons with Alzheimer disease have many more, which serves to make the diagnosis.
BP6 739–740   PBD6 1329–1333

44. **(A)** The brain stem shows linear midline hemorrhages, called Duret hemorrhages. The acute bacterial meningitis led to brain swelling with edema and subsequent herniation with Duret hemorrhages in the pons. Although not seen here, an infection could organize with scarring of foramina to produce a noncommunicating hydrocephalus, or it might scar the vertex and impair reabsorption of CSF at the arachnoid granulations to produce a communicating hydrocephalus. Abscess is not a common accompaniment to meningitis, although some cases of meningitis may arise when an abscess in paranasal or mastoid air cells extends to the cranial cavity. The small meningeal vessels do not bleed due to inflammation caused by a meningitis. Laminar necrosis could occur after brain death, but this finding is not specific for meningitis.
BP 716   PBD 1298

45. **(C)** Such a tumor in this location is also known as a cerebellopontine angle tumor. Schwannomas in this location arise from the eighth cranial nerve and therefore are also called acoustic neuromas. Most schwannomas are benign, slow-growing tumors that can be resected. Meningiomas are rare at this location. Astrocytomas involve the hemispheres of adults and the cerebellum of children most often. Medulloblastomas likewise typically arise in the cerebellum of children. Ependymomas arise in the ventricular system, often the fourth ventricle.
BP6 743   PBD6 1352

46. **(B)** The location in the cerebral hemispheres and the presence of necrosis with pseudopalisading are characteristic of an aggressive brain tumor called glioblastoma multiforme. This is the most malignant form of glioma. These neoplasms can infiltrate widely within the CNS, particularly along white matter tracts. The prognosis is poor. Metastases generally are found at the gray-white junction and are multiple. Medulloblastomas and cystic astrocytomas are childhood neoplasms of the posterior fossa. Primary CNS melanomas are rare.
BP6 732   PBD6 1343–1345

47. **(E)** He has AIDS dementia complex late in the course of his HIV infection. HIV-1 produces an encephalitis that is characterized by a collection of reactive microglial cells (i.e., "microglial nodules"). HIV-1–infected mononuclear cells, particularly macrophages, can fuse to form the multinucleate cells. These are seen in association with microglial nodules. Plaques of demyelination are typical for multiple sclerosis. Senile plaques and tangles are typical for Alzheimer disease, something he is unlikely to manifest at his age. Lacunar infarcts refer to small cavitary infarcts resulting from arteriolosclerosis of the deep penetrating arteries and arterioles. Such arteriolar lesions occur in those with long-standing hypertension and are unlikely to be found in a 37-year-old male. Spongiform change suggests Creutzfeldt-Jakob disease, a rapidly progressive dementia unrelated to HIV infection.
BP6 730   PBD6 1320–1321

48. **(B)** Spina bifida is the mildest form of neural tube defect. There is defective closure of vertebral arches with intact meninges and spinal cord. A radiograph may demonstrate its presence in up to 20% of the population. The Dandy-Walker malformation is detected by ultrasonographic evidence for a cyst in the region of the fourth ventricle along with agenesis of cerebellar vermis. Tuberous sclerosis is a rare disease with firm hamartomatous "tubers" in the cortex. In Arnold-Chiari malformation, there is a small posterior fossa and extension of the cerebellum into foramen magnum, along with a lumbar meningomyelocele. Meningomyeloceles are open neural tube defects.
BP6 724   PBD6 1300–1302

49. **(E)** He has acute bacterial meningitis. In his age group, the most common organism is *Haemophilus influenzae*. The gram-positive cocci of *Streptococcus* are more likely to be seen in an adult. The gram-negative diplococci of *N. meningitidis* are seen in young adults. The short, gram-positive rods of *L. monocytogenes* appear sporadically or in epidemics from food contamination. The gram-negative bacilli of *Escherichia coli* are most often seen in neonates. With these clinical and CSF features, it is very unlikely that bacteria are not present in CSF.
BP6 725–726   PBD6 1315

50. **(A)** The progressive and symmetric nature of his disease is classic for amyotrophic lateral sclerosis (ALS). The muscles show a denervation type of grouped atrophy from loss of upper motor neurons. The "bulbar" form of ALS involves mainly cranial nerve nuclei and has a more aggressive course. Huntington disease presents with abnormal movements, not weakness, and there can be associated dementia over time. However, mental function is preserved with ALS. The demyelinating plaques of multiple sclerosis can produce a variety of motor signs and symptoms over time, but symmetry is not part of this disease. Guillain-Barré syndrome usually follows a viral infection and manifests with a rapidly progressive ascending motor weakness. Parkinson disease is characterized by rigidity and involuntary movements, not muscular weakness.
BP 741–742   PBD6 1338–1339

51. **(A)** Germinal matrix hemorrhage is the most common cause for intraventricular hemorrhage in premature infants. The germinal matrix, composed of highly vascularized tissue with primitive cells, is most prominent between 22 and 30 weeks' gestation. Hemorrhages within this area readily occur with common neonatal problems such as hypoxemia, hypercarbia, acidosis, and changes in blood pressure. Hemorrhages in the germinal matrix can extend into the cerebral ventricles and from there into the subarachnoid space. Smaller hemorrhages can resolve without sequelae. With larger hemorrhages, organization of the blood in the aqueduct of Sylvius or the fourth ventricle or foramina of

Luschka may obstruct the flow of CSF, thus producing hydrocephalus. Down syndrome babies may have vascular malformations that can bleed into the parenchyma. The bilirubin staining of kernicterus does not result in scarring. CMV can cause considerable necrosis of the brain parenchyma but not hemorrhage. Medulloblastomas are tumors of childhood (not typically of infancy) that could cause obstruction of CSF flow.
BP6 725-726   PBD6 1302

52.   **(D)** There is an aneurysm in the circle of Willis and extensive subarachnoid hemorrhage. The hemorrhage occurs at the base of the brain because the berry aneurysms involve the circle of Willis and its branches. The vasospasm caused by the leakage of blood can lead to ischemia that further complicates the course. A glioblastoma often has extensive necrosis with some hemorrhage, but remains intraparenchymal. Thromboembolic infarctions can be hemorrhagic, because the embolus does not completely occlude the vessel, but the hemorrhage is localized. Rupture of bridging veins occurs at the vertex beneath the dura, producing a subdural hematoma. Hypertensive hemorrhages most often occur in basal ganglia, in pons, and in cerebellum from rupture of small arteries with hyaline arteriolosclerosis, and the blood typically remains intraparenchymal.
BP6 720   PBD6 1311-1312

The Eye

PBD6 Chapter 31 - Diseases of the Eye

1. Pain in the right eye for several days prompts a 29-year-old female to seek medical attention. A slit-lamp examination with the use of fluorescein dye reveals a dendritic ulcer on the right cornea. The most probable cause for this finding is

O (A) Trachoma
O (B) Herpes simplex virus infection
O (C) Carcinoma in situ
O (D) Cytomegalovirus (CMV) infection
O (E) Vitamin A deficiency

2. A 31-year-old male has increasing difficulty seeing at night but has no problems during the day. Several years later, his daytime visual acuity is decreasing as well. Funduscopic examination reveals a branching reticulated pattern to the retina; a pale, waxy-appearing optic disc; and attenuation of retinal blood vessels. These findings are most characteristic for

O (A) Macular degeneration
O (B) Hypertensive retinopathy
O (C) Retinitis pigmentosa
O (D) Proliferative retinopathy
O (E) Arteriosclerotic retinopathy

3. A newborn male is diagnosed with unilateral retinoblastoma. Molecular analysis of the enucleated tumor cells reveals loss of both normal alleles of the *Rb* gene. In comparison, skin fibroblasts of the patient do not show any abnormality at the *Rb* locus. Which of the following statements regarding his clinical appearance is most accurate?

O (A) A predisposition to develop this tumor was inherited by this patient.
O (B) His sibs have an increased risk for developing retinoblastoma.
O (C) He is at increased risk for developing osteosarcomas in later life.
O (D) Both copies of the *Rb* gene were lost because of mutations in retinoblasts.

O (E) He is at a high risk for developing retinoblastoma in the other eye.

4. A 63-year-old woman has carried a diagnosis of type I diabetes mellitus since the age of 18. She has had increasing difficulty with vision for the past decade. Which of the following pathologic findings is most likely?

O (A) Corneal stromal dystrophy
O (B) Retrolental fibroplasia
O (C) Granulomatous uveitis
O (D) Capillary microaneurysms
O (E) Papilledema

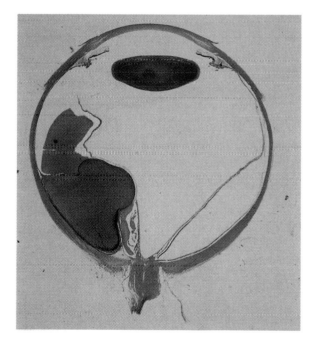

5. An enucleated eye is shown here in transverse section. The patient is a 61-year-old female. The disease process that produced this appearance is most likely

O (A) Granulomatous uveitis
O (B) Uveal melanoma

○ (C) Toxoplasmosis
○ (D) Malignant hypertension
○ (E) Ocular trauma

6. A 50-year-old male suffers a penetrating injury to his left eye because he was not wearing protective goggles while ripping plywood on his table saw at home. The wood splinter is removed, and there appears to be a partial uveal prolapse, but he still has vision in the left eye. Three weeks later, he has loss of accommodation, photophobia, and blurred vision in his right eye, and choroidal infiltrates are seen on funduscopic examination. The most likely diagnosis is

○ (A) Undiagnosed trauma
○ (B) Aspergillosis
○ (C) Sarcoidosis
○ (D) Fuchs dystrophy
○ (E) Sympathetic ophthalmia

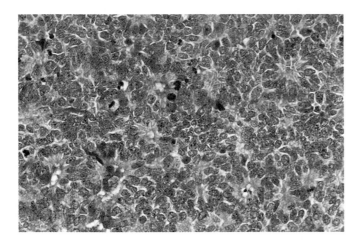

7. The microscopic appearance of a mass from the left eye of a 3-year-old boy shown here is most characteristic for which of the following neoplasms?

○ (A) Metastatic adenocarcinoma
○ (B) Retinoblastoma
○ (C) Squamous cell carcinoma
○ (D) Astrocytoma
○ (E) Melanoma

8. A 62-year-old female has decreasing vision. Funduscopic examination reveals deepening of the optic cup with excavation. Otherwise, the retina appears normal. The disease that led to these findings should have been detected by screening

○ (A) Serum glucose
○ (B) Serum cholesterol
○ (C) Homocystine in urine

○ (D) Blood pressure
○ (E) Intraocular pressure

9. Examination of the eyes of a 5-year-old child with mental retardation reveals Brushfield spots (i.e., speckled irides from ringlike foci of iris hypoplasia surrounding relatively normal iris stroma). Hypertelorism is also present. The child most likely has

○ (A) Trisomy 18
○ (B) Hydrocephalus
○ (C) Tay-Sachs disease
○ (D) Trisomy 21
○ (E) Adrenoleukodystrophy

10. A 6-year-old child has decreased vision. Examination of the eye demonstrates diffuse punctate inflammation of the cornea along with pannus extending as a growth of fibrovascular tissue from conjunctiva onto the cornea. A corneal scraping examined microscopically reveals lymphocytes, plasma cells, and neutrophils along with scattered corneal epithelial cells that have cytoplasmic inclusion bodies. The most likely infectious agent that led to these findings is

○ (A) Herpes simplex virus
○ (B) Treponema pallidum
○ (C) Cytomegalovirus
○ (D) Rubella
○ (E) Chlamydia trachomatis

11. Findings on funduscopic examination of a 68-year-old male include arteriolar narrowing, flame-shaped hemorrhages, cotton-wool spots, and hard, waxy exudates. These findings most strongly suggest that he has

○ (A) Chronic hypertension
○ (B) Retinitis pigmentosa
○ (C) Advanced atherosclerosis
○ (D) Diabetes mellitus
○ (E) Cerebral edema

12. A 30-year-old male has severely impaired vision in both eyes. His brother is similarly affected. However, both parents are normal. Examination reveals diffuse cloudiness of the anterior stroma with aggregates of gray-white opacities in the axial region of the corneal stroma. He undergoes corneal transplantation. The diseased corneas demonstrate basophilic deposits in the stroma that stain positively for acid mucopolysaccharides. The best diagnosis is

○ (A) Cataracts
○ (B) Keratomalacia
○ (C) Macular dystrophy
○ (D) Pterygium
○ (E) Trachoma

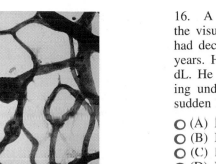

13. This figure shows a special preparation of human retina removed from a patient who died of chronic renal failure. The changes seen in the retina are most characteristic of which of the following?

○ (A) Systemic lupus erythematosus
○ (B) Malignant hypertension
○ (C) Diabetes mellitus
○ (D) Amyloidosis
○ (E) Polycystic kidney disease

14. An 8-year-old child has markedly decreased visual acuity as a consequence of keratomalacia. The patient has severe keratinization of all mucous membrane epithelia, including cornea and conjunctiva, and has xerophthalmia. These findings are most often a consequence of

○ (A) Herpes simplex virus infection
○ (B) Vitamin A deficiency
○ (C) Congenital rubella syndrome
○ (D) Trachoma
○ (E) Sjögren syndrome

15. A baby is born prematurely at 32 weeks' gestation and requires intubation and positive pressure ventilation with 100% inspired oxygen to treat hyaline membrane disease. The baby survives and is discharged home on the 23rd day of life. Two months later, the mother notices that the baby does not appear to respond visually to her presence. The baby is examined and found to have evidence of

○ (A) Keratomalacia
○ (B) Retrolental fibroplasia
○ (C) Macular degeneration
○ (D) Cataracts
○ (E) Retinitis pigmentosa

16. A 70-year-old male suddenly lost the upper half of the visual field in his right eye. Before this event, he has had decreasing visual acuity in both eyes for the past few years. His fasting serum glucose concentration is 165 mg/dL. He has been obese for decades. Which of the following underlying pathologic processes best accounts for the sudden loss of vision on the right?

○ (A) Retinitis pigmentosa
○ (B) Macular degeneration
○ (C) Dendritic corneal ulcer
○ (D) Uveal melanoma
○ (E) Retinitis proliferans

17. A 76-year-old woman has decreasing vision, mainly in a central pattern, involving both eyes. On funduscopic examination, the retinal pigment epithelium appears atrophic and depigmented. These findings are most typical for

○ (A) Retinitis pigmentosa
○ (B) Proliferative retinopathy
○ (C) Retinal detachment
○ (D) Macular degeneration
○ (E) Retrolental fibroplasia

18. Long-term high-dose glucocorticoid therapy is required for a patient with systemic lupus erythematosus complicated by severe lupus nephritis. This is most likely to eventuate in which of the following ocular complications?

○ (A) Background retinopathy
○ (B) Macular degeneration
○ (C) Granulomatous uveitis
○ (D) Cataracts
○ (E) Corneal stromal dystrophy

19. Retinal detachment is most likely to be a complication of which of the following conditions?

○ (A) Macular degeneration
○ (B) Glaucoma
○ (C) Retinitis pigmentosa
○ (D) Cataracts
○ (E) Diabetic retinopathy

20. A 78-year-old woman has increasing difficulty with vision that is worse on the right side. She cannot see clearly when looking straight ahead because of cloudiness and opacification, so that she cannot read printed material. Vision is better peripherally. Which of the following pathologic processes is most likely to have occurred?

○ (A) Retinal macular degeneration
○ (B) Keratomalacia
○ (C) Sympathetic ophthalmia
○ (D) Glaucoma
○ (E) Nuclear sclerosis of the lens

21. A 54-year-old male has had some decreasing visual acuity on the right side. The ophthalmologist notices a 15-mm choroidal mass on funduscopic examination. A week later, the patient experiences a sudden loss of vision in his

right eye "as though someone pulled a window shade down halfway." The condition that best accounts for these findings is

○ (A) Uveal melanoma
○ (B) Diabetic retinopathy
○ (C) Sarcoidosis
○ (D) Glaucoma
○ (E) CMV infection

ANSWERS

1. **(B)** The most common cause of corneal ulcers is infection by herpes simplex virus. Such ulcers can perforate through to the globe, making them a medical emergency. Some chronic herpetic corneal infections cause localized opacity. Lymphocytes and plasma cells are present along with viral inclusions in the corneal epithelial cells. Trachoma, an infection seen most often in children, produces inflammation leading to extensive corneal and conjunctival scarring. A carcinoma in situ produces a white, shiny lesion (i.e., leukoplakia). CMV rarely causes corneal lesions. It can cause retinitis in congenital infections and in states of immunodeficiency in adults. Vitamin A deficiency leads to keratomalacia with scarring.
PBD6 1362–1363

2. **(C)** Retinitis pigmentosa can be inherited in a variety of patterns, and progression of disease is variable. Night blindness due to loss of rod photoreceptors is an early symptom. Later, the cones begin to degenerate as well, producing blindness. Macular degeneration is seen in the elderly. Vascular changes are seen with hypertensive and arteriosclerotic retinopathies. Neovascularization is a feature of diabetic proliferative retinopathy.
PBD6 1370–1371

3. **(D)** This is a sporadic form of retinoblastoma because the somatic cells of the patient have normal *Rb* genes. Both mutations must have arisen in the retinoblasts. This patient did not inherit susceptibility to develop retinoblastoma, because both copies of *Rb* gene are normal in unaffected somatic cells (i.e., fibroblasts). If he had inherited one copy of the mutant (or deleted) *Rb* gene, all the cells in the body would have only one normal copy of the *Rb* gene. The patient's sibs are at no increased risk for developing retinoblastomas, and he is at no increased risk of developing osteosarcomas. For similar reasons, the risk of developing a second retinoblastoma in the other eye is also not greater than that for the population in general.
PBD6 1372

4. **(D)** Formation of capillary microaneurysms is a common presenting clinical sign with background diabetic retinopathy. Generally, the retinopathy begins to develop at least 15 to 20 years after the original diagnosis of diabetes mellitus (type I or type II) is made. Corneal stromal dystrophies are typically inherited conditions. Retrolental fibroplasia is a complication of high-dose oxygen therapy for

neonates. Granulomatous uveitis can be produced by a variety of conditions such as sarcoidosis and sympathetic ophthalmia. Papilledema results from increased intracranial pressure.
BP6 571   PBD6 1369–1370

5. **(B)** The patient has a pigmented uveal mass with retinal detachment. After skin, the eye is the most common site for melanoma. This is the most common intraocular malignancy in adults. Granulomatous uveitis can occur from sarcoidosis, but the inflammation does not produce a large mass lesion. Toxoplasmosis can produce small foci of inflammation but not a mass. Hypertensive retinopathy can produce small hemorrhages. Ocular trauma may lead to sympathetic ophthalmia with inflammation but no mass effect.
PBD6 1365–1367

6. **(E)** Sympathetic ophthalmia is an unusual but devastating complication of penetrating ocular trauma that results from the release of an antigen from one eye that results in an inflammatory reaction in the opposite eye. The traumatized eye must be removed before inflammation begins in the opposite eye to avoid this complication. Trauma alone cannot produce this spectrum of findings. Infection with *Aspergillus* is unlikely to become disseminated in a nonimmunocompromised person and is not typically associated with traumatic lesions. Sarcoidosis can affect the eye, but lesions in the choroid are uncommon. Fuchs dystrophy is an inherited condition that affects the corneal endothelium.
PBD6 1364–1365

7. **(B)** Retinoblastoma is the most common malignant ocular neoplasm of childhood. Histologically, clustering of cuboidal or short columnar cells around a central lumen is characteristic. These clusters are sometimes called Flexner-Wintersteiner rosettes. This tumor can spread to the orbit or along the optic nerve. Adenocarcinomas and squamous cell carcinomas are uncommon childhood neoplasms. Gliomas may affect the optic nerve in a child, but the microscopic pattern does not include the rosettes shown. Melanomas of the eye are seen in adults and have spindle or polygonal cell patterns.
BP6 212–213   PBD6 1372–1373

8. **(E)** She has glaucoma. Increased intraocular pressure is believed to cause the loss of nerve fibers, resulting in a characteristic cupped excavation of the optic disc. Because there are no obvious early signs or symptoms, screening is important for detection. Glaucoma has several causes, and a variety of medications are used to treat it. Hyperglycemia suggests diabetes mellitus, which can increase the risk for glaucoma. An increased cholesterol level suggests an increased risk for arteriosclerotic diseases. Homocystinuria is a rare condition that also increases the risk for atherosclerosis. Hypertension can produce a retinopathy.
PBD6 1374–1375

9. **(D)** A variety of ocular abnormalities are associated with Down syndrome, but they tend not to be severe.

Trisomy 18 can produce hypertelorism, but abnormalities of the iris occur infrequently. Hydrocephalus affects the cerebral hemispheres, which atrophy. The neuronal degeneration of Tay-Sachs disease results in severe neurologic abnormalities in infancy, and the affected person may have a cherry red macula. Adrenoleukodystrophy produces predominantly white matter disease of the brain.
PBD6 1360

10.   **(E)** Trachoma is one of the world's major causes of blindness. The initial inflammation is followed by progressive scarring of the conjunctiva and cornea. Herpetic keratitis can result in ulceration and scarring, and herpesviruses have intranuclear inclusions. Congenital *T. pallidum* infections result in an interstitial keratitis. CMV, one of the herpesviruses, is a rare ocular infection in children. It gives rise to prominent intranuclear inclusions. Congenital rubella, which is now a rare disease because of immunization, produces a retinopathy.
PBD6 1361–1362

11.   **(A)** Hypertensive retinopathy results from long-standing hypertension, with progressive changes that begin with generalized narrowing of the arterioles and proceed to the changes seen in this case. Retinitis pigmentosa is an inherited condition that may begin later in life (but usually earlier) and produces a waxy pallor to the optic disc. Arteriosclerotic retinopathy has vascular changes, including arteriovenous nicking and hyaline arteriolosclerosis with "copper-wire" and "silver-wire" arterioles. Diabetic retinopathy can have a variety of findings, including capillary microaneurysms, cotton-wool spots, arteriolar hyalinization, and more severe changes of proliferative retinopathy with neovascularization. Cerebral edema may result in papilledema.
PBD6 1370

12.   **(C)** Most of the several forms of inherited corneal stromal dystrophy are autosomal dominant. However, the most severe is macular dystrophy, and this disease has an autosomal recessive form of inheritance. It is essentially a form of mucopolysaccharidosis confined to the cornea. Cataracts are seen most often in the elderly and result from opacifications of the crystalline lens. Keratomalacia can be a consequence of vitamin A deficiency. A pterygium is a localized area of basophilic degeneration of conjunctival epithelium that extends onto the cornea. Trachoma is caused by infection with *C. trachomatis*.
PBD6 1363

13.   **(C)** The microaneurysms in the retinal vessels are seen in persons with diabetes mellitus. Several other changes can also occur in diabetes, including hemorrhages, arteriolar hyalinization, cotton-wool spots, neovascularization, and fibroplasia. All other conditions listed can also cause renal failure, but retinal microaneurysms are not seen.
PBD6 1369–1370

14.   **(B)** Keratomalacia and xerophthalmia are characteristic of vitamin A deficiency. This is the most common cause for preventable blindness in children worldwide.

In adults, hypovitaminosis A may lead to night blindness. The most serious abnormality associated with congenital rubella is retinopathy. Trachoma, caused by *C. trachomatis*, results in conjunctival and corneal scarring as a consequence of the inflammation. Dry eyes can result from lacrimal gland involvement with Sjögren syndrome. This is seen in older persons.
BP6 248–249   PBD6 1361

15.   **(B)** Retrolental fibroplasia results from oxygen toxicity to the immature retinal vasculature, leading to neovascularization of the retina with ingrowth into the vitreous. In some cases, scarring continues to retinal detachment. Keratomalacia is a feature of vitamin A deficiency, which takes longer to develop. Macular degeneration is a disease of the elderly. Cataracts are also seen in older persons. Retinitis pigmentosa can be inherited in a variety of patterns with a variable onset from childhood through older age.
PBD6 1368–1369

16.   **(E)** The clinical features suggest retinal detachment. Retinitis proliferans is a late stage of proliferative retinopathy associated with diabetes mellitus. The neovascularization results in a membrane with fibrosis that increases traction on the retina, leading to sudden detachment. Macular degeneration is a common cause of decreased vision in the elderly but not of retinal detachment. Dendritic corneal ulceration suggests infection with herpes simplex virus. Uveal melanomas may lead to retinal detachment, but they are not a feature of diabetes mellitus. Retinitis pigmentosa is an inherited, degenerative condition that is not related to diabetes mellitus.
BP6 571   PBD6 1370

17.   **(D)** Macular degeneration is most often an age-related condition and is the most common cause of decreased vision in the elderly. An absence of retinal vessels in the center of the macula may contribute to this disease, because the retina has high metabolic demands. The disease may result in fibrous metaplasia with scarring of the macular region with permanent loss of central vision. Retinitis pigmentosa is an inherited disorder that produces a characteristic waxy pallor to the optic disc. Proliferative retinopathy is characterized by neovascularization of the retina. Retrolental fibroplasia is a complication of high-dose oxygen therapy for neonates (often premature).
PBD6 1371

18.   **(D)** Cataracts of crystalline lens are an important complication of systemic therapy with glucocorticoids. Cataracts can be caused by aging, diabetes mellitus, glaucoma, ultraviolet light, or irradiation. Retinopathy is most often a feature of diabetes mellitus or hypertension. Macular degeneration is a disease of aging. Granulomatous uveitis occurs with sarcoidosis. Stromal dystrophies are inherited conditions that affect the cornea.
PBD6 1367–1368

19.   **(E)** In patients with diabetes mellitus, neovascularization with scarring and retraction of vitreous collagen leads to traction on the retina and may lead to detachment.

Macular degeneration with an absence of retinal vessels in the center of the macula may result in fibrous metaplasia with scarring of the macular region and permanent loss of central vision. The increased intraocular pressure of glaucoma is not a risk for retinal detachment. Retinitis pigmentosa leads to loss of rod and cone cells. Cataracts involve the crystalline lens.
PBD6 1371–1372

20. **(E)** Nuclear sclerosis of the lens gives rise to cataracts in aging persons. This change causes opacification due to compression of the lens fibers in the central (nuclear) portion of the lens. Macular degeneration also occurs in the elderly and results in loss of central vision, but it does not cause cloudiness. Sympathetic ophthalmia in one eye follows trauma to the other eye. Glaucoma results from increased intraocular pressure and damages the optic nerve, but it is not characterized by loss of central vision.
PBD6 1367–1368

21. **(A)** Uveal melanomas can involve the choroid, the iris, or the ciliary body. They are often pigmented. In addition to causing retinal detachment, as in this case, they may cause choroidal hemorrhage or macular edema. Retinal detachment can occur with diabetic retinopathy, but there is no mass effect. Choroidal and corneal granulomatous inflammation can occur with sarcoidosis, but retinal detachment does not occur. Glaucoma is characterized by increased intraocular pressure. CMV infection can produce focal lesions from inflammation, but retinal detachment is uncommon.
PBD6 1365–1367